Essentials of Neurology

Essentials of Neurology

Lord Walton TD MA MD DSc FRCP
Warden, Green College, Oxford;
Honorary Consultant Neurologist, Oxford District Hospitals;
Former Professor of Neurology, University of Newcastle upon Tyne

SIXTH EDITION

CHURCHILL LIVINGSTONE
EDINBURGH LONDON MELBOURNE AND NEW YORK 1989

CHURCHILL LIVINGSTONE
Medical Division of Longman Group UK Limited

Distributed in the United States of America by Churchill
Livingstone Inc., 1560 Broadway, New York, N.Y. 10036, and
by associated companies, branches and representatives
throughout the world.

First edition (Published by Pitman Publishing Limited) 1961
Second edition (Published by Pitman Publishing Limited) 1966
Third edition (Published by Pitman Publishing Limited) 1971
Fourth edition (Published by Pitman Publishing Limited) 1975
Fifth edition (Published by Pitman Publishing Limited) 1982
Sixth edition (Published by Churchill Livingstone) 1989

ISBN 0-443-03986-0

British Library Cataloguing in Publication Data
Walton. Lord, *1922–*
    Essentials of neurology. — 6th ed.
    1. Man. Nervous system. Diseases.
    I. Title
    616.8

Library of Congress Cataloging in Publication Data
Walton, John Nicholas.
    Essentials of neurology / Lord Walton. — 6th ed.
        p. cm.
    Includes bibliographies and index.
    1. Nervous system — Diseases. 2. Neurology. I. Title.
    [DNLM: 1. Nervous System Diseases. WL 100 W239e]
RC346.W25 1989
616.8 — dc20
DNLM/DLC
for Library of Congress   89–7087
                                              CIP

Produced by Longman Singapore Publishers (Pte) Ltd
Printed in Singapore

Preface to the Sixth Edition

In the preface to the fifth edition of this book I remarked that developments in neurology during the preceding five years, along with the comments and advice of those who read and reviewed the first four editions, had necessitated substantial changes in the text though the general structure of the book remained the same. All previous editions were published by Pitman Books Ltd; after that company was taken over by Churchill Livingstone of the Longman Group, I had several discussions about the future of the book with the publishers in the light of a number of professional opinions upon the fifth edition which had been obtained by Pitman and in consideration of published reviews. We agreed first that the time had come to restructure the book and to present it in a totally different format, deleting much outdated material. It was further agreed that in view of the burgeoning developments in clinical neurology and neuroscience which had taken place in the six years since the last edition had appeared, substantial additions to the text and many new illustrations would be required. It has been our deliberate intention to aim this edition at post-graduate students in medicine and neurology studying for higher diplomas, such as the MRCP (UK), even though we hope that the book will continue to prove useful to undergraduate medical students wishing to read a somewhat more comprehensive text than those primarily directed at a student audience. We also noted that reviewers had generally concluded that it would be more sensible to include advice on treatment and management of individual neurological disorders in those chapters of the book devoted to them, rather than in a separate chapter on treatment; this change has therefore been made. However, some general comments on management and rehabilitation which are in my view appropriate to the study of neurology as a whole and which were previously included in the chapter on treatment have now been covered in the introductory part of the book in order to set the scene for the individual commentaries upon treatment which follow. Clearly, too, it has been necessary to include much more material on advances in

neurochemistry, neuropharmacology, neuroimmunology, neurophysiology and other aspects of fundamental neuroscience, though the emphasis of the book continues to be predominantly clinical. Above all, improvements in diagnostic techniques and particularly in neuroimaging have required extensive revisions in the text, the addition of much new material and of many new illustrations of CT scanning and MR imaging.

In the preparation of this edition, Dr M.D. O'Brien, physician for nervous diseases at Guy's Hospital in London, has given me tremendous help, has added substantial material to the book and has been intimately involved in the revision of all of the chapters and in providing many new illustrations. I wish to pay a very great tribute to the outstanding work he has done in assisting and supporting me. Though many of the major revisions have been mine and I accept full responsibility for them, I am deeply grateful to Dr O'Brien for the splendidly lucid and original contributions and additions which he has made, and for the many new and excellent illustrations he has provided.

I also wish to acknowledge with gratitude the permission so gladly given by many authors, editors and publishers who have allowed me to reproduce in this volume portions of text and illustrations which have appeared elsewhere. Thus in certain parts of the book I have drawn in abbreviated form upon some sections of the ninth edition of *Brain's Diseases of the Nervous System* written by myself and published by Oxford University Press, and elsewhere I have quoted extensively from the second edition of my *Introduction to Clinical Neuroscience*, published by Baillière Tindall. I am especially grateful to Mr John Manger of Oxford University Press and Mrs Katharine Hinton of Baillière Tindall for their willingness to agree to this arrangement. A number of illustrations have also been reproduced from those books and some have come from the fifth edition of *Disorders of Voluntary Muscle*, edited by myself and published by Churchill Livingstone. The Guarantors of Brain and Baillière Tindall have agreed to the reproduction of

v

illustrations from *Aids to the Examination of the Peripheral Nervous System*. Some illustrations appeared in previous editions of the book and their sources were acknowledged at the time. Several were provided by my former colleagues in Newcastle, Drs G.L. Gryspeerdt, Arnold Appleby and D.D. Barwick, as well as by Miss B.P. Longley, and photographic reproductions were made in the Audio-Visual Centre of the University of Newcastle upon Tyne. Others have been taken from *A Physiological Approach to Clinical Neurology* by J.W. Lance and J.G. McLeod and I am grateful to them and to Butterworths for permission to reproduce them, as I am to Drs H.D. Patton, J.W. Sundsten, W.E. Crill and P.D. Swanson from whose volume *Introduction to Basic Neurology*, published by Saunders USA, a number of other illustrations have been taken. Dr Ronald Melzack and Professor Patrick Wall and the American Association for the Advancement of Science, as well as Penguin books, have allowed me to reproduce two illustrations dealing with pain mechanisms. Dr W.N. Mann kindly agreed that I should include figures reproduced from drawings by himself first published in *Conybeare's Textbook of Medicine*. Professor Peter Kennedy gave me permission to publish a table from his book *Infections of the Nervous System*, jointly edited with Johnson and published by Butterworths, and Dr J.P. Patten generously allowed me to include a redrawn version of an illustration previously published by himself in his book *Neurological Differential Diagnosis*, published by Harold Starke Ltd. Several illustrations originally published in the second edition of *Atlas of Clinical Neurology* by J.D. Spillane and J.A. Spillane and subsequently reproduced in *Brain's Diseases of the Nervous System* have also been included, as well as a table published by Dr David Warrell in the second edition of *The Oxford Textbook of Medicine*. I am also grateful to Professors J.A. Simpson and P.S. Harper for their agreement to my using illustrations from the chapters which they contributed to *Disorders of Voluntary Muscle*. And I must again thank Dr O'Brien for the many new illustrations, particularly of radiological topics, which he has contributed and which were supplied by the Department of Radiological Sciences, UMDS (Guy's) and the Department of Neuroradiology, Guy's–Maudsley Neurosurgical Unit and prepared in the Department of Medical Illustration of Guy's Hospital.

Finally, I wish to express my very deep indebtedness to my secretary, Rosemary Allan, who has shouldered the immense burden of work involved in the course of rewriting and totally restructuring this edition, in typing the very large number of additions and inserts and in so expertly preparing the reference lists at the end of the individual chapters. I am also grateful to the staff of Churchill Livingstone for all of their help and co-operation during its preparation and publication.

Oxford, 1990   J. W.

Preface to the First Edition

Although there can be no absolute distinction between diseases of the nervous system and those which affect other organs or systems of the human body, by convention the clinical science of neurology embraces those many disorders which affect the functioning of the central and peripheral nervous system. This book has been written in order to help the undergraduate or postgraduate student to learn the principles of neurological diagnosis and treatment. It is hoped that it will also assist the practising physician in his management of patients suffering from this variety of illness.

The first ten chapters of the book are devoted to a consideration of the cardinal symptoms and signs of neurological disease, to the mechanism of their production and the various pathological changes which may produce these clinical manifestations. In this review of the principles of neurological diagnosis, brief mention is made of investigative methods, some simple and others highly specialised, but only in sufficient detail to indicate to the student or practitioner the indications for employing these methods, their failings and their dangers, and the information which they are likely to divulge. The ensuing chapters contain brief descriptions of specific syndromes of nervous disease, taking into account the general principles previously stressed. Exhaustive descriptions of pathological changes and of differential diagnosis are omitted and the reader will look in vain for lists and tables of diseases and syndromes. Nor will he find detailed analyses of the physiological mechanisms by which symptoms and signs are produced. Since this work is based upon clinical methodology, scientific premises are only mentioned when absolutely necessary for an understanding of clinical principles. The intention has been to make this a book which can be read by the student who wishes to obtain a composite picture of neurological illness, but can also be used for reference if need be. Each chapter is concluded with a list of references to other volumes in which more detailed information can be found and from which the reader can obtain further references to original sources of information, should he wish to consult them.

The book ends with a general review of therapeutic measures which are of value in the field of neurological medicine, but only those appropriate to general practice are considered fully, while more specialised techniques receive mention sufficient only to indicate which patients should be referred to a specialist for these measures to be undertaken.

In preparing this book, I am conscious of the debt I owe to those from whom I learned the principles of neurological diagnosis and management and I wish particularly to thank Professor F. J. Nattrass, Sir Charles Symonds, Dr E. A. Carmichael, Dr Raymond D. Adams and Dr H. G. Miller for the help and encouragement they have given me in the past. No textbook is written without reference to other volumes. I have obtained help particularly from *An Introduction to Clinical Neurology* by Sir Gordon Holmes, Sir Russell Brain's *Diseases of the Nervous System* and the chapters by Dr R. D. Adams in Harrison's *Principles of Internal Medicine*, and wish to express my indebtedness to the authors and publishers concerned. I must also thank the many authors and publishers concerned. I must also thank the many authors and publishers who have given permission for the reproduction of stated illustrations. I am also grateful to Dr A. E. Clark-Kennedy for his helpful advice and to Dr Peter Nathan, Dr J. B. Foster and Dr David Poskanzer for their valuable criticisms of the manuscript. The work of preparing the typescript was performed by Miss Shirley Whillis and Miss Rosemary Allan, and many of the illustrations were prepared by Miss M. Mustart of the Department of Photography, King's College, Newcastle upon Tyne. I also wish to thank Mr D. K. C. Dickens and the staff of the Pitman Medical Publishing Company Ltd. for their enthusiastic and willing co-operation in the production of this volume.

Newcastle upon Tyne, 1959   J.W.

Contents

1. Some general principles in neurology

The nervous system of the individual cannot be considered in isolation, for without an adequate supply of oxygen and of nutrients, which depend in turn upon efficient circulatory and respiratory activity, the nervous system cannot survive. The converse is also true, for the activity of the autonomic nervous system exercises a profound and continuing influence upon the behaviour of the heart and circulation, upon respiratory activity, upon the gastrointestinal system, and upon the endocrine glands. These complex and important interrelationships, upon which the normal functioning of the human body depends, have been elucidated increasingly by anatomical and physiological studies; their understanding requires an appreciation of those homeostatic mechanisms already familiar to readers of this volume. But there are still many problems which defy comprehension. Upon what, for instance, does the ability of the brain to control thought processes depend? Disordered activity of the mind is often present when modern techniques fail to show any abnormality of brain structure or function; and the influence of the mind upon visceral function can also be profound.

Mental disorders can both initiate and accentuate symptoms of physical disease, while conversely some organic diseases are regularly accompanied by psychological manifestations. These important relationships must be recognised by the physician who deals with sick people. Diseases are not independent entities; it is the patient who suffers from the disease who is real and who shows a personal and individual reaction to it. The pattern of his illness depends upon many factors, for the pathological process is influenced by his genetic constitution, by the condition of other bodily organs apart from that which is primarily affected, and by his state of mind.

Many physical disorders of the nervous system regularly produce a consistent series of symptoms and physical signs independent of the personality and constitution. The syndrome resulting from division of one median nerve, for instance, is not significantly modified by the patient's mental state. But if the nerve lesion is incomplete, due perhaps to transient compression, the severity of the resultant symptoms and the rate of recovery can be influenced by factors independent of the physical process concerned with the restoration of normal conduction in the damaged nerve fibres. Much can depend, for instance, upon the nature of the lesion; if it was an industrial injury, involving a claim for financial compensation, the patient's disability may be out of proportion to the residual organic deficit.

Many functions of the nervous system, such as those concerned with speech, with seeing and hearing, with the control of movement and with the appreciation of sensation, are subserved by the passage of nervous impulses along pathways which have been clearly delineated. These functions can be disordered if there is a fault in development (a congenital defect). They may also become abnormal through a pathological process, whether it is the result of inherited factors (genetically-determined illness) or whether it is acquired. The lesions so produced will give rise to symptoms and signs depending upon their situation and character and the functions of the pathways which they involve; many subsequent chapters of this book deal with these functions, the means by which abnormalities can be recognised, the lesions responsible localised and their nature determined. The aim of this introduction is to indicate that the clinical effects of these processes are not immutable, and that the resultant disease can be greatly influenced by the personality and constitution of the individual and by the mental state. Some patients are born physically and mentally less perfect than others and yet show no obvious defect; but constitutionally they are less capable of resistance to stress, and are seriously disturbed by environmental influences which would leave others unaffected. The possible effects of fatigue, of ageing processes, and of other contributory influences which cannot easily be quantified, must also be considered. Are the headaches which the patient describes due to emotional tension or to

1

an intracranial tumour? Are his suspicions that he is suffering from malignant disease well-founded or is he suffering from cancerophobia? Do his insomnia and his anxiety symptoms depend upon constitutional inadequacy and a low resistance to stress, or are they the result of underlying physical disease?

We must also consider the use of the term 'functional' as commonly utilised in medicine to identify the nature of a patient's illness, since its use is a common cause of misconception. It is reasonable to regard as functional disorders those diseases in which the function of some bodily organ is disordered, but in which there is no recognisable pathological change in the organ concerned, whether structural or biochemical. In neurology, 'idiopathic' epilepsy would be a good example, though it is likely that in this and many other states of altered function, some biochemical or structural abnormality is present which cannot be recognised with techniques at present available. But the term 'functional disorder', as conventionally used, is not generally applied to such diseases, but rather to symptoms and signs which result from a disordered state of mind. Thus when a physician says that a symptom is functional, he usually means that it has no known physical cause and, by implication, that he believes its origin to be psychological. For instance, headaches due to anxiety or nervous tension are 'functional', and so too is loss of the voice (hysterical aphonia) in the young singer about to face her first professional engagement. In other words, anxiety reactions, symptoms resulting from mental or emotional fatigue, and those due to a subconscious desire to escape from stress (hysteria) are usually included in this category. It would be incorrect, however, to classify as such deterioration of intellectual function (dementia) which results from physical disease of the brain.

Functional disorders, therefore, are conditions in which symptoms and signs result not from physical disease, but from mental processes, whether conscious or subconscious. These mental processes may in turn influence the body's physical functioning; the increased heart rate, perspiration and insomnia which commonly accompany anxiety are examples. Hence, the clinical use of the term 'functional', if not strictly correct semantically, can usefully be employed, provided the doctor appreciates its meaning, and does not regard this as a final diagnosis. For if a disorder is accepted as 'functional' one must decide whether it is due to conscious anxiety, whether it is hysterical, or whether it could even be psychotic. The distinction between organic and functional disease can be one of the most difficult differential diagnoses in medicine. Even when there is clear evidence of physical disease, symptoms and signs are often accentuated or distorted by concurrent psychological factors.

THE FOUNDATIONS OF NEUROLOGICAL DIAGNOSIS

In order to forecast the outcome of an illness and to advise treatment, accurate diagnosis is usually necessary. In diseases of the nervous system, the physical signs often indicate the anatomical localisation of the lesion or process responsible for disordered function, while the history of the illness, revealing the evolution of the patient's symptoms, generally suggests the nature of the pathological process.

Hence the intelligent interpretation of physical signs demands an adequate knowledge, first, of neuroanatomy. This does not imply that the student must be familiar with the minutiae of neuroanatomy. He should, however, know which areas of the cerebral cortex control certain major functions, such as those of speech, the control of movement, and the appreciation of visual and somatic sensation. He must also be familiar with the general topography of the cerebral hemispheres, brain stem, spinal cord, peripheral nerve and muscle and with the organisation of the autonomic nervous system, especially in relation to the situation of the more important cranial nerve nuclei and the pathways traversed by the main motor and sensory pathways. Knowledge of anatomy alone, however, is not enough, for one must also understand the normal functions of these structures before being able to decide that these are disturbed. Later chapters discuss disorders of the motor, sensory and other systems and how these are recognised, how they are produced, and how the responsible lesion can be localised and identified.

Most symptoms and signs resulting from nervous disease are positive or negative. **Positive symptoms** are those produced by irritation or stimulation of a part of the nervous system, causing it to behave abnormally; focal epilepsy resulting from irritation of or pressure upon the motor area of the cerebral cortex is an example. **Negative symptoms**, by contrast, are those produced by temporary or permanent loss of function, so that an activity or ability, normally present, is lost; paralysis of a limb is one such symptom. Hughlings Jackson's **law of dissolution** said that those functions and skills most recently acquired during the processes of evolution and training are the first to be lost in brain disease, while primitive activities and instincts survive longer. A similar principle applies to temporary disturbances of cerebral function produced, say, by anaesthetics or other drugs. Thus a naturalised foreigner sometimes reverts to using his native tongue during recovery from anaesthesia, and only when recovery is more complete can he utilise the language of his adopted country. To take another example, man differs from the higher primates in his ability to move individual fingers and to use opposition of the thumb to the other fingers in order to perform fine and deliberate movements. This can be called the 'precision grip'; the primate possesses only the 'power grip', produced by flexion of all the fingers. In an early lesion of the appropriate area of the motor cortex or of its efferent corticospinal or pyramidal fibres in man the 'precision grip' is impaired, as is discrete movement of the individual fingers, at a time when the 'power grip' still seems normal. Similarly, in the leg, movement of the toes is affected early.

Disordered function depends not only upon the situation of pathological change, but upon its severity, its extent and the effects it has upon contiguous nervous tissue and upon interconnected though anatomically remote structures in the nervous system. Thus an acute lesion may affect more of the brain than its anatomical extent would lead one to expect, for around its edge the activity of the surrounding nervous tissue is disturbed by oedema and vascular changes. Furthermore, an acute lesion can produce a state of 'shock' or temporary dissolution of function in related areas of the brain or spinal cord. This is seen in the patient with a hemiplegia which is initially flaccid, later spastic, or in one with an acute spinal lesion; the limbs below the level of the lesion are initially flaccid and totally paralysed but later, as shock wears off, spasticity resulting from bilateral lesions of the corticospinal (pyramidal) tracts develops. By contrast, lesions of equal extent, but of slower development, produce fewer symptoms and physical signs, as it is only those structures which are actively invaded or destroyed whose function is disturbed; the surrounding tissues have more time to adapt to the presence of the lesion. Other forms of adaptation also occur, particularly in the cerebral cortex, for here a function which has been lost through a cortical lesion may be 'adopted', though usually much less efficiently, by another area of the brain. Such adaptation occurs more readily in children than in adults, for the younger the patient the greater the flexibility of cerebral organisation. In the spinal cord, there is less opportunity for this type of reorganisation than in the brain, for the nervous pathways are more stereotyped and less complex. In the peripheral nerves opportunities for adoption of functions in this way are almost non-existent, but these nerves are able to regenerate effectively following injury, while effective regeneration does not occur within the spinal cord or brain.

PATHOLOGICAL REACTIONS IN THE NERVOUS SYSTEM

Pathological changes in the nervous system can be classified into four broad groups, namely, **focal lesions**, which cause a localised disturbance of function; **multi-focal lesions**, simultaneously involving many parts of the nervous system; **diffuse or generalised disorders**, whether of infective, metabolic, toxic or other aetiology, which affect nervous and supporting elements throughout the nervous system; and **system diseases**, in which the pathological process shows a predilection for a particular functional unit or system, such as the motor system. Some focal and multifocal lesions and diffuse disorders affect nervous tissue by accident and are not primarily neurological diseases. Thus cerebral vascular disease, which can produce a focal cerebral lesion, such as an infarct, is usually a complication of hypertension and/or atherosclerosis, and multifocal cerebral metastases often complicate extracerebral cancer, while the diffuse pathological changes in the brain in syphilis represent only one component of the changes relating to infection of the entire human organism. In the system disorders by contrast, as in motor neurone disease, there is an as yet undefined factor which causes the pathological process to be virtually confined to motor nerve cells or motor pathways. The tissues of the nervous system also vary in their susceptibility to many noxious influences. Thus ischaemia affects nerve cells more severely than fibres, while plaques of demyelination, as in multiple sclerosis, have a much greater effect upon white matter. There are also differences in the effects of ischaemia, compression and various toxins upon nerve fibres, depending upon their calibre and myelination and upon whether they conduct motor or sensory impulses.

These pathological processes, and particularly the focal lesions, can also be subdivided on an aetiological basis. Virtually every lesion of the nervous system will be embraced by one of the following headings:

1. Congenital (developmental disorders)
2. Traumatic (physical or chemical (toxic) injury)
3. Inflammatory $\left\{\begin{array}{l}\text{infective} \\ \text{allergic or postinfective} \\ \text{(autoimmune)}\end{array}\right.$ $\left\{\begin{array}{l}\text{acute} \\ \text{subacute} \\ \text{chronic}\end{array}\right.$
4. Neoplastic $\left\{\begin{array}{l}\text{benign} \\ \text{malignant}\end{array}\right.$ $\left\{\begin{array}{l}\text{primary} \\ \text{secondary}\end{array}\right.$
5. Vascular
6. Degenerative
7. Metabolic and endocrine.

1. Congenital or developmental disorders

Most important central nervous lesions of congenital origin are clearly apparent as disorders of anatomical development and configuration; examples are anencephaly, hydrocephalus due to stenosis of the aqueduct of

Sylvius, and meningomyelocele. Arteriovenous malformations or angiomas, which may develop in the brain or spinal cord, are also of developmental origin. These malformations are also benign neoplasms, just as craniopharyngiomas, which are certainly neoplasms, arise initially from developmental remnants of Rathke's pouch.

2. Trauma

Trauma to the nervous system, as elsewhere, produces necrosis, haemorrhage and subsequent scar formation, the scar consisting of proliferated neuroglial cells and fibrils (gliosis) and of mesenchymal fibrous tissue derived from fibroblasts in the supporting tissue of the blood vessels.

3. Inflammation

Among the acute inflammatory disorders are the meningitides which produce typical changes of inflammation and exudation in the meninges. Meningitis can also cause superficial degeneration in the underlying nervous tissue or more extensive ischaemic changes in the nervous parenchyma resulting from an obliterative endarteritis of blood vessels which traverse the subarachnoid space. **Pyogenic infection** of the brain substance or spinal cord begins as a diffuse suppuration, but localisation and abscess formation generally follow with capsule formation.

Most so-called neurotropic **viruses**, such as those which cause viral encephalitis and anterior poliomyelitis, are polioclastic, i.e. they show an affinity for nerve cells; inflammatory changes, with perivascular cellular infiltration, and degeneration with phagocytosis (neuronophagia) of nerve cells, are therefore seen in the grey matter of the brain and spinal cord. Sometimes inclusion bodies are found within the nucleus or cytoplasm of infected cells. The herpes zoster virus shows a particular affinity for cells of the posterior root ganglia. **Syphilis**, despite its decreasing incidence, is still an important chronic infection. The meningovascular form gives meningeal inflammation and endarteritis of cerebral and spinal arteries; in general paresis there is degeneration of nerve cells, gliosis and minimal inflammatory changes in the cerebral cortex; in tabes dorsalis gliosis and meningeal fibrosis occur at the entry zone of the posterior spinal nerve roots with secondary ascending degeneration of the posterior columns. Gummas of the brain are now very rare. In **allergic or postinfective encephalomyelitis**, in contrast to the virus infections, inflammatory changes are largely confined to the white matter, where perivascular collections of inflammatory cells and loss of myelin are found.

The pathological changes in this disease show some resemblance to those seen in the **demyelinating diseases** of unknown aetiology, such as multiple sclerosis, in which there is patchy loss of myelin throughout the white matter of the brain and spinal cord. This primary lesion, in which axons are initially preserved, is eventually replaced by a glial scar.

4. Neoplasia

Most **benign tumours** affecting the central nervous system are extracerebral and extramedullary, lying outside the brain or spinal cord, though within their bony encasements. The two commonest are the meningioma, arising from arachnoidal cells, and the neurofibroma or neurilemmoma, which grows from the sheath of Schwann of the cranial nerves, spinal roots or peripheral nerves. These neoplasms compress and distort but do not invade nervous tissue. The gliomas are the principal **malignant tumours**; these are invasive growths whose relative malignancy depends upon whether the principal constituent cell is a relatively mature astrocyte or one of its more rapidly multiplying primitive precursors. Metastatic malignant neoplasms are also common; cancer of the lung, breast and kidney and the malignant melanoma are among those which most often metastasise to the brain. Secondary deposits, often seen at the junction of the white and grey matter, are sometimes single but much more often multiple. Less commonly these deposits, or plaques of reticulosis, involve the meninges; if this occurs in the spinal canal, or if a vertebral body has collapsed following malignant infiltration, spinal cord compression can result.

5. Vascular disorders

These are common. Bleeding into the subarachnoid space produces aseptic meningeal inflammation and sometimes a degree of meningeal organisation or arachnoiditis results. Chronic subarachnoid bleeding can produce haemosiderosis of the meninges. Haemorrhage into the nervous parenchyma causes an area of necrosis which is eventually walled off by gliosis and fibrosis; if it is small the necrotic area is absorbed and a scar results, but more often a cavity filled with clear straw-coloured fluid containing bilirubin is left. An infarct, too, shows central ischaemic necrosis. Within 24 hours, activated microglial cells (the histiocytes or scavengers of the nervous system) invade the necrotic area and become distended with the fatty remnants of necrotic myelin. A minute infarct, produced by embolic occlusion of a tiny cortical or a deep (perforating) artery, may consist of little more than a small cluster of activated microglial cells or a tiny cavity, whereas a large one will show an extensive central area of necrosis surrounded by distended phagocytes ('gitter' cells) and proliferating astrocytes. A large area of infarction may eventually be represented by a contracted glial scar or by a larger cavity, while multifocal infarction sometimes gives many multiple small cavities or lacunes ('status lacunosus').

6. Degenerative disorders

There are many disorders of the nervous system whose aetiology is at present unknown, but in some of which specific neuropathological changes are seen. In motor neurone disease, for instance, the cells of the motor nuclei of the brain stem, the spinal anterior horn cells, and the pyramidal tracts show progressive degeneration; in Huntington's chorea there is selective degeneration of the caudate nucleus and of nerve cells in the frontal cortex. But in these and in many other disorders, although the anatomical distribution of pathological change is well-defined, their nature and cause is little understood.

7. Metabolic disorders

Anoxia affects particularly the cells of the deepest layer of the cerebral cortex, the Ammon's horn area of the hippocampus and the cerebellar Purkinje cells, while deficiency of vitamin B_{12}, as in subacute combined degeneration of the spinal cord, damages selectively the posterior columns and pyramidal tracts. Many other metabolic disorders which seriously derange nervous function produce relatively little pathological change, although in hypoglycaemia the changes resemble those of anoxia, while in hepatic failure there is astrocytic proliferation, particularly in the basal ganglia. The pathological changes in many forms of **polyneuropathy** are also non-specific, consisting either of segmental loss of myelin, beginning in the region of the nodes of Ranvier (demyelinating neuropathies), or of swelling and fragmentation of axons in the peripheral nerves (axonal neuropathies).

CONSTITUTION AND HEREDITY

In considering the aetiological factors responsible for a patient's illness it is easy to overlook important genetic influences. Many neurological disorders, and particularly some referred to above as being 'degenerative' in character, are inherited in a strictly Mendelian manner. A disease resulting from a dominant gene situated on one of the autosomes, an autosomal dominant trait, is passed on by an affected individual to half his or her children of either sex if penetrance or expressivity of the gene is complete. Examples of disorders which are inherited in this way are Huntington's chorea and facioscapulohumeral muscular dystrophy. A recessive gene, carried on an autosome, however, can only produce its effect if paired with a similar gene lying on the other chromosome of the pair. Such a trait, autosomal recessive, can only come to light, therefore, when two unaffected heterozygotes marry, and hence there is usually no previous history of the disease in the family, unless there has been intermarriage between relatives (consanguinity). In such families, the likelihood is that the disease will affect one in four of a series of brothers and sisters (a sibship); Friedreich's ataxia, hepatolenticular degeneration and most forms of spinal muscular atrophy are examples.

A recessive gene can produce an effect, however, if situated on the unpaired portion of the X-chromosome; such a condition occurs in males and is carried by apparently unaffected females. It is then known as a sex-linked or X-linked recessive character; the disease may have affected maternal uncles and now appears in half the male children of a female carrier. Diseases inherited in this manner include red-green colour blindness, haemophilia and the Duchenne and Becker types of muscular dystrophy. Some female carriers may show minor clinical manifestations. Any inherited disease can, of course, appear anew in a family if a previously normal gene has undergone a process of spontaneous change or mutation.

Apart from diseases which are clearly inherited by these genetic mechanisms, there are many other nervous disorders in which genetic influences are important, though less clearly defined. In epilepsy and multiple sclerosis, for example, more than one member of a family is affected more often than could be accounted for by chance, though no clear pattern of inheritance emerges. From time to time, too, one finds families in which several individuals have died from cerebral tumour or subarachnoid haemorrhage. Furthermore, there is some evidence that an individual's emotional and physical constitution may influence his susceptibility to certain infections or other neurological disorders. An increasing number of diseases, such as multiple sclerosis, myasthenia gravis and narcolepsy, have been shown to be related to the histocompatibility (HLA) antigen constitution of the individual. One must therefore consider not only the environmental, but also the constitutional influences which may have a bearing upon each patient's disease.

TREATMENT AND MANAGEMENT IN NEUROLOGY—SOME GENERAL PRINCIPLES

Whereas the preceding pages have dealt with the foundations of neurological diagnosis, it is the treatment of the patient's disease and not diagnosis itself which is, or should be, the ultimate aim. While accurate diagnosis may be an essential first step before appropriate therapy can be recommended, this is not invariable and there are some patients suffering from nervous disease in whom the correct management is clear even though diagnosis remains obscure. In a case of progressive dementia arising in the presenium, for instance, there may be no certain means of deciding whether the illness is due to Alzheimer's disease or to some other cause. Provided, however, that treatable conditions such as general paresis, vitamin B_{12} deficiency and frontal meningioma have been excluded, management then depends upon the patient's behaviour and social circumstances. If he is placid and manageable, despite his dementia and associated incontinence, and if he has a capable wife or other relatives, the situation should be explained to them and he should be cared for at home with suitable sedative drugs and nursing and social assistance. But if, on the other hand, he is violent or disturbed in his behaviour, if he lives alone, or if his relatives are frail or incompetent, there may be no alternative but to arrange his admission to a mental hospital.

Treatment is not merely a matter of prescribing drugs, and of seeing that they are properly administered (a problem often more difficult than the simple act of writing a prescription). It also involves management of the individual and of his relatives. When should the patient be treated and nursed at home and when in hospital? How far should special investigations be pursued, particularly if they are unpleasant or potentially dangerous? Are they to be carried out because of possible benefit to the patient, or merely to satisfy the doctor's curiosity? Will the results of the test influence the patient's management? How much should he be told of the nature and prognosis of his illness, and how much information should be given to his family? When is it necessary to ask for a second opinion? These are questions which continually arise in clinical practice and are not easily answered in the pages of a textbook. The ability to solve these problems with tact, patience and understanding stems not only from a knowledge of disease, but also from experience of patients as individuals and of their personalities, emotional reactions and family background. So diverse may be the personal and domestic circumstances of two patients suffering from identical illnesses, that although the correct pharmacological treatment is similar, the appropriate management when considered in more general terms may be quite different.

The first important lesson that the student must learn is that his value as a doctor does not depend merely upon his ability to diagnose illness and to prescribe appropriate drugs, but also upon the way in which he manages sick people and their relatives. The second is that while there are many incurable neurological illnesses, none are untreatable.

While it is clear that many neurological disorders can now be cured or benefited by pharmacological or surgical means, even in those in which the basic pathological process is relatively uninfluenced by any treatment at present available, substantial improvement in the patient's symptoms or in his attitude to his disease can often be achieved with drugs or physical methods. Often, too, it is of great help to the patient if the doctor can do no more than give an accurate forecast of the natural history and eventual outcome of the illness. In inherited conditions, one must also be able to give appropriate advice about the prospect of affection of other members of the family, if this information is sought, and particularly if the parents of an ill child are considering adding to their family. If, on the other hand, they already have other children, it may be wise not to reveal this prospect at the outset, perhaps until the parents become aware of it themselves. It is also wise in cases of progressively crippling illness, to keep some hope alive by referring to the research being done upon the chronic neurological diseases and by saying that these are not incurable conditions, but rather diseases for which no cure has yet been found. It is, however, equally important to be sure that the hopes of the patient and his relatives should not be unduly raised only to be shattered by subsequent events.

Physiotherapy and rehabilitation

Physiotherapy plays an important part in treating many neurological disorders. Thus when disease results in a partial or complete paralysis of a limb, or of more than one limb, appropriate physiotherapeutic treatment must be instituted as soon as possible. Its purpose is to help the patient to make the best possible use of the available power in the affected limb if the paralysis is partial, and to prevent muscular contractures, stiffening and deformity if it is complete. When paralysis is almost total, whether it be flaccid (a lower motor neurone lesion, or an upper motor neurone lesion during the stage of spinal shock) or spastic (upper motor neurone lesion), the first essential is that passive movements of the affected muscles are carried out repeatedly through the maximum range at all affected joints. This action will maintain the elasticity of the muscles, will prevent the development of contractures and may, if spasticity is present, help in modifying the enhanced muscular tone. Later, once voluntary power begins to return, active movements are encouraged, first with support or positioning of the limb to nullify the effect of gravity and later against resistance. Repeated isometric contraction is particularly valuable. In a patient with a hemiplegia following cerebral thrombosis, for instance, this process may be very slow, requiring great patience and continual encouragement on the part of the physiotherapist and nurse (and the relatives), and confidence and determination from the patient. Nearly all hemiplegic patients are eventually helped to walk, although in many, little useful function in the paralysed fingers is regained. The help of a physiotherapist is also essential in patients with respiratory paralysis, as skilful positioning will not only help the patient to expectorate secretion which might otherwise obstruct the bronchi, but will also help him to make the best possible use of ventilatory capacity which he regains.

Rehabilitation is important not only in restoring to useful activity those patients who are recovering from any illness causing paralysis, but may also be of inestimable value in some individuals suffering from chronic neurological diseases. Thus in patients with cerebellar ataxia, Fraenkel's walking exercises, in which the patient learns to walk along a line or to follow foot-prints drawn on the floor, may be helpful. Programmed exercises, if utilised with enthusiasm and persistence, and combined with vigorous passive movements, are also of value in the rehabilitation of the paraplegic, and in the education of children with cerebral palsy. They may even produce improvement in patients with diseases such as multiple sclerosis and Parkinsonism, in whom there is hope of remission or arrest. On the other hand, physiotherapeutic treatment is not always indicated in other remorselessly progressive disorders such as motor neurone disease; it may be disappointing to the patient and frustrating for the physiotherapist, as the disease progresses rapidly enough to nullify any temporary benefit which may result from the treatment. However, in spinal muscular atrophy in childhood, in which the disease process often seems to arrest spontaneously, exercise plays an important role in maintaining or even improving power in those muscles which retain a nerve supply and in preventing or correcting contractures. Swimming is particularly helpful in such cases. Much the same is true in cases of muscular dystrophy, since, although the disease is progressive, regular moderate exercise may help to slow the rate of deterioration; it is also of benefit in such cases to demonstrate to the parents of affected children the passive movements (dorsiflexion of the ankle, extension of the knees) which they can employ to delay the onset of contractures and the attention to posture or the use of appliances which can help prevent scoliosis.

There are many appliances which can compensate for disability and aid the physiotherapist. Thus in the patient who is beginning to walk after a disabling illness and even in some who are deteriorating slowly, walking machines, walking tripods, crutches, calipers and walking-sticks, may all be required at some stage to give the patient support and confidence. Night splints applied to a spastic or paralysed limb can be useful in preventing contractures, while in a patient with foot drop, a caliper and spring fitted to his shoe or a light plastic moulded splint to prevent the toe from dragging will improve walking considerably. Similarly, a 'cock-up' forearm splint will be required in a patient with wrist drop. In obtaining for his disabled patients appropriate appliances and invalid aids, the neurologist is dependent upon the advice of his colleagues in rehabilitation medicine and upon the help of physiotherapists and occupational therapists.

Occupational therapy

The occupational therapist plays an invaluable role in helping patients with chronic progressive neurological diseases and those recovering slowly from disabling disorders of the nervous system (including head injury). As days and weeks of comparative monotony slip by, with improvement which may at first be imperceptible, particularly to the patient, he or she must be kept occupied and interested. Not only is constant encouragement needed, but time spent in appropriate activities is not only an antidote for despondency but also helps to improve the power and co-ordination of the limbs. Occupational therapists are especially skilled in assessing the effects which a particular disability may have upon the patient's daily life and in designing tasks and mechanical aids which may help him to overcome or compensate for his disability. This treatment is of especial value to the disabled housewife in assisting her to adjust to her disability in the performance of domestic tasks, but is also invaluable in the rehabilitation of the wage-earner as well as in the management of the seriously disabled. Television and organised sports (such as archery for the paraplegic) are also excellent for morale in appropriate long-stay hospitals. Considerable ingenuity may be demanded of the doctor who is supervising the slow recovery of a patient who has been ill in his own home, but domiciliary occupational therapy is also helpful.

Speech therapy

The speech therapist is another important member of the team of those concerned in the treatment and rehabilitation of neurological cases. Much of her time is spent in the painstaking education of children who are born with defective speech or who begin to speak in an abnormal way. Two important categories are the deaf child and the child with severe cerebral palsy. While considerable improvement may be expected in these with patient training, complete recovery may be achieved within a few years in children with dyslalia. Stammering can also be improved in some cases, for example by teaching the use of syllabic speech. But speech therapy is also useful in patients suffering from dysarthria and more particularly aphasia as a result of disease of the brain (as after cerebral vascular accidents). With the aid of patient re-education, recovery can be accelerated and is in the end much more complete, provided the patient is capable of enthusiastic co-operation.

The management of the 'incurable' case

So many chronic neurological disorders are relatively uninfluenced by any form of treatment that sufferers from them often present difficult problems in management. The specialist and more particularly the general practitioner must often mobilise all his reserves of patience, tact and human understanding in dealing with these problems. As mentioned above, physiotherapy is often of temporary benefit and many appliances and invalid aids are available to assist patients in compensating for and adjusting to their disabilities. But when the patient, despite his efforts and those of his doctors, sees himself deteriorating it is not surprising that he often becomes despondent. To strike the right note of encouragement, of sympathy combined with firmness, to offer a glimmer of hope without unjustifiable optimism, and to think of something new to say to the patient and his relatives at each weekly visit; these are the problems which often strain the doctor's resources. When to tell the patient the truth about his condition? When to encourage his desire for yet another opinion and when to dissuade him? What to tell his relatives and what to withhold? These are questions to which no definitive answers are available as so much depends upon the patient's personality, his responsibilities and his domestic circumstances.

The correct course of action can only be chosen in the light of experience and there can be few circumstances in which the doctor's judgement is more important. Some patients demand and deserve to be told the truth and their resolve and resistance is strengthened by knowing the facts of the situation, however gloomy, while others prefer at least partial ignorance and seem curiously lacking in insight to the end. Some are helped by sedative or antidepressive remedies when despair deepens, others regard their illness as a challenge, and triumph in every minor victory over disability. It is only to be expected that some patients should resort to unorthodox forms of treatment when orthodox medicine has failed. While it is the doctor's duty in such a case to advise his patients against accepting potentially dangerous or inappropriate remedial measures, particularly if this involves a financial outlay he can ill afford, the physician who regards this deviation upon the part of his patients as being a personal affront or evidence of loss of faith in his ability shows lack of understanding.

When it becomes clear that the illness is drawing towards its close management is guided by a few simple principles. The most important are that pain and suffering should be relieved, and emotional distress alleviated by all available means, so that the patient is made as comfortable as possible. The question as to whether he should be nursed at home or in hospital during this terminal period depends upon many variables, including the efficiency and devotion of his relatives and the nature of his illness. If there is no reason to suppose that the nursing and medical care which the patient would receive in hospital would be in any way superior to that he is obtaining at home, it is better that he should remain in familiar surroundings. But even in the best circumstances there are occasions when, because of confused or irrational behaviour, incontinence and the like or intolerable strain upon relatives, admission to the hospital cannot be avoided.

Of the drugs which are available for the relief of pain and suffering in a terminal illness, morphine and its analogues are unquestionably the best, but sedatives such as the benzodiazepines are often required in addition, while phenothiazines and/or antihistamines too are often helpful, as they not only potentiate the action of many other drugs but also help to relieve the nausea and vomiting which are often troublesome features. If the patient dies peacefully in reasonable comfort, and his relatives have been well-informed and know that everything possible, from both the medical and nursing standpoint has been carried out, the doctor can be satisfied that his duty has been done.

CONCLUSIONS

A systematic approach to each patient with symptoms suggesting disease of the nervous system is an essential preliminary to accurate diagnosis. The question should first be asked, **where** is the lesion or system process responsible for these symptoms and signs? Is it extracerebral in the skull or meninges, in the cerebral cortex, in the white matter, in the brain stem or cerebellum? Or if the clinical picture indicates, say, a disorder of the spinal cord or of the lower motor neurone, is the lesion in the spinal column, the meninges, the spinal cord, the spinal roots, plexuses, peripheral nerves, motor end-plates or muscles? And in each of these situations, **what** is the lesion or process? Could it be congenital, traumatic, inflammatory, neoplastic, degenerative or metabolic?

What influences are constitutional factors playing in its genesis? Is there disease in the heart, great vessels, lungs or other organs which could be responsible? Are emotional or psychological factors responsible for any part of the patient's disability? While in many cases the answers to some of these questions are self-evident it is well that they should be asked, since it is only through such a comprehensive approach to patients with neurological disease that the doctor will eventually acquire the skill and experience which will allow him to discard the irrelevant and to concentrate upon those salient facts which lead to accurate diagnosis.

Diagnosis in specific or in general terms once achieved, with the support, when necessary, of various tests or investigations (see Ch. 3), then treatment, whether by pharmacological, surgical or other physical means becomes the objective, as a part of overall management. Detailed commentaries upon methods of management of individual diseases and symptom-complexes will be given in the chapters which follow, but the part to be played by counselling and the many other supportive methods referred to above, especially in chronic progressive or other disabling diseases, must never be overlooked.

REFERENCES

Adams J H, Corsellis J A N, Duchen L W 1984 Greenfield's neuropathology, 4th edn. Arnold, London

Adams R D, Victor M 1985 Principles of neurology, 3rd edn. McGraw-Hill, New York

Davison A N, Thompson R H S 1981 The molecular basis of neuropathology. Arnold, London

Emery A E H 1983 Elements of medical genetics, 6th edn. Churchill Livingstone, Edinburgh

Matthews W B 1975 Practical neurology, 3rd edn. Blackwell, Oxford

Rosenberg R N 1986 Neurogenetics: principles and practice. Raven Press, New York

Swash M, Kennard C (eds) 1985 Scientific basis of clinical neurology. Churchill Livingstone, Edinburgh

Walton J N 1985 Brain's diseases of the nervous system, 9th edn. Oxford University Press , Oxford

Walton J N 1987 Introduction to clinical neuroscience, 2nd edn. Baillière Tindall, London

2. The symptoms and signs of disease in the nervous system

In neurology, as in any branch of medicine, prognosis and treatment usually depend upon accurate diagnosis, while diagnosis, in turn, stems from an elucidation of symptoms and signs, combined with information obtained from appropriate investigations. In some nervous disorders such as epilepsy and migraine, a careful appraisal of the patient's symptoms is all-important in diagnosis, and physical examination is essentially negative. Conversely, in many other diseases, the history is uninformative and all depends upon a meticulous neurological examination. Usually, however, the history and examination are mutually interdependent, one throwing light upon the significance of the other. The physical signs may identify the anatomical situation of a lesion responsible for a patient's illness, while the evolutionary pattern of its symptomatology indicates the nature of the pathological process. So many individual symptoms and signs may result from nervous disease that a planned approach to each individual patient is needed; an approach so designed that major manifestations of illness which may at first seem irrelevant are not overlooked, but are fitted into place so that the patient and his disease are viewed as a whole. In this chapter an attempt is made to describe the framework of neurological diagnosis and management.

Diagnosis is not, however, an end in itself. The doctor is assessed by his patients, who justify his professional existence, not upon his flair for diagnosing rare diseases, but upon his understanding of their needs, of their hopes and fears and of the intensely personal problem which their illness presents. Sometimes fears of cancer or of insanity play an important role in contributing to the patient's symptoms; these factors can be consciously suppressed, but are yet of aetiological significance. Furthermore, the correct management of two identical cases of disabling disease of the nervous system can be very different if the sufferers differ widely in attitude, emotional constitution and domestic environment. There are many chronic and crippling progressive disorders of the nervous system which continually pose serious problems of management to patient and doctor. These conditions require of the doctor much tact, sympathy and understanding, as well as diagnostic expertise and ingenuity in changing circumstances. Ability to communicate clearly, meaningfully and sensitively with the patient and his relatives is also fundamental. These skills are not learned from textbooks but are derived from continuing contact with patients and their relatives, not only in hospital, but in their homes. Diagnosis is only the beginning, and need not necessarily be strictly accurate for management to be correct, provided the general nature of the patient's disease is recognised. But there are also many conditions, such as meningitis, subdural haematoma and spinal tumour, in which diagnosis must be made early if death or severe disability is to be avoided.

SOME USEFUL TERMS IN NEUROLOGY

Several terms, largely derived from Greek and Latin, are in common use in neurological medicine. Thus the prefix 'a-' means absence of, the prefix 'dys-' disturbance of; 'hyper-' means increased and 'hypo-' decreased. If the Greek suffix '-phasis' is taken to denote conceptual skills involved in speech function, then 'aphasia' is used to denote loss of this function, 'dysphasia' when the disorder of function is less severe. Similarly aphonia is loss of the ability to phonate, anarthria means inability to articulate and dysarthria slurring or indistinct articulation. Atrophy of muscles means wasting and hypertrophy enlargement, while hypoaesthesia (often shortened to hypaesthesia) is used to identify reduced sensation, while hyperpathia (much preferred to the semantically inaccurate hyperalgesia) is taken to indicate an abnormal, unpleasant and increased sensitivity to sensory stimuli.

In much the same way, ataxia means unsteadiness or lack of co-ordination, apraxia loss of motor skills. The suffix '-plegia' means paralysis and '-paresis' weakness. Thus a monoplegia is a paralysis of one limb, a monoparesis weakness of one limb. Similarly a hemiplegia means paralysis of one arm and leg on the same side of the body, tetraplegia or quadriplegia paralysis of all four limbs, and paraplegia paralysis of the lower limbs only. The term diplegia is often used to identify a form of spastic weakness of all four limbs but usually affecting the lower limbs more severely than the upper.

TAKING THE HISTORY

Some introductory principles

The principles of history taking in neurological disease do not differ from those applicable to any branch of medicine. This is, however, of particular importance in neurology and contributes to over 80% of the evaluation of patients with neurological disease. More errors of diagnosis are made from failure to take a proper history than from any other single cause. The history is often the only source of information, since patients commonly present in the very early stages of a disease when there may be symptoms but no signs. In addition, many neurological disorders are episodic, so that the patient is entirely normal between attacks; this is especially true of two of the most common conditions affecting patients attending a neurology clinic, namely migraine and epilepsy.

The history must be structured because patients do not know what is important and what is not. A fine balance must therefore be drawn between allowing the patient to express his or her problem in his own words, while at the same time structuring the interview with judicious guiding questions in such a way as to get all the necessary information. It may be helpful to consider that all histories have a shape. They start at one point in time and the problem may be maximal at onset or may evolve in some way to a maximum. The pace of this evolution gives valuable information about the nature of a condition. For example, there are many causes of a hemiplegia but one that comes on at a stroke is likely to have a vascular origin, while one that evolves slowly over weeks is more likely to be due to a space-occupying lesion. The patient may be seen at a time when the problem is still evolving or it may be that the problem has evolved to its maximum, then remaining unchanged for a period of time before improving. The patient may make a full recovery from an event or be left with some persisting deficit. To determine the 'shape' of a history therefore requires precise details of the onset, the pace of evolution, the duration for which the problem was at its worst and the degree of deficit at that time and the pace of recovery. Conditions which produce episodic deficits such as some migrainous auras, focal epileptic seizures, transient ischaemic attacks and multiple sclerosis may all produce similar manifestations, but the time course of each of these events is often entirely different and a detailed history is usually all that is required to differentiate them.

As well as obtaining a detailed account of an event or a typical event of many, it is also necessary to obtain information about the frequency of similar events over a period of time. In conditions like migraine and epilepsy, the patient may have had many similar attacks over a number of years. The attacks sometimes occur in clusters, as in periodic migrainous neuralgia (see p. 56), or there may be clustering of attacks around the time of menstruation, or they may occur at random. Not only is this information about the spacing of attacks very useful in determining the nature of the condition, but it is also essential in determining how serious and disabling a problem the condition presents to the patient and serves as a baseline for comparison in assessing the effect of treatment. Patients often have difficulty in remembering how seriously disabling their condition was before treatment, particularly if the treatment is not completely effective.

Many individuals have difficulty in remembering the precise details of the onset of their symptoms; if this happened suddenly at a specific time instead of evolving slowly, it is often helpful to ask for precise details about the day of the week, the time of day and the activity in which they were engaged when symptoms began, as this serves to cue the patient's memory about the onset and often provides very useful information.

There are many circumstances in which the patient is unable to give a full history; this commonly occurs in patients with dementia or confusional states as well as in those with epilepsy. In these circumstances it is imperative to obtain an account from a witness. It may then become apparent that the patient's mental deterioration has been slowly evolving over some years; and in patients with epilepsy, details of exactly what happens when they are unconscious can give valuable information about the nature of the attack.

The structured history

It is usual to begin by listing the **principal symptoms** of which the patient complains and then to give, in chronological order, a description in his own words of how they developed. Judicious questions may be needed to restrain the garrulous and cut short irrelevancies, as well as to expand and clarify individual points. It is easy to forget that most patients are not medically trained; to them, opinions previously expressed by Dr X, or the fall a few weeks ago may seem much more important than the transient blurring of vision, say, apparently unconnected with the present complaint, which occurred three years before. Hence, once the patient has given his story, amplified by judicious guidance and prompting, one must ask **leading questions** which have been avoided assiduously at an earlier stage so as not to present the suggestible patient with additional symptoms which he may profess. These should relate to some of the principal symptoms of nervous disease, each of which will later be considered individually. Has there been, for instance, any pain or headache, any loss or impairment of consciousness, either brief or prolonged? Have there been any visual symptoms, such as impairment of sight or diplopia, or has the patient noticed any alteration in speech or swallowing? Are memory, behaviour and concentration unimpaired, has he had deafness, tinnitus, giddiness or unsteadiness, or involuntary movements of the head, trunk or limbs? Usually, too, it is wise to enquire specifically about weakness, paralysis or clumsiness of the limbs (though few patients would overlook such striking symptoms) and about numbness, tingling, pins and needles or other unusual sensations. Finally, enquiry should be made as to whether control of the vesical or anal sphincters and/or of sexual function has been impaired and whether there have been other more general symptoms such as breathlessness, weight loss (or gain), anxiety, depression, sleeplessness, anorexia or vomiting.

Having elicited in this way one or more symptoms, it is usually clear that this knowledge alone is insufficient. If the complaint is of headache, for instance, much more is needed. Where in the head is it situated, and does it spread? What is its character? When does it or did it begin? How long does it last and how often does it occur? Is there any warning of its onset? Does anything precipitate it or make it worse once it has begun, and does anything relieve it? This kind of enquiry may be applied, with minor modifications, to almost any symptom of nervous disease, but should not be learned by rote. An inquisitive approach in which each symptom is scrutinised and analysed in detail is better. Such critical enquiry and appraisal is more revealing and profitable to both doctor and patient than a carefully ordered routine learned by heart. On the other hand, the enquiry must be comprehensive. While the experienced physician may reach the heart of the problem with a few well-chosen questions, there are no short cuts for the beginner. This is one of the most important lessons to learn. If history taking is at first slow and laborious, growing experience, and experience alone, will teach which symptoms may safely be discarded as irrelevant and which are of crucial importance.

With increasing experience, if a detailed history of the problem has been obtained, the number of routine systematic enquiry questions can often be considerably reduced. However, it is always useful to ask about appetite and weight; the patient who says that his appetite is very poor but that his weight is increasing gives useful information about his emotional status. It is also useful to ask about sleep habits; if the patient sleeps badly it is important to know whether there is difficulty in going to sleep, staying asleep or whether there is a tendency to wake early and whether this problem is recent or of long standing. Enquiry should also be made about allergies as this may have a direct effect on treatment. It is also necessary to know what, if any, drugs are being taken at the time; if this is uncertain, additional medication should not be prescribed except in an emergency because possible interactions cannot be evaluated. It is also necessary to ask women in the child-bearing age whether or not they are taking the combined contraceptive pill; women should also be asked brief details of their menstrual history. Careful enquiry about tobacco and alcohol consumption and about the use of potentially addictive drugs or about habits such as glue sniffing should be tactfully included as these may each be associated with neurological problems.

Having dealt with the history of the patient's present illness one must then enquire as to his **previous health**. The patient should be asked what previous accidents, operations or illnesses they have had in their lives and this enquiry may reveal relevant information which the patient had not thought appropriate to mention. Many people forget about previous illnesses and it is sometimes helpful to cue their memory by asking if they have ever been in hospital or to a hospital out-patient clinic. It is also useful to know about the patient's educational standard and what occupations he has followed. Is he married, with a family, or does he live alone? Are his domestic circumstances satisfactory or are there financial and/or personal difficulties? And what is known about his physical and emotional constitution? Has he been physically active, athletic and extraverted, or studious, retiring and introspective? Was he excessively nervous or over-protected as a child, did he wet the bed or walk in his sleep, and has he changed his employment frequently? What are his interests and hobbies, and have these changed of late? Questions of this type can be very rewarding, eliciting answers which reveal deterioration in intellect, change in personality, or life-long psychopathy and failure of adjustment to the demands of society.

It is also helpful to the doctor to know about the patient's occupational history. This may, for example, give evidence of past exposure to toxic chemicals which can damage the nervous system; alternatively the symptoms resulting from the illness may have caused loss of time from work or other problems in his employment. Often the development of a neurological problem precludes continued employment, as, for example, does epilepsy in a heavy goods vehicle driver; the prospect of losing his job may have a profound effect on the patient's attitude.

Finally, the family history can be very important, as some neurological disorders are clearly inherited, while in others inherited predisposition plays a part. If the patient is thought to have a developmental or hereditary disease, a detailed family history is imperative; and if further cases of disease come to light, then a pedigree should be drawn. If no such suspicion arises, then it is only necessary to enquire about first degree relatives.

Important diseases of other systems should also be noted in other family members; for instance, a strong family history of coronary artery disease may suggest that atherosclerosis of the cerebral, rather than of the coronary arteries, accounts for the patient's symptoms.

Clearly this guide to history taking can only give a broad outline of general principles. It is, however, worth emphasising the great importance of a full history, both in reaching a diagnosis and in the subsequent management of the patient, when considering all relevant factors including his job, his environment and his personal and family background. The time taken to establish a proper history at the patient's first consultation is never wasted and often avoids a succession of errors, both in diagnosis and in management.

THE NEUROLOGICAL EXAMINATION

Many schemes for examining the nervous system have been recommended and most are satisfactory, provided they are complete and carefully itemised. The outline given below is of a method for examining the nervous system which the author has found satisfactory in practice. A full examination so performed is admittedly time-consuming, but once it has been learned and practised assiduously, experience will teach which parts of it may be discarded or abridged in any individual case. However, when experience is limited, attempts to abbreviate the process lead to inevitable and important oversights.

The mental state

Disease of the brain may have a profound effect upon behaviour and awareness, so that accurate assessment of the patient's mental state is of great importance. Individual symptoms and signs will be considered in later chapters; it is therefore unnecessary at this stage to define terms but brief outlines are given of some common abnormalities.

First, the patient's state of awareness must be assessed. Is he comatose or semicomatose, confused or disorientated, or is he alert and well orientated in time and in place? Secondly, is his mood normal, or is he euphoric, elated, depressed, anxious or agitated? Thirdly, are his behaviour and social adjustments normal or is he anti-social and amoral, dirty in his habits and blandly unconcerned? Does he show disordered thought processes with ideas of persecution (paranoia) or other delusions, or are there visual or auditory hallucinations? These questions can usually be answered through observation and by questioning the patient, but simple tests of a more formal nature may be needed in order to assess memory and intellect and the powers of abstract thought.

Quantitative assessment of intellectual function requires the application of specific tests by a trained clinical psychologist; among those most commonly used are the Wechsler Adult Intelligence Scale (and the comparable scale for children) with their many modifications. It is, however, possible to carry out simple bedside tests which give useful qualitative information about a patient's memory and intellectual function. The following tests are often used in this context:

Memory:

a. Immediate recall. This is tested by the digit retention test. The patient is asked to repeat a random series of numbers forwards and backwards. Normal individuals should achieve 6 or 7 numbers forwards and 3 or 4 numbers backwards.

b. Short-term memory. This is tested with the 5 minute memory test. A patient is given a number of items to remember; a name and an address is a convenient form. It is usual to add an entirely different item from this, such as the name of a flower. The patient is asked to repeat these items immediately and again at 5 minutes. The number incorrect is recorded.

c. Long-term memory. The patient is asked to give details of his past life or, where appropriate, details of national or international importance in the past which they might reasonably be expected to remember. This item depends considerably on social and educational background. Often it is useful to ask for the names of Prime Ministers or US Presidents.

Simple arithmetic. A number of simple additions, multiplications or divisions can be used but the serial 7s test is commonly used. The patient is asked to subtract 7 from 100 and to continue to do so. The time taken and the number of errors made are recorded.

Learning. The ability to learn can conveniently be tested with the Babcock sentence. The patient is asked to repeat the sentence until he can do so without error. The version of the Babcock sentence most commonly used is: 'One thing a nation must have to be rich and great is a large, secure supply of wood'. Most subjects can learn this in three attempts and more than four is abnormal.

Abstract ideas. This can be tested by asking the meaning of proverbs such as 'A rolling stone gathers no moss' or 'People in glass houses should not throw stones'. Patients with early dementia or some with psychosis may only be able to give a literal meaning to these proverbs and may not have any idea of the underlying concept.

Current events. Asking the patient about recent news items gives some idea of their awareness and perception, whether they read newspapers and are capable of understanding the published news or that on television or radio.

Praxis and gnosis and the body image

Praxis is the ability to perform purposive skilled movements; if this function is impaired, skills most recently acquired may be the first to be lost. The patient should be asked to perform movements of moderate complexity, such as those involved in dressing, in shaving, in opening a box of matches and striking one or in constructing a model with toy bricks. If a patient without obvious motor weakness or sensory impairment cannot perform such movements, this may indicate a disorder of praxis, known as apraxia.

Gnosis is the ability, following the reception of sensory stimuli, either visual or tactile, to recognise the nature and significance of objects. This usually relates to articles in the patient's environment, but may also be concerned with the parts of his own body. The patient may be asked to interpret humorous drawings or pictures which tell a story, or to identify objects, such as coins placed in the hands. He is also asked to identify parts of his or the examiner's body, for example, one ear, a knee or individual fingers. His awareness of his own body and of its relationship to extrapersonal space is known as the body image and loss of awareness of a part of that image is a form of agnosia or impairment of gnosis.

Speech

The function of speech may be subdivided into the higher or cortical control of speech, and the lower level mechanisms responsible for phonation and articulation. Reading (understanding of the written word) and writing (expression by means of the written, rather than the spoken word) are closely related to speech function, as is the ability to calculate. Inability to express one's thoughts in words when the peripheral mechanisms of articulation are intact, and understanding of the spoken word is preserved, is known as motor, expressive, non-fluent or Broca's aphasia; while failure to understand the spoken word is called sensory, receptive, fluent or Wernicke's aphasia. These and related functions are most easily tested by asking the patient to name a series of common objects of progressive difficulty (hand, mouth, pen, radiator, spectacles, stethoscope, etc.) and by giving simple commands, or by asking simple questions. A patient with slight motor aphasia may be accurate in his speech but yet hesitant and at a loss for simple words, while one with sensory aphasia may fail to obey commands or name simple objects or may use totally inappropriate words in his reply to questions (see Ch. 5). When his answers have been recorded the patient should then be asked to read, interpret and perhaps paraphrase a short passage from a book, to write from dictation, to copy a sentence and to write down his name and address and some of his outstanding symptoms. The ability to do a number of simple sums should also be tested.

A patient with complete paralysis of the articulatory muscles is well able to understand and interpret the spoken and written word and to express himself fluently in writing. If he cannot make a sound (phonation) this is called aphonia, but if a sound is uttered and cannot be moulded into words, this sign is entitled anarthria. Complete anarthria is rare, but slurring or indistinctness of speech (dysarthria) is much more common. The patient should be asked to repeat some set phrases if dysarthria is suspected; 'British constitution' and 'Methodist episcopal' are good examples in common use.

The skull and skeleton

Inspection and palpation of the skull is an essential part of the neurological examination. The size and shape of the skull and any asymmetry should be noted, as should the presence of any abnormal bony protuberances or points of tenderness. Auscultation in the temporal fossae and over the globes of both eyes should also be carried out while the patient holds his breath, so that the presence or absence of a **cranial bruit** or murmur may be recorded. Auscultation for such a bruit over the carotid, vertebral and subclavian arteries in the neck is also necessary; rarely a bruit can be heard over the vertebral column (a spinal bruit). Cranial bruits are often heard in normal children but if unilateral are more likely to be significant. In adults one must be sure that a bruit heard in the neck is not being conducted from the heart (as in aortic stenosis). In the remainder of the skeleton, any bony deformities (abnormal spinal curvature, pes cavus, etc.) should be noted as should limitation of movement in the spine (cervical, dorsal or lumbar) or in limb joints. Restricted straight leg raising with pain down the back of the thigh may be due to meningeal irritation (Kernig's sign) or to compression of one of the nerve roots which form the sciatic nerve, as by a prolapsed intervertebral disk (Lasègue's sign).

The special senses

The sense of **smell** (the olfactory nerves) should be tested in each nostril independently with the other occluded. Camphor, coffee, peppermint and oil of cloves are convenient test substances.

Taste should be tested on either side of the tongue. Testing on the anterior two-thirds is feasible in clinical practice, on the posterior third almost impossible, though often attempted. The four modalities of taste which can be recognised are sweet (sugar), salt (salt), bitter (quinine) and sour or acid (vinegar). The tongue should be protruded and dried and held with gauze while a fine brush dipped in a solution of one of the test agents is applied to its surface. The patient is then asked to point to one of four cards on which these four modalities are given. Taste sensation from the anterior two-thirds of the tongue is carried in the chorda tympani (facial nerve) and from the posterior one-third in the glossopharyngeal nerve.

Vision (the optic nerves)

In testing vision it is customary first to test the **visual acuity** in each eye independently, the other being covered. Usually, Snellen's test types are used, and the patient is asked to read, at a distance of 6 m, letters on the card. Each line of type is numbered and the acuity is recorded as 6 over the number of the lowest line of type which can be read accurately; for instance, 6/6 is normal. If the patient normally wears spectacles it is reasonable to record acuity when they are worn, so-called corrected acuity. A pinhole may be used if there is a refractive error and spectacles are not available. The test is appropriate to distance vision, while near vision may be tested with Jaeger's reading card, in which case acuity is expressed as from J1 to J6, J1 being normal, J6 severely impaired acuity. The cards approved by the London Faculty of Ophthalmologists use N6 for normal reading acuity (to correspond to 6/6 for normal distance acuity) and N12, N24, N36, etc., when reading acuity is progressively impaired. When vision in one or both eyes is so severely impaired that none of the test types can be seen, one records that sight is limited to 'counting fingers', 'hand movements' or 'light perception only', whichever is the case. In patients who claim to be blind and in whom hysteria is suspected, it is helpful to see whether blinking occurs at the threat of a blow.

Colour vision is rarely impaired by disease, but colour-blindness is present from birth in about 8% of males and in occasional females, being inherited as an X-linked recessive trait. This function is tested most satisfactorily with the Ishihara charts with which full instructions are supplied.

The **visual fields** must also be tested, first by confrontation. The patient and examiner sit face to face and the patient is instructed to gaze steadily at the bridge of the examiner's nose. One eye is covered and a test object (such as a hat-pin with a white head) is brought into the patient's field of vision from all angles, the patient being instructed to say 'now' whenever it first comes into view. The procedure is then repeated with the other eye. In this way, gross defects in the peripheral visual fields can be detected and must then be confirmed by accurate charting on a perimeter. Even the perimeter, however, is insufficiently accurate to plot in full the important area of central vision, the area around the fixation point, subserved by the macular area of the retina. To examine this area, especially if small scotomas (small areas of visual loss) are to be detected, central vision should be charted on the Bjerrum screen. Patients with central scotomas, due to disease of the macula or of the nerve fibres from this area, may have greatly reduced visual acuity and may be unable to read, even though the peripheral fields as charted with a perimeter are full. The visual field for large objects is larger than for small, and more extensive for white objects than for red; a scotoma for red is sometimes detected before one for white can be found.

The **optic discs and fundi** are next inspected, after dilatation of the pupils with homatropine if necessary. The optic disc is normally faintly pink in colour, but its temporal half is paler than the nasal. A deep physiological cup into which the vessels enter can give a mistaken impression of pallor of the central and temporal areas of the disc until a pink rim of normal-appearing disc is seen to its temporal side. Some blurring of the nasal margin is common in normal individuals and sometimes only the extreme temporal margin is clear-cut. In papilloedema (swelling of the optic nerve head), not only are the disc margins blurred and sometimes impossible to define, but the vessels are 'heaped up' in its centre, no physiological cup is present, the veins are distended, and there may even be haemorrhages and exudates in the surrounding retina. In optic atrophy, by contrast, the disc is flat and dead-white in colour with clearly-defined and often irregular margins. In that type of optic atrophy often seen in multiple sclerosis, the temporal half of the disc may be strikingly pale (temporal pallor). In examining the fundus, abnormal pigmentation, patches of retinal degeneration, haemorrhage, exudates and vascular changes (arterial narrowing, 'nipping' of veins at arteriovenous crossings, micro-aneurysms) or any other abnormality should be noted and described if present.

Any abnormal position of the globe of either eye, such

as proptosis (asymmetrical protrusion), exophthalmos (uniform protrusion), or enophthalmos (sunken eye) must also be recorded, as must the state of the **eyelids and pupils**. Drooping of the eyelids, or ptosis, may be seen, or alternatively lid-lag, revealing white sclera above the cornea on downward ocular movement. The size, equality or otherwise, and regularity of the pupils should now be examined, along with the response to shining a bright light into the eye; the effect upon the other pupil (the consensual reaction) as well as the direct reaction should be noted. Changes occurring on accommodation-convergence, when transferring the gaze rapidly from a distant to a near object, such as a finger placed a few inches from the eyes, should also be tested. The afferent pathway for the pupillary reflex to light is in the optic nerve, the efferent pathways are in the parasympathetic constrictor fibres of the oculomotor nerve and in the dilator fibres of the ocular sympathetic.

Ocular movements (controlled by the oculomotor, trochlear and abducent nerves) must now be examined. The patient is asked to follow an object, such as a finger or hat-pin, which is moved quickly from right to left and then up and down in front of the eyes. If diplopia (double vision) occurs in any direction of gaze, this is noted, as well as the position of the two images in relation to one another. When diplopia is present, noting which image disappears when each eye is covered in turn is helpful in identifying the external ocular muscle which is weak or paralysed, as the false image is projected in the direction in which the paretic muscle would normally move the eye. Any deviation of the ocular axes during movement should be recorded as well as the occurrence of nystagmus, an oscillatory or rotatory movement which can be a very important physical sign. If present, its character and direction should be noted, as well as the ocular movements which produce it. Sometimes it is not the movement of one or other eye which is defective, but movement of the two together, either laterally, upwards or downwards, is impaired. These movements are necessary for the maintenance of binocular vision. Such defects of conjugate ocular movement have considerable localising value and should also, if present, be carefully defined. Similarly, the ability to converge the ocular axes when watching an object approach the bridge of the nose, may be lost in disease and should be examined.

Hearing and labyrinthine function (The auditory and vestibular nerves)

A crude clinical assessment of a patient's **hearing** can be obtained by recording the distance at which a whispered voice or the ticking of a watch can be heard by each ear,

with the other temporarily occluded. If comparison with a normal subject suggests that one or both ears is deaf, one must then determine whether this is due to disease of the middle ear (conduction deafness) or of the cochlea or auditory nerve (nerve, perceptive or sensorineural deafness). This may be done with a 256-frequency tuning fork. Normally air conduction is better than bone conduction and in nerve deafness this principle is still true though hearing by either means may be greatly diminished; in middle-ear deafness, by contrast, bone conduction is better. In **Rinne's test**, a vibrating tuning fork is applied to the mastoid process and when the sound is no longer heard the fork is held at the external auditory meatus; the normal and those with nerve deafness will still hear it, while those with middle-ear deafness will not. While performing this test the contralateral ear must be occluded. Even if this is done, the results of the test are easily misinterpreted as the sound produced when the fork is applied to one mastoid process is often heard in the contralateral ear even when the ipsilateral one is totally deaf. In **Weber's test** the vibrating fork is applied to the vertex; normal individuals hear the sound equally in the two ears, while patients with nerve deafness hear it louder in the normal ear, in contrast to those with conductive deafness to whom it seems louder in the affected ear. Accurate measurement, however, depends upon audiometry (Ch. 3).

Clinical assessment of **labyrinthine** function can be difficult, but in patients with vertigo it is reasonable to alter suddenly the position of the head to see if this produces nystagmus or vertigo. For instance, a patient may be asked to lie down suddenly and the head is then turned sharply to one or other side. This test is particularly useful in those who complain of giddiness brought on by change in posture. Caloric tests, mentioned in Chapter 3, are important in testing the function of the labyrinths and of central vestibular connexions.

The motor system

Foremost in examining the motor system in the patient who can walk, is observation of the **gait**. Some neurological diseases cause striking abnormalities, many of them distinctive. The hemiplegic patient drags or circumducts his weak and spastic leg, while the arm is commonly flexed at the elbow and lies across the abdomen; the patient with a spastic paraparesis, by contrast, shows a stiff and clumsy mode of progression, in which both feet seem to drag along the ground. The festinant gait of parkinsonism is even more striking; the patient shuffles with short hurried steps, the head bowed and the back bent, as if continually having to press forwards to prevent himself from falling on his face. By contrast, the individual with cerebellar ataxia walks on a wide base, the feet far apart; he staggers from side to side and if asked to stop suddenly or to turn round he may be very unsteady and may even fall. He finds heel–toe walking ('tandem' walking in the USA) difficult if not impossible. Equally characteristic is the 'clopping' or slapping gait of the patient with unilateral or bilateral foot-drop resulting from weakness of the foot dorsiflexors, while the waddle, protuberant abdomen and accentuated lumbar lordosis of one with pelvic girdle weakness due to muscular dystrophy (or to other forms of myopathy or spinal muscular atrophy) is also virtually pathognomonic. Another important abnormality is the high-stepping unsteady gait of sensory ataxia, as in tabes dorsalis; the patient slaps his feet down hard as if he is not sure where they are in space.

Having observed the gait one must also note any **abnormalities of posture** or **involuntary movements**. These are abnormalities which cannot be corrected, and movements which cannot be prevented, by willed effort on the patient's part. If involuntary movements are seen, their situation, nature, amplitude, rhythmicity and frequency should be assessed. It is also important to observe whether postural changes are permanent or temporary and whether they are influenced by volitional activity.

Next comes detailed examination of the **neuromuscular system**. It is customary first to inspect the muscles of the cranium, trunk and limbs, for **atrophy** (wasting or reduction in muscular bulk), **hypertrophy** (muscular enlargement) or **fasciculation** (involuntary twitching of isolated bundles of muscle fibres). Next, contractures or irreversible shortening of muscles and tendons, possibly resulting in skeletal atrophy or deformity, should be looked for before going on to examine muscular **power**.

Beginning with the **motor cranial nerves**, the muscles of mastication (temporals, masseters and pterygoids), supplied by the motor division of the fifth or trigeminal nerve, are tested by asking the patient to clench the teeth or to move the jaw from side to side against resistance while the bulk and firmness of the muscles on the two sides are compared. The function of the seventh or facial nerve is first assessed by inspecting the face for asymmetry and then by asking the patient to close the eyes tightly and to show the teeth. Inability to bury the eyelashes adequately on one side may be significant. while differences in power between the upper and lower facial muscles should be noted. If emotional movement of the face, as in smiling, is normal, but volitional movement on command is impaired, this may be important. If the uvula moves to one side on saying 'ah', this implies weakness of the opposite side of the soft palate, possibly resulting from a lesion of the vagus nerve. Similarly, atrophy and weakness of one trapezius and

sternomastoid can imply disease of the ipsilateral spinal accessory nerve, while atrophy and fasciculation of the tongue and deviation to one side when it is protruded indicate a lesion of the twelfth or hypoglossal nerve on the side to which the tongue protrudes.

In testing the **power of the trunk and limb muscles**, most can be tested individually if necessary. Rational application of simple anatomical knowledge will indicate how this can be done, but unless there is striking atrophy of single muscles or muscle groups, so detailed an examination is rarely necessary. In a routine examination it is usual to test representative groups, which are contracted against resistance from the examiner; such muscles are those concerned in abduction of the shoulder, flexion and extension of the elbow, extension and flexion of the fingers (the grip) in the upper limbs. The upper and lower abdominal muscles may be compared in the recumbent patient by noting whether the umbilicus deviates upwards or downwards on lifting the head. In the lower limbs hip flexion, flexion and extension at the knee, and dorsi- and plantar-flexion at the ankle are usually tested.

No single method of assessing the power of individual muscles is perfect in view of subjective variations from one examiner to the next, but that given in the Guarantors of Brain's pamphlet *Aids to the Examination of the Peripheral Nervous System* 1986 is most widely used and gives numerical gradings from 5 to 0 to identify degrees of power as given below:

0   No contraction
1   Flicker or trace of contraction
2   Active movement, with gravity eliminated
3   Active movement against gravity
4   Active movement against gravity and resistance
5   Normal power

Grades 4−, 4 and 4+ may be used to indicate movement against slight, moderate and strong resistance respectively.

If examination reveals weakness of one or more major muscle groups it may then be necessary to examine in detail the power of individual muscles in order to determine whether the pattern of weakness indicates, for instance, disordered function of a single peripheral nerve or nerve root. Details of methods of examination of all of the limb and trunk muscles are outside the scope of this volume. However, methods of testing a number of representative muscles are illustrated in Figures 2.1–2.6. In clinical practice muscle power is examined not only to identify weakness of individual **muscles** but also weakness of specific **movements**. Thus in upper motor neurone lesions (see Ch. 9) shoulder abduction, elbow flexion and fine finger movement are selectively affected early in the upper limbs, hip flexion and individual toe movement in the lower.

Sometimes it is also necessary to test for muscular **fatigability**. In patients with myasthenia gravis an initial contraction (say of deltoid in abducting the shoulder) may be powerful, but if the movement is repeated several times it becomes progressively weaker. By contrast, in **myotonia** muscular contraction may be powerful, but on relaxing (say after making a fist) the fingers 'uncurl'

abnormally slowly. Direct percussion of a myotonic muscle gives a 'dimple' which slowly disappears; this phenomenon must be distinguished from myoidema, a localised ridge which forms after a direct blow upon a muscle belly and which is usually seen in malnourished, cachectic, or hypothyroid patients.

The **tone** of the limb muscles is next tested by noting and comparing the resistance which the muscles show to passive movement at the shoulder, elbow, knee and ankle

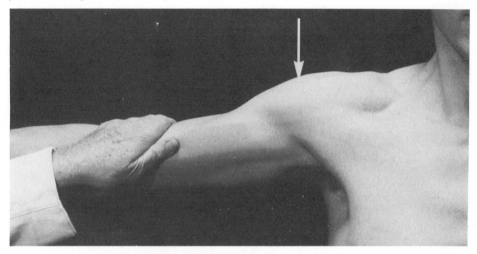

Fig. 2.1 Shoulder abduction. Deltoid (axillary nerve; **C5**, C6). The patient is abducting the upper arm against resistance. *Arrow*: the anterior and middle fibres of the muscle can be seen and felt.

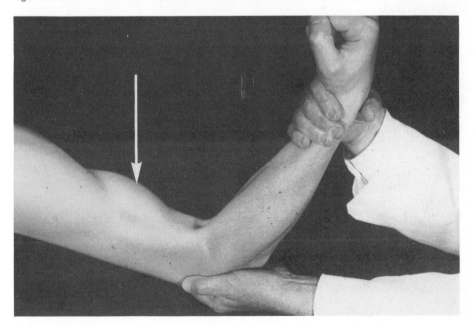

Fig. 2.2 Elbow flexion. Biceps (musculocutaneous nerve; C5, C6). The patient is flexing the supinated forearm against resistance. *Arrow*: the muscle belly can be seen and felt.

joints. This can be a difficult assessment as some patients find it almost impossible to relax the limb being tested and try to help by carrying out the movements themselves. If tone is reduced (hypotonia) the limbs are limp, 'floppy' and excessively mobile with little resistance, but if it is increased (hypertonia) they may be spastic, when there is a severe initial resistance which suddenly 'gives' (clasp-knife rigidity); alternatively tone can be increased throughout the entire range of movement (plastic or lead-pipe rigidity); or intermittently normal and in-

creased (cog-wheel rigidity). In spastic limbs, a muscle which is being stretched may show the phenomenon of **clonus** (rapid intermittent involuntary contraction and relaxation); this may be seen best at the ankle on sudden dorsiflexion of the foot, at the knee on pushing sharply against the upper border of the patella, and occasionally on sudden extension of the fingers.

Tests for **co-ordination** are next needed in order to seek signs of cerebellar disease. The patient is asked to touch his nose and the examiner's finger alternately, with

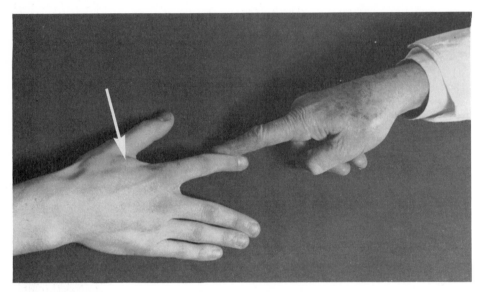

Fig. 2.3 Abduction of the index finger. First dorsal interosseous muscle (ulnar nerve; C8, **T1**). The palm and fingers are flat upon a table. The patient is abducting the index finger against resistance. *Arrow*: the muscle belly can be felt and usually seen.

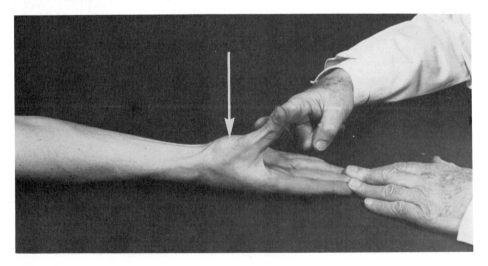

Fig. 2.4 Thumb abduction. Abductor pollicis brevis (median nerve; C8, **T1**). The patient is abducting the thumb at right angles to the palm against resistance. *Arrow*: the muscle belly can be seen and felt.

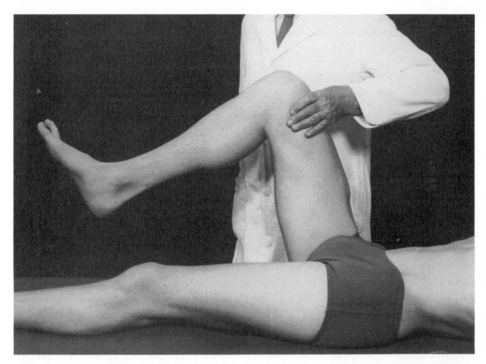

Fig. 2.5   Hip flexion. Iliopsoas (branches from L1, 2 and 3 spinal nerves and femoral nerve; **L1, L2**, L3). The patient is flexing the thigh against resistance with the leg flexed at the knee and hip.

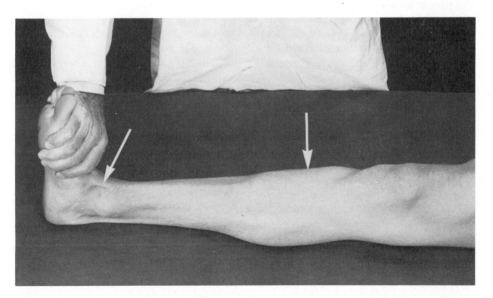

Fig. 2.6   Dorsiflexion of the foot at the ankle. Tibialis anterior (deep peroneal nerve; **L4**, L5). The patient is dorsiflexing the foot against resistance. *Arrows*: the muscle belly and its tendon can be seen and felt.
(Figures 2.1–2.6 are reproduced from Guarantors of Brain 1986 with the permission of the authors and publishers.)

the tip of his index finger, and any tremor or past-pointing should be noted. In the lower limbs, the heel-knee test, in which the heel of one foot is placed on the opposite knee and then moved smoothly down the shin, is used. Other valuable tests for the clumsy inco-ordinate movements of cerebellar disease include rapid tapping with the fingers or toes on the opposite limb or a convenient surface, 'playing the piano' on a table top, or rapid alternating pronation and supination of the hands and forearms; clumsiness in performance of the latter test, one of the least useful, is called dysdiadochokinesis.

There are several **primitive reflexes**, which, present in the newborn, disappear with maturation but may persist in infants with cerebral palsy; some also reappear in adults suffering from diffuse degenerative brain disease. The tonic neck reflex is elicited by turning the head and neck to one side; extension of the limbs occurs on the side towards which the head is turned. In the normal infant this reflex is no longer obtainable after the sixth month; it is typically present in adults with severe cerebral or brain stem lesions giving a 'decerebrate state'. The grasp reflex is one in which stroking the palm of the hand along the base of the fingers produces involuntary grasping, which becomes firmer as withdrawal is attempted. In the adult this indicates a contralateral frontal lobe lesion. The sucking reflex of the normal neonate and the closely-related snout reflex (a pout or snout evoked by a sharp tap on the closed lips) may reappear in adults with diffuse brain disease or with bilateral corticospinal tract lesions in the upper brain stem or above. In normal adults the contraction of both orbicularis oculi muscles (blinking) induced by a tap on the centre of the forehead above the nose (the glabellar tap sign) quickly habituates if the tap is repeated, but in patients with parkinsonism the blinking continues to occur rhythmically in time with the taps. For the interpretation of infantile automatisms (including the Moro, 'placing', and parachute reactions) the reader is referred to texts on paediatric neurology.

Of particular value in assessing the integrity of the brain stem in comatose patients are the **oculocephalic** and **oculovestibular reflexes**. When the eyelids are held open and the head is rotated from side to side or if it is flexed, the eyes show conjugate deviation away from the direction to which the head is moved. They return rapidly to the midline even if the head remains rotated or flexed. This oculocephalic reflex (the doll's head phenomenon) may be lost in severe pontine lesions, as is the oculovestibular reflex (nystagmus elicited by irrigation of the external auditory meatus with cold or warm water).

Finally, the **deep and superficial reflexes** should be tested. First the jaw jerk is elicited by placing a finger across the patient's chin, with the mouth slightly open and then tapping sharply downwards on the finger. A brisk contraction of the masseters is a positive jaw jerk, which is present in about 10% of normal individuals but is exaggerated when there is bilateral corticospinal tract disease in the upper brain stem. In the upper limbs, the biceps jerk is elicited by a blow on a finger placed across the biceps tendon with the elbow flexed; the radial jerk by a brisk tap on the tendon of the brachioradialis as it traverses the lateral aspect of the lower end of the radius; and the triceps jerk by tapping the tendon of the triceps just above its insertion into the olecranon, again with the elbow flexed. To produce a finger jerk the examiner's fingers are tapped as they lie in contact with the palmar aspect of the tips of the patient's partially flexed fingers. Like the jaw jerk, the finger jerk is present in some normal individuals and in some who are tense; if it is present only on one side, however, this may be significant. Concomitant flexion of the terminal phalanx of the thumb when the finger jerk is elicited usually indicates that this reflex is exaggerated. Similar flexion of the terminal phalanx of the thumb occurring when the terminal phalanx of the middle finger is flicked sharply downwards between the examiner's finger and thumb (Hoffmann's sign) may also indicate corticospinal tract dysfunction, particularly if present on one side only. In the lower limbs, the knee jerk is elicited by a blow on the patellar tendon with the knee in a semiflexed position, while the ankle jerk is obtained by tapping the tendo Achilles while the foot is dorsiflexed passively. Sometimes reinforcement (Jendrassik's manoeuvre) is needed to bring out these reflexes; the patient is asked to grip an object or to clasp the hands firmly when any tendon is about to be tapped.

Turning to the superficial reflexes, the first to be tested are usually the abdominals; brisk strokes are made downwards and inwards in each quadrant of the abdomen with a sharp instrument such as the point of a pin and the umbilicus should move towards the stimulus. The cremasteric reflex is less valuable clinically; it comprises an upward movement of the ipsilateral testis on stroking the inside of the thigh. The superficial anal reflex consists of contraction of the external sphincter when the skin around the anus is stroked. Finally, a most important reflex is the plantar response. A firm stroke is made along the sole from the heel to the base of the fifth toe, along the outer side of the foot. Plantar-flexion of all the toes is a flexor or normal response, while dorsiflexion of the great toe with plantar-flexion and 'fanning' of the other toes is the extensor or Babinski response.

When it is necessary to assess the integrity of the parasympathetic outflow from the second and third sacral segments of the spinal cord, it may be necessary to elicit the anal sphincter reflex (contraction of the internal sphincter around an examining finger) or the bulbocavernosus reflex (contraction of bulbocavernosus elicited by pinching the glans penis).

When examining the deep tendon and abdominal reflexes the patient should be resting comfortably and the muscles being tested should be relaxed. Furthermore it is best to compare each reflex on one side of the body with the corresponding one on the opposite side, observing any asymmetry of response. Conventionally, each reflex is recorded as $-$, $+$, $++$ or $+++$ depending upon its activity, while the plantar responses are recorded as $\downarrow$ (flexor), $\Uparrow$ (equivocal) or $\uparrow$ (extensor).

The sensory system

It is usual to test the different modalities of sensation independently, as they follow different pathways in the spinal cord and brain. The perception of pain may conveniently be tested by pinprick and that of touch with a fine wisp of cotton wool. Each form of sensation can be tested quantitatively by applying painful stimuli of graduated weight (algesiometers) or hairs which are calibrated so that a particular force is required to bend them (von Frey hairs). Such refinements are, however, unnecessary in clinical practice. Abnormalities of sensory perception should be sought on the face, trunk and limbs, by exploring representative areas with these two types of stimuli; the corneal reflexes, evoked by touching each cornea with a fine wisp of cotton wool, should also be compared. If an area of diminished pain sensation (hypalgesia) or touch sensation (hypaesthesia) is discovered, or even one of apparent hypersensitivity (hyperpathia), this should be outlined by applying repetitive stimuli from within to without the area and vice versa, asking the patient to say when any change occurs. The area or sensory change should then be charted on a drawing of the human body, each modality being recorded separately. If pain loss is found, then temperature perception should be tested within the same area, using test-tubes filled with hot and cold water.

The finer and more discriminative aspects of sensibility should also be tested. Thus the patient may be asked to identify objects placed in the hands when his eyes are closed, or figures drawn on the skin. He is also asked to state the direction of movement each time the terminal phalanx of a finger or the great toe is moved passively upwards or downwards and any defects in position and joint sense, so elicited, must be recorded. In the normal individual, movements of 1 mm are easily appreciated. The appreciation of vibration should also be tested with a 128-frequency tuning fork over bony prominences such as the sternum, elbow, knuckle, anterior superior iliac spine, patella and external malleolus. The ability to perceive whether the tips of the fingers or the soles of the feet are being touched with one or two points may also be noted. The normal threshold for two-point discrimination on the tips of the fingers is 2–3 mm, while on the sole of the foot it is 2–3 cm. Another useful test for minor defects of sensation is to touch similar points on opposite limbs, sometimes independently and sometimes together, while asking the patient to say which has been touched. A patient who can feel perfectly stimuli applied independently may only feel the stimulus on one side when both are touched at the same time. This phenomenon is known as tactile inattention.

Testing of sensory function carries many pitfalls for the unwary and needs much practice and experience before it can be accurately performed. One reason is that many suggestible individuals readily produce spurious areas of cutaneous sensory loss, and hypalgesia is one of the commonest neurological signs of hysterical origin. Furthermore, some less intelligent patients find it difficult to understand what is required of them, while the more intelligent may find sensory changes which are more dependent upon unintentional variation in intensity of stimulus than upon organic disease.

Signs of disease in other systems

The human body cannot function as an isolated nervous system and neurological manifestations often result from dysfunction in other systems. Cerebral infarction, for instance, can follow cardiac infarction, a brain abscess may be due to bronchiectasis, otitis, or paranasal sinusitis, while a confusional state can result from uraemia due to renal disease, from pernicious anaemia or from liver failure. Hence even though the patient's symptoms and signs indicate nervous disease, examination of the patient as a whole must be no less assiduous, for the principal clue to the nature of the patient's illness may lie elsewhere.

DISCUSSION AND DIFFERENTIAL DIAGNOSIS

A full clinical history and a physical examination recorded in meticulous detail will be of no value unless they can be interpreted and it is upon this interpretation that treatment may depend. It is at this stage that experience plays the greatest part, but experience can only be acquired if the student or young doctor learns to sift the accumulated data, discarding the irrelevant and tabulating the significant. He must therefore apply his powers of inductive and deductive reasoning in order to decide first the situation and secondly the nature of the pathological changes responsible for the patient's disease. He must be expected to tabulate in order of likelihood the possible diagnoses which he is considering, and must then decide which ancillary investigations, if any, are required in order to establish whichever is correct. For the history and examination are but a means to an end, the end being diagnosis, upon which management of the patient must depend.

REFERENCES

Adams R D, Victor M 1985 Principles of neurology, 3rd edn. McGraw-Hill, New York

Bickerstaff E R 1980 Neurological examination in clinical practice, 4th edn. Blackwell, Oxford

Gordon N, Schutt W 1976 Paediatric neurology for the clinician. Spastics International Medical Publications, Heinemann, London

Guarantors of Brain 1986 Aids to the examination of the peripheral nervous system. Baillière Tindall, London

Holmes G 1968 An introduction to clinical neurology, 3rd edn, revised by Matthews W B. Livingstone, Edinburgh

de Jong R 1979 The neurologic examination, 5th edn. Hoeber, New York

Klein R, Mayer-Gross W 1957 The clinical examination of patients with organic cerebral disease. Cassell, London

Mayo Clinic, Section of Neurology 1981 Clinical examinations in neurology, 5th edn. Saunders, Philadelphia

Paine R S, Oppé T E 1966 Neurological examination of children. Clinics in Developmental Medicine, 20/21. The Spastics Society and Heinemann, London

Spillane J D, Spillane J A 1982 An atlas of clinical neurology, 3rd edn. Oxford University Press, London

Walton J N 1985 Brain's Diseases of the nervous system, 9th edn. Oxford University Press, Oxford

3. Investigation of the patient with neurological disease

In considering the ancillary investigations which are used as aids to diagnosis in a patient whose symptoms and signs suggest a disorder of the nervous system it is important to appreciate that symptoms of neurological dysfunction may result from disease in another part of the body. The patient must therefore be viewed as a whole if he is not to be subjected to a series of unpleasant tests designed to demonstrate a primary nervous disease, when the lesion responsible may be in some other organ far removed from the brain and spinal cord. A second principle too often forgotten is that investigations should be planned to give the maximum required information about the patient's illness with the least possible discomfort and risk.

In many patients with neurological disorders there is no need for investigations either for diagnosis or for guidance on management. Migraine, for instance, is a condition in which the diagnosis is usually made on the history alone and in which ancillary tests are rarely needed. In other cases, investigations should be designed to establish or exclude the diagnoses which are suggested by the patient's symptoms and signs. It is reasonable to begin by carrying out the simpler tests which the doctor can do himself, before proceeding, if still in doubt, to the more difficult investigations which need specialised apparatus and skilled technical help. Ethical considerations must always be considered in assessing potential risks on the one hand against the information which may be derived from investigation on the other. A useful criterion is whether the result of the test is likely to be important in determining management; and patients must be fully informed about the risks of any investigation, so that they can give informed consent to the procedure.

GENERAL MEDICAL EXAMINATION AND IN-VESTIGATIONS

There are many disease processes which are confined to the nervous system, but many disorders of other systems affect the nervous system and can present with neurological symptoms and/or signs. Conversely, neurological problems are often associated with symptoms and signs of dysfunction of other systems so that evaluation of neurological problems often involves the investigation of other systems. For example, the nervous system may be directly involved by a systemic disease such as systemic lupus erythematosus or tuberculous meningitis in miliary tuberculosis; metastases to the brain may be the first manifestation of a carcinoma elsewhere; some 'pure' neurological syndromes may be a complication of disease elsewhere such as subacute combined degeneration of the cord due to vitamin B_{12} deficiency or the non-metastatic cerebellar syndrome that may be the presenting feature of an occult neoplasm.

Cardiovascular system

Investigation of the cardiovascular system is a necessary part of the evaluation of all patients with cerebrovascular disease, numerically the commonest group of neurological disorders. Examination of the pulse may reveal an abnormal rate; thus too rapid a pulse may be a sign of thyrotoxicosis, but is more likely to be a manifestation of anxiety. Bradycardia is common in fit, young, athletic subjects, but may also indicate myxoedema, medication with beta blockers or digoxin, or even heart block. Bradycardia may also occur in comatose patients with raised intracranial pressure due to compression of medullary centres. Irregularity of the pulse is usually of more importance than its rate. Atrial fibrillation is associated with a significant risk of emboli from thrombus in the left atrium and some other changes of rhythm are also associated with similar risk. A normal pulse does not exclude an arrhythmia as a possible cause of a cerebrovascular event and it may be necessary to undertake prolonged monitoring to demonstrate intermittent periods of abnormal rhythm. Abnormalities of the peripheral pulses may give a useful indication of the extent of degenerative vascular disease, but palpation of the carotid arteries is of limited value as only the common carotid can be reliably felt. Bruits may be heard over sites of atheromatous narrowing, notably at the carotid bifurcation, over the subclavian arteries in the neck and over the femoral arteries.

Hypertension is the most important treatable cause of cerebral vascular disease and the blood pressure should always be recorded. If there is any history suggestive of syncope or symptoms related to change in posture, the blood pressure should be recorded both standing and lying to detect and measure any postural fall. It may also be necessary to record the blood pressure in both arms to demonstrate lesions at the aortic arch or in the subclavian arteries. Doppler ultrasonic angiography may be very helpful in elucidating signs found in this way. If a cardiac source of emboli is suspected, in addition to clinical examination of the heart and electrocardiography (ECG) it may be necessary to proceed to echocardiography. Some neurological diseases can in turn produce quite profound cardiac changes; the ECG is usually abnormal after subarachnoid haemorrhage and striking abnormalities of rate and rhythm may be found in the Guillain-Barré syndrome; cardiac arrhythmia is one of the causes of sudden death in the latter condition so that patients should be carefully monitored in the early stages of the illness.

Gastrointestinal and hepatic systems

There are relatively few neurological disorders associated with abnormalities of the gastrointestinal tract. Subacute combined degeneration of the cord due to vitamin B_{12} deficiency and associated with gastric achlorhydria, which may be demonstrated by a zylose tolerance test and the Schilling test, is a well-known example. B_{12} deficiency may also develop in intestinal blind loop syndromes, often in association with other manifestations of malabsorption. Rarely it is seen in vegans who refuse to consume any animal products. Both the liver and the nervous system are affected by alcohol so that the features of cirrhosis may be found in patients with alcoholic peripheral neuropathy, Wernicke's and Korsakov's syndromes and in those with alcoholic cerebellar degeneration. Hepatic or portal-systemic encephalopathy produces a characteristic clinical picture (see p. 324) of which a 'flapping' or 'wing-beating' tremor of the outstretched hands (asterixis) is often a feature. Some inborn errors of metabolism such as Wilson's disease may also affect both the liver and the brain.

Respiratory system

Acute pulmonary infections causing respiratory insufficiency may cause an acute confusional syndrome, especially in the elderly, and may present in this way. Headache and drowsiness are also common symptoms of alveolar hypoventilation, however caused. Anoxic episodes due to sleep apnoea may also present as episodes of confusion and may remain undiagnosed without an eyewitness account. A number of neurological diseases may profoundly affect respiration. Patients with severe myasthenia gravis may require periods of ventilation as may patients in the acute stage of the Guillain-Barré syndrome, and many subacute neuromuscular disorders can cause slowly progressive respiratory insufficiency.

Genitourinary system

Renal disease may be the cause of hypertension; occasionally the first clinical manifestation is the development of headaches, and papilloedema with haemorrhages may be found on examination. A disturbance of bladder control is a common and important feature of many neurological conditions affecting the neuraxis from the medial part of the frontal lobes to the cauda equina. Many such patients require extensive genitourinary investigation including specialised examinations such as video cystometrography.

Examination of the urine may give valuable and sometimes diagnostic information, as, for example, in patients with diabetes, who may present in the neurological clinic with a mononeuritis, polyneuritis or amyotrophy. Myelomatosis with Bence-Jones proteinuria can present with spinal cord compression. *Polyuria* is occasionally a functional or psychiatric symptom, but if much urine of low specific gravity is passed, it may indicate diabetes insipidus due to a disorder of the hypothalamic-pituitary axis. *Albuminuria* and *the abnormal cells* and *casts* in the urine may indicate primary renal disease causing uraemia and drowsiness, or hypertension and consequent cerebral symptoms. Alternatively, minimal albuminuria with some red cells may be due to embolism (as in subacute bacterial endocarditis) or diffuse arterial disease (as in polyarteritis nodosa) and these conditions also give neurological manifestations. A number of biochemical tests also give useful information. Thus *bilirubin* in the urine may be an expression of liver disease, in which episodes of confusion and disturbed behaviour may occur, while a dark port-wine coloured urine which goes darker on standing is indicative of *porphyria*, a condition in which confusion, abdominal pain and peripheral neuropathy occur. Estimation of *sodium and potassium output* can also be of value in patients suffering from intermittent attacks of flaccid muscular paralysis, for some have a nephritis causing excessive salt loss and consequent hypokalaemia, while others, in whom there is a diminished output of sodium, may have attacks of paralysis caused perhaps by excessive adrenal aldosterone secretion.

Haematology

A full blood picture has become a routine examination for almost all patients, and that includes patients with neurological disease. A high haematocrit is associated with increased blood viscosity and this may be an important factor in patients with stroke. This applies not only to the very high haematocrit that occurs in polycythaemia rubra vera, but also in the less marked hyperhaematocrit of patients with pulmonary disease, also seen in heavy smokers. Although anaemia by itself produces little in the way of neurological symptoms or signs, it can certainly aggravate a wide range of neurological problems. The erythrocyte sedimentation rate (ESR) is seldom affected in primary disorders of the nervous system but is a useful non-specific test for many systemic disorders and very high rates of the order of 80–100 mm/hour are commonly found in the collagen-vascular or connective tissue diseases such as polyarteritis nodosa, systemic lupus erythematosus (SLE) and giant cell arteritis. These conditions may present with cerebrovascular events, such as an encephalopathy in the case of SLE, stroke (rarely) in cranial arteritis, or with peripheral neuropathies. Dermatomyositis is nearly always associated with a high ESR as are myeloma and the lymphomas which may involve the nervous system. Central nervous system involvement with leukaemia is quite common in children, especially in some of those who had previously been effectively treated.

The endocrine system

Neurological conditions can have a profound effect on the endocrine system, mostly through abnormalities in the region of the hypothalamus and pituitary. A range of 'pituitary function tests' is appropriate in patients presenting with lesions in this area. These include measurement of thyroxine (T4), tri-iodothyronine (T3), thyroid stimulating hormone (TSH) and thyroid releasing hormone (TRH). Sensitive versions of these tests are particularly useful in patients presenting with dysthyroid ophthalmoplegia. The serum prolactin is markedly elevated in prolactinomas and often shows an elevation after acute events such as attacks of grand mal epilepsy. The serum cortisol and ACTH can be measured; the cortisol should show a marked diurnal variation which disappears in patients with cortisol secreting tumours (basophil adenoma) and the circulating cortisol level cannot be suppressed with dexamethasone. More sophisticated tests of the hypothalamic-pituitary axis may sometimes be necessary, including the insulin stress test and growth hormone assays.

Inappropriate antidiuretic hormone (ADH) secretion sometimes occurs in a wide variety of neurological disorders which affect the hypothalamic-pituitary system; thus it commonly occurs in the basal meningitides such as tuberculous meningitis, sarcoidosis and carcinomatosis, but may also occur after head injury.

Biopsy techniques

These can be of great value in the investigation of suspected nervous disease; in certain cases, skin, liver, rectal or renal biopsy and other methods commonly used in general medicine may be applicable. *Lymph node biopsy* may be indicated if a reticulosis involving the nervous system is suspected and bone marrow examination may also be required when leukaemia, myeloma or other haematological disorders are being considered.

Muscle biopsy has, however, a more immediate relevance to neurological medicine as this method can be very useful in deciding whether muscular weakness and wasting is due to a disease of the motor nerves (neuropathy) or of the muscles (myopathy), and in identifying the nature of the myopathic affliction. It may also be of help in the diagnosis of 'connective tissue' disease and particularly of polyarteritis nodosa. Sural *nerve biopsy* is occasionally of use in investigating cases of peripheral neuropathy, while *brain biopsy* is utilised in the diagnosis of cerebral tumour or (less often) in suspected diffuse degenerative or metabolic disease; these techniques have relatively restricted clinical applications.

In some rare inherited disorders of the nervous system in which specific enzymatic abnormalities have been detected, these can be identified in skin fibroblasts or white blood cells in culture; similar techniques applied to amniotic cells obtained by *amniocentesis* can be used for antenatal diagnosis with a view to therapeutic abortion on eugenic grounds. *Chorionic villus biopsy*, which can be performed at an earlier stage of pregnancy than amniocentesis, is being used increasingly for these purposes and in order to use gene-specific probes capable of detecting, for example, diseases such as Duchenne muscular dystrophy in the fetus.

THE CEREBROSPINAL FLUID (CSF)

Formation and composition

From experimental work carried out in the early part of this century it was found that the choroid plexuses of the cerebral ventricles play an important part in forming the cerebrospinal fluid. Blockage of the aqueduct of Sylvius was found to cause a striking dilatation of the lateral and third ventricles, due to the continued production of cerebrospinal fluid for which there was no longer an outlet (obstructive hydrocephalus). From these observations and from the fact that hydrocephalus could follow blockage of the sagittal sinus and was then presumed to result from impaired reabsorption of the fluid (communicating hydrocephalus), the classical view of CSF formation and circulation evolved. According to this view, the fluid is formed in the choroid plexuses, not by simple diffusion or dialysis but by a process of active secretion; that secreted in the lateral ventricles then passes through the foramina of Monro, the third ventricle, the aqueduct and fourth ventricle, to enter the basal cisterns of the subarachnoid space through the foramina of Magendie and Luschka. It then flows upwards over the surface of the cerebral hemispheres, while some flows down into the spinal subarachnoid space; reabsorption into the blood stream then occurs through the arachnoidal villi which protrude into the sagittal and other venous sinuses. Work on the passage of radioactive substances into the CSF has confirmed that this mechanism of secretion and reabsorption operates and the mean rate of formation is about 0.35 ml/min. In addition there is a constant process of dialysis, with exchange of chemical constituents between the CSF and blood, occurring across the arachnoid membrane at all levels. Large molecules cannot enter the fluid as they are unable to pass the vascular endothelium which effectively constitutes the blood-brain barrier, but there is a rapid exchange of substances of small molecular weight between the CSF and the extracellular fluid of the central nervous system. Thus in some ways the CSF acts as a 'sink' in preventing the extracellular fluid from achieving true equilibrium with the blood plasma. The composition of the ventricular fluid is very different from that in the lumbar subarachnoid space and many constituents of the lumbar fluid are added to it by diffusion across the spinal arachnoid membrane.

The CSF acts as a cushion protecting the brain and cord against external pressure waves. It has no nutritional function but removes metabolites from the nervous system, and through its hydrogen ion concentration (its pH is in equilibrium with that of the extracellular fluid of the brain) it influences the respiratory volume and rate, cerebral blood flow and other aspects of cerebral metabolism.

The total volume of cerebrospinal fluid in the normal adult is between 100 and 130 ml. The fluid is clear and colourless; it contains less than four white blood cells per mm^3 and all of these are lymphocytes. The protein

Table 3.1 Normally accepted values relating to CSF obtained at lumbar puncture

Pressure (at lumbar puncture)	50–200 mmH$_2$O
Volume	100–130 ml
Cells: adults	0–4 mononuclears
infants	0–20 mononuclears
Total proteins (mostly albumin)	0.15–0.45 g/l
Globulin	0–0.06 g/l
Glucose	0.50–0.85 g/l

content of the lumbar fluid is 0.15–0.45 g/l, the respective values for ventricular and cisternal fluid being 0.05–0.15 g/l and 0.15–0.25 g/l; most of the protein present is albumin. Normally, too, the fluid contains 0.50–0.80 g glucose and 120–130 mEq chloride (expressed as NaCl) per litre. The plasma concentration of glucose is about twice that of the CSF. The concentrations of these and other substances in the CSF are given in Table 3.1. Thus the protein content of the fluid is low when compared with that of the blood serum, the sugar level is also lower than in the serum, while the chloride is higher. Sodium, potassium, urea and some drugs such as sulphonamides, pass freely into the fluid and are there found in concentrations equal to that in the serum, whereas other substances such as antibodies, salicylates, penicillin and streptomycin pass into it in relatively minute quantities even if the serum concentration is high. Bromide, too, is found in the lumbar CSF in only about one-third the concentration in which it is present in the blood. Clearly, therefore, the entry of many chemicals into the CSF is a selective matter and does not depend upon a simple process of diffusion across a semipermeable membrane. Disease, and particularly inflammation of the arachnoid, may influence this process and in some cases of meningitis, penicillin, say, and bromide enter the fluid more easily.

Lumbar puncture

Cytological and chemical examination of the CSF is of great value in neurological diagnosis and specimens of fluid are most easily obtained by lumbar puncture, which is usually a comparatively simple and safe procedure though never to be undertaken lightly. The exploring needle is inserted into the lumbar subarachnoid space below the termination of the spinal cord, and as the roots of the cauda equina are pushed aside by the needle, the risks of damage to nervous tissue are negligible. The investigation is, however, dangerous if the intracranial pressure is high, and particularly if an intracranial tumour is present, since reduction in the fluid pressure in the lumbar subarachnoid space can result in impaction of the cerebellar tonsils in the foramen magnum or of the medial aspects of one or both temporal lobes between the brain stem and the edge of the tentorium cerebelli, with fatal results. Hence papilloedema is a contraindication and lumbar puncture should also be avoided if the patient's symptoms suggest that the intracranial pressure is raised; should manometry reveal that the pressure is unexpectedly high, it is wise to remove only a few drops of fluid. Even this precaution, however, will not always avoid cerebellar or tentorial herniation, as persistent leakage of fluid can occur through the hole in the spinal dura mater left by the exploring needle. This mechanism, with consequent reduction of the intracranial pressure below normal, is probably the cause of the common post-lumbar-puncture headache.

In carrying out lumbar puncture, the patient should lie horizontally on the left side with his neck firmly flexed, the knees drawn up to the chin and the trunk flexed but not rotated. The skin of the back is cleaned with a suitable antiseptic; a line is then drawn down the spinous processes of the vertebrae and another joining the highest points of the iliac crests. This line usually crosses the spine of the fourth lumbar vertebra and the needle may be inserted either in the intervertebral space above or in the one below this line. Full aseptic precautions are essential; the operator should wear a mask and sterile gloves, and the lumbar puncture outfit, including needles, stylets and manometer, should have been auto-claved. Harris's or similar needles are satisfactory. After infiltration of the skin and subcutaneous tissue with local anaesthetic (e.g. 1% lignocaine) the needle is then inserted with its stylet in position and is passed horizontally inwards in a slightly cephalad direction. It passes through the interspinous ligaments and then encounters the resistant ligamentum flavum. After penetrating this ligament resistance suddenly lessens as the needle enters the subarachnoid space. The stylet is now removed from the needle and the fluid drips out slowly. Care must be taken not to insert the needle too far, as a vertebral vein may then be punctured or an intervertebral disc can be damaged.

It is usual to measure the pressure of the fluid by attaching a manometer to the needle and the height of the fluid column in mm of CSF is measured when it ceases to rise in the upright tube. The normal pressure in the recumbent adult is 50–200 mm of fluid; when he is sitting upright the pressure in the lumbar subarachnoid space is about 200-250 mm. It is important that the patient is lying comfortably relaxed during this procedure. Coughing or straining causes an increased pressure in abdominal veins and consequently in the vertebral veins, thus raising the CSF pressure. Similarly, if there is a free communication between the cerebral and lumbar subarachnoid spaces, a temporary increase in the intra-cranial pressure is reflected in the manometer. Such an increase may be produced by compressing one or both internal jugular veins in the neck, thus reducing venous outflow from the cranium. In carrying out this procedure, known as **Queckenstedt's test**, there is usually a sharp rise in pressure to 300 mm or more, with an equally rapid fall when the pressure is released. If there is a block to the free passage of fluid in the subarachnoid space, then no rise in pressure occurs during the manoeuvre, while if the block is partial the rise and fall are both abnormally slow. This test has been used to diagnose thrombosis in one lateral sinus when digital compression of one jugular vein produces a rise in pressure but no rise occurs on the affected side; it has also been used to demonstrate a block in the spinal canal. But the increasing sophistication of radiological techniques such as myelography and angiography and the relative imprecision of Queckenstedt's test, which gives too many false negative results to be reliable, has meant that it has been largely discarded in clinical practice except where neuro-radiological facilities are not immediately available. Even in such circumstances, if a spinal tumour with cord compression is suspected, the patient should be transferred immediately to a neurosurgical unit as withdrawal of CSF below the block may increase the neurological deficit.

After pressure readings have been taken it is then usual to collect fluid in two separate sterile and chemically clean test-tubes or other appropriate containers. One specimen is used for bacteriological, the other for cytological and chemical studies. When the examination is complete, the stylet is reinserted into the needle, it is withdrawn and the track is sealed by a simple dry dressing. Failure to obtain fluid (a 'dry tap') may mean that the puncture has been performed incorrectly or vertebral disease may have narrowed the interspace; if the first puncture is unsuccessful, another attempt should be made in the interspace above or below. A genuine 'dry tap', when the needle is in the subarachnoid space but no fluid can be withdrawn, even on suction, means either that the space is blocked at a higher level or that the lumbar sac is filled by a neoplasm or developmental lesion such as a lipoma.

Cisternal and lateral cervical puncture

Cisternal and lateral cervical puncture are more difficult and dangerous procedures than lumbar puncture, since if the needle is inserted too far into the cisterna magna, the lower part of the medulla oblongata is pierced. Similarly, the cord may be damaged in lateral cervical puncture if the needle is introduced at the wrong angle. Hence these methods are only used if lumbar puncture is impossible owing to spinal deformity, if contrast medium is to be injected to define the upper level of a spinal lesion causing a block, if it is necessary to compare the chemical constitution of the lumbar and cisternal fluids, or if intrathecal injections of therapeutic agents are to be given and there is a block in the spinal subarachnoid space. These techniques, unlike lumbar puncture, should only be performed by a skilled operator working in a specialised unit, preferably with fluoroscopic control.

Ventricular puncture

Direct needle puncture of a lateral cerebral ventricle is sometimes necessary in order to relieve symptoms of increased intracranial pressure prior to an operation for intracranial tumour, or in order to inject air for ventriculography. Rarely, when there is inflammatory exudate in the subarachnoid space and lumbar or cisternal puncture do not produce a free flow of CSF, this route is used to administer antibiotics. In infants the ventricles can be entered directly by a needle inserted in the lateral angle of the fontanelle which is then passed through the cerebral substance. In older children and in adults, cranial burr-holes must first be made. In view of its potential hazards, this technique is one for the specialist.

Examination of the cerebrospinal fluid and some common abnormalities

Pressure

An increase in the CSF pressure above 200 mm in a relaxed, recumbent patient usually implies raised pressure inside the cranium. This is usually due to an increased brain volume, either produced by oedema alone, as in benign intracranial hypertension (pseudotumour cerebri) or by a lesion such as a tumour, abscess or haematoma, which is often associated with oedema. A moderate rise occurs in patients with severe arterial hypertension. An unusually low pressure is much less significant if there is no other evidence of spinal block, and is generally of no diagnostic value. A syndrome of intracranial hypotension has been postulated as an explanation of this finding, but the evidence that such a condition exists is dubious, although dehydration, as in a 'hangover', may temporarily reduce CSF pressure.

Naked-eye appearance

Turbidity of the fluid usually indicates a polymorphonuclear pleocytosis; excessive lymphocytes, even in large number, rarely give visible changes. Some specimens of fluid which contain an excessive quantity of protein may

clot on standing; a fine cobweb-like **fibrin deposit** appearing after a few hours also implies an increased protein content; it is seen in tuberculous meningitis and less commonly in poliomyelitis and meningovascular syphilis. Frank **blood** in the CSF may be present owing to puncture of a vertebral vein by the exploring needle, in which case the contamination of the fluid becomes less as it flows; if two test-tubes are filled, the second is less stained than the first, and if the specimen is centrifuged the supernatant fluid is clear. Uniform blood-staining is, however, seen in subarachnoid haemorrhage or if a primary cerebral haemorrhage has extended to the subarachnoid space; in such cases, the supernatant fluid, after centrifuging, generally shows a yellow colouration or **xanthochromia**. A faint colour, generally orange, appears within four hours of a subarachnoid bleed and is then due to the presence of oxyhaemoglobin; within 48 hours the deep yellow colour of bilirubin appears. This colour may persist for six weeks after a haemorrhage but usually disappears in from two to three weeks. Xanthochromia is also seen in CSF with a very high protein content (as in spinal tumour), in some patients with subdural bleeding, and in others who are deeply jaundiced.

Cytology

Total cell counts are made from unstained fluid. Methylene blue is used to stain the white cells for a differential count. A number of counting chambers are available including the Fuchs-Rosenthal chamber and the Neubauer chamber. Staining is usually good enough for red cells, lymphocytes and polymorphonuclear leucocytes to be identified. Tumour cells, yeasts and other abnormal cells are occasionally found but require specialised cytological techniques and skilled scrutiny for their recognition and interpretation.

A small number of **red cells** may be present due to the trauma of the puncture but if they persist in several specimens this can indicate a cerebral infarct, a haemorrhage approaching the surface of the brain, or bleeding into the subdural, as distinct from the subarachnoid space; the possibility of minor leakage from an intracranial aneurysm must also be considered. An increase in **white cells** generally implies inflammation in the meninges and this can be primary, as in meningitis, or secondary to diffuse cerebral disease, as in encephalitis. In general, polymorphonuclear leucocytes predominate in pyogenic infections such as coccal or influenzal meningitis and many thousands of cells may be present per mm^3 of fluid. As the condition resolves, so the polymorphs are gradually replaced by lymphocytes in decreasing numbers. In a case of cerebral abscess, without obvious meningitis, it is usual to find between 20 and 200 cells/mm^3 of which most are polymorphs. In tuberculous meningitis there is a polymorphonuclear reaction at the beginning of the illness but within a few days the pleocytosis is generally entirely mononuclear (lymphocytes and histiocytes) and usually of from 200 to 1000 cells/mm^3. Meningovascular syphilis generally gives a mononuclear pleocytosis of up to 200 cells/mm^3, but some polymorphonuclears are present in the more acute cases; patients with tabes dorsalis rarely show an excess of cells in the fluid, but in patients with general paresis counts of from five to 50 lymphocytes/mm^3 are usual.

In viral infections such as encephalitis, lymphocytic meningitis and poliomyelitis, a moderate lymphocytic reaction, up to 1000 cells/mm^3 is general, but in poliomyelitis a number of polymorphs, and even a predominance, may be seen in the first few days of the illness.

A slight pleocytosis, nearly always of lymphocytes, can also be found in many miscellaneous conditions, including cerebral tumour (primary or secondary), cerebral infarction, venous sinus thrombosis and multiple sclerosis. Only rarely in these conditions does the count exceed 40 to 50 cells/mm^3. In subarachnoid haemorrhage, too, the aseptic meningitis produced by blood in the CSF excites a moderate lymphocytic pleocytosis, and the number of white cells present is proportionately greater than would be expected from the number of red cells found. In occasional cases of intracranial tumour, particularly medulloblastomas in childhood, neoplastic cells, which look very like lymphocytes, are present in the fluid in comparative profusion. Specialised cytological techniques are sometimes helpful in identifying other varieties of tumour cells and are particularly valuable in diagnosing carcinomatosis of the meninges. Even with precise modern cytological techniques, malignant cells are detected in the fluid in only 10% of cases of glioma and 20% of patients with intracranial metastases. Immunofluorescent techniques of examining fresh or cultured cells obtained from CSF are being increasingly used in the rapid diagnosis of viral encephalitis.

Chemical abnormalities

Protein. An increase in the protein content of the CSF is one of the commonest abnormalities discovered in neurological practice and also one of the most difficult to interpret. A rise to 0.5–5.0 g/l is usual in inflammatory disorders of the meninges such as meningitis and a lesser increase persists after the pleocytosis is no longer present; this is also true of poliomyelitis, in which disease a rise in protein without an increase in cells is sometimes seen only four or five days after the onset. A moderate increase, usually to about 1.0 g/l or less may be found in encephalitis, cerebral abscess, cerebral infarction, neurosyphilis (excluding tabes dorsalis), intracranial venous sinus thrombosis and multiple sclerosis. A similar moderate rise is common in patients with intracranial gliomas and metastases but extracerebral neoplasms such as meningiomas often give a higher value and the protein content of the fluid is usually well over 1.0 g/l in a patient with an acoustic neuroma. Particularly high values for CSF protein, often to as much as 10 g/l, are found in patients with postinfective polyneuropathy (the Guillain-Barré syndrome), and in these cases there is usually little or no pleocytosis ('dissociation albuminocytologique'). Virtually the only other circumstance in which similarly high readings are found in the lumbar CSF is in cases of spinal block, usually due to a spinal neoplasm, but occasionally resulting from vertebral collapse and angulation, extra-dural tumour or abscess, or arachnoiditis, which may be of undetermined aetiology, but sometimes follows chronic (especially tuberculous) meningitis. Often this fluid with a high-protein content is xanthochromic, and these signs, combined with a Queckenstedt test indicating a block, constitute Froin's syndrome. Minor degrees of spinal cord compression without complete block, as in cervical myelopathy due to spondylosis, show less striking rises in the protein content of the fluid, rarely to above 1.0 g/l. A moderate rise usually below that value is also found sometimes in patients suffering from a recent prolapse of an intervertebral disc, either lumbar or cervical.

Albumin–globulin ratio. In the normal CSF the albumin–globulin ratio is approximately 8:1 but in many of the inflammatory conditions referred to above there is a selective rise in globulin. Various techniques of electrophoresis, immunoprecipitation and immunoelectrophoresis are now being used not only to estimate γ-globulin as a fraction of total CSF protein but also to fractionate IgG, IgA, IgM and IgD. These methods have shown that the total γ-globulin content of the fluid is usually raised in such diseases as multiple sclerosis, neurosyphilis and subacute sclerosing panencephalitis but it is necessary to show that there is a relative rise in γ-globulin so it is usual to express the results of this test as the IgG/albumin ratio. The normal range lies between 0.07 and 0.21 with a mean of 0.13. Ideally, this ratio should be expressed as a ratio of the concentrations of IgG and albumin in the blood to show that the increased γ-globulin is not derived from blood but is generated within the nervous system. The demonstration of oligoclonal bands by CSF protein immunoelectrophoresis is an abnormal finding, strongly suggestive of inflammatory disease; these bands are found in over 90% of patients with multiple sclerosis.

Sugar. Sugar disappears completely from the CSF in pyogenic meningitis. A moderate fall to about 0.20–0.45 g/l occurs in tuberculous meningitis and in meningeal carcinomatosis, unlike lymphocytic meningitis where the sugar remains normal.

Chlorides. The chlorides in the CSF run parallel to those in the blood and are therefore reduced in patients who have vomited frequently. For this reason they are usually low in tuberculous meningitis, but this has no diagnostic value.

Microbiological examination

If turbid CSF is removed, a smear should be stained with Gram's stain and examined for microorganisms and another specimen cultured. In pneumococcal, staphylococcal, streptococcal and influenzal meningitis the causal organisms are usually profuse in a direct smear, but meningococci may be difficult to find and culture. Tubercle bacilli should also be looked for in preparations stained by the Ziehl-Nielsen or auramine techniques and may be found in cases of tuberculous meningitis after an assiduous search, particularly if a fibrin 'web' can be examined. If no bacilli are found, confirmation of the diagnosis depends upon finding the organisms on culture on Lowenstein-Jensen slopes or guinea-pig inoculation, but these measures take about six weeks. In some cases of chronic meningitis, special culture media (e.g. Sabouraud's medium for cryptococcosis and Korthof's for leptospirosis) are required for the identification of some rare infections. Virological studies carried out on CSF tend to give results only when the illness is over but are useful even at this stage in establishing the nature of the organism responsible for some obscure infections of the nervous system. However, newer techniques of immunofluorescent staining for viral antibodies have added precision to early diagnosis. Serological tests for syphilis such as the Wassermann and Kahn reactions, which might be negative in blood and positive in the CSF, have now been abandoned in favour of more specific tests, so that negative VDRL, treponema immobilisation and fluorescent treponema antibody absorption (FTA/ABS) reactions in the blood virtually exclude neurosyphilis.

ELECTROENCEPHALOGRAPHY (EEG)

Electroencephalography is a technique of recording the electrical activity of the brain through the intact skull. Electrodes are applied to the scalp and the potential changes so recorded are amplified and presented for interpretation as an inked tracing on moving paper. Machines in common use have eight, sixteen or more channels so that the activity from many different areas of the head can be recorded simultaneously. The technique is simple and harmless and may give valuable diagnostic information, particularly in patients with suspected epilepsy or encephalitis.

In the normal adult the dominant electrical activity in the EEG from the post-central areas is usually a sinusoidal wave form with a frequency of 8–13 Hz. This is the alpha rhythm; it commonly disappears on attention, as when the eyes open. Normally there is often some faster or so-called beta activity (14–22 Hz) in the frontal regions; this is accentuated by barbiturates and sometimes by anxiety. In young infants the EEG is dominated by generalised slow activity of delta frequency (up to 3.5 Hz); gradually during maturation this is replaced by theta activity (4–7 Hz) and subsequently by the alpha rhythm. Theta activity disappears last from the posterior temporal regions, particularly on the right side, and the record is usually fully mature, showing no theta activity, by the age of from 12 to 14 years. During drowsiness and sleep in the normal adult, theta activity and later delta activity reappear. Some common EEG appearances are illustrated in Figure 3.1.

The EEG is of particular value in the diagnosis of **epilepsy**, though the interictal record may be normal. In **petit mal** it often shows regular, rhythmical, generalised outbursts of repetitive complexes, each consisting of a spike and a delta wave (spike-and-wave), and recurring at a frequency of about 3 Hz. In idiopathic or 'centrencephalic' **major epilepsy**, the inter-seizure record may show brief generalised outbursts of spikes or sharp waves, or of mixed spikes and slow activity (an irregular spike-and-wave discharge). In patients suffering from **focal epilepsy**, including **temporal lobe or 'psychomotor' attacks**, there are often spikes, sharp waves or rhythmical outbursts of slow (delta or theta) activity arising in the epileptogenic area of cortex. Unfortunately, a single record taken in an epileptic patient is often normal; positive findings are commoner in children and less common the older the patient. Many other patients show non-specific abnormalities, such as excessive temporal theta activity, a finding often attributed to immaturity in the broadest sense. Hence, it may be necessary to take repeated recordings or to use various **activation techniques** in order to uncover epileptic discharges. Overbreathing for from two to three minutes is particularly effective in evoking the discharges of petit mal, while photic stimulation (repetitive light flashes of variable frequency) can also bring out epileptic discharges. A sleep record may show an abnormality that is not apparent while the patient is awake, since temporal spikes or sharp waves often appear in early sleep. It is better, if possible, to allow the patient to sleep naturally, perhaps helped by sleep deprivation the night before, than to give sedation which alters the recording. In some cases, and particularly when the patient's symptoms are sufficiently severe for surgical treatment to be contemplated, recordings are made from underneath the medial surface of the temporal lobe by inserting a needle electrode to lie in contact with the basi-sphenoid.

Prolonged EEG monitoring may also give very useful information, particularly in determining whether the patient has epilepsy or pseudoseizures. A 24-hour recording can be made using a portable tape recorder; since these devices have four to eight channels, it is convenient to use one of these for the timer and another for

simultaneous ECG recording in case cardiac arrhythmia accounts for the patient's attacks. More useful information still is obtained from telemetry which allows the recording of many more channels and this is often combined with simultaneous video recording, using split-screen devices, so that the EEG tracing can be compared directly with the patient's behaviour. In addition to its value in patients with epilepsy, the other principal use of the EEG is in patients with encephalitis and/or metabolic brain disease. The EEG is always abnormal with widespread slow activity, usually asymmetrical in the early stages. Such abnormalities, with a CT scan which is

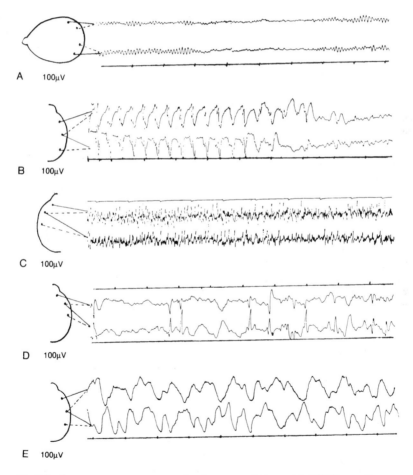

Fig. 3.1 Some common appearances in electroencephalographic (EEG) recordings. **A** A normal alpha rhythm recorded from both occipital regions and disappearing (in the centre of the recording) when the eyes are open. **B** A 3 Hz spike-and-wave discharge of petit mal epilepsy, recorded in this illustration from the right temporal region. **C** High-frequency discharges (mainly muscle artefact) recorded from the left fronto-temporal region during a major epileptic seizure. **D** A right anterior-temporal focus of spike discharge in a patient suffering from temporal lobe epilepsy. **E** A focus of high-amplitude delta activity seen in the right mid-temporal region in a patient suffering from a cerebral abscess in this situation.

usually normal, are strongly indicative of an encephalitis or metabolic encephalopathy. Some forms of encephalitis, notably herpes simplex encephalitis, may produce a characteristic EEG, with a burst-suppression pattern starting in one temporal lobe, the bursts becoming further apart over the next few days to be followed by marked attenuation of all activity. Burst-suppression means regularly recurring single high amplitude slow waves (bursts) separated by periods of comparative electrical silence (suppression). A similar sequence follows in the other temporal lobe, usually after a few days. The EEG may therefore suggest a diagnosis and is useful in following the patient's progress. A similar but generalised burst-suppression pattern occurs in subacute sclerosing panencephalitis (SSPE) and in some patients with Creutzfeldt-Jakob disease.

The EEG in children can be difficult to interpret; focal abnormalities are much more common and do not necessarily imply an underlying structural abnormality. A grossly abnormal record with high voltage spike, sharp and irregular slow activity, often called hypsarrhythmia, may be found in records from infants with so-called infantile spasms (see p. 80).

It can be concluded that a single routine EEG is of limited value, but should generally be performed, using simple activation techniques if necessary, in most patients suspected to be suffering from epilepsy. If epileptic discharges are found in the record this will support the diagnosis and the nature of the discharge may help in choosing appropriate treatment. Negative findings, however, do not exclude this diagnosis. The more difficult techniques should be reserved for use in intractable or problem cases or those in which confirmation of the diagnosis is particularly important, e.g., for, medicolegal reasons.

The EEG is also of limited value in the diagnosis of **focal cerebral lesions**. A relatively acute lesion of one cerebral hemisphere usually gives a focus of delta activity in or around the area of the lesion. It is not the lesion itself which produces this abnormal discharge, but the changes which it has produced in the surrounding brain. A **cerebral abscess** usually produces a very slow discharge of high amplitude, and similar though less striking abnormalities result from **tumour, haemorrhage, local injury** or **infarction**. A **subdural haematoma** is another condition which may be revealed by the EEG, as such cases often show a unilateral suppression of the alpha rhythm and some irregular slow activity on the affected side. While the EEG was regularly used in the past as an aid to diagnosis of such intracranial space-occupying lesions, if only because the more precise radiological methods were more risky and uncomfortable for the

patient, the advent of the CT and MRI scans (see below) have meant that the EEG is not an appropriate investigation if any of these lesions are suspected.

Tumours in the posterior fossa or deeply situated lesions near the midline often give paroxysmal outbursts of theta or delta activity at the surface, but these changes are by no means specific as they occur in patients with many diffuse cerebral disorders including **meningitis** and **subarachnoid haemorrhage** or conditions causing **disorders of cerebral metabolism** such as anoxia, uraemia, hyperglycaemia, hepatic encephalopathy or pernicious anaemia. Similar non-specific abnormalities are found in patients who are confused or comatose from any cause. Perhaps the diffuse so-called triphasic waves of hepatic encephalopathy may be somewhat more specific, if not diagnostic.

The EEG is of little value in **psychiatric diagnosis** although anxious and obsessional patients often show excessive frontal fast activity, while individuals with severe personality disorders (psychopaths) and children with **behaviour disorders** have typically immature records with excessive temporal slow activity, particularly on the right side posteriorly. Patients with **organic dementia** often show a dominant rhythm of theta rather than alpha frequency; this is in a sense a reversion to the childhood pattern and may even occur in ageing without dementia; it is certainly not specific.

Hence the EEG has considerable value in the diagnosis of epilepsy and encephalitis and of certain uncommon brain diseases in which relatively specific abnormalities are found; it is less useful in the investigation of patients with suspected intracranial tumour or cerebrovascular disease.

EVOKED POTENTIAL RECORDING

The increased sophistication of electrophysiological techniques and of equipment for stimulating and recording, as well as the introduction of small computers and microprocessors, has resulted in the increasing utilisation of techniques of evoked potential recording in neurological diagnosis. The basic principles of all such techniques are similar and it is now possible to record visual evoked responses, auditory evoked responses, somatosensory evoked responses, brain stem crossed acoustic responses and descending cortical motor neurone evoked responses. The EEG is recorded with standard EEG electrodes over the relevant part of the cortex and the appropriate stimulus is applied. This stimulus evokes a time-locked response in the cortex which is far too small to be identified against the random background EEG activity. However, if repeated stimuli are given and the tracing is averaged by computer, the random EEG activity cancels out and the time-locked response is enhanced and can be identified. Any delay can be measured and implies a slowing of transmission in the pathway concerned; this has proved, for example, to give a useful indication of central demyelination. The delay in conduction from one eye compared to the other therefore indicates delay in that optic nerve and is strong evidence of a retrobulbar neuritis in the past, even if the patient has been unaware of it. These tests are useful in demonstrating the presence of multiple lesions and therefore in supporting a clinical diagnosis of multiple sclerosis. Descending motor pathways can be stimulated electrically but magnetic induction is proving to be a more satisfactory clinical method. Evoked response audiometry has proved particularly useful in investigating childhood deafness.

ECHO-ENCEPHALOGRAPHY

Ultrasound has been used in neurological diagnosis for over 30 years. A number of simple and relatively inexpensive machines are available commercially which pass an ultrasonic beam horizontally through the intact skull and an 'echo' is recorded from midline structures (the 'A' scan). A 'shift' of the midline can readily be demonstrated and this method, which carries no risk to the patient, is of value in confirming rapidly the presence of a space-occupying lesion in or overlying one cerebral hemisphere. Thus, the method can be used for rapid screening of patients in whom, for instance, a subdural or extradural haematoma or a cerebral tumour is suspected. This technique has been largely superseded by CT scanning.

GAMMA-ENCEPHALOGRAPHY

Scanning of the radioactivity recorded over the skull surface following the intravenous injection of a suitable isotope (^{99}Technetium pertechnetate is commonly used) has been widely employed in neurological and neurosurgical units as an aid to the diagnosis of intracranial lesions. Following intravenous injection, the radioactive tracer remains in the vascular compartment with only a small amount of sequestration. Labelling of tissues therefore occurs only when there is a significant breakdown in the blood-brain barrier, as may occur in vascular lesions and tumours. This technique has been superseded by CT scanning, but it may be of value in demonstrating multiple intracranial lesions where metastases are suspected and it may show a subdural haematoma quite

clearly at a time when it is isodense on a CT scan and therefore difficult to see.

ISOTOPE CISTERNOGRAPHY

The circulation of CSF can be demonstrated by isotope cisternography. A small amount of isotope-labelled material is injected by lumbar puncture. ^{99m}TC-labelled EDTA or ^{113m}Indium are commonly used though the latter is preferred because of its longer half-life. Gamma camera pictures of the head are then taken, usually at 6, 24 and 48 hours. In normal subjects the tracer can be seen to pass up to the cisterna magna and then to follow the normal circulation of CSF around the brain stem, up through the Sylvian fissures and over the surface of the hemisphere to be absorbed into the longitudinal sinus. An obstruction to this pathway, usually at the tentorial hiatus or at the longitudinal sinus, causes the isotope to enter the ventricles and to remain there for 48–72 hours, and this is the typical picture of communicating hydrocephalus. In patients with large ventricles due to cerebral atrophy, the tracer often enters the ventricles in the first 24 hours, but by 48 and 72 hours it is distributed uniformly over the surface of the brain, so that a 24-hour scan is unsatisfactory in differentiating atrophy from communicating hydrocephalus. This technique has also proved to be helpful in detecting fistulous communications between the subarachnoid space and the middle ear or paranasal sinuses such as may occur after head injury, otitis media or sinusitis.

SINGLE PHOTON EMISSION COMPUTERISED TOMOGRAPHY (SPECT)

The technique of computerised tomography can be applied to gamma-emitting isotopes and a computerised map of the brain can be developed. The resolution of these machines is rather poor with isotopes currently available, but it is possible to measure blood flow changes in relatively large areas and to obtain tomographic pictures which correspond to the more usual isotope brain scan. The definition is not sufficiently good for most clinical purposes and the technique is at the moment largely used for research.

STUDIES OF PERIPHERAL NERVE AND MUSCLE FUNCTION

Many methods of electrodiagnosis are in common use to study peripheral nerve function. It has long been known that motor nerves respond to an applied electrical current of brief duration (faradism) and that muscle, even when it has lost its motor nerve supply, will contract, though sluggishly, in response to a long-duration current (galvanism). In Erb's **reaction of degeneration** (R.D.) there is loss of the response to faradism and retention of that to galvanism, a finding which implies denervation. However this classical method did not indicate whether this was partial or complete; to overcome this difficulty, the method was replaced by the charting of **strength-duration** (S.D.) curves which were more quantitative but have now been superseded by electromyography.

Electromyography (EMG)

Electromyography (Fig. 3.2) is a technique of recording the electrical activity produced by muscle at rest and during contraction. Surface electrodes can be used but are only useful for physiological studies, in determining, for instance, which muscles contribute to a particular movement, or for recording the frequency of involuntary movements (e.g. tremor). For most diagnostic work, bipolar concentric needle electrodes are inserted into the muscle being tested; the electrical activity is then passed through a high-gain amplifier and is presented for interpretation both on an oscilloscope screen and in a loudspeaker. Sometimes the visual trace is more valuable, sometimes the auditory pattern, but the combination is more valuable than either alone. **Normal voluntary muscle** is electrically silent at rest, but on contraction motor unit potentials are seen and appear in increasing number and frequency as contraction increases, to give a continuous trace across the screen and a low-pitched rumble in the loudspeaker. These potentials are smooth, monophasic, diphasic or triphasic waves, each about 5–8 ms in duration and about 1 mV in amplitude. They are generally known as motor unit action potentials, as it was once thought that each resulted from the contraction of all of the muscle fibres innervated by one anterior horn cell and its axon (a motor unit). It is now known that these potentials are due to the contraction of only a few component fibres of the motor unit which happen to be close to the recording electrode (a 'sub-unit').

When a muscle **loses its nerve supply**, spontaneous **fibrillation** or contraction of individual muscle fibres begins within 14 to 21 days and the related electrical activity can be recorded from the relaxed and resting muscle; it takes the form of a series of repetitive small spikes on the screen and produces a ticking noise in the loudspeaker. If the muscle has lost only a part of its nerve supply, some motor unit potentials will still appear on attempted contraction, but the pattern of voluntary effort will be much reduced. During re-innervation after nerve regeneration complex polyphasic potentials of long duration appear, so-called **recovery potentials**; their long duration is due to the fact that regenerating nerve sprouts, which re-innervate previously denervated muscle fibres, conduct at different rates. Hence in patients with disease of the motor neurone at any point from the anterior horn cell to the motor end-plate the EMG will show spontaneous fibrillation and a **reduced pattern** of motor units on voluntary effort. When the lesion is in the anterior horn cells some of the surviving motor unit action potentials may be unusually large, up to 5 mV in amplitude and 10 ms in duration ('**giant' units**); this is because collateral axonal sprouts from surviving neurones may 'adopt' and re-innervate some denervated muscle fibres. Sometimes in disorders of the anterior horn cell there are also spontaneous **fasciculation potentials** which look like normal motor unit potentials but are recorded from the resting muscle, while if there is nerve or nerve root irritation, groups of two or three motor unit potentials may be recorded, again from a muscle which is apparently at rest. Clinically, fasciculations may be seen through the skin, but fibrillation cannot be seen as the contractions of individual muscle fibres are too small. Fibrillation can, however, be seen in the denervated tongue.

In **primary diseases of muscle**, such as muscular dystrophy, the pattern is different. Spontaneous activity such as fibrillation is scanty or absent, and on volition the motor unit potentials are seen to be broken-up, **polyphasic** and of **short duration**. Hence the pattern is complex and spiky and the noise in the loudspeaker is a crackling sound, like hail on a tin roof. The phenomenon of **myotonia** also gives a characteristic EMG; chains of oscillations of high frequency are seen which give a typical 'snarling' or 'dive-bomber' sound in the loudspeaker.

The technique of **single fibre electromyography** involves the use of a special needle with a very fine tip which records from only a very small area. This type of electrode can be used to record contraction of individual fibres. It is particularly useful in patients with abnormalities of the neuromuscular junction. An axon, derived from one anterior horn cell, divides within muscle so that each terminal branch innervates a single muscle fibre. If the terminal branch of one fibre is slightly longer than that to an adjacent fibre, the impulse will take longer to travel down this longer branch and the fibre will therefore contract a few milliseconds later than its neighbour. Since these impulses are derived from a single impulse initiated more proximally, the time interval between these two contractions is constant, so that if the activity of the first fibre is used to trigger a sweep on the EMG oscilloscope, the contraction of the second fibre appears at a time-locked interval after the first. If there is some disturbance of neuromuscular function, the second

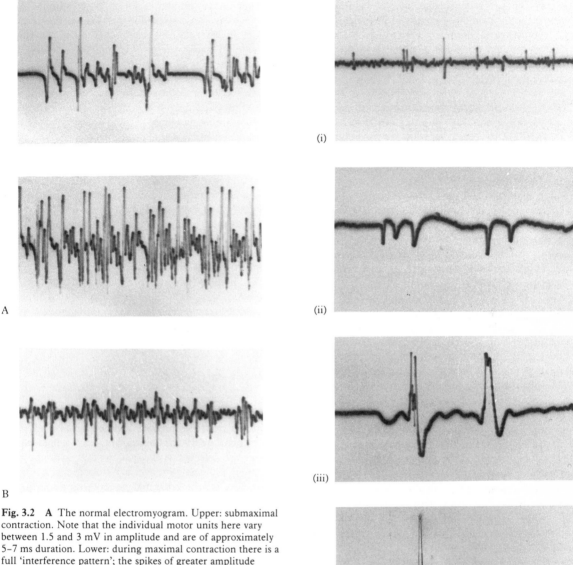

(i)

(ii)

(iii)

(iv)

A

B

C

Fig. 3.2 A The normal electromyogram. Upper: submaximal contraction. Note that the individual motor units here vary between 1.5 and 3 mV in amplitude and are of approximately 5–7 ms duration. Lower: during maximal contraction there is a full 'interference pattern'; the spikes of greater amplitude represent action potentials derived from motor units lying relatively close to the recording electrode, while those of lower amplitude are derived from motor units lying some distance away. **B** The electromyogram in myopathy. The constituent motor units are greatly reduced in amplitude and duration and many are polyphasic. **C** The electromyogram in denervation. From top to bottom:

(i) Spontaneous fibrillation; this is recorded from relaxed resting muscle: the individual potentials measure no more than about 100 µV in amplitude and are about 1 ms duration.

(ii) Positive sharp waves (saw-tooth potentials) also recorded from relaxed resting muscle; this phenomenon is occasionally seen in denervated muscle.

(iii) Fasciculation potentials firing spontaneously, also recorded from relaxed resting muscle in a patient with motor neurone disease; these potentials are morphologically indistinguishable from motor unit action potentials.

(iv) A giant motor unit action potential of approximately 5 mV in amplitude occurring during volitional activity in a patient with motor neurone disease. (Figures 3.2 A-C kindly provided by Dr R. Weiser) fibre may contract at a variable interval later than it should, though it cannot, of course, contract earlier; it may not contract at all. If the first fibre is still used to trigger the sweep and repetitive stimulation is used, the response from the second fibre is seen to occur at variable times after the first and this movement is known as jitter. And if, during repeated muscular contraction, whether voluntary or electrically induced, the second potential disappears, this is known as **blocking** and may indicate either a failure of conduction in the nerve branch concerned, or more probably a failure of neuromuscular transmission at its motor end-plate, as in myasthenia gravis. The measurement of these phenomena has proved to be of considerable diagnostic value.

The electromyogram is thus of considerable value in neurological diagnosis. It is of particular use in investigating peripheral nerve injuries and in studying cases of muscular wasting and weakness in which it is especially helpful in distinguishing disease of the muscle from that of the motor nerves.

Nerve conduction

By stimulating a motor nerve at two separate points along its course (Fig. 3.3) and by recording the motor unit potentials so produced from an appropriate muscle, it is possible to measure the stimulus–contraction interval in each case and hence to calculate the rate of conduction of the impulse along the nerve. For accurate recording the temperature of the limb must be carefully controlled. Nerve conduction is slowed in some forms of polyneuropathy and the technique can also be utilised to localise focal lesions in nerves, such as compression of the median nerve in the carpal tunnel, of the ulnar nerve at the elbow or of the common peroneal nerve at the neck of the fibula. Thus, if one applies a supramaximal stimulus to the median nerve in the cubital fossa and records the muscle action potential evoked in the abductor pollicis brevis, a similar action potential can then be obtained by stimulating the nerve at the wrist. By measuring the stimulus–contraction latency in each case and the distance between the stimulating electrodes, the conduction velocity in the forearm segment of the nerve can be calculated. If the nerve is compressed in the carpal tunnel then 'terminal latency' (normally 4 m/s or less) is increased.

The normal conduction velocity in the adult is 50–60 m/s in the median, ulnar and radial nerves and 45–50 m/s in the common peroneal. In demyelinating peripheral neuropathies conduction is markedly slowed, while in those due to axonal degeneration the surviving axons conduct at a normal rate but the amplitude of the evoked muscle action potential is reduced. Measurement

of the conduction velocity in sensory fibres, stimulated by ring electrodes on a digit and picking up the sensory volley by an electrode over the nerve trunk, is also widely used for diagnosis. These techniques involve the measurement of sensory nerve action potential (SNAP) amplitude and latency in such nerves as the median and ulnar in the upper limbs and the common peroneal and sural in the lower, and test the integrity of the nerve distal to the dorsal root ganglion.

If one refers to the action potential recorded from, say, the calf muscles on stimulation of the sciatic nerve as the M-response, there is a second wave form of longer latency which follows it and is called the H-reflex. This results from the fact that the stimulus applied to the trunk of the nerve also produces an afferent volley in the sensory fibres of the nerve and this volley reflexly excites anterior horn cells in the same segment of the cord to send a further action potential down their axons to produce this second muscle action potential. A somewhat similar wave form can be seen in the small muscles of the hands after stimulation, say, of the ulnar nerve and is called the F-wave. Measurement of these wave forms and of their latencies can give information about conduction velocity in proximal segments of the respective nerves.

Motor end-plate dysfunction

If repetitive supramaximal shocks are applied to the ulnar nerve at the elbow at 3–5/s and the evoked motor action potential is recorded from the hypothenar muscles, then in a patient with myasthenia gravis in whom these muscles are affected it is usual to find a progressive decrement in the amplitude of the evoked response. This abnormality can be corrected temporarily by an intravenous injection of edrophonium hydrochloride (Tensilon®); a similar decrement usually occurs at fast rates (50/s) of stimulation which produce a muscle tetanus. By contrast, in the myasthenic-myopathic (Lambert-Eaton) syndrome (see p. 300), the evoked potential is initially of low amplitude and a striking increment in amplitude is obtained at fast stimulation frequencies. Weakness in this condition is little influenced by edrophonium but may be corrected by guanidine hydrochloride.

Increased jitter and blocking in single fibre electromyography are more sensitive indicators of abnormalities of neuromuscular transmission.

RADIOLOGY

Radiological methods are among the most helpful and widely-used of all the ancillary techniques used in neurological diagnosis. While final diagnosis often

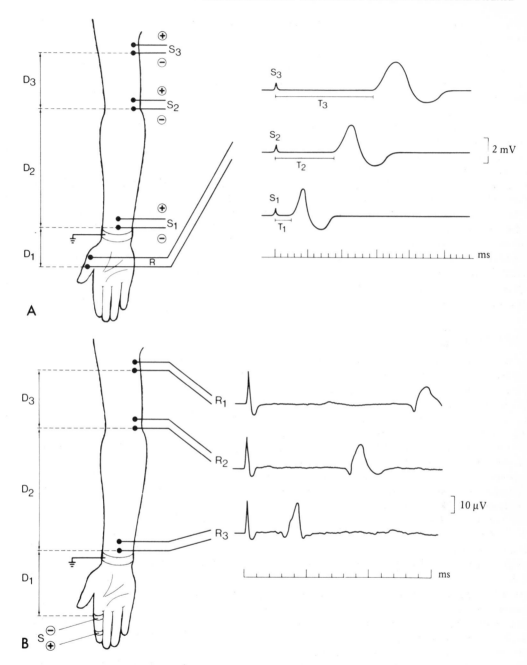

Fig. 3.3 **A** Diagrammatic representation of the technique of measuring maximum motor conduction velocity in the median nerve. **B** Diagrammatic representation of the technique for measuring maximum sensory conduction velocity in the median nerve by orthodromic stimulation.
(Reproduced with permission from Bradley 1974)

depends upon highly specialised methods involving computerised tomography or the use of contrast media, each of these techniques, which will be considered below, is time-consuming, expensive and some are disturbing to the patient. It must therefore be remembered that valuable and even conclusive information can sometimes be obtained from plain radiographs of the skull and/or spine and even of other parts of the body. Thus in patients with a clinical picture suggestive of intracranial tumour, or in others with a subacute meningitic illness, it is important to X-ray the chest, as in one case a bronchogenic carcinoma may be revealed suggesting a metastatic intracranial lesion, while in another the appearances of pulmonary tuberculosis may be discovered. In other cases changes in the skeleton will cast light upon the significance of neurological symptoms and signs as, for instance, in cases of prostatic carcinoma or multiple myelomatosis.

Straight radiography of the skull

It is usual to take routine anteroposterior and lateral views of the skull, while in most specialised centres an anteroposterior view is also taken with the brow depressed some 35° so that the petrous temporal bones become visible (Towne's view), and another of the skull base. Stenver's view is also utilised to examine the petrous temporal bone. Usually the **skull vault** is first examined to see if there is reasonable uniformity of bony thickness or whether there is any **erosion** or **bony overgrowth** (as may result from a meningioma) or **abnormal vascular markings** due to dilatation of the middle meningeal artery which is supplying a meningeal tumour or vascular malformation. Sometimes, as in carcinomatosis or myelomatosis, there are multiple areas of **bony rarefaction** in the skull vault or there is a general thickening or 'woolliness' of the bone as in Paget's disease. In young children, hydrocephalus due to any cause gives **separation of the cranial sutures** and a characteristic 'beaten copper' mottling of the bone. However, the latter appearance is so often seen in normal individuals, even in adult life, that in itself it is not diagnostic. Fractures of the vault are, of course, noted if present, and it is also wise to examine the frontal, maxillary sphenoidal and ethmoid paranasal sinuses for opacities which would suggest infection or neoplasia. **Hyperostosis** of the inner table of the frontal bone is not uncommon but has no definite pathological significance.

The **base of the skull** is next examined, first in the lateral projection. Here the relationship of the upper **cervical spine** to the **foramen magnum** is observed and it is noted whether there is any protrusion of the odontoid

process of the axis above Chamberlain's line which joins the posterior margin of the hard palate to the posterior lip of the foramen magnum. If the odontoid does show above this line, or if there is an abnormal tilt of the body of the atlas implying invagination of the basi-occiput, then **basilar impression**, which may give important neurological symptoms and signs, is present. Another important structure in the skull base visible on the lateral projection is the **sella turcica**. Its size and shape and the integrity and density of the anterior and posterior clinoid processes which form its lips are noted. In patients with primary pituitary neoplasms the sella is expanded or ballooned and partially decalcified. In those with suprasellar lesions the sella is also expanded, but is shallower and flattened and there is often erosion of the clinoid processes. Moderate flattening and expansion of the sella with decalcification of the posterior clinoid processes may occur in any patient with increased intracranial pressure whether there is a lesion near the sella or not.

Also to be noted on the lateral projection is the presence or absence of **intracranial calcification**. If present, such calcification is then more accurately localised in anteroposterior views, or sometimes by stereoscopic lateral projections. In about 50% of adults, and even in some normal children, the **pineal gland**, which lies above and behind the sella, is calcified and may even measure up to 0.5 cm in diameter. If the gland is calcified it is important to measure its distance from the inner table of the skull at either side on anteroposterior radiographs, as lateral displacement may indicate the presence of a space-occupying lesion in one cerebral hemisphere. Other intracranial structures which occasionally calcify in the normal individual are the choroid plexuses, the falx cerebri and the petro-clinoid ligaments. **Pathological intracranial calcification**, if mottled in type and suprasellar in situation, usually indicates a craniopharyngioma, but many other intracranial tumours, including meningiomas, gliomas and oligodendrogliomas, occasionally show a fine spidery pattern of calcification. Fine curvilinear lines of calcification are rarely seen in the wall of a large aneurysm, while calcific stippling or even dense calcification may occur within a haematoma or in an arteriovenous angioma. Rare causes of intracranial calcification include hamartoma, cysticercosis (calcified cysts), toxoplasmosis (mottling in the basal ganglia) and hypoparathyroidism (also in the basal ganglia). A form of calcification outlining clearly the gyri of one occipital and/or parietal lobe is seen in diffuse cortical angiomatosis associated with a port-wine naevus of the face (the Sturge-Weber syndrome).

In anteroposterior, Towne's, Stenver's and the basal views, a most important feature to look for is **enlargement** or erosion of cranial exit foramina. **Sclerosis and over-growth of bone** may also occur, particularly in the wings of the sphenoid, in patients who have a meningioma in this region. It is also usual to examine carefully the optic foramina, superior orbital fissures, and internal auditory meati. A funnel-shaped erosion of the internal auditory meati, revealed by Towne's and Stenver's views, is characteristic of acoustic neuroma. The basal view may reveal bony erosion due to malignant infiltration of the base of the skull or enlargement of one foramen spinosum due to a meningioma producing dilatation of one middle meningeal artery.

Radiology of the spinal column

In examining radiographs of the spine we are concerned first with changes in the **vertebrae** themselves, secondly with the **intervertebral discs** and thirdly with the **intervertebral foramina**. It is usual to carry out anteroposterior and lateral views to study the vertebrae and discs, but to examine the intervertebral foramina, oblique views are needed. Lateral views in flexion and extension may be necessary to show instability and subluxation. In the vertebrae themselves one may observe **congenital abnormalities** such as **fusion** of several vertebral bodies (if in the cervical region this is called the Klippel-Feil syndrome) or **spina bifida**, either of which may be responsible for, or associated with, neurological signs. Fracture, fracture-dislocation, Paget's disease, osteomyelitis, neoplasia, either benign or malignant, of vertebral bodies, any one of which can give vertebral collapse and spinal cord compression, are generally revealed by routine X-rays. **Bony erosion** and, in particular, enlargement of the relevant intervertebral foramen is typically seen, often with the extraspinal soft tissue shadow of a dumb-bell tumour, in cases of spinal neurofibroma. Less striking but of equal diagnostic importance is a **variation in interpedicular distance**. The distance between the vertebral pedicles is large in the cervical region, diminishes to a minimum in the mid-dorsal region, and then expands again in the lumbar region, corresponding to the cervical and lumbar enlargements of the spinal cord. If successive interpedicular distances are measured and one or more measurements fall outside the expected arithmetical progression, particularly if the medial aspects of the pedicles are flattened, this indicates an expanding lesion within the spinal cord or spinal canal in this region. Dorsal meningiomas may produce no more radiological change than this, whereas neurofibromas commonly give bony erosion as well. Measurement of the **anteroposterior diameter** of the spinal canal is also of value, particularly in the cervical region; an unduly wide canal is seen, for instance, in some cases of syringomyelia. A narrow canal may be congenital and can contribute to the early development of a myelopathy in patients with cervical spondylosis, or may be acquired due to hypertrophy of apophyseal joints, usually in the lumbar region; this is one cause of lumbar canal stenosis.

In a patient with an acute **intervertebral disc prolapse**, radiographs of the spine are often normal or reveal simply narrowing of the disc space concerned. The prolapsed disc is not itself radio-opaque. If one or more disc protrusions have been present for months or years, the margins of the prolapsed tissue gradually become calcified, giving posterior (and often anterior) **osteophyte formation** at the upper and lower borders of the contiguous vertebrae. As the prolapsed tissue often projects laterally as well, osteophytes also tend to encroach upon the intervertebral foramina and this change is shown on oblique views. A combination of changes of this type, which are most often found in the cervical and lumbar regions, is referred to as **spondylosis**.

Computerised tomography (CT scan)

The introduction of this technique in the early 1970s has transformed the practice of clinical neurology, especially in relation to the diagnosis of intracranial lesions.

The first apparatus commercially available, developed by Dr (now Sir) Godfrey Hounsfield of Bristol, was manufactured by the British company, EMI Ltd, and hence the earliest records were often called Emiscans. The method involves the rotation of an X-ray tube around the skull with the simultaneous rotation of a detector on the opposite side of the head. The detector records the amount of X-rays transmitted and a computer calculates the X-ray absorption of small volumes of brain (voxels). The size of a voxel varies from machine to machine, but usually measures 1 mm × 1 mm × 9 mm, the 9 mm being the thickness of the slice in the axial plane. Thin slices down to 1.5 mm can be made for high-definition pictures of small areas such as the pituitary fossa, but this exposes the patient to considerably greater irradiation. The X-ray absorption of each voxel is shown two-dimensionally and is then known as a pixel. Problems with resolution occur close to interfaces between structures of widely differing X-ray absorption such as brain, CSF and bone where part of a voxel is bone and part is CSF; the pixel shows an average between the X-ray densities and this partial volume effect blurs the image. Modern machines use a variety of multiple X-ray generators and detectors which considerably reduce the scanning time. Unenhanced scans cause no discomfort and are harmless, the total exposure to X-rays simply corresponding to that involved in taking a series of routine skull X-rays. Confused or restless patients and children may require sedation as the head must be held still during the recording.

Using this technique the brain parenchyma, ventricular system, the CSF cisterns, the pineal, falx cerebri, brain stem, cerebellar hemispheres, orbital contents and even individual intracranial arteries can be visualised. In general, most neoplasms can be seen as areas of increased density unless their centre is necrotic or cystic when a rim of dense tumour around a translucent area is seen, an appearance which may resemble that of an abscess. Areas of haemorrhage, too, usually show typical increased density, whether in the extradural, subdural, sub-arachnoid or ventricular spaces or within the brain substance. Infarcts are generally apparent as areas of reduced density, as are plaques of demyelination, while cerebral atrophy can be diagnosed when the cortical sulci are widened and the ventricles enlarged. The appearance of many lesions can be enhanced following intravenous injection of contrast material. An iodinated water-soluble contrast medium is used (such as Urographin®). This outlines the vascular pool and, therefore, may show arteriovenous malformations and aneurysms. The con-trast material also passes the blood-brain barrier where this is damaged and may enhance the appearance of malignant brain tumours, some infarcts and haemor-rhages. A normal CT scan is illustrated in Figure 3.4.

The CT scan is, however, rather less successful in identifying lesions in the posterior fossa than in the cerebral hemispheres. For a lesion to be visualised it must have a density different from that of the surrounding brain and must be 5 mm or more in diameter. Nevertheless the diagnostic yield of this technique is far greater than that of any of the contrast methods (to be mentioned below) upon which neurologists and neurosurgeons were compelled to rely before its introduction.

Contrast methods

Before the advent of the CT scan, the methods most often used in the diagnosis of intracranial lesions were first the outlining of the cerebral ventricular system with air or oxygen either by injection through a lumbar puncture needle (**air encephalography or pneumoencephalo-graphy**) or by **ventriculography**, which involved inserting a needle into one lateral ventricle via a burr-hole in the skull vault. Sometimes for greater diagnostic accuracy air

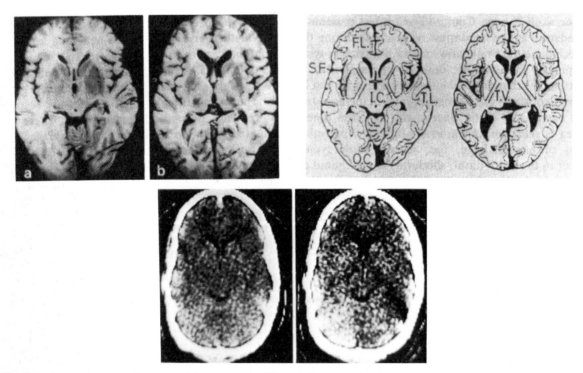

Fig. 3.4   A normal computerised transaxial tomogram (a CT scan) above, showing the cerebral ventricular outlines at different sagittal planes, as seen in the brain slices (top left) and the diagram (top right). F.L. = frontal lobe; S.F. = Sylvian fissure; I.C. = internal capsule; T.L. = temporal lobe; O.C. = occipital cortex; T.V. = third ventricle; T = temporal horn.

ventriculography was followed by the injection of an oily or a water-soluble contrast medium into the ventricular system. Air encephalography was usually performed in patients in whom intracranial tumour, communicating ('low-pressure') hydrocephalus or cortical atrophy were suspected but in whom there were no symptoms or signs of increased intracranial pressure which contraindicated lumbar puncture, while ventriculography was felt to be needed in patients with suspected posterior fossa tumours or in those with suspected neoplasia in one or other cerebral hemisphere in whom angiography and the gamma scan had given inadequate or conflicting information. Now, in centres where the CT scan is available, these investigations have been abandoned.

Cerebral angiography, however, whether by injection or catheterisation of the carotid or vertebral arteries or of the aortic arch, continues to be a useful investigation providing some information which the CT scan cannot reveal. Thus in cases of intracranial haemorrhage or infarction it may reveal an aneurysm or angioma as a cause of the haemorrhage and/or occlusion or stenosis of an intracranial or extracranial artery or vein. And in some patients with intracranial neoplasia the pattern of the vascular supply of the tumour can give a useful indication of its pathology.

In the investigation of suspected spinal cord compression, **myelography** using water-soluble contrast media, or, less commonly, air or oxygen, injected by lumbar puncture, remains the method of choice, but may with time become less necessary as the use of magnetic resonance imaging (MRI) (see below) increases. The basal cisterns can be clearly seen on CT scans if the contrast material is run up into the head and this may be a very useful method of outlining small acoustic neuromas as the internal auditory meati are clearly defined by this technique. It is the method of choice for outlining small non-vascular extramedullary lesions in the posterior fossa. **Spinal cord angiography**, achieved by injecting contrast medium into the aorta, is also useful in demonstrating arteriovenous angiomas of the cord.

Now that the CT and MRI scans give so much information without risk or discomfort, the need for invasive investigations has diminished greatly. Thus now, even more than in the past, it should be stressed that those uncomfortable and sometimes potentially hazardous investigations should only be performed if the information which they yield cannot be obtained in any other way.

Cerebral angiography

Cerebral angiography is nowadays always carried out via catheterisation of the femoral artery. A fairly large catheter is required in order to inject sufficient contrast material to obtain adequate opacification of the ascending aorta and its major branches. Finer catheters are used for selected injection into the innominate or common carotid arteries and the vertebral arteries and these may be advanced into the external or internal carotid arteries if selective injection of these vessels is required. The use of direct puncture of the carotid or vertebral arteries has been largely abandoned because of the increased risk of complications.

Following injection, a rapid series of films is taken in the anterior, posterior and lateral planes. Oblique views are sometimes required to visualise the origin of aneurysms or to outline the sagittal sinus. Subtraction techniques considerably enhance the value of cerebral angiography. A plain film of the head, taken in the same plane, is subtracted from the angiographic film, thus leaving the outline of the vessels only and eliminating the images of bone and soft tissues. Small vessels can be clearly seen by this technique, particularly where they overlie and are obscured by bone in the normal angiogram. Magnification views also make interpretation of some angiograms easier.

Angiography is particularly valuable in the diagnosis of **vascular lesions**. Thus **intracranial aneurysms** (Fig. 3.5) and **arteriovenous angiomas** (see p. 258) are readily demonstrated and localised; the technique must be used

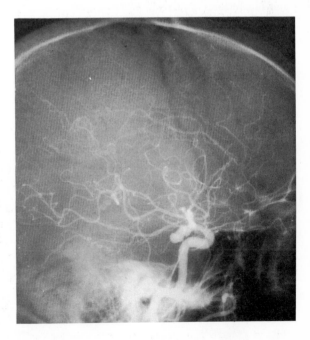

Fig. 3.5 A supraclinoid aneurysm arising at the junction of the right internal carotid and posterior communicating arteries.

with some caution in cases of presumed cerebral ischaemia or infarction because of the danger of complications, but in many such cases obstruction or **stenosis of
the internal carotid artery** (Fig. 3.6), or of other major
vessels in the neck or cranium are clearly demonstrated.
Subdural haematoma, too, can be diagnosed with confidence, by finding an avascular area beneath the vault of
the skull in the anteroposterior view (see p. 203). With
the introduction of CT scanning, arteriography is no
longer used for the localisation of tumours, but it may add
valuable information about the vascular supply and the
vascularity of space-occupying lesions (Fig. 3.7).

Myelography

Myelography is a valuable method of localising lesions
which compress or distort the spinal cord. It is usual to
inject contrast medium into the lumbar subarachnoid
space and then to observe its flow up and down the spinal
canal under the screen (fluoroscope) on tilting the
patient. Anteroposterior and lateral radiographs are also
taken at intervals. It is only necessary to use cisternal
injection when there is a block beyond which contrast
medium injected in the lumbar region will not pass and
information is required concerning the upper limit of the
lesion. The investigation has few complications with the
use of recently introduced non-ionic water-soluble contrast material, though there is a slight risk of precipitating
epileptic seizures in susceptible individuals.

An **extramedullary neoplasm** will almost always be
localised accurately on myelography, either by the presence of a block or by a characteristic filling defect in the
column of contrast medium (see p. 262). Expansion of
the spinal cord, indicative of an **intramedullary neoplasm**, or of **syringomyelia** can also be demonstrated,
while an outline of abnormal vessels in patients with
spinal vascular malformations may also be seen. It is of

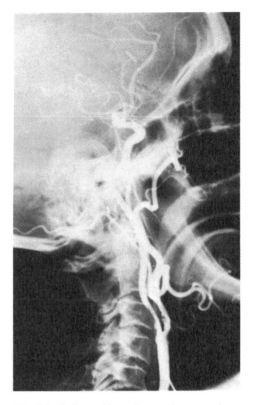

Fig. 3.6 Left carotid arteriogram demonstrating
stenosis at the origin of the internal carotid artery.

particular importance to carry out myelography with the
patient in the supine as well as in the prone position,
especially when the foramen magnum area is being
examined, as supine views may demonstrate descent of
the cerebellar tonsils (a Chiari anomaly) or, less commonly, arachnoiditis around the foramen magnum, disorders
with which the syndrome of syringomyelia is generally

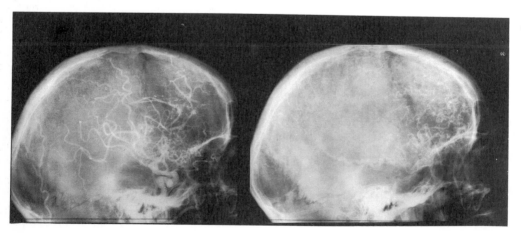

A

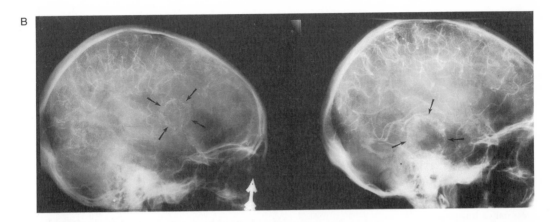

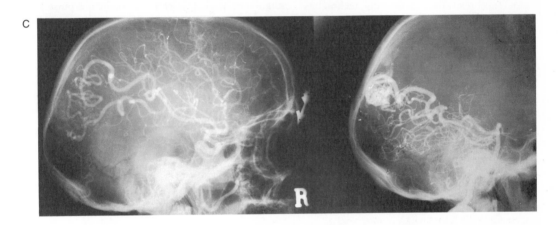

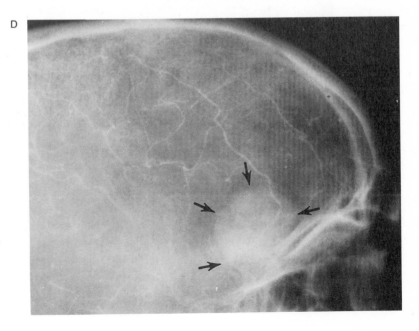

Fig. 3.7 **A** A pathological circulation in a large frontal lobe glioma. **B** Left carotid angiogram (left) showing a vascular metastasis in the fronto-parietal region (arrows). Right carotid arteriogram of the same patient (right) showing a similar lesion in the right temporal lobe. **C** An occipital arteriovenous angioma supplied by both the carotid (left) and vertebral (right) systems. **D** A subfrontal meningioma showing a typical 'blush' (arrows) in the late arterial phase. (Reproduced with permission from Walton 1985).

associated. **Prolapsed intervertebral discs** and spondylotic changes are demonstrated best in lateral views, when indentations in the contrast column are seen opposite the disc space or spaces concerned (see p. 290); lateral protrusions may result in a failure of certain root sleeves to fill, and this is seen best in the anteroposterior view. Myelography is an essential preliminary to any operation performed for the relief of spinal cord compression, as clinical signs in themselves are never sufficiently accurate for exact localisation of the lesion, which usually lies several segments above the level suggested by clinical signs such as the upper border of sensory loss.

Magnetic resonance imaging (MRI)

This is another major advance in imaging techniques recently introduced, and it has the great advantage over normal CT scanning that the patient is not subjected to X-irradiation. Anatomical detail is very well shown, particularly the difference between grey and white matter, and it does not suffer from the partial volume effect problems of the CT scan in the posterior fossa (Fig. 3.8). Very good pictures can be obtained of the spinal cord and cervical and lumbar roots so that it is likely that this technique will eventually replace myelography, particularly as it can show both extrinsic and intrinsic lesions, including, for example, a syrinx (see p. 197).

The patient lies in a strong magnetic field; satisfactory pictures can be obtained with magnetic fields of 0.5–1.5 tesla, but the higher field strengths are required for spectroscopy. This magnetic field aligns a small number of protons. These protons are then displaced from this alignment with a brief radio-frequency pulse. As the protons spin back into magnetic alignment they give off a

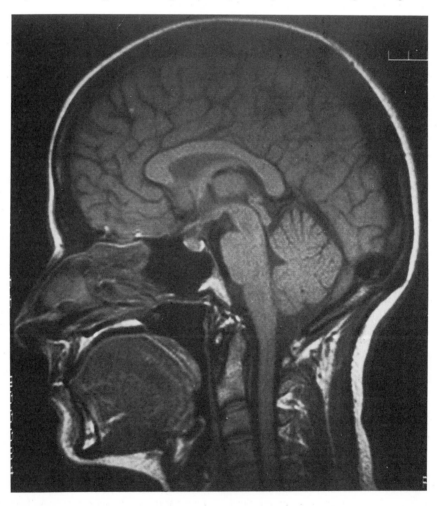

Fig. 3.8 Normal sagittal MRI, T1 weighted.

weak radio-frequency signal which can be recorded. The signal can be resolved into two vectors, in line with the magnet (T1) and at right angles to this (T2). Computerised tomographic techniques can then be used to construct a picture in any plane. Different pictures can be obtained by varying the repetition time of the radio-frequency signal (TR) and also by varying the time from the pulse to the echo (TE). Short TR and TE produces a T1 weighted image which largely shows proton density and, therefore, the distribution of water; this gives the best anatomical pictures. A long TR and TE gives a T2 weighted image which often gives more information about the pathology of a lesion.

Positron emission tomography (PET)

In the same way that computerised tomographic scans can be obtained from the transmission of X-rays through the head (transmission tomography) so similar pictures can be obtained by the use of positron-emitting radio isotopes (emission tomography). These isotopes are produced in a cyclotron and used to label naturally occurring products such as glucose with ^{18}F or water and carbon dioxide with ^{15}O. A number of ligands can be prepared in a similar way. These are introduced to the patient either by injection or inhalation and the radio isotopes are then detected by external counting. Computerised tomographic techniques allow maps to be produced, although with far less definition and resolution than with X-ray CT scanning or MRI. However, it is the only technique which can show simultaneously cerebral blood flow, cerebral blood volume and cerebral glucose uptake. The oxygen extraction ratio and cerebral metabolic rate for oxygen can also be calculated. The use of ligands can be used to follow the metabolism of neurotransmitters and other metabolic activities in the brain.

These techniques require complex and expensive equipment as well as an on-site cyclotron. A large team of specialists is required to operate such a system and it is not surprising, therefore, that relatively few such centres exist throughout the world. PET scanning has not made a major contribution to clinical management and remains largely a research tool.

THE SPECIAL SENSES

Visual and oculomotor function

Methods of examining the visual apparatus which are part of the routine neurological examination have been described in Chapter 1. These include testing of the visual acuity, charting of the peripheral and central visual fields, examination of the pupils, of the ocular movements and ophthalmoscopy. The principles of visual evoked potential recording have also been mentioned (see p. 34).

Slit-lamp examination is occasionally helpful in neurological diagnosis, either for detecting early cataract, or in looking for the peripheral corneal pigmentation which occurs in Wilson's disease (the Kayser-Fleischer ring).

Recording of ocular muscle imbalance on a **Hess's chart** is also valuable in the investigation of cases of diplopia, since repeated recordings may give an objective assessment of the patient's progress.

Ophthalmodynamometry, a technique of measuring the pressure in the retinal arteries by applying a simple instrument to the globe of the eye, is occasionally helpful in the diagnosis of occlusion of the internal carotid artery, as the ophthalmic artery is a branch of the internal carotid and retinal artery pressure on the affected side is reduced.

Fluorescein retinal angiography is helpful in confirming the presence of early papilloedema and in elucidating other ocular fundal lesions. It may also be useful to elicit **optokinetic nystagmus** by rotating a striped drum or unrolling a piece of vertically-striped cloth in front of the patient's eyes, first in one direction and then in the other, as this reflex response gives valuable information about the integrity of the visual pathways.

Auditory and vestibular function

Simple tuning-fork tests for assessing auditory function are described in Chapter 2. For a more accurate assessment of degrees of deafness **audiometry** is necessary. Each ear is tested independently and sounds of different frequencies are used, produced by an electronic instrument which gives pure tones. At each frequency, the intensity of sound (measured in decibels) is increased until the patient can just hear it. Thus the degree of deafness, if any, which is present in each ear can be measured and it can also be determined whether it affects all frequencies. Evoked response audiometry is especially useful in children.

In disease of the cochlear end organ (as in Ménière's syndrome), the phenomenon of **recruitment** may occur. This means that impaired hearing in the affected ear decreases progressively as the intensity of the stimulus is increased so that eventually it is heard equally loudly in the unaffected and diseased ears. Recruitment does not occur in patients with lesions of the auditory nerve (e.g. acoustic neuroma).

Vestibular function can be tested by **caloric tests**. The head is tilted backwards 60° so that the lateral semicircular canal is vertical and the ear is then irrigated with cold water (at 30°C). This produces nystagmus with the quick phase to the right if the left ear is irrigated or vice versa. The test is then repeated using warm water (44°C), when the quick phase of the nystagmus occurs in the opposite direction, that is to the side of the ear being tested. The two ears are stimulated independently and the total duration of the nystagmus obtained in each of the four tests is recorded. The accuracy of recording may be improved by **electronystagmography**. In lesions of the peripheral vestibular system (Mènière's disease) or of the vestibular nerve, stimulation of the affected labyrinth by caloric tests either produces no nystagmus at all or else its duration is greatly reduced (**canal paresis**). This finding is often of diagnostic value. In some patients with lesions of the brain stem or of the temporal or parietal lobes of the contralateral cerebral hemisphere, the duration of the nystagmus occurring to the side opposite to the cerebral lesion is reduced, whether it is produced by warm water in one ear or cold in the other. This finding, known as **directional preponderance**, is not due to a labyrinthine lesion but to a lesion of the central pathways which are responsible for conducting and recording labyrinthine stimuli. In stuporose or comatose patients a modified caloric test, involving only the injection of cold water into the internal auditory meati, to see whether nystagmus is evoked, often gives valuable evidence as to the integrity of the vestibular nuclei and is thus invaluable in the diagnosis of brain stem dysfunction and of 'brain death'.

PSYCHOLOGICAL TESTING

Simple tests of intellectual function have been described in Chapter 1. Many methods for assessing intelligence and personality are available. Detailed consideration of these psychometric tests is beyond the scope of this volume, but they are widely used to assess objectively the mental changes which occur in organic neurological disease. The Wechsler-Bellevue series are particularly valuable in confirming the presence of early dementia and in assessing degrees of deterioration. A comparison of verbal and performance tests will sometimes reveal specific defects in the utilisation of language or in the execution of skilled motor activity which may not be immediately apparent on routine clinical examination. In neurological medicine these tests are most helpful in confirming objectively subjective impressions of early intellectual deterioration. Other tests designed for the assessment of personality rather than intellect, such as the Rorschach ink-blot test, have more application to psychiatry than to neurology.

REFERENCES

Bradley W G 1974 Disorders of peripheral nerves. Blackwell, London
Dubowitz V, Brooke M 1988 Muscle biopsy: a practical approach, 2nd edn. Saunders, London
Fishman R A 1980 Cerebrospinal fluid in diseases of the nervous system. Saunders, Philadelphia
Kiloh L G, McComas A J, Osselton J W 1981 Clinical electroencephalography, 4th edn. Butterworth, London
Kimura J 1983 Electrodiagnosis in diseases of nerve and muscle. Davis, Philadelphia
Krayenbuhl H A, Yasargil M G 1972 Cerebral angiography, 3rd edn. Butterworth, London
Mayo Clinic 1981 Clinical examinations in neurology, 5th edn. Saunders, Philadelphia
Moseley I 1988 Magnetic resonance imaging in diseases of the nervous system. Blackwell, Oxford
Oldendorf W H 1980 The quest for an image of the brain. Raven Press, New York
Ramsey R C 1977 Computed tomography of the brain. Advanced exercises in diagnostic radiology, Vol 9. Saunders, Philadelphia
Rosenberg R N, Heinz R 1984 Neuroradiology. The clinical neurosciences, Vol 4. Churchill Livingstone, New York
Shapiro R 1975 Myelography, 3rd edn. Year Book Medical Publishers, Chicago
Walton J N 1985 Brain's diseases of the nervous system, 9th edn. Oxford University Press, Oxford
Walton J N (ed) 1988 Disorders of voluntary muscle, 5th edn. Churchill Livingstone, Edinburgh
Weisberg L A, Nice C, Katz M 1978 Cerebral computed tomography. Saunders, Philadelphia
Wood J H (ed) 1980 Neurobiology of the cerebrospinal fluid. Plenum Press, New York

4. Pain

Pain is one of the most common and disturbing of human experiences. While it has many causes, the appreciation of painful sensations depends upon the stimulation of pain-sensitive nerve endings in the skin muscles, skeleton, blood vessels, viscera and membranes, and upon the conduction of nerve impulses into the central nervous system where the sensation enters consciousness. The central pathways along which impulses conveying painful sensations travel and the effects of disease of the central nervous system upon its appreciation will be considered in Chapter 10. In this chapter some common neurological syndromes of which pain is a prominent symptom are mentioned, with particular reference to its pathophysiology. Some general principles relating to methods of relieving pain are also described.

Individuals vary widely in their response to painful experiences, some remaining relatively impassive when experiencing sensations which produce in others an intense reaction. This individuality in emotional responses to painful stimuli means that although the threshold stimulus intensity required to produce pain (the pain threshold) is relatively constant, the reaction to painful stimuli which exceed this threshold intensity may be specific to the individual and can even vary in the same patient, depending upon circumstances.

RECEPTORS

Types of sensory receptor are described in Chapter 10. It is now known that while individual cutaneous sensory receptors are most sensitive to a particular form of natural stimulation, this specificity is not absolute and other types of stimuli may also excite the endings concerned (Iggo 1985). Those responsive to painful stimuli are called nociceptors; they are excited by higher intensity, potentially damaging stimuli.

Nociceptors, which are innervated either by small myelinated ($A\delta$) or non-myelinated (C) afferent fibres, have small receptive fields. Some are mechanical and are excited by very firm pressure or by penetrating the skin with a sharp object; those responsible for pain sensation are often called fine C-terminals. Others are thermal or mechanothermal receptors, innervated by C-fibres; they can be excited by severe mechanical stimuli but are principally responsive to high skin temperatures (i.e: 42°C or above), well above the normal threshold (about 40°C) that stimulates warm thermoreceptors. Algogenic chemicals such as bradykinin, 5-HT and prostaglandins E_1 and E_2 produced in the skin during inflammation either excite or enhance the excitability of C-nociceptors.

PAINFUL SENSATIONS: THEIR RECORDING AND MODULATION

As mentioned above, painful stimuli applied to the skin stimulate specific nociceptors, which respond to stimuli of such intensity that they 'threaten to damage the skin' (Iggo 1985), just as thermoreceptors respond to warm and cold stimuli. Painful sensations are then conveyed by $A\delta$ or C fibres to the posterior horn of grey matter to synapse with interneurones. In the so-called **gate theory** of Melzack & Wall (Figs. 4.1 and 4.2) it was proposed that interneurones in the substantia gelatinosa of the spinal cord exercise a modulating effect upon sensory input before this activates the first central transmission (T) cells in the dorsal horn of the cord which in turn stimulate central mechanisms responsible for response and perception. Tonic activity in small C fibres is thought to keep open the 'gate' and allows the onward transmission of painful sensation. Activity in large A fibres, by contrast, is essentially inhibitory and tends to close the 'gate'. The final discharge from the T cells and the perception of pain is thus dependent upon the relative activity in large and small fibres. Counter-irritation, as by scratching or rubbing, increases large fibre discharge and so reduces pain.

Wall (1985) has suggested that in future we shall need to modify the classical view that nerve impulses which signify the presence of injury are reliably transmitted by specified and automatic relay cells. He suggests that at least four different modifying mechanisms may generate chronic and intractable pains, as follows:

1. With a latency of milliseconds, combinations of afferent signals and of descending controls operate a rapid and powerful gate control.

2. With a latency of minutes, impulses in C fibres change the excitability of peripheral endings and of spinal cord circuits.

3. With a latency of days, chemical transport in C fibres from areas of damage further modifies cord connectivity with the disappearance of inhibitors and an expansion of receptive fields.

4. With a latency of weeks or months, anatomical degeneration produces secondary changes in deafferented cells with atrophy, but also sprouting and abnormal firing patterns.

On the basis of this theory, so-called **hyperalgesia**, better called **hyperpathia**, can be explained by an excessive continuing stimulation of C fibres, keeping the gate open, or by a selective loss of A fibres, reducing inhibition. Similarly, the phenomenon of referred pain (see below) can be explained by central summation effects, as there is a widespread, diffuse monosynaptic input to the T cells, often from relatively distant efferents. (**Hypalgesia** is the term used to imply diminished pain sensation.)

The role of the cerebral cortex in the perception and localisation of pain remains to be considered. Cortical lesions which impair the ability to localise touch sensation similarly disrupt the faculty of localising painful stimuli. There are few cortical neurones which show any selective response to painful stimuli. Electrical stimulation of the sensory cortex fails to evoke painful sensations, though similar stimulation of cells in the posterior thalamus and intralaminar reticular substance may do so. The receptive fields of the latter cells are immense and would appear to be incapable of recording spatial information, even though it seems that the perception of pain occurs at this level. It is probable that the localisation of painful stimuli recorded by nociceptors with high stimulus thresholds depends upon the simultaneous activation of other contiguous receptors of lower threshold which, with their central pathways, have precise localising capabilities. In other words the ability to localise painful sensations appears to depend, at least in part, upon the fact that nociceptive stimuli such as pain invariably stimulate other nearby receptors concerned with touch. It is now thought, in addition, that the simultaneous stimulation of mechanoreceptors by noxious stimuli plays a part in pain localisation. These views receive support from clinical evidence which shows that patients with lesions of the lemniscal system do not localise pain well.

SOME RECENT DEVELOPMENTS IN THE NEUROPHARMACOLOGY OF PAIN

Many neurones concerned with pain perception possess morphine (or other opiate) receptors with which mor-

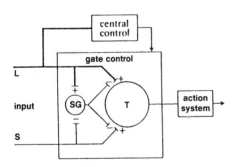

Fig. 4.1   Schematic diagram of the gate-control theory of pain (Mark I). L, the large-diameter fibres; S, the small-diameter fibres. The fibres project to the substantia gelatinosa (SG) and first central transmission (T) cells. The inhibitory effect exerted by SG on the afferent fibre terminals is increased by activity in L fibres and decreased by activity in S fibres. The central control trigger is represented by a line running from the large-fibre system to the central control mechanisms; these mechanisms, in turn, project back to the gate-control system. The T cells project to the action system. +, excitation; −, inhibition. (Reproduced with permission from Melzack & Wall 1965)

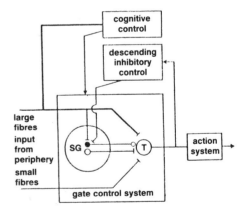

Fig. 4.2   The gate-control theory (Mark II). The new model includes excitatory (white circle) and inhibitory (black circle) links from the substantia gelatinosa (SG) to the transmission (T) cells as well as descending inhibitory control from brain stem systems. The round knobs at the end of the inhibitory link implies that its actions may be presynaptic, postsynaptic, or both. All connections are excitatory, except the inhibitory link from SG to T cell. Reproduced with permission from Melzack & Wall 1982)

phine and its analogues combine to produce their analgesic effects. The cells of the periaqueductal grey matter of the brain stem seem to possess many such receptors, and it is believed that this area is a principal site of action of such analgesic drugs. It is thought that the action of morphine upon neurones in this region produces analgesia by activating a descending serotoninergic system which inhibits the transmission of pain sensation in the spinal cord, but the exact mechanism of this action is still poorly understood. The brain produces its own endogenous analgesic in the form of a pentapeptide called encephalin, which has an action similar to morphine. The naturally-occurring C-fragment of β-lipotropin (also called β-endorphin) contains the encephalin sequence and has been isolated from the pituitary. It has been shown to have a particularly powerful analgesic effect when administered intraventricularly in animals. The part played by encephalin and by the endogenous ligands which are formed when it is combined with various cerebral lipoproteins in those disorders of the central nervous system that produce abnormalities of pain perception remains to be clarified. However, it is now known that one important action of encephalin is to inhibit the release of substance P, which is believed to be a neurotransmitter/neuromodulator of nociceptive primary afferent neurones. In the dorsal spinal cord encephalin-containing interneurones make axo–axonic synapses with the central projections (laminae I and outer II) of these primary afferent neurones. Encephalin released from these interneurones inhibits the release of substance P from the primary afferents by presynaptic inhibition.

TYPES OF PAIN AND THEIR CAUSATION

Analysis of the pain which follows cutaneous stimulation has shown that it has two components, the first immediate and the second delayed. These two forms of the sensation are probably conveyed by nerve fibres which conduct at different rates. A sensation of deep pain is also experienced after stimulation of deeper structures such as tendons, blood vessels and the periosteum. Painful lesions of the muscles or viscera sometimes give pain in the overlying skin, or else this symptom can be experienced in a cutaneous area which is comparatively remote (referred pain). Such painful sensations are felt as if they were coming not from the viscus involved but from the body surface. This apparent error in localisation is systematic and not random, as the reference is always to the dermatomes innervated by the same dorsal roots that supply the diseased viscus. Afferent pain fibres from the myocardium enter the T1–T5 dorsal root ganglia, and myocardial pain is therefore referred to the anterior chest wall and down the inner aspect of the left or of both arms. Similarly, pain fibres from the diaphragm travel in the

phrenic nerve (C3–C4) so that diaphragmatic pain is often referred to the C3 and C4 dermatomes in the neck and shoulder.

Many different types of lesion or pathological process can give rise to pain, through stimulation of pain-sensitive nerve endings in the diseased organ or organs. Trauma and inflammation are two of the most important causes of cutaneous pain, while pain of skeletal origin is often similarly produced. Malignant disease, including metastases in bone, can also be very painful. Visceral pain, particularly that arising in the abdominal organs, most often results from excessive contraction of smooth muscle, giving rise to the passage of pain-carrying impulses along afferent fibres accompanying sympathetic nerves. Distension of hollow organs or inflammation of their enveloping membranes (such as the peritoneum) can also be painful. In the latter case the impulses are carried by somatic afferents. Pain arising in skeletal muscle is commonly due to prolonged overactivity, cramp or fatigue, though repeated activity of a muscle with an inadequate blood supply (ischaemic work) can also be responsible. This principle applies also to cardiac muscle (angina of effort).

The sensory nerve fibres and central structures concerned in the reception and appreciation of painful stimuli are themselves sensitive to inflammation or irritation. There are a number of other pain-sensitive structures within the cranium and spinal canal. Pain is thus a relatively common symptom of disease of the nervous system.

THE RELIEF OF PAIN

Pain is a common symptom of nervous disease, and the doctor is often called upon to choose an appropriate remedy for its relief. Much depends upon its severity, its situation and its cause. Musculoskeletal pain which is relatively mild and not due to serious organic disease can be relieved by the local application of heat, or by immobilisation, while relief of tension headache is most often achieved not with analgesic drugs but with sedatives given to relieve emotional stress. Indeed there is evidence that tricyclic antidepressant drugs and/or tranquillisers, such as the phenothiazines, may themselves possess some analgesic properties. Certainly they have an adjuvant effect when given along with analgesic remedies, through relief of the overlay of tension, depression and anxiety which so often accompanies persistent pain.

Drug treatment

Generally, however, if the cause of the pain cannot be eliminated immediately, analgesic remedies are indicated in order to produce symptomatic relief. A detailed commentary upon the very large number of analgesic drugs now available would be out of place in a textbook of neurology; methods of treatment have been comprehensively reviewed by Bonica (1986). Broadly, the drugs available are classified into the non-narcotic and narcotic groups. The efficacy of aspirin and other non-narcotic remedies in relieving headache, arthritis or muscular pain and mild to moderate pain caused by other conditions has been appreciated for nearly a century. Aspirin remains one of the best analgesic drugs but must be avoided in childhood because of the risk of precipitating Reye's syndrome and hence, in the young, paracetamol is to be preferred. Many other non-steroidal anti-inflammatory agents (NSAIDs), which are also useful analgesics, are now available and, like aspirin, generally act by inhibiting the synthesis of prostaglandins, which are pain-producing substances synthesised in injured or inflamed tissue and which sensitise nociceptors. NSAIDs also potentiate the effect of narcotic drugs and are often given in combination with codeine in order to relieve moderate pain or along with morphine or other potent narcotics for the relief of severe pain.

Of the narcotic remedies, morphine remains the best, and has long been accepted as the standard of reference against which all other narcotics are compared. Given by month or by injection, it produces pain relief for 3–5 hours. About 20–25 narcotic drugs are currently in use, some being semi-synthetic derivatives of morphine, others wholly synthetic compounds. Generally all of these remedies produce similar side-effects (sedation, confusion, nausea and vomiting, constipation and depressed respiration) but the existence of so many different narcotic drugs available for pain relief is justified by the fact that some patients appear more prone to side-effects with some such remedies than are others.

All of the more powerful analgesics are drugs of addiction and should therefore be used sparingly. These powerful remedies are nevertheless appropriate when pain is either post-operative or the result of injury from which rapid recovery is expected or when it is due to a self-limiting illness in which analgesics are only required for a few days or at the most a few weeks. The fear of tolerance, physical dependence and of addiction has meant that some doctors and nurses have prescribed narcotic remedies in inadequate doses and many patients have similarly feared to take adequate doses, when prescribed, for similar reasons. There is no excuse for giving too little of these remedies in acute self-limiting conditions, as physical dependence does not develop in less than several weeks of continuous administration in high dosage, while true addiction may take much longer. And in patients with fatal, painful disorders such as terminal malignant disease, these risks can generally be ignored. Neverthe-

less, the guiding principle must be to give the minimum dose necessary to achieve adequate pain relief as often, and for as long, as may be needed. When the duration of the illness is likely to be measured in months, it is unwise to begin treatment with these remedies, unless the patient's expectation of life is short, either because of the nature of the disease, or on account of his age. In younger patients suffering chronic pain, it is important to persist with less powerful analgesics or to employ physical or surgical methods for its relief, for the patient may readily become addicted to the more powerful remedies.

As mentioned above, there are many adjuvant remedies which help in pain relief. These include the antidepressants which, as well as counteracting depression, decrease insomnia; phenothiazines and other tranquillisers which relieve tension and anxiety and have a muscle relaxant effect; antihistamines which potentiate the effect of narcotics; anticonvulsants which are particularly valuable in treating trigeminal and some other varieties of neuralgia; and corticosteroids, which are potent anti-inflammatory remedies and which also, for example, diminish cerebral oedema, thus relieving the headache of increased intracranial pressure.

Physical methods

Some traditional techniques of relieving pain may still have a useful role. Thus rest, temporary immobilisation and the application of local heat are often helpful in musculoskeletal pain, while manipulation of stiff, painful joints, or of the spinal column after, say, intervertebral disc prolapse is valuable in certain cases; and local corticosteroid injections are still invaluable in the treatment of 'frozen' shoulder or tennis elbow, to quote but two examples. Repeated percussion with a rubber mallet of painful neurones in an amputation stump may still help to relieve intractable phantom limb pain, but the use of electrical vibrators or of cooling ethyl chloride sprays in, for example, the treatment of post-herpetic neuralgia has now been largely supplanted by newer methods such as transcutaneous electrical nerve stimulation (TENS), a technique which has been found to give short-term relief in 70–80% of patients with localised pain and long-term relief in 15–30% (Bonica 1986). Acupuncture and electroacupuncture are thought to work similarly by 'closing the gate' in the posterior horn of grey matter or by activating supraspinal descending inhibitory systems.

In more severe and intractable cases dorsal column stimulation, using an electrode implanted surgically over the posterior column of the spinal cord or via a needle inserted into the epidural space, has been found to be helpful; even more effective in appropriate cases, but necessitating highly skilled surgical technique, is stimulation via an electrode implanted stereotactically into the thalamus or hypothalamus or into the peri aqueductal or periventricular grey matter in a patient under local anaesthesia.

Regional analgesia with injected local anaesthetic agents is also of benefit in some patients with localised pain, and repeated injections sometimes give relief for far longer than the local anaesthetic agent can have been presumed to last. Epidural anaesthesia is one such technique which, if repeated on several occasions, sometimes gives longer and longer relief after each so-called 'block' with ultimately long-lasting relief presumed to be due to the cessation of self-sustaining activity in various neuronal loops in the neuraxis, which is thought to be associated with some chronic pain states. The injection into the spinal subarachnoid or epidural space of narcotic agents has also been shown to relieve pain for 16–24 hours, and repeated injections delivered through a narrow indwelling catheter have also been used.

Regional neurolysis using alcohol (which destroys both motor and sensory nerves) or phenol (which has a more selective effect upon sensory fibres carrying nociceptive impulses) has also been widely used either for direct injection into appropriate cranial or peripheral nerves or through subarachnoid injection in order to destroy selectively appropriate spinal sensory roots or spinal nerves. The latter technique is still widely employed but carries a significant risk of complications, including sphincter dysfunction when lumbosacral injections are used. Some workers use thermocoagulation or alternatively freezing (cryotherapy) to produce similar effects, especially in procedures on the Gasserian ganglion in the treatment of trigeminal neuralgia. Recently neuroadenolysis of the pituitary gland, involving the injection of alcohol into the sella turcica via a needle introduced via the nose and the sphenoid sinus, has been shown to be effective in relieving severe and diffuse pain due to malignant disease, but the risk of complications such as cerebro-spinal fluid rhinorrhoea and diabetes insipidus is not insubstantial, depending upon the skill and experience of the operator.

A variety of psychological techniques including relaxation training, biofeedback, operant conditioning and hypnosis have also been used by pain therapists but their effect is greatest in patients with so-called 'learned pain behaviour', i. e. in those whose pain is largely or wholly psychologically determined, and in pain of physical origin the benefit of these methods is less obvious and largely adjuvant to other established techniques.

In the last resort, operative division of nerves, sensory roots or central pain pathways may have to be employed. The techniques available include sympathectomy (for causalgia), neurectomy (of individual sensory nerves), spinal dorsal rhizotomy (which has the unfortunate side-effect of deafferentation of the part of the body concerned, a problem only partially overcome by the use of selective nerve fibre division), cranial sensory rhizotomy, percutaneous differential thermal rhizotomy, spinothalamic tractotomy, percutaneous cervical cordotomy, cranial stereotactic surgery and even psychosurgery (which does not relieve pain but renders it more bearable by lessening the patient's concern and his emotional reaction to it). The choice of the appropriate method(s) to be employed in any patient whose chronic pain is not relieved by less destructive techniques is a matter for the expert and has fully justified the establishment of specialised 'pain clinics' in most major hospitals.

HEADACHE

Headache is produced by the stimulation of pain-sensitive structures within the cranium or in the extracranial tissues of the head and neck. Sensitive extracranial structures include the occipital, temporal and frontal muscles, the skin of the scalp, the arteries which traverse the subcutaneous tissue, and the periosteum. The cranial bones themselves are insensitive. Within the skull the sensitive areas are the meninges, particularly the basal dura mater and that forming the walls of the venous sinuses, as well as the large arteries at the base of the brain which form the circle of Willis and its branches. Most of the cerebral substance itself is insensitive to stimuli which are painful if applied to appropriate receptors.

One of the commonest causes of **headache of extracranial origin** is tension. **Tension headaches** are typically occipital, but sometimes frontal, in situation, and result from continuous partial contraction of muscles attached to the scalp. Usually these headaches come on towards evening when the patient is tired; the posterior neck muscles are often tender and the pain may be relieved by rest if the patient can be taught to relax properly. The headaches of so-called **eye-strain** are probably similar in aetiology; if an uncorrected visual refractive error is present, then the continuous effort required to compensate for this defect also causes tension, producing headaches which are relieved by appropriate spectacles. Headache of purely **psychogenic origin**, of the type which occurs in neurotic, hypochondriacal or hysterical individuals, is often vertical in situation and is typically described in over-elaborate terms, perhaps in order to impress; a common example is to say that the top of the head feels as if it were being lifted off. Often such patients also experience true tension headaches towards the end of the day. Headaches described as being like 'a sense of pressure' or like 'a tight constricting band' are usually of this type and many depressed patients complain of headaches occurring in the mornings when depression is often at its worst.

Disorders of the **extracranial arteries** can also give rise to headache and indeed the symptoms of migraine, which will be discussed below, may be attributed in part to alterations in calibre occurring in the branches of the external carotid artery. Other 'vascular' headaches, such as that of a 'hangover', or of hypertension, can probably be attributed at least partly to dilatation of extracranial rather than intracranial arteries. The pain of temporal or cranial arteritis is also extracranial in origin, being due to inflammatory changes in the temporal arteries. Other causes of extracranial headache are **paranasal sinusitis** and **middle-ear disease** in which the pain results either from the increasing tension of pus in a confined space or from spread of inflammation to the bone and its coverings.

Headache of intracranial origin is due to inflammation, compression, and distortion of or traction upon the pain-sensitive meninges and blood vessels within the skull. Such headaches are usually felt in the frontal or occipital regions or both, though a unilateral lesion sometimes produces a unilateral headache, say, in one or other temple. When this is the case it can be assumed with reasonable confidence that the lesion concerned lies upon the same side of the head as that upon which the headache is felt.

The headache of **diffuse meningeal inflammation**, as in meningitis, subarachnoid haemorrhage and following pneumoencephalography, is generally severe, continuous and unvarying and associated with neck stiffness. Like that of **increased intracranial pressure**, whether resulting from a single space-occupying lesion or from diffuse brain swelling or hydrocephalus, it is typically made worse by sudden movements of the head, by stooping, or by coughing and straining. Each of these increases the distortion of pain-sensitive structures already present, either through movement, or through a sudden brief increase in intracranial pressure produced by delaying the outflow of venous blood from the cranium. Typically this type of headache is throbbing in nature, probably due to the transmission of arterial pulsation to tissues already under increased tension. It is often present on waking but tends to improve as the day wears on. If a cerebral abscess or tumour is the cause, then vomiting and papilloedema may also occur.

A headache similar in character to that described above is due to a similar mechanism in cases of **reduced intracranial pressure**, in which there is again traction upon pain-sensitive arteries and meninges. This is the basis of the **post-lumbar puncture headache** which is presumed to be due to continued leakage of CSF through the hole in the spinal dura left by the exploring needle. The headache of dehydration has a similar cause and it

was once thought that a clinical syndrome of **intracranial hypotension**, characterised by this type of headache, occurs spontaneously; this now seems very improbable and the pressure in the spinal theca on lumbar puncture may be low in healthy patients who make no complaint of headache. Dehydration caused by the diuretic effect of alcohol probably contributes to the 'hangover' headache. A benign syndrome of '**cough headache**' does however occur in which severe headache, typically of 'intracranial' type, accompanies coughing. While some such patients have emphysema and are presumed to have an unusually large increase in intracranial pressure during coughing owing to delayed venous return to the heart, others have no evidence of severe chest disease and in them the aetiology of the syndrome is obscure. While the possibility of intracranial tumour should always be considered in such patients, many cases of this type carry an excellent prognosis, though little can be done to relieve this symptom except to advise avoidance of the circumstances which induce coughing.

Migraine (see below) is believed to be the most typical variety of **vascular headache** but severe throbbing headache (other than that of raised intracranial pressure) can be a feature not only of subarachnoid haemorrhage but also of malignant hypertension. Headache of similar nature can also complicate uraemia, may follow general anaesthesia or severe infections and is also experienced by patients with chronic CO_2 intoxication (as in alveolar hypoventilation) or mountain sickness. Sudden prostrating headache mimicking subarachnoid haemorrhage has been well described in patients taking monoamine-oxidase inhibitors on eating cheese or drinking red wine and has been attributed to nitrite in frankfurter sausages. Syndromes of 'benign coital cephalalgia', prevented by propranolol, and of 'benign exertional headache', controlled by indomethacin, have also been described. All vascular headaches can be accentuated or precipitated by alcohol.

Migraine

Migraine is one of the commonest neurological disorders and may also be one of the most disabling. It occurs in both sexes, but is more common in women, and generally begins in adolescence or early adult life, often in patients who have had bilious attacks in childhood. Rarely migrainous headaches begin first at the time of the menopause, usually in hypertensive women, and attacks are particularly liable to occur during or just before the menstrual periods. Often there is a strong family history of the condition, while it has been thought, probably erroneously, to occur most often in the more intelligent and industrious, though intense and obsessional, members of the community. Attacks of migraine tend to be more frequent during or after episodes of emotional stress.

Migraine has been defined as a paroxysmal unilateral headache, preceded by visual and sensory phenomena and accompanied or followed by nausea and vomiting. While this description fits a 'typical' case, there are many patients with undoubted migraine in whom no visual or sensory aura is ever experienced and in whom the headache is never one-sided. Its paroxysmal occurrence is its most important feature. Some patients experience an aura alone, without subsequent headache but with vague malaise only, in some attacks.

The pathophysiology of the migrainous headache was, until recently, thought to be well understood. The initial disturbance is believed to be one of vasospasm in the extra- and intra-cranial arteries and their branches, often on one side of the head, and this is followed some 10 to 30 minutes later by a dilatation of the same vessels. The arterial constriction is responsible for the symptoms of the aura, the dilatation for the headache. The aetiology of these alterations in vascular tone, however, remains obscure. It is also puzzling that the aura may sometimes persist when the headache is severe; that the aura may suggest ischaemia of one cerebral hemisphere with the headache occurring over the contralateral hemisphere; and that cerebral blood flow may be generally rather than focally diminished in an attack. A possible association with Leao's 'spreading depression' which can be recorded in the electroencephalogram has been postulated. Allergy to chocolate and other foodstuffs has been well documented in a minority of patients. There is evidence of excessive fluid retention in the body before each attack, followed by a subsequent diuresis, a finding which has suggested a metabolic or endocrine cause. Biochemical studies have revealed an increased urinary excretion of 5-hydroxindolacetic acid (5-HIAA) during attacks, suggesting an intermittent release of 5-hydroxytryptamine (serotonin) into the circulation. A disorder of the blood-brain barrier rendering the cerebral circulation vulnerable to the effects of circulating vasoactive substances such as substance P and serotonin has also been suggested. Paroxysmal headaches of migrainous type may be prominent in patients harbouring intracranial arteriovenous angiomas or even aneurysms, but in these individuals the headache is usually strictly unilateral, occurring on the same side of the head as the vascular anomaly; the reason for this association is not known.

Usually the migrainous attack begins soon after waking. A visual aura is the most common, resulting from spasm of the retinal arteries or of branches of the posterior cerebral artery supplying one or both occipital lobes. The patient then experiences either a hemianopic field defect, a less well-defined scotoma or rarely transient blindness, jagged lines ('fortification spectra'), or bright dancing or shimmering lights (teichopsia) in one half-field. Alternatively a sensory aura, with paraesthesiae (tingling, numbness and pins and needles) in the corner of the mouth and in the arm, or less commonly in the leg on the same side, may occur, presumably due to spasm of those branches of the middle cerebral artery which supply the sensory cortex. In a few patients the aura (vertigo, diplopia, bilateral paraesthesiae, often around the lips) suggests that the hind-brain rather than the fore-brain circulation is involved (basilar artery migraine) and sometimes fainting occurs—either during the aura or at the height of the headache. Attacks of epilepsy occur in sufferers from migraine slightly more often than can be accounted for by chance. Rarely there is actual transient weakness of one arm and leg (hemiplegic migraine) or paresis, of one oculomotor nerve (ophthalmoplegic migraine); however, some patients with the latter condition have an aneurysm of the internal carotid artery compressing the nerve trunk within the cranium. Exceptonally, hemianopia, hemiparesis, ophthalmoplegia or other neurological signs can persist as permanent sequelae of a severe attack due to cerebral infarction (so-called 'complicated migraine'). Hemiplegic migraine is commonly familial, with recovery from the unilateral paresis following each attack in the affected family members.

As the aura passes off the headache usually begins and mounts in intensity; why some patients experience an aura after the headache has developed is difficult to explain. The headache can be unilateral and frontal (above one or other eye), bifrontal, bioccipital, or generalised. Sometimes it is comparatively mild, though accompanied by lassitude and depression, but more often it is prostrating, and there is photophobia, so that the patient must lie down in a darkened room. Typically the headache lasts all day, passing off after a night's sleep, but sometimes it wanes in an hour or two. Alternatively, it may persist, though with diminishing intensity, for a few days or even for as long as a week. Characteristically it is accompanied by nausea, sometimes by vomiting and occasionally by retching. There are some individuals who never have an aura, and others who occasionally have it without headache; indeed numerous variants occur. 'Bilious attacks' in childhood are almost certainly migrainous, while some believe that the same is true of recurrent abdominal pain or cyclical vomiting in children and adolescents.

Attacks of migraine can be mild and infrequent, occurring once every few months and having only a nuisance value, but in other cases they are severe and prostrating, occurring every few days, and causing serious disability. A temporary exacerbation with frequent attacks often accompanies a paramenopausal depressive illness.

The **treatment of migraine** falls clearly into three categories, prevention, treatment of the attack and prophylaxis.

Prevention through the avoidance of aggravating or precipitating factors can be very effective and is to be preferred to drug therapy whenever possible. Many patients can identify a single factor which may precipitate attacks but are often puzzled by the fact that it does not always do so. This is probably because more than one factor is required and they are only able to identify one of these. The commonest cause of an increase in the frequency or severity of migraine attacks in young women is use of the combined contraceptive pill. This is not necessarily contraindicated in migraine unless the patient has a fixed aura, in which case there is a real risk of permanent neurological sequelae arising due to infarction. The progesterone-only pill does not seem to be associated with this problem. In middle-aged men the commonest cause is the development of hypertension. The menopause is frequently associated with a change in the pattern of migraine, sometimes aggravating the condition; less often there is a marked improvement. The form which first develops in post-menopausal women may be particularly intractable. Unfortunately aggravation does not respond to hormonal treatment. Some patients can identify specific factors which will precipitate an attack; these include certain food substances, particularly cheese, chocolate, eggs, liver, cured meat, pickled herring, and citrus fruits as well as alcohol. Bright or flickering lights precipitate migraine in a few patients but this is not usually a consistent factor. Some patients only have their migraine attacks at weekends, either because of relief of stress or because they stay in bed much later at weekends than during the week. Many of these precipitants are easily dealt with and it is well worth making enquiries about the circumstances of a patient's migraine in order to try to avoid situations in which an attack is likely to occur.

Treatment of the acute attack is often disappointing unless the treatment can be taken very early. Patients who wake with an attack often find treatment ineffective for this reason. Simple treatment includes soluble aspirin, preferably taken with 10 mg of metaclopramide as the absorption of aspirin is shown to be markedly impaired during an attack; metaclopramide results in normal or even rapid absorption of aspirin and indeed of other medications since the failure of absorption seems to be related to gastric stasis. Ergotamine tartrate can be extremely effective in some patients if taken early enough, but in others it seems to make the nausea and vomiting worse. Ergotamine is available in sublingual preparations, it can be swallowed, there are aerosol preparations for inhalation which result in very rapid absorption and it is also available by suppository which is particularly suitable for patients who vomit repeatedly. It is often useful to combine the ergotamine with an antiemetic such as prochlorperazine which may be taken by mouth or by suppository or given by injection. In the occasional patient who has very severe attacks but at long intervals, a single large dose of a tranquilliser such as diazepam may help the patient to sleep off the attack.

Prophylaxis is probably the most effective treatment and is indicated in all patients who have frequent attacks. Most of the effective drugs work by modifying vascular reactivity. Very small doses of **clonidine** (0.05 mg t.d.s.) can provide very effective prophylaxis in some patients; the drug seems to act by modifying the reactivity of vascular smooth muscle. **Beta-adrenergic blockade** with propranolol or metoprolol can also be very effective, but must not be used in patients who also have asthma. **Tricyclic antidepressant drugs** have an effect on migraine which cannot be entirely explained by their antidepressant effect, though this can be extremely useful in patients in whom anxiety and depression are major aggravating factors, especially at about the time of the menopause. Often quite small doses can be effective and it is worth starting with small doses of dothiepin or amitriptyline and increasing the dose as appropriate since some patients are intolerant of these drugs. The **serotonin antagonist** methysergide is extremely effective in migraine, but the risk of pericardial and retroperitoneal fibrosis has meant that it is now restricted to only the most severe and intractable patients. These risks are minimised if the dose is kept below 3 mg a day for no more than 6 months at a time. Another antagonist, pizotifen, is also very effective and needs to be given in a dose of 3 mg a day for more than 3 weeks to produce its full effect. Weight gain due to appetite stimulation can be a problem in some patients. **Non-steroidal anti-inflammatory drugs** may also be effective in some patients with migraine, probably through the inhibition of prostaglandins. Naprosyn has been shown to be effective. A number of **calcium channel blockers** have been developed in recent years and some of these seem to have a beneficial effect on migraine, whereas others actually cause headache. It is likely that newer preparations and further clinical trials will define the role of this group of drugs in the management of migraine.

The most important point to recognise in prophylactic treatment is that it is impossible to predict the response in any individual case. Patient trial and error using the many alternative remedies mentioned above often pays dividends.

Periodic migrainous neuralgia (cluster headache)

In this condition, episodes of severe and continuous pain occur, often intensely burning or boring in character, in, around or behind one eye or in the cheek, forehead and temple. These attacks occur in bouts lasting a few weeks or months and during a bout the patient suffers one or several attacks, lasting from 15 minutes to several hours, each day. Not uncommonly the attacks recur at the same time of day or night and may waken the patient from sleep. There is often suffusion of the conjunctiva and blocking of the nostril on the affected side during the attacks. The aetiology of this condition, which has been variously referred to as **histamine headache**, **ciliary neuralgia**, or **cluster headache**, is unknown, but it has some affinities with migraine and has been called periodic migrainous neuralgia. To avoid confusing the condition with migraine (as its management is different), the term 'cluster headache' is now generally preferred. Attacks can be precipitated by alcohol and other vaso-dilators.

Treatment with ergotamine tartrate preparations (see p. 56) given regularly two or three times daily once a bout begins has been shown to be effective in controlling the attacks. Dihydroergotamine (1–2 mg two or three times a day) has been, until recently, the most favoured remedy, with methysergide or pizotifen being used in intractable cases, and there is now increasing evidence that the prostaglandin inhibitor indomethacin (50–200 mg daily) is also worthy of a trial when other remedies are ineffective. However, it seems that the latter remedy is more effective in chronic paroxysmal hemi-crania (which resembles cluster headache but occurs mainly in women who experience about 15 short severe attacks daily and not usually at night) and in benign exertional headache (throbbing headache precipitated by exertion such as running and usually occurring in males). Treatment should be given regularly until the bout is over; this can only be assessed by gradually withdrawing the drug to see whether the attacks recur. If they do not, no further treatment is needed until the next bout begins. An interesting and important development has been the discovery that lithium salts, given in a sufficient dose (usually lithium carbonate 800 mg initially) to produce a blood level of 0.7–1.2 mmol/l, have a powerful and as yet unexplained prophylactic effect.

FACIAL PAIN

Pain in the face is a common symptom which presents formidable difficulties in understanding and interpreta-tion. Whereas it sometimes results from local causes such as maxillary sinusitis, neoplasia of the maxilla, mandible or soft tissues, caries, dental abscess, impacted wisdom teeth or parotitis, it can also be due to many pathological lesions involving the trigeminal nerve, its branches and central connexions. Thus a plaque of demyelination or a syrinx (cavity) in the brain stem can give a continuous

unilateral facial ache through irritation of the central connexions of the trigeminus, as may a tumour (acoustic neuroma, meningioma, nasopharyngeal carcinoma) or aneurysm which compresses the Gasserian ganglion or the intracranial portion of the fifth cranial nerve. Sim-ilarly, herpes zoster of this ganglion, which tends to affect particularly the ophthalmic division, gives severe and continuous pain in the eye and forehead. Even more frequent, however, are the syndromes of intermittent facial pain, including trigeminal neuralgia and atypical facial neuralgia. In differential diagnosis it is useful to note that pain provoked by hot or cold foods or liquids is almost invariably of dental origin, while that of paranasal sinusitis is often accentuated by stooping, coughing or exertion and there may be local tenderness over the affected sinus.

Trigeminal neuralgia (Tic douloureux)

Trigeminal neuralgia is an intermittent, brief, lancin-ating pain in the face, confined to the area innervated by one trigeminal nerve, and often evoked by facial move-ment or by touching the skin. It is slightly more common in females and is most often seen after middle-age, particularly in the elderly, though it rarely occurs in early adult life.

The aetiology of the 'idiopathic' form of the syndrome is still uncertain though the condition is sometimes a symptom of multiple sclerosis, resulting from a plaque of demyelination at the point of entry of the trigeminal root into the brain stem; rarely it is the first symptom of a posterior fossa tumour, such as an acoustic neuroma lying in one cerebello-pontine angle. In young and middle-aged patients it is particularly important to seek for such an underlying lesion using CT and, where possible, MRI scanning in order to discover whether or not an angle tumour or plaque of demyelination is present. Sometimes in such cases, alternatively or in addition, CSF examina-tion or CT cisternography may be wise. Its increasing incidence in the elderly gave rise to the suggestion that ischaemia of the trigeminal nerve or ganglion, resulting from atherosclerosis, might be the principal aetiological factor, but recent studies have strongly suggested that many, if not most, cases are due to compression or kinking of the sensory root due to an ectatic intracranial artery.

The pain of tic douloureux is typically sudden, excru-ciating and brief, 'like the stab of a red-hot needle'; a continuous pain in the face, or one lasting for several minutes, is not tic douloureux, though some patients have a background of dull aching between paroxysms. The pain does not extend outside the area supplied by the trigeminal nerve, nor does it cross the midline. It can occur in the distribution of any one or all of the divisions of the trigeminus; if the ophthalmic division alone is involved, it may be called **supraorbital neuralgia**. Its intensity can be judged from the apparently involuntary spasm of the facial muscles on the affected side and the agonised expression which accompany each attack. The patient often holds a hand in front of the face to protect it and will not allow it to be touched as he knows that movement, as in speaking, chewing, touching the face (especially so-called 'trigger zones' which vary from patient to patient), or in shaving or washing, may provoke an attack. Neurological examination is rarely informative, though slight objective diminution of sensory perception is very rarely found on the affected side of the face. A slightly atypical history, perhaps with lack of spontaneous remission, dull background pain or a slightly impaired corneal reflex on the affected side may suggest that the condition is symptomatic of an underlying organic lesion.

Characteristically, tic douloureux is a periodic disorder. It occurs in bouts lasting several weeks or months, during which the pain occurs with variable frequency and severity. Long remissions of weeks, months or even years separate the bouts but these remissions tend to become progressively shorter. The condition, though intensely distressing, is essentially benign, and does not shorten life, though a few patients are driven to suicide to find relief from their agony. Fortunately, the response to drug treatment is usually good. Carbamazepine (100–200 mg three or four times daily, depending upon the response and upon tolerance) is the most effective remedy, but baclofen (30–80 mg daily) is a useful alternative in some cases. In patients failing to respond it was usual to inject the Gasserian ganglion with alcohol or phenol or to use osmolytic neurolysis or radiofrequency coagulation of the ganglion, and these methods may still be useful in frail, elderly patients who show an inadequate response to drug treatment and who are judged unfit for major surgery. In other cases it was usual in the past to recommend partial or total surgical division of the sensory root via a middle fossa approach but exploration of the posterior fossa is now preferred as it is often possible to find an artery which is compressing the root, to dissect it free and to separate it from the root with gelfoam, thus avoiding the necessity of root section and the permanent facial sensory loss which inevitably follows the destructive operation.

Atypical facial neuralgia

Apart from the local causes of facial pain mentioned above, other painful syndromes of intermittent character can affect the face. One of these is migrainous neuralgia (cluster headache) which has already been considered.

Costen's syndrome is a condition in which a severe shooting pain radiates down the lower jaw or into the temple whenever the patient chews. It differs from trigeminal neuralgia in that chewing is the only 'trigger' which produces the pain, and touching the face, for instance, has no effect. It is due to dental malocclusion with arthrosis of the temporomandibular joint, resulting in compression of branches of the auriculotemporal nerve in the neighbourhood of the joint. The pain can be relieved by building up the 'bite'.

A common form of **atypical facial pain** is an intermittent but long-lasting pain of aching character which affects the cheek and upper jaw and occurs almost without exception in young and middle-aged women. In such a case it is wise to exclude dental sepsis, sinusitis and other organic lesions, but investigations are almost always negative. This type of pain, which often responds poorly to treatment, is generally believed to be a manifestation of psychiatric illness, particularly depression or anxiety. Unquestionably the pain is sometimes improved by psychotherapy, by tranquillisers and/or antidepressive drugs or even by electroconvulsion therapy, but in some patients it is intractable. This is one of the many varieties of psychogenic regional pain in which 'learned pain behaviour' (Tyrer 1986) plays an important part. Whereas in most cases there is positive evidence of psychiatric disturbance, the pathogenesis of this condition is poorly understood. Attempts made to relieve the pain by cervical immobilisation or by sectioning the greater auricular nerve have no rational basis, and this troublesome condition remains difficult to manage.

GLOSSOPHARYNGEAL NEURALGIA

This rare condition resembles trigeminal neuralgia as the pain occurs in periodic bouts and is brief and lancinating. It occurs in the tonsillar fossa, back of throat and larynx and may radiate to the ear on the affected side. Swallowing is the usual precipitant. Recent evidence suggests that in many cases, as in trigeminal neuralgia, the condition is due to compression or kinking of the glossopharyngeal nerve intracranially by an aberrant artery. While the drugs which work in trigeminal neuralgia (see above) may relieve this condition too, surgical exploration of the posterior fossa with release or division of the affected nerve is usually curative.

PAIN IN THE SPINAL COLUMN AND LIMBS

While many skeletal and ligamentous lesions produce pain in the spinal column, some lesions of the nervous system also cause spinal pain. Diffuse inflammatory conditions like ankylosing spondylitis, or metabolic disorders producing osteoporosis, may give dull aching pain involving the greater part of the spine, while osteomyelitis of a vertebral body or a metastasis in one or more vertebrae give severe and continuous pain localised to the affected area. As a secondary effect distortion and deformity of the bony architecture can occur, resulting in compression of the spinal cord (this is in general painless) or of spinal roots (giving pain in the distribution of the root concerned). Similarly, lesions of the spinal cord and its roots, whether intramedullary (e.g. multiple sclerosis, syringomyelia), intrathecal (meningioma, arachnoiditis) or extradural (prolapsed intervertebral disc) can irritate or compress sensory tracts or fibres or nerve roots, producing similar pain. And a neoplasm such as a neurofibroma which begins by producing pain due simply to compression of its parent spinal root, may later grow sufficiently large to erode the vertebral body, giving a dull continuous 'skeletal' type of pain in the affected spinal area. Furthermore root irritation often produces a 'protective' spasm of the overlying spinal muscles and this spasm may itself be painful, while the muscles concerned become tender. Voluntary contraction of these muscles will then increase the pain, as will nervous tension.

NERVE AND NERVE-ROOT COMPRESSION

When nerve fibres or trunks which transmit pain-carrying impulses are compressed or irritated, whether in the spinal cord, spinal roots or peripheral nerves, an unpleasant continuous, burning pain, often accompanied by painful spontaneous sensations (dysaesthesiae), is produced. If fibres concerned with touch and proprioception run in the same nerve, then associated paraesthesiae (tingling, numbness, pins and needles) also occur. Some of these features are due to direct nerve irritation, others to ischaemia. Paradoxically, vasodilatation due to warmth can so increase the volume of the nerve being compressed that its blood supply is further reduced and the pain is made worse, while vasoconstriction due to cold will also increase ischaemia and the symptoms. Pain due to compression of a peripheral nerve is referred to the skin area from which it receives sensory fibres. Similarly, root pain radiates throughout the dermatome of the root concerned, but deep muscular pain due to the same cause may be more widepread, corresponding broadly to the muscles supplied by the homologous motor root. Root pain has other special characteristics; thus it is affected by sudden spinal movements which would be likely to displace the root or the lesion which is compressing it. Similarly a sudden increase in CSF pressure, as in coughing or straining, will cause a sharp, shooting paroxysm of pain in the appropriate distribution. When

such symptoms persist, the trunks of peripheral nerves which contribute to the sensory root or roots involved often become tender on pressure.

CAUSALGIA

Causalgia is a peculiarly unpleasant burning type of continuous pain which may foliow peripheral nerve injuries, or, much less often, root lesions, particularly those in which severance of a nerve has been incomplete and some regeneration has occurred. It is most common in the hand and arm but does occur occasionally in the leg; it is most frequent after median and ulnar nerve lesions. A very similar syndrome rarely follows local anaesthesia (especially mandibular block) given for dental treatment and has been called dental causalgia. The skin area in which spontaneous pain occurs is usually shiny and perspires excessively; the patient will not allow the skin to be touched as this greatly accentuates the pain. Although the exact mechanism of this syndrome is not fully understood autonomic pathways clearly play an important role, as blocking or section of somatic sensory nerves from the skin area concerned do not always relieve the pain, but sympathectomy is usually effective. Chemical sympathectomy produced by the injection of local anaesthetic into the stellate ganglion or by the intra-arterial injection of guanethidine is useful in determining whether surgical sympathectomy is likely to be effective.

PHANTOM-LIMB PAIN

After amputation of a limb (or removal of an ear or some other member) sensations may be experienced for several months or years suggesting that the part concerned is still in situ. Not infrequently, pain of a curiously unpleasant and intolerable nature, resembling causalgia in many respects, develops in the phantom member. Usually such patients are found to have plexiform neuromas in the amputation stump, resulting from regeneration of fibres from the severed ends of peripheral nerves, and digital compression of such a neuroma will reproduce the patient's spontaneous pain. Repeated percussion, injection of local anaesthetic agents, or finally, if all else fails, excision of the neuroma may relieve the pain.

POST-HERPETIC NEURALGIA

Pain in the distribution of the affected root, whether it be the ophthalmic division of the trigeminus, or a cervical, dorsal or lumbar posterior root, is a striking feature of herpes zoster. In younger patients the pain generally resolves within a few weeks, but in the elderly severe continuous pain may persist for years afterwards. The pain appears to depend upon the reception of sensory stimuli from the skin area concerned, as in the early stages it can sometimes be relieved by subcutaneous infiltration of local anaesthetic. However, relief is often only temporary and it seems that progressive central facilitation occurs in pain pathways with persistent opening of the 'gate' (see p. 49), for eventually the pain continues to occur apparently spontaneously, despite division of peripheral pathways. The pain can be so intolerable that some patients are driven to suicide. Eventually in most cases spontaneous improvement occurs, but nevertheless the condition is difficult to manage. Even powerful analgesics often seem only to blunt the pain; but physical methods (electrical vibration, cooling sprays, TENS) have been used with some success in order to close the 'gate'.

THALAMIC PAIN

Spinal cord lesions which affect the spinothalamic tracts sometimes produce pain in the limbs and this is often accompanied by burning dysaesthesiae and by sensations of either warmth or coldness. Similarly, a lesion of the thalamus itself (usually an infarct, rarely a tumour) can cause severe pain in the contralateral face, arm and leg. So-called thalamic pain is intense, burning and continuous in character and has other peculiarly unpleasant qualities, often described by the patient with such adjectives as 'tearing' or 'grinding'. Typically it is felt around the angle of the mouth and cheek and in the affected hand and foot. Pain of this type is fortunately rare as it is relatively unaffected by any but the most powerful analgesics. Neurosurgical measures occasionally utilised in such cases are mentioned above.

CONCLUSIONS

Headache and pain in the face, spine and limbs are among the most common symptoms of nervous disease. A rational approach to differential diagnosis and treatment depends upon a working knowledge of the anatomy of the sensory pathways and of the pathophysiology of pain. The patient must also be assessed as an individual so that the importance of emotional factors in the genesis of his symptoms, as well as the significance of his emotional reaction to the pain he is experiencing, may be taken into account.

REFERENCES

Baskin N H, Appenzeller O 1980 Headache. Major problems in internal medicine, Vol XIX (Smith L H Jr, series ed) Saunders, Philadelphia
Bonica J J 1986 Pain. In: Walton J, Beeson P B, Bodley Scott R (eds) Oxford Companion to medicine. Oxford University Press, Oxford
Dalessio D J (ed) 1980 Wolff's headache and other head pain, 4th edn. Oxford University Press, New York
Hopkins A 1987 Headache: problems in diagnosis and management. Major problems in neurology, Vol 15 (Walton J, series ed) Saunders, London
Iggo A 1985 Sensory receptors in the skin of mammals and their sensory functions. Revue Neurologique (Paris) 10: 599
Lance J W 1982 The mechanism and management of headache, 4th edn. Butterworth, London
Melzack R 1973 The puzzle of pain. Penguin Education, Harmondsworth
Melzack R, Wall P D 1965 Pain mechanisms: a new theory. Science 150: 971
Melzack R, Wall P D 1982 The challenge of pain. Penguin, Harmondsworth
Pawl R P 1979 Chronic pain primer. Year Book Publishers, Chicago
Peatfield R 1986 Headache. Clinical medicine and the nervous system, No 1 (Conomy J P, Swash M, series eds). Springer, Berlin
Tyrer S P 1986 Learned pain behaviour. British Medical Journal 292: 1
Wall P D 1985 Future trends in pain research. In: Iggo A, Iversen L L, Cervero F (eds) Nociception and pain. Philosophical Transactions of the Royal Society B3O8: 217
Walton J N 1987 Introduction to clinical neuroscience, 2nd edn. Baillière Tindall, London

5. Disorders of language and speech, apraxia and agnosia

To understand how speech and language are developed and controlled and how they may be disordered is difficult for many students. Even more difficult are the functions of praxis and gnosis, the first concerned with the performance of complex willed movements, the second with the recognition of sensory information (visual, auditory and tactile). Certainly the anatomical and physiological organisation of these functions is complex and not fully understood. And yet, an appreciation of some simple basic principles may bring clarity to this difficult field. First one must understand the way in which speech, language and other higher cerebral functions are acquired and developed before considering how they can be disordered by disease.

THE ORGANISATION OF SPEECH AND LANGUAGE

The young infant takes his first step towards the acquisition of language function when he begins to associate specific sounds with particular objects in his environment. These sounds are subsequently organised into words which are symbols used to identify the objects concerned. Nouns, therefore, are first acquired, and subsequently conceptual or abstract powers of thought are developed in the utilisation of adjectives, verbs and adverbs to qualify these nouns or to describe activities instead of things. As the psychological concept of a word symbol develops, so the proprioceptive sensory impulses derived from the muscles of articulation come to be unconsciously associated with the expression of the word concerned, so that the child learns that a group of movements of the larynx, palate, lips and tongue will result in the vocalisation of this word. Gradually, as additional words are acquired, these symbols lose some importance as individual entities but acquire new significance or meaning from their association with other words. In this way meaningful phrases and sentences are built up. When the child begins to read, visual symbols take their place alongside the appropriate sounds and, in writing these same symbols acquire new associations in proprioceptive sensations derived from the fingers of the writing hand. Words acquire new and abstract meanings and are utilised not only for the communication of thoughts to others, but also for so-called 'internal language' or the conscious logical process of abstract thought. Not all thought is verbal; some depends upon the construction of visual or auditory images within the mind, but the more complex problems are generally dealt with by the thinker in verbal form. The scientist or the musician may, by contrast, think in terms of mathematical or chemical formulae or of musical sounds, but these too are symbols, either auditory or visual, which are comparable to the written or spoken word. It is clear from the very large number of different languages in use throughout the world that the actual sound is unimportant; it is the learned association of a sound with a particular meaning that constitutes language, so that learning a foreign language entails learning new associations.

It follows that many sensory and motor activities are concerned in understanding and producing words, whether spoken or written. Thus in order to speak a sentence, the individual must first formulate the thought he wishes to express, then choose the appropriate words (a choice which depends upon his acquired knowledge of what these symbols mean), and then control the motor activity of the muscles of phonation and articulation. This process involves the reception and correlation of proprioceptive sensory impulses from the muscles concerned. If the message is to be written rather than spoken, motor and sensory impulses from the hand are also involved. Similarly, in understanding speech, whether spoken or written, the accurate reception of auditory or visual stimuli is essential before the symbols received can be interpreted. A simple schema outlining the anatomical areas and mechanisms concerned with the control of speech and language is given in Figure 5.1.

Language function is almost entirely lateralised to one hemisphere, usually called the dominant hemisphere.

This is the left hemisphere in practically all right-handed people, who constitute about 93% of the population. Of the remaining 7% who are left-handed, the left hemisphere remains dominant for language in more than 50%. Sensory information containing language can reach the left hemisphere from many sources, though spoken and written language are much the most common. It is possible to transmit language by other visual and auditory forms such as semaphore and morse code or by tactile stimulation as is used in reading braille. In whatever form language is communicated, it can only be interpreted in

Wernicke's area which is situated at the posterior end of the superior temporal gyrus and extends to part of the angular gyrus; it is virtually contiguous with the auditory cortex. A lesion in this area affects the patient's ability to attach a meaning to any form of language input and this is known as Wernicke's aphasia (see below).

A patient's ability to understand the written or spoken word may also be affected before this sensory information reaches Wernicke's area. Assuming that the patient's vision is normal and that the visual information reaches the visual cortex, the symbols may be clearly seen by the

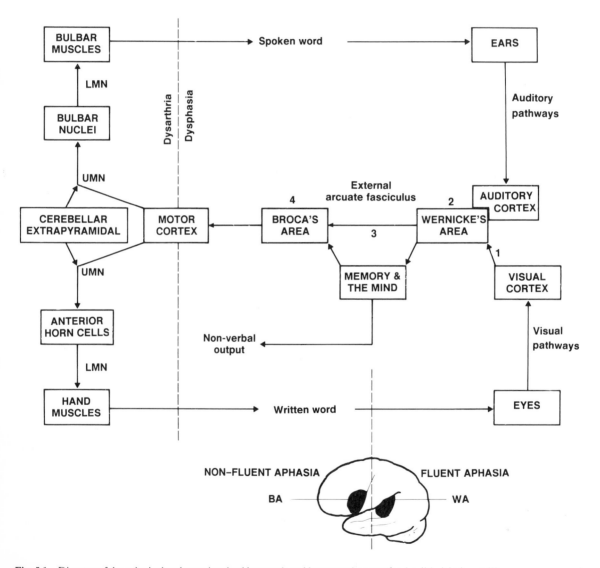

Fig. 5.1 Diagram of the principal pathways involved in speech and language (see text for details). A lesion at (1) causes a pure word-blindness or dyslexia. A lesion at (2) causes a Wernicke's aphasia. A lesion at (3) causes a conduction aphasia, and a lesion at (4) causes a Broca's dysphasia. BA = Broca's area; WA = Werricke's area.

subject but cannot be interpreted as language until that information reaches Wernicke's area from the left occipital cortex and across the corpus callosum from the right occipital cortex. A lesion in this pathway causes dyslexia, so that the patient cannot attach a meaning to the symbols that he can see, but since the auditory pathways are intact, the patient can understand the spoken word without difficulty. This is a not uncommon clinical finding and is usually associated with a right homonymous hemianopia. It is due to a lesion in the left parieto-occipital region affecting the fibres from the left occipital pole and those crossing in the corpus callosum from the right occipital pole.

The analogous defect in which the spoken word cannot be comprehended, but patients can read normally, is exceptionally rare because there is bilateral representation of sounds above the auditory nuclei in the brain stem and because the auditory cortex is so close to Wernicke's area that a lesion causing this problem would need to affect not only the auditory cortex of the dominant hemisphere, but also the crossing fibres from the other auditory cortex.

The other principal centre of language function in the dominant hemisphere is Broca's area, situated in the lateral part of the frontal cortex, just above the Sylvian fissure and anterior to the motor strip. This area is responsible for the initiation of all speech output, either to the cortical areas for the bulbar muscles in the case of speech, or to the cortical centres responsible for the control of hand movement in writing. Wernicke's area and Broca's area are directly connected via the external arcuate fasciculus so that it is possible for a subject to repeat a phrase parrot fashion or read aloud without necessarily any comprehension. Clearly there are very many complex connections between these two areas which enable a subject to hear a question, understand its meaning, search the memory for the appropriate answer which can then be delivered in a number of different forms; the response does not have to be verbal. Similarly, central thought processes can initiate a language output, though it is uncertain whether such internal speech requires normal function of Wernicke's area.

Aphasia

Wernicke's aphasia (sensory, receptive, posterior or fluent aphasia)

A patient with a lesion in Wernicke's area shows a partial or complete failure to understand the meaning of words heard or seen. Since there is no defect of speech output, spoken or written speech is usually fluent and voluble but may be inappropriate, partly because the patient is unable to monitor his or her own speech. The fluent verbal output is associated with normal intonation and often with literal and verbal paraphrases and neologisms. Mild forms of this condition are often missed and the patient is thought to be confused because he makes a fluent but inappropriate answer to a question. Most patients with marked Wernicke's aphasia have relatively large lesions involving the posterior part of the temporal lobe and often the inferior parietal lobe and anterior occipital lobe.

Broca's aphasia (motor, expressive, anterior or non-fluent aphasia)

Patients with Broca's aphasia are much more easily recognised because of the striking difficulty with speech they demonstrate even though they fully understand what is being said and can easily make non-verbal responses. Since the auditory feedback mechanism is functioning normally, the patient can hear that a mistake is being made as soon as it occurs and will therefore try to correct the error almost before the incorrect word has been completed. In its severest form the patient may completely lose the power to speak at all, whereas milder forms may cause just a hesitancy of speech. Once again, the lesions responsible for this are often surprisingly large and may also give disordered articulation (see dysarthria). Usually, the expression of language in written form is also impaired (agraphia).

Other forms of aphasia

A number of less common aphasia syndromes have been described and it is convenient to consider these as disconnection syndromes.

Pure word blindness (alexia (total) or dyslexia (partial)) is the inability to understand the written word despite normal vision and is due to a lesion affecting the pathway between the occipital cortex and Wernicke's area.

Pure word deafness is more of a concept than a reality and no very satisfactory case has ever been reported; it would be due to a lesion disconnecting the auditory cortex from Wernicke's area.

Conduction dysphasia is due to a lesion of the pathway (the arcuate fasciculus) connecting Wernicke's area to Broca's area so that a patient finds it difficult to read aloud or write fluently to dictation, but can understand the written and spoken word and can write and speak without difficulty.

Nominal (amnestic) dysphasia, a difficulty in naming objects, is not really a separate entity although this phenomenon is prominent in some aphasic subjects;

however, asking a patient to name objects and parts of objects is a good general test for language disorders.

Broca's and Wernicke's areas both lie in that part of the cerebral cortex supplied by the middle cerebral artery; since vascular disease is the commonest cause of dysphasia, most patients have a mixture of language difficulties and pure syndromes are relatively rare. A combination of Broca's and Wernicke's aphasia is usually called **global aphasia**.

Other lesions of association pathways (interconnecting areas concerned with language) can produce fractional disorders of speech. **Agraphia**, an inability to write, is simply a form of expressive aphasia (as mentioned above) and occurs in lesions near Broca's area, but can also result from a lesion of association pathways when spoken speech is unimpaired. Similarly, **alexia** can occur, usually with agraphia, as a result of focal lesions in the angular or supramarginal gyri of the dominant parietal lobe. **Acalculia**, or the inability to calculate, is a closely related phenomenon; the patient cannot appreciate the symbolic significance of figures rather than of letters and words; a similar disorder may derange the understanding of musical or scientific symbols.

Examination of a patient with aphasia

It is possible to test all the forms of language input against all the forms of language output and thus the integrity of all the various pathways involved. For example, reading aloud tests the visual input to Wernicke's area and output in the form of speech. Asking a patient a question tests the auditory input and speech output and involves central connections with memory. Similarly a patient may be asked to write to dictation or to write answers to written questions. The function of Wernicke's area can be assessed separately from that of Broca's area by asking for a non-verbal output, as, for example, by asking the patient to make a particular movement in response to a command.

THE NEUROMUSCULAR CONTROL OF SPEECH

There are two essential processes, namely phonation and articulation, by which the voluntary musculature converts the thought conceived in the cerebral cortex into the spoken word. Phonation, or the production of sound, results from the controlled passage of a column of air across the vocal cords, and the sound so produced resonates in the sounding-box of the larynx and pharynx. The sound is then modified by movements of the lips, tongue and palate which subserve the function of articulation.

DYSARTHRIA

Complete loss of speech due to a disorder of the neuromuscular mechanisms controlling articulation is known as **anarthria**, which is rare, but **dysarthria**, or impaired articulation, is relatively common. The speech of a dysarthric patient is slurred and indistinct, but his use of words is appropriate and his understanding unimpaired. Dysarthria can result from a lesion anywhere in the motor pathway from the motor cortex to the muscles responsible for articulation which include those of the face, the larynx and pharynx, and the jaw and tongue, as well as lesions of those systems which modify the activity of the main motor pathways including the extrapyramidal and cerebellar systems.

Cortical lesions. A lesion at the highest level in the motor pathway can cause a speech dyspraxia causing dysarthria; this may occur in acute unilateral lesions in the dominant hemisphere, usually associated with more obvious Broca's aphasia.

Upper motor neurone lesions. Except for a short time after acute lesions such as a stroke, or in cases of Broca's aphasia described above, unilateral upper motor neurone lesions do not cause persisting dysarthria unless both corticospinal pathways are involved, since the upper motor neurone control of bulbar muscles is bilateral. Dysarthria due to upper motor neurone lesions is always associated with other features of a pseudo-bulbar palsy such as emotional lability, difficulty in swallowing with nasal regurgitation, a spastic slow-moving tongue and brisk facial and jaw reflexes. The causes include congenital diplegia, double hemiplegia due to vascular disease, degeneration of the upper motor neurone pathways in motor neurone disease, multiple sclerosis and multiple lacunar infarcts associated with hypertension.

Lower motor neurone lesions causing dysarthria are associated with other features of a bulbar palsy including wasting of the tongue and fasciculation as well as difficulty in chewing and swallowing and nasal regurgitation of fluids. Causes include bulbar poliomyelitis, syringobulbia and motor neurone disease (progressive bulbar palsy), all of which affect the lower motor neurones in the medulla. A motor neuropathy affecting the bulbar nerves may occur in diphtheria and the Guillain-Barre syndrome.

The neuromuscular junction. Dysarthria is common in patients with myasthenia gravis, due to fatigability of the muscles of articulation (see p. 297), but does not usually occur in the Lambert-Eaton syndrome.

Disorders of muscle. Dysarthria can occur both in acquired myopathies such as polymyositis and in the genetically-determined muscular dystrophies, particularly those involving the facial muscles such as facioscapulohumeral dystrophy. Palatal weakness, if present, imparts a marked nasal quality to speech.

Cerebellar lesions. Dysarthria due to inco-ordination of the muscles of articulation is a striking feature of lesions of the cerebellum and its connections and is therefore common in patients with multiple sclerosis. In very severe cases, marked slurring and separation of syllables (so-called scanning speech) is characteristic. Profound dysarthria with disequilibrium but no nystagmus and little or no limb ataxia is characteristic of central cerebellar and some degenerative lesions.

Extrapyramidal lesions. Dysarthria is common in patients with Parkinson's disease (flat, monotonous speech) and may also occur in other disorders of the extrapyramidal system including Huntington's chorea, Wilson's disease and those forms of torsion dystonia which affect the muscles of the face and neck.

Although lesions in all these sites may produce specific forms of dysarthria that can be recognised, it is unreliable to try and make a diagnosis based on the sound alone, particularly where there is more than one cause of dysarthria such as combined upper motor neurone and cerebellar deficits in a patient with multiple sclerosis. It is also unnecessary in most cases, since the associated clinical features give a clear indication as to the cause of the difficult articulation.

MUTISM

Mutism is a total inability to speak, sometimes seen in a person without any demonstrable organic disease of the central nervous system. It can occur in psychotic patients (e.g. schizophrenia) and is an occasional manifestation of hysteria. Mutism combined with the loss of volitional movement of the trunk and limbs occurring in a patient who nevertheless appears to be conscious (akinetic mutism or 'the locked-in syndrome' can be a rare result of an upper brain stem lesion.

APHONIA AND DYSPHONIA

Patients with aphonia (total loss of the ability to phonate) or dysphonia (disordered phonation) are still able to articulate, so that they speak in a whisper. While aphonia may be the result of disease of the larynx (laryngitis, tumour or paralysis of the vocal cords) it is most often an hysterical manifestation, the unconscious motivation usually being an attempt to escape from stress. It is necessary to inspect the vocal cords in order to establish the diagnosis of hysterical aphonia and to exclude organic disease, but apart from a history of previous hysterical manifestations or of recent stress, the most

useful diagnostic pointer is that the patient can still phonate when coughing.

SPEECH DISORDERS IN CHILDHOOD

Developmental disorders of speech form a small but important group of disorders in which accurate diagnosis is important as many affected children are wrongly regarded as mentally retarded and many respond to appropriate treatment.

Deafness

The totally deaf child remains mute unless properly trained, as the normal channel for acquiring speech (i.e. through hearing) is not available. Usually the diagnosis becomes apparent when it is noted that the child, who has caused concern to his parents through failure to speak, also fails to respond to external noise. High-tone deafness is more difficult to diagnose, as the child with this condition does acquire speech, though this is unintelligible to any but his parents as he fails to utilise those vowel sounds and consonants (e.g. *e* and *t*) which depend upon high tones for their recognition. Audiometry will confirm the diagnosis.

Developmental dysarthria

Dysarthria in childhood can be a manifestation of local developmental abnormalities such as cleft palate, or of cerebral palsy, in which case there are usually other neurological signs. There is, however, a small group of children with inco-ordinate or clumsy movements of the tongue and palate as the only neurological abnormality. The condition is due to a congenital apraxia of articulation. These cases respond well to long-continued speech therapy.

Developmental aphasia

Congenital **word-deafness** or auditory imperception is a rare speech defect in which the patient fails to acquire normal speech function, is not deaf, as he responds to sounds, yet shows no interest or attention when spoken to. After several years many patients acquire a vocabulary of their own which, though meaningful to them, is incomprehensible to all except their nearest relatives. Their speech is difficult to distinguish from that associated with high-tone deafness except by audiometry.

Developmental dyslexia also occurs in various degrees of severity, being commonest in left-handed children; it can occur sporadically or be inherited as a dominant trait. It seems to be due to a defect in the establishment of speech function in one or other cerebral hemisphere, and is often associated with 'mirror-writing' (writing from right to left with reversals of words and letters, as if viewed in a mirror). The printed word is wrongly pronounced, a dictated word wrongly spelt and writing is usually abnormal. It occurs in children who are in other respects intelligent. Many normal children, particularly in families in which one or other parent is left-handed or ambidextrous, pass through a temporary phase of 'mirror-writing', at least of certain letters, when first learning to write.

Stammering

Stammering is a disorder of articulation characterised by the repetition of sounds or syllables and by prolonged pauses which punctuate speech. It is much more common in boys than in girls. Dentals (*t, d*), labials (*p, b*) and gutturals (*k*) are the sounds which seem most difficult to pronounce, and severe facial grimacing can accompany the attempt to utter words containing these letters. While many have suggested that this condition is psychogenic, others believe that, like dyslexia, it has an organic basis and it may be related to an incomplete localisation of speech function in one or other cerebral hemisphere. It can be present from the age of two or three years, but often begins at the age of six to eight when a child who has previously spoken fluently is beginning to read and write. While many stammerers seem shy and introspective, this mental attitude is most probably the result rather than the cause of their disability. There is no evidence that stammering is a result of acquired organic brain disease, though it may develop for the first time in some adults with mild Broca's aphasia. It is more properly regarded as a disorder of the organisation and establishment of speech function. It can often be controlled to some extent by the use of syllabic speech.

MANAGEMENT OF SPEECH DISORDERS

Comprehensive assessment and management of these various speech and language disorders in both adults and children can be undertaken by speech therapists, who are in the best position to advise on appropriate treatment and upon the use of the many types of communication aids now available. These may, for example, be of particular value for patients with severe dysarthria, as may occur in motor neurone disease. Speech therapists may also be very helpful in advising patients with feeding and swallowing disorders, as too are occupational therapists and physiotherapists in appropriate cases.

APRAXIA

Apraxia is the inability to carry out an organised voluntary movement despite the fact that the motor and sensory pathways concerned in the control of the movement are intact. In other words the difficulty is not due to paralysis, ataxia or sensory loss. Thus a patient who is asked to put out his tongue may be completely unable to do so on request, though a moment later he will spontaneously lick his lips. Hence the condition can be regarded as a loss of acquired motor skills, or an inability to reactivate those nervous pathways in which the memory and technique of specific movements (**praxis**) have been recorded. It can be considered to be a defect of the 'association' areas or fibres concerned with volitional motor activity. The supramarginal gyrus of the dominant parietal lobe appears to contain an important cell-station in this organisation of movement, and lesions of this area commonly produce bilateral apraxia. A lesion between this cortical area and the motor cortex of the left cerebral hemisphere will lead to an apraxia of the right limbs, while a lesion of the corpus callosum dividing those fibres which are passing to the right motor cortex will give rise to a left-sided apraxia.

Apraxia of the lips and tongue is relatively common (orofacial apraxia), while in the extremities apraxic disturbances may be revealed as an inability to dress or undress (**dressing apraxia**) or to construct models from blocks or letters with matches (**constructional apraxia**). Dressing apraxia is usually associated with lesions of the non-dominant parietal lobe, constructional apraxia with dominant hemisphere lesions. Apraxia of gait occasionally results from bilateral frontal lobe lesions, and may be associated with dementia (see communicating hydrocephalus). Oculomotor apraxia involving eye movements has also been described.

AGNOSIA

Visual, auditory and tactile stimuli are perceived in the occipital, temporal and post-central areas of the cortex, respectively, as crude physical phenomena which only acquire significance when related to past sensory experiences which have been collated and 'stored' as sensory memories in the appropriate association areas of the cortex. This process of recognising the significance of sensory stimuli is known as **gnosis**. Lesions of these association areas may impair this faculty of recognition, even though the primary sensory pathway is intact; the syndrome so produced is called **agnosia**. Visual agnosia is an inability to recognise objects seen, in a patient who is not blind; auditory agnosia is a failure to appreciate the significance of sounds in a patient who is not deaf (a condition which closely resembles Wernicke's aphasia). A patient with tactile agnosia (often called **astereognosis**) cannot identify objects which he feels. Usually an agnosic defect involves only vision or hearing or touch in isolation, so that a patient who cannot recognise a pen, and may not even see that it is an object with which to write (unlike the patient with nominal aphasia) will name it at once if it is placed in his hand, while conversely one with tactile agnosia will identify visually the object which was unrecognised when he held it.

THE BODY IMAGE

A constant stream of sensory impulses from the special senses, skin, muscles, bones and joints informs us of the condition and situation of the parts of our body in relation to each other and in relation to our external environment. From these stimuli we build up almost unconsciously an image of our body which is continually varying. Certain parts of the body such as the hands and mouth play such important roles in our everyday activity, and are so well endowed with highly-developed sensory receptors, that their share of the body image is proportionally much greater than, say, the small of the back. A skilled craftsman or the driver of a motor vehicle may become so attuned to the use of his tools or vehicle that in a sense these become a part of his body image and he then unconsciously relates himself plus the tool or vehicle and not himself alone to his environment. This concept of the body image is 'stored' in the association areas of the parietal lobes, and when the performance of motor skills is included it becomes clearly related to the function of praxis mentioned above. Some lesions of the parietal lobe tend to distort the body image so that the patient is unable to distinguish right from left (**right–left disorientation**). He may neglect the opposite side of his body and the whole of extrapersonal space on that side (**autotopagnosia**) while he may even deny that there is anything wrong with the contralateral limbs (**anosognosia**) and sometimes attempts to throw them out of bed. The term 'anosognosia' is sometimes used to describe denial of other gross neurological manifestations. Often the patient with a parietal lobe lesion will perceive normally sensory stimuli applied independently to the two sides of the body, but if bilateral stimuli are simultaneously applied, one may be ignored (**tactile inattention**).

It has been said that disorders of the body image occur only with lesions of the non-dominant parietal lobe, but this may be due to the fact that in lesions of the dominant

hemisphere they are obscured by aphasic, apraxic or other defects. Commonly, because of the contiguity of important association areas in the dominant parietal lobe, multiple defects occur, thus **Gerstmann's syndrome** is a combination of right–left disorientation, finger agnosia (an inability to identify individual fingers) and constructional apraxia. Acalculia and/or dyslexia are also common in such cases and the lesion responsible usually involves the angular gyrus.

DEVELOPMENTAL APRAXIA AND AGNOSIA

Specific learning defects other than developmental dyslexia (see p. 65) have been recognised increasingly in recent years and appear to be the result of either minimal brain damage due to birth injury or defective physiological organisation of cerebral dominance. The term 'minimal cerebral dysfunction' is sometimes applied to this group of syndromes. In contradistinction to the dyslexics, these 'clumsy children', who are often wrongly regarded as being mentally retarded, and who often demonstrate minor choreiform involuntary movements, generally show a higher verbal than performance level on the Wechsler intelligence scale for children. Defects of sensory perception as well as of skilled motor activity may be recognised in these children, who often improve to some extent as they grow older; but many require patient individual tuition in the particular skills (e.g. writing) in which they are defective.

REFERENCES

Adams R D, Victor M 1985 Principles of neurology, 3rd edn. McGraw-Hill, New York. Section V, Ch. 22

Benson D F 1985 Language and its disorders. In: Swash M, Kennard C (eds) Scientific basis of clinical neurology. Churchill Livingstone, Edinburgh

Critchley M 1953 The parietal lobes. Arnold, London

Critchley M 1964 Developmental dyslexia. Heinemann, London

Critchley M 1970 Aphasiology. Arnold, London

Critchley M 1975 Silent language. Butterworth, London

Geschwind N 1974 Selected papers on language and the brain. Reidel, Dordrecht, Holland

Gubbay S S 1975 The clumsy child. Major problems in neurology, Vol 5 (Walton J, series ed). Saunders, London

Kertesz A 1986 Language, cognition and higher cerebral function. In: Walton J, Beeson P B, Bodley Scott R (eds) Oxford Companion to medicine. Oxford University Press, Oxford

Morley N 1972 The development and disorders of speech in childhood, 3rd edn. Livingstone, Edinburgh

Walton J N 1985 Brain's Diseases of the nervous system, 9th edn. Oxford University Press, Oxford

6. Disorders of consciousness

Consciousness is a state or faculty which almost defies definition. It implies a state of awareness of one's self and of one's surroundings, and its contents include a variety of recurring sensory experiences combined with emotions, ideas and memories which are the product of thought processes. While it is clear that the cerebral cortex plays an important role in maintaining and determining the content of the conscious state, cortical mechanisms of motor or sensory activity are by no means autonomous and can be activated or suppressed through the activity of the reticular substance and by hypothalamic mechanisms. This reticular–hypothalamic complex exercises important influences upon the state of awareness and it is evident that disturbances of consciousness which are observed in clinical neurological practice are largely dependent upon lesions, either functional or structural, of these areas of the brain or the pathways which connect them to the cerebral cortex.

The term **arousal** refers to a state of wakefulness which is simply the converse of **sleep**, while various disorders of consciousness are labelled **clouding of consciousness**, **stupor** and **coma**. In this chapter we shall consider briefly the pathophysiology of consciousness and normal and pathological variations in the conscious state.

The thalamo-cortical projection system consists of specific thalamic nuclei which project to specific sensory cortical areas, but in addition there are non-specific thalamic nuclei (the intralaminar, septa or midline and ventricular thalamic nuclei) which act as pacemakers of cortical activity. These in turn are controlled by neurones of the **reticular activating system** (Fig. 6.1) which are situated in the **reticular formation** in the core of the pons and midbrain, extending into the posterior hypothalamus. A downward projection of this system into the medulla includes the centres which control respiration and vasomotor tone, and yet other parts of it are concerned with control of temperature and gastrointestinal secretion. Experimental work in animals has shown that electrical stimulation of this system causes arousal, while destructive lesions cause unconsciousness. Sim-

ilarly, anaesthetic and hypnotic drugs selectively depress its activity, while stimulant drugs have the opposite, facilitatory effect upon it.

Plum & Posner (1980) summarised certain principles of importance in the pathophysiology of consciousness as follows:

1. Lesions which destroy the reticular formation below the lower third of the pons do not produce coma.
2. Above this level a lesion must destroy both sides of the paramedian reticulum to interrupt consciousness.
3. The arousal effects of reticular stimulation upon behaviour and the EEG, are separable in that bilateral lesions of the pontine tegmentum producing coma may be associated with a normal 'waking' EEG.

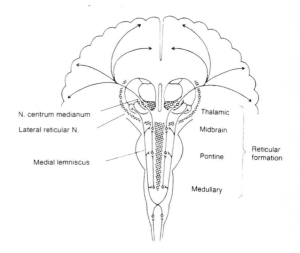

Fig. 6.1 The ascending reticular activating system. The reticular formation extends rostrally to include the lateral reticular nucleus of the thalamus, the midline and intralaminar nuclei, and part of the centrum medianum, which project diffusely to the cerebral cortex as the unspecific afferent system, responsible for the maintenance of consciousness. The reticular formation of medulla, pons and midbrain receives collaterals from ascending specific sensory pathways.
(Reproduced with permission from Lance & McLeod 1981.)

4. Sleep is an active physiological process, not a mere failure of arousal and is clearly separable from stupor and coma.

5. Sleeping and waking can occur in man even after total bilateral destruction of the cerebral hemispheres.

Hence a lesion or dysfunction of the reticular system will only produce stupor or coma if it:

a. affects both sides of the brain stem;
b. is located between the lower third of the pons and the posterior diencephalon; and
c. is either of acute onset or large in its extent.

SLEEP

Sleep can be regarded as a periodical physiological depression of function of the parts of the brain controlling consciousness. The EEG shows that as sleep deepens there is a transition from normal alpha waves to a phase of bursts of more rapid waves (spindles) and then the development of slow random waves. This is so-called slow-wave, orthodox or non-REM sleep. It can be divided into four stages according to EEG criteria (Fig. 6.2). Stage I is drowsiness and the EEG shows largely theta and beta frequencies. Stage 2 is light sleep with more theta

activity and some K-complexes and sleep spindles. Stage 3 is moderate sleep in which delta activity appears and K-complexes predominate. Stage 4 or deep sleep is dominated by delta activity at around 2 Hz for more than 60% of the record. An additional phase of sleep is the rapid eye movement stage (REM) during which most dreams occur. Although this is a deeper stage of sleep than Stage 4 of non-REM sleep as measured by the arousal threshold, the patient appears to be in relatively light sleep with irregular heart and respiration rates and occasional twitchy movements of limbs or facial muscles, hence the term paradoxical sleep. Paradoxical sleep occurs shortly after falling asleep and is usually followed sequentially by the stages of orthodox sleep before a fairly quick transition back to a period of REM sleep, after which the cycle starts all over again. These cycles occur every 50–90 minutes throughout the night with a predominance of orthodox sleep in the first part of the night and of REM sleep during the latter part of the night. These relationships, cycle times and time spent in each stage of sleep vary with age and are disturbed in a wide range of neurological disorders. Insomnia, particularly in the elderly, is usually associated with brief awakenings and with a reduced proportion of paradoxical sleep. In drug withdrawal syndromes (e.g. delirium tremens), the pa-

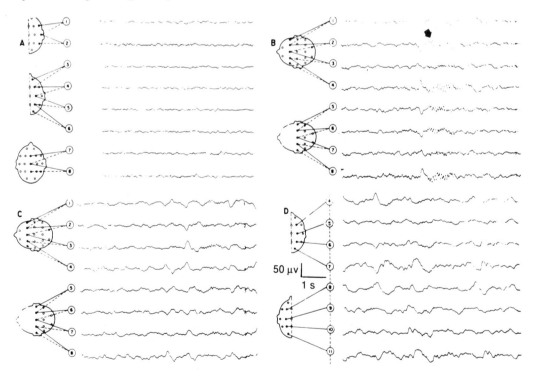

Fig. 6.2 Sequential EEG records showing (**A**) Stage I, (**B**) Stage II, (**C**) Stage III, and (**D**) Stage IV of slow-wave sleep. The arrow in **B** illustrates sleep spindles. (Reproduced with permission from Patton et al 1976.)

tient alternates between wakefulness and fitful sleep of which up to 100% is paradoxical. Barbiturate anaesthetics produce EEG changes similar to those accompanying normal sleep. Though sleep-like states can be induced by electrical stimulation of an area in the diencephalon, it is an oversimplification to regard this as a 'sleep centre'.

During sleep not only is consciousness lost, but certain bodily changes occur. The pulse rate, blood pressure and respiratory rate fall in orthodox sleep but rise in the paradoxical phase; the eyes usually deviate upwards (but show rapid bursts of conjugate movement in the paradoxical phase), the pupils are contracted, but usually react to light, though slowly; the tendon reflexes are abolished and the plantar reflexes may become extensor.

Recent neuropharmacological studies are also relevant. Neurones of the brain stem median raphe contain large quantities of 5-hydroxytryptamine (5-HT) and lesions here in animals give insomnia which can be reversed by giving a 5-HT precursor. Drugs such as p-chlorphenylalanine which block 5-HT synthesis decrease both REM and 'slow-wave' sleep. Destruction of norepinephrine (NE)-containing neurones of the locus coeruleus suppresses REM but not 'slow-wave' sleep, while reserpine, which depletes both 5-HT and NE, gives insomnia, but if a 5-HT precursor is then given 'slow-wave' sleep is re-established but REM sleep is not.

Many disorders of sleep are known, some of which are semi-physiological and of no serious significance, while others are due to organic lesions involving the midbrain and hypothalamus.

Sleep paralysis is a condition in which the patient, when falling asleep, or more often on waking, finds himself unable to move a muscle, though motor activity returns immediately if he is touched. This experience can be very alarming, but movement generally returns within a minute and the condition is of no serious significance. Another related disorder may take the form of so-called **hypnagogic hallucinations**, a series of visual or other hallucinations which are of brief duration, though often terrifying in character, and which occur as the patient is falling asleep. Presumably this condition is due to persisting activation of cortical association areas; **night terrors** in children are probably similar. **Nocturnal myoclonus** (hypnagogic jerks), a sudden jerk of the musculature which occurs as the patient is drifting into sleep, is also physiological and results from a sudden transient reactivation of the motor system. Myoclonic jerks occurring repeatedly in sleep, however, must often be regarded as pathological, as some such patients develop epileptic seizures.

Insomnia occurs so frequently in the elderly that it is again difficult to know when it becomes pathological. In younger patients it is usually the result of anxiety, an emotional disturbance which clearly influences the reticular–hypothalamic system. Depression is a common cause of early morning wakening. It is important to realise that many patients have unrealistic expectations and it is quite common for patients who claim to sleep badly actually to sleep quite normally but to become very anxious if they awaken even for short periods during the night. The widespread use of hypnotics and sedatives is to be deplored, particularly because both dependence and tolerance are usual. The cause of insomnia should be determined and, if this is due to some identifiable short-term and non-recurring problem such as a bereavement, emotional upset or illness, a short-acting benzodiazepine may be the appropriate treatment, but this should be stopped as soon as possible and preferably given intermittently to reduce the risk of dependence. More chronic insomnia should not be treated by regular hypnotics and is more often due to anxiety, depression, and drug abuse including alcohol. When due to depression, patients are better treated with a tricyclic drug than with a hypnotic. In all these conditions, barbiturates should be avoided and short-acting benzodiazepines preferred such as temazepam or triazolam. However there are a few patients in whom these are ineffective and who require the longer acting nitrazepam, though because of its potential daytime 'hangover' effect this is not recommended for long-continued routine administration.

Somnambulism or sleep-walking is also related to emotional stress and can be regarded as a reactivation of complex co-ordinated muscular movements occurring while consciousness remains impaired.

Narcolepsy is another relatively common disorder which results from a functional disturbance within the reticular–hypothalamic system. Patients with this condition experience attacks of almost irresistible sleep which develop during the day, most often in the afternoons. Such sleep is usually immediately of the REM type and in many such patients the REM/ non-REM ratio of nocturnal sleep is abnormal. The desire to sleep can be resisted if the patient moves around, but if he sits down the somnolence is overwhelming and he falls asleep, usually only for a few minutes, but sometimes for several hours. He can, however, be aroused with ease, as from normal sleep. Males are affected more often than females and the condition usually begins in adolescence or early adult life. There is a strong association with HLA DR2. Narcolepsy is treated with central nervous system stimulants. The smallest effective dose should be used and it is preferable not to give a stimulant drug later than the mid-afternoon because it may keep the patient awake at night. Treatment should be started with mazindol 2 mg in the morning and the dose may be increased by the addition of

1–2 mg at lunchtime. Pemoline may also be used and if these fail or become ineffective, methylphenidate may be substituted (methylphenidate is available in the United Kingdom on a named patient basis). In more resistant cases it may be necessary to prescribe dexamphetamine sulphate. All these drugs tend to become ineffective after a while and it may be necessary to change from one to another periodically. Many patients who experience such attacks also suffer from **cataplexy**, a name given to episodes of sudden loss of tone in the voluntary muscles, which cause the patient to go 'weak at the knees' and even to slump suddenly to the ground; he may be unable to move for several seconds or even for as long as a minute. These attacks are commonly precipitated by sudden emotion such as laughing, crying, fear or excitement. The condition can be regarded as a transient inactivation of that part of the reticular substance controlling motor activity and is again an exaggeration of the physiological reaction as normal people sometimes become 'weak with laughter'. The tricycle drug clomipramine is very effective in the treatment of cataplexy, often in quite small doses of around 30 mg a day.

Idiopathic hypersomnolence is often confused with narcolepsy but is different in its clinical and electrophysiological features (sleep is immediately of the orthodox or non-REM type). This condition of pathological daytime drowsiness is not uncommon and in a sense suggests that the 'set' of the reticular activating system is more towards depression than towards arousal of consciousness. Affected patients often sleep abnormally heavily during the night and may easily fall into a heavy and prolonged sleep during the day. Serotonin antagonists such as dimethylsergide are often helpful in treatment, whereas drugs which are effective in the narcolepsy-cataplexy syndrome (see above) are not.

Organic lesions, whether neoplastic or inflammatory, in the region of the third ventricle and hypothalamus or upper brain stem, rarely give rise to symptomatic narcolepsy, but more often they produce **hypersomnia**, in which the patient sleeps for long periods, is difficult to rouse and may then be confused for some time. Periodic hypersomnia with megaphagia (excessive appetite) is a disorder of unknown aetiology (the Kleine-Levin syndrome) most often seen in adolescent males and often associated with hypersexuality; it is thought to be due to hypothalamic dysfunction (see p. 322). Certain other lesions of the midbrain and contiguous areas, and particularly those of encephalitis lethargica, produce **reversal of the sleep rhythm**, so that the patient sleeps by day but is awake and restless at night. These disorders cease to be physiological variants and are closely related to the pathological states of stupor and coma which result from structural or metabolic disorders affecting similar areas of the brain.

STUPOR AND COMA

There is a continuum of impaired consciousness from fully conscious and alert to deep coma. This ranges through drowsiness, stupor, light coma and deep coma. The drowsy patient can be fully aroused, if for only short periods of time. The stuporose patient cannot be fully aroused, but can be 'woken up' even if not to normality. The patient in light or semi coma responds to painful stimuli, but does not recover consciousness, whereas patients in deep coma do not respond to any stimuli. The Glasgow coma scale devised by Teasdale & Jennett quantifies the level of consciousness according to four grades of eye opening, five of verbal response and five of motor response. This scale is easy to apply at the bedside and can be used for sequential assessment:

1. Eye opening
Spontaneous	4
To speech	3
To pain	2
None	1

2. Verbal response
Orientated	5
Confused	4
Occasional words	3
Sounds but no words	2
None	1

3. Best motor response
Obeys commands	5
Localises painful stimulus	4
Flexes to painful stimuli	3
Extends to painful stimuli	2
No response	1

Mechanisms of stupor and coma

While coma can result from many conditions (see Table 6.1, p. 74) some of which are lesions or diseases of the brain, while others are generalised metabolic disorders, the disturbance of consciousness whether due to a structural or a biochemical lesion, is produced by disordered function in the reticular system.

There are certain important principles, however, which govern the production of stupor or coma as a result of supratentorial or infratentorial mass lesions (Fig. 6.3).

While diffuse cerebral oedema can cause compression of the upper brain stem through symmetrical downward pressure, a localised space-occupying lesion or unilateral oedema (say after extensive infarction) produces a similar effect upon the reticular substance either as a consequence of uncal herniation through the tentorial hiatus or, less often as a result of herniation of cerebellar tonsils through the foramen magnum. Cingulate gyrus herniation beneath the falx cerebri, by contrast, produces its effects by compressing the anterior cerebral vessels, thus increasing frontal lobe oedema. In uncal herniation, compression of the trunk of the third nerve against the free edge of the tentorium often gives unilateral pupillary dilatation, followed by ptosis and ultimately a complete third nerve palsy. Persisting uncal herniation can give rise to haemorrhages in the median raphe of the brain stem causing irreversible coma. Subtentorial lesions, by contrast, may compress the brain stem directly or else may cause either upward displacement of the midbrain and cerebellum through the tentorial notch or downward cerebellar tonsillar herniation. Any form of herniation

may be accentuated with disastrous effects if cerebrospinal fluid is removed by lumbar puncture. Destructive brain stem lesions (e.g. infarction), on the other hand, cause coma through direct damage to the reticular formation, as do inflammatory processes such as encephalitis, while meningitis combines with the effects of inflammation to give a marked increase in intracranial pressure. Ischaemia and hypoxia also affect the reticular substance directly, while post-epileptic stupor depends upon a temporary suppression of synaptic transmission in this system and/or in the pathways connecting it to the cortex.

Examination of the unconscious patient

Neurological examination of the unconscious patient is rather different from that normally employed, since there is no co-operation from the patient, so that the examination is necessarily rather abbreviated, though some additional specialised tests may be necessary.

Fundi. The fundi should be examined for papilloedema, which would indicate raised intracranial pressure and the surrounding retina for subhyaloid haemorrhages, perhaps indicating a subarachnoid haemorrhage.

Pupils. The pupillary responses are valuable in the assessment of the unconscious patient, and midriatic drugs, often used to obtain an adequate view of the fundi, should be used with extreme caution in unconscious patients as the paralysis of the pupil which they produce eliminates a valuable source of information. In midbrain lesions the pupils may be of median size and unreactive to light. Lesions of the pontine tegmentum, such as a pontine haemorrhage, give small fixed pupils. Cerebral anoxia causes pulpillary dilatation. A fixed dilated pupil on one side is often indicative of a third nerve palsy on that side, usually the result of herniation of the medial temporal lobe through the tentorial hiatus.

Ocular movements. The optical axes are usually divergent in unconscious patients without any eye movement disorder. Massive hemisphere lesions may result in deviation of the head and eyes towards the side of the lesion, due to the unopposed effect of the opposite hemisphere, whereas pontine lesions cause conjugate deviation of the eyes to the opposite side. The oculocephalic reflex or doll's eye movement is elicited by rapid rotation of the head to one side and then the other, or up and down; the eyes deviate away from the direction of movement as if maintaining fixation, but there is of course no visual fixation and the reflex is not dependent on normal vision as it persists in completely blind individuals. The reflex depends on vestibular and proprioceptive pathways to the brain stem oculomotor

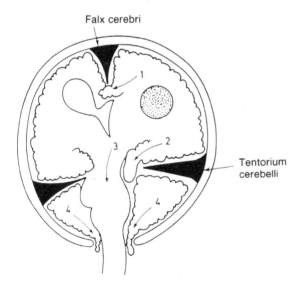

Falx cerebri

Tentorium cerebelli

Fig. 6.3 Effect of expanding supratentorial lesions on cerebral structures. The cingulate gyrus may be herniated beneath the falx cerebri (cingulate herniation) (1), a portion of the temporal lobe may be compressed between brain stem and margin of tentorial notch (2), or the brain stem may be displaced downwards through the tentorial opening (central herniation) (3). In expanding infratentorial lesions, or after injudicious lumbar puncture in the presence of raised intracranial pressure, the cerebellar tonsils may herniate through the foramen magnum (4).
(Reproduced with permission from Lance & McLeod 1981.)

nuclei. Absence of doll's eye movements is therefore indicative of a brain stem lesion. The caloric response is a more powerful stimulus of similar pathways. Ice-cold water is infused into the external auditory meatus; this stimulates movement of the endolymph and in normal conscious subjects would produce nystagmus but in the unconscious patient it produces tonic deviation of the eyes. The absence of a response indicates a severe brain stem lesion.

Gag and cough reflexes. These are mediated through the medulla.

Respiration. Respiratory effort may be depressed by drug overdose and a wide range of abnormal respiratory patterns may occur with pathological lesions at various levels in the brain and brain stem. These include Cheyne-Stokes respiration, central neurogenic hyperventilation, apneusis, cluster breathing and ataxic breathing. The pathophysiology of these patterns of respiration has been reviewed by Plum & Posner (1980).

The motor system. Power cannot be tested in the unconscious patient, but the position of limbs may be important. Flexion and adduction of the arm with flexion of the wrists and fingers and extension of the leg is known as **decorticate rigidity** and indicates a lesion of the corticospinal pathways usually at or above the internal capsule. Marked increase in tone with the arms held stiffly extended and adducted with extension of the legs and feet is known as **decerebrate rigidity** and is usually indicative of a more widespread lesion and lesions below the internal capsule. The reflexes are pathologically brisk and the plantar responses extensor.

Sensation. Only the response to painful stimuli can be assessed and this forms part of the Glasgow coma scale (see above). **The head** should be examined for signs of recent or past injury and **the tongue** for scars resulting from previous fits. The smell of alcohol on **the breath** or of acetone (in diabetic coma) or foetor (in uraemic or hepatic coma) may be of diagnostic value. **Cervical rigidity** will suggest either meningitis, cerebellar herniation or subarachnoid haemorrhage, while **a bruit** over the cranium or in the neck may indicate a vascular malformation or arterial stenosis. In **the skin** cyanosis (in respiratory insufficiency), a cherry-red colour (in carbon monoxide poisoning—though this colour is only really striking at autopsy), purpura (in various blood diseases), the typical changes of Addison's disease or hypothyroidism or scars of previous injections (in drug addicts) may give clues to the cause of the coma.

Clearly, examination of other systems to exclude diseases of the heart, lungs, liver and kidneys is obligatory in any comatose patient and this includes standard investigations of the functions of these systems.

Differential diagnosis of coma

The **differential diagnosis** of the causes of coma (Table 6.1) is a difficult but common clinical problem. Where an adequate history is available from friends or relatives the diagnostic problem is often eased, but when a patient is found comatose and no accurate history of the onset is available, diagnosis may bristle with difficulties. Thus **head injury**, an important cause, is generally identified by the history; even if this is lacking there is usually some external evidence of laceration or contusion. In cases of **subdural haematoma**, however, the causal injury may have been trivial and the patient may gradually have become increasingly drowsy over a period of weeks or months. Some such patients are stuporose rather than comatose. In **subarachnoid haemorrhage** a history of sudden onset with headache and neck stiffness, and the presence of blood-stained CSF are revealing; however, the clinical picture of **primary cerebral haemorrhage** is not dissimilar, though in such cases a profound hemiplegia is usually present from the onset. When **cerebral thrombosis** is the cause, the onset is generally more gradual with less severe clouding of consciousness, though if the infarct is extensive, the patient can be

Table 6.1 The common causes of stupor and coma (Reproduced from Walton 1987 and modified from Plum & Posner 1980.)

Supratentorial lesions (causing upper brain stem dysfunction)
Cerebral haemorrhage
Massive cerebral infarction
Extradural haematoma
Subdural haematoma
Cerebral tumour
Cerebral abscess

Infratentorial lesions (compressing or destroying the reticular formation)
Pontine haemorrhage
Posterior fossa tumour
Cerebellar haemorrhage
Cerebellar abscess
Brain stem infarction

Metabolic process or other diffuse lesions
Anoxia
Hypoglycaemia
Deficiency disorders
Renal or hepatic failure
Disorders of electrolytes and/or ionic equilibrium
Poisoning, intoxications
Infectious or autoimmune disorders
Meningitis
Encephalitis
Head injury, including concussion and contusion
Post-epileptic states

comatose and hemiplegic, a clinical picture which differs little from that of cerebral haemorrhage. The onset of **cerebral embolism** is of course abrupt, and there is often clinical evidence of a source of emboli, generally in the heart (mitral stenosis, bacterial endocarditis, cardiac infarction). **Encephalitis** and **meningitis** are usually accompanied by fever, and the patient's comatose state is usually the end-result of an illness which has lasted for a day or two or longer, with headache, neck stiffness (in meningitis particularly), drowsiness and confusion. In such individuals, CSF examination is of the greatest importance. Similarly, sudden coma is uncommon in patients suffering from **cerebral tumour**, many of whom have experienced previous headache, focal fits or the gradual development of paralysis and papilloedema will often be present. In patients with **cerebral abscess**, too, the onset is generally gradual and there will often be an evident focus of infection in the middle ear, nasal sinuses, skin or lung. The relatively uncommon **hypertensive encephalopathy** is generally recognised through the retinal changes of malignant hypertension combined with the blood pressure reading. Recognition of the stupor or coma which follows an attack of **epilepsy** rests upon a history of previous fits.

Turning to toxic and metabolic causes of coma, **anoxia** will generally be identified by a history of carbon-monoxide poisoning, whether from coal gas, a coke brazier or exhaust fumes, or by a history of partial drowning, difficult general anaesthesia or chronic pulmonary insufficiency. **Acute alcoholism** will be suspected from the smell of alcohol on the breath and confirmed by urine or blood-alcohol estimation. However, intoxicated patients are particularly liable to suffer head injury, while cerebral vascular catastrophes sometimes occur during an alcoholic debauch. Deep, hissing, 'acidotic' respiration with acetone in the breath, glycosuria and ketonuria, will usually establish a diagnosis of **diabetic (hyperglycaemic) coma**, while a pale, sweating and flaccid patient with bilateral extensor responses may be shown by blood-sugar estimation to be suffering from **hypoglycaemia** due either to insulin administration or to a tumour of the pancreatic islet cells. Patients with **uraemia** tend to have a deep acidotic breathing like that of diabetic coma, but the breath has a uriniferous smell, and hypertension, retinal changes and albuminuria are usually present. **Liver disease** is easily overlooked as a cause of coma, but the patient will often have shown the characteristic 'flapping' tremor of the outstretched hands, and there may be jaundice, dark urine and stigmata of hepatic cirrhosis such as 'liver palms' and cutaneous spider naevi.

Other rare causes of a comatose state include **malaria, heat stroke** (as in athletes competing in hot countries),

Addison's disease, myxoedema and **hypopituitarism**. In the latter two conditions, **hypothermia** is a common cause of coma and the rectal temperature may be less than 36°C. Finally, **drug intoxication** must also be remembered as an increasingly common cause of a type of coma which may show no specific clinical features, especially if **barbiturates, psychotropic drugs or anticonvulsants** have been taken, say, in an attempt to commit suicide. **Salicylates**, by contrast, tend to produce a characteristic deep cyanosis with acidotic breathing, while **opiates** give characteristic pin-point pupils and paracetamol usually causes liver damage. However, in any patient with coma of unknown cause, when no history is available, poisoning should be considered and the patient's belongings should be searched for a container which may have held the offending tablets. Blood and urine samples should always be taken on admission and kept for subsequent drug analysis.

THE DIAGNOSIS OF BRAIN DEATH

This problem has assumed increasing importance in recent years, first because of the increasing difficulty of deciding in patients with brain damage whether it is justifiable to maintain life indefinitely with assisted respiration and other supportive measures, and secondly because of the difficult question of deciding when it may be concluded that the cerebral lesion is irreversible, that cardiac arrest is imminent, and that preparations may be made to remove viable organs for subsequent transplantation.

This topic has been a fertile source of national and international dispute, but there is now reasonably general agreement that the British criteria adopted by the Department of Health on the advice of the Conference of Royal Colleges and Faculties of the United Kingdom are reliable, and these are given below. It is recommended that in any individual case diagnosis according to the criteria should be confirmed by two experienced doctors acting independently and that the tests should be repeated after a 24-hour interval before the decision is made to discontinue life support systems and to remove organs when appropriate. It is unnecessary to carry out an EEG since this may show some activity in the presence of irreversible brain stem damage or alternatively it may be isoelectric in patients with drug overdosage.

The following are the conditions and criteria laid down:

Conditions under which the diagnosis of brain death should be considered

1. The patient is deeply comatose.

  a. There should be no suspicion that this state is due to depressant drugs.
  b. Hypothermia as a cause of coma should have been excluded.
  c. Metabolic and endocrine disturbances which can be responsible for or can contribute to coma should have been excluded.
2. The patient is being maintained on a ventilator because spontaneous respiration had previously become inadequate or had ceased altogether.
  a. Relaxants (neuromuscular blocking agents) and other drugs should have been excluded as a cause of respiratory inadequacy or failure.
3. There should be no doubt that the patient's condition is due to irremediable structural brain damage. The diagnosis of a disorder which can lead to brain death should have been fully established.

Diagnostic tests for the confirmation of brain death

All brain stem reflexes are absent:

  (i) The pupils are fixed in diameter and do not respond to sharp changes in the intensity of incident light.
  (ii) There is no corneal reflex.
  (iii) The vestibulo-ocular reflexes are absent.
  (iv) No motor responses within the cranial nerve distribution can be elicited by adequate stimulation of any somatic area.
  (v) There is no gag reflex or reflex response to bronchial stimulation by a suction catheter passed down the trachea.
  (vi) No respiratory movements occur when the patient is disconnected from the mechanical ventilator for long enough to ensure that the arterial carbon dioxide tension rises above the threshold for stimulation of respiration.

DELIRIUM AND CONFUSION

There are many physical illnesses which are accompanied by mental symptoms of varying degree, most of which present as **clouding of consciousness**, with or without other more specific manifestations. These disorders are the **symptomatic psychoses**. They occur not only as a result of cerebral lesions but also in many infective and metabolic disorders. These are not primarily diseases of the nervous system but they may affect profoundly its function, even without producing histological changes in the brain identifiable by present techniques. The lack of awareness which results may be no more than the minimal disinterest and 'fuzziness' in the head which accompanies mild influenza, but it can take the form of a severe psychotic reaction with grossly disturbed con-

sciousness and bizarre disorders of thought. There is evidence that the type of reaction an individual shows may depend at least partly upon his previous personality and emotional constitution.

Delirium is a term used to identify a state of severely clouded consciousness in which the patient is disorientated in time and place, and his attention span is brief. His thought processes are disordered so that he cannot appreciate his present circumstances and relate them to past experience; he may be living in a fantasy world peopled by the products of his imagining. Hence delusions or false imaginary ideas are frequent, as are hallucinations, usually visual, which can be vividly real and may result in an intense fear reaction with restless or even violent behaviour. Fluctuation in the mental and physical state is common, so that periods of shouting and restlessness alternate with others of apparent somnolence, punctuated by muttering. Commonly speech is slurred. Drowsiness is often worst during the day while the patient becomes excited, hallucinated and uncontrollable at night. The stage of true delirium is often preceded by one of restlessness and irritability, insomnia, lack of concentration and pathological brightness or euphoria, a stage which may last for hours or days, depending upon the cause. Often there are also motor manifestations; the patient is tremulous, and spontaneous twitching or jerking of the voluntary musculature occurs, even in sleep. A return to restful sleep may be the first sign of resolution of the delirium, but even after apparent recovery, delusions may persist and often have a paranoid character, encompassing ideas of persecution or ill-treatment.

Delirium classically occurs in patients with chronic alcoholism after a debauch or after alcohol withdrawal and is then known as **delirium tremens**. The condition which follows withdrawal of barbiturates, benzodiazepines or amphetamine in patients habituated to these drugs is often similar, and can also be characterised by the occurrence of drug-withdrawal convulsions. Less severe delirious states, differing only in detail but not in overall pattern, are seen in patients with encephalitis or meningitis, in severe infections such as septicaemia or typhoid fever, in metabolic disorders such as liver disease and pernicious anaemia, in some cases of bronchogenic carcinoma without cerebral metastases, after treatment with ACTH or steroids and in many other disorders. Mild delirium is common in febrile illness in childhood, particularly at night.

When mental disturbances are less striking but yet the patient shows fluctuations in awareness, with incoherence of thought and variable disorientation ('where am I'), but usually without frank delusions or hallucinations, the condition is often called **confusion** or a **confusional** state, of mild, moderate or severe degree. This differs from delirium only in detail and indeed these disorders merge with one another so that the delirious patient generally passes through a phase of confusion during recovery. In recovery from a head injury causing coma, for instance, the patient may be delirious and later confused as consciousness slowly returns. Hence some authorities have suggested that the term confusion should be dropped and the condition referred to as **subacute delirium**. Other terms utilised to identify these disorders include toxic-infective psychosis, metabolic or exhaustion psychosis, or organic reaction state, as these disorders are essentially mental reactions resulting from organic disease which is disordering brain function. From the standpoint of convenient clinical usage it is probably justifiable to retain the term 'delirium' to identify the severe disturbance and 'confusion' the less severe, provided it is appreciated that there is no essential difference between the two.

CEREBRAL IRRITATION

In addition to the manifestations of delirium or confusion which occur in patients with diffuse brain disease such as meningitis, encephalitis and subarachnoid haemorrhage, these individuals often show a typical behaviour pattern which is characteristic of so-called 'cerebral irritation'. They lie curled up on one side in bed, often with their eyes away from the light, and resent being disturbed, so that they may pull back the bedclothes when the doctor attempts to remove them. If the meninges are inflamed, neck stiffness will generally be apparent as well.

TRANSIENT DISORDERS OF CONSCIOUSNESS

One of the commonest problems which a doctor is asked to solve is to determine the significance of brief disorders of consciousness, often referred to as 'blackouts'. Are these fits or faints, that is, are they epileptic or syncopal or, less commonly, of metabolic or emotional origin? No distinction can be more important for social and occupational reasons and, at times, none can be more difficult to make with confidence.

Epilepsy

Epilepsy is the clinical manifestation of abnormal electrical activity of the brain. Everybody is potentially epileptic and would have a fit given sufficient stimulus. There is, however, a wide range of epileptic thresholds and it is probably the epileptic threshold which is genetically determined. Some people have very low thresholds and are very susceptible to epilepsy and some

people have very high thresholds and are therefore highly resistant to epilepsy. This concept explains why a space-occupying lesion such as a meningioma may present with epilepsy in some patients several years before the development of neurological deficit, and in other patients presents much later with neurological deficit and without epilepsy. Similarly, some patients recover from severe head injury without epilepsy and other patients develop epilepsy following quite minor injury. According to this concept, patients with the lowest epileptic threshold would have idiopathic generalised epilepsy and patients with a slightly higher threshold would only develop epilepsy if there was a focal area of damage in the brain which would give rise to the abnormal electrochemical activity. Whether or not this remained a focal disturbance or spread to become a more generalised disturbance would depend on the epileptic threshold of the surrounding brain.

The pathophysiology of epilepsy is not fully understood. Theoretically, it could arise as an result of an increase in activity of excitatory mechanisms or a decrease in the activity of inhibitory systems, or indeed a combination of these two. There are numerous neurotransmitters involved in both these processes, but γ-aminobutyric acid (GABA) is the most widely distributed inhibitory neurotransmitter and the glutamate-aspartate system is a widely represented excitatory system. Some disturbance of relative balance of these neurotransmitters may be the basis of epilepsy.

It is convenient on clinical grounds to divide patients with epilepsy into two broad groups, viz. idiopathic and symptomatic epilepsy, though these probably form a continuous spectrum. Patients with idiopathic epilepsy show no evidence of an organic brain lesion and their attacks do not have a focal onset. The abnormal electrical activity is a generalised phenomenon and one explanation for this is that it results from a disturbance in the deep grey matter of the brain and has therefore been referred to as central or centrencephalic epilepsy (Fig. 6.4). In symptomatic epilepsy, the attacks are a symptom of organic brain disease. To some extent this difference is artificial because patients who develop epilepsy as a result of fever, diffuse degenerative brain disease, anoxia, toxaemia, hypoglycaemia, hypocalcaemia or drug withdrawal, particularly of alcohol, are all likely to have a low epileptic threshold. Another group of patients with symptomatic epilepsy has some form of focal brain lesion such as an infarct, an abscess, a tumour or brain damage due to trauma, and the epileptic activity arises in this abnormal area. What occurs following such a focal epileptic disturbance depends on the resistance of the brain to the spread of the epileptic discharge. If this resistance is low and spread is rapid, a focal lesion will

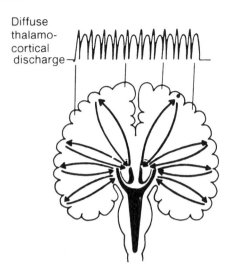

Diffuse
thalamo-
cortical
discharge

Fig. 6.4 Diffuse thalamocortical discharge, associated with impairment of consciousness. This may be triggered by extension of epileptic activity from a cortical focus (secondary centrencephalic epilepsy) or may occur spontaneously in patients with the centrencephalic trait of petit mal epilepsy. (Reproduced with permission from Lance & McLeod 1981.)

Table 6.2 Some important causes of symptomatic epilepsy. (Modified from *Brain's Diseases of the Nervous System*, 9th edition (Walton, 1985) by kind permission of the publishers.)

Local causes
a. Focal intracranial lesions:
    Intracranial tumour; cerebral abscess; subdural haematoma; angioma or haematoma.
b. Inflammatory and demyelinating conditions:
    Meningitis; all forms of acute and subacute encephalitis; toxoplasmosis; neurosyphilis; multiple sclerosis; cerebral cysticercosis.
c. Trauma:
    Perinatal brain injury and/or haemorrhage; head injuries of later life.
d. Congenital abnormalities:
    Congenital diplegia; cerebral malformations.
e. Degenerations and inborn errors of metabolism:
    The cerebral lipidoses; diffuse sclerosis and the leucodystrophies; encephalopathies of infancy and childhood, including 'infantile spasms'; phenylketonuria and other inborn errors; tuberous sclerosis and other phacomatoses; Pick's disease; Alzheimer's disease; progressive myoclonic epilepsy; subacute spongiform encephalopathy; Creutzfeldt-Jakob disease.
f. Vascular disorders:
    Cerebral atheroma, intracranial haemorrhage, thrombosis, embolism; eclampsia and pre-eclampsia; hypertensive encephalopathy; cerebral complications of 'connective tissue' or 'collagen' diseases; polycythaemia; intracranial aneurysm; acute cerebral ischaemia from any cause.

General causes
a. Exogenous poisons:
    Alcohol; absinthe; thujone; cocaine; strychnine; lead; chloroform; ether; insulin; amphetamine; camphor; leptazol; picrotoxin; antihistamines; intrathecal penicillin; pyridoxine analogues; some amino acids; local anaesthetics such as lignocaine; water-soluble contrast media such as metrizamide; organophosphorus and organochlorine compounds used as insecticides, and fluoracetic acid derivatives; amine-oxidase inhibitors, imipramine and its derivatives and *withdrawal* of alcohol, barbiturates and other drugs.
b. Anoxia:
    Asphyxia; carbon monoxide poisoning; carbon dioxide intoxication; nitrous oxide anaesthesia; profound anaemia.
c. Disordered metabolism:
    Uraemia; heaptic failure; water intoxication; high fat intake; porphyria; hypoglycaemia; hyperpyrexia; alkalosis; hyperkalaemia; pyridoxine deficiency.
d. Endocrine disorders:
    Parathyroid tetany; idiopathic hypoparathyroidism and pseudohypoparathyroidism; hypo-adrenalism; pituitary dysfunction; hyperthyroidism and myxoedema.
e. Conditions associated particularly with childhood:
    Rickets; acute infections ('febrile convulsions').

give a generalised convulsion with immediate loss of consciousness and no obvious localising features; while if the resistance is high, the epileptic manifestations will remain localised to the appropriate area of the body (focal epilepsy) or may only spread a short distance across the cortex (Jacksonian epilepsy) without necessarily producing any loss of consciousness. Some of the more important causes of symptomatic epilepsy are listed in Table 6.2.

However desirable an aetiological classification may be, in practice it is usually necessary to use a clinical classification which depends on the characteristics of the attack. Of all these different varieties, from the management aspect, it is important to identify two special groups. The first includes patients with true petit mal since both the prognosis and the drug management of this condition are different from those of the other forms of epilepsy. Secondly, it is important to identify patients with a focal abnormality since many of these patients will require specialised investigations, particularly if the epilepsy starts later than the second decade. An up-to-date clinical classification of the types of epileptic seizures is given in Table 6.3.

Focal epilepsy (partial or local seizures)

Focal epilepsy may result in a great variety of epileptic manifestations because the pattern of the seizures depends on the area of the brain affected by the organic lesion whether it be a tumour, a scar of previous injury, or any other pathological change, and upon the direction of spread of the epileptic discharge. Focal epilepsy always implies the presence of a localised cerebral lesion, even though in some cases techniques of investigation at present available are inadequate to demonstrate its na-

Table 6.3 The clinical classification of epileptic seizures. (Adapted from the Commission on Classification and Terminology of the International League Against Epilepsy (ILAE).)

1. Focal Seizures (partial or local)
   a. Simple focal seizures (no impairment of consciousness):
      focal motor
      focal motor with march (Jacksonian)
      somatosensory
      special sensory (simple or complex hallucinations)
      autonomic features
   b. Complex partial seizures (with impairment of consciousness);
      any of the above simple focal seizures which are followed by impairment of consciousness and may evolve to generalised tonic-clonic seizures. NB: The focal nature of these attacks may not be evident clinically and consciousness may be lost at onset

2. Generalised seizures
   a. Absence attacks (petit mal and its variants)
   b. Myoclonic seizures
   c. Clonic, tonic and clonic-tonic seizures
   d. Atonic seizures

ture. In such cases, the EEG may show focal spike or sharp-wave discharges, or localised slow activity.

If the lesion lies in or near the motor cortex, then the attack usually consists of intermittent rhythmical (clonic) jerking of a hand and arm and this may spread to the face or leg, depending upon which part of the cortex is involved. It is this spread of epileptic activity which is known as a Jacksonian march or Jacksonian epilepsy. The attack usually subsides in seconds or minutes but may be prolonged, exceptionally to hours or even days (epilepsia partialis continua) and may be followed by transient weakness of the affected member (Todd's paralysis). Though consciousness is often clouded during the attack it is sometimes unimpaired throughout. So-called *adversive attacks* with turning of the head and eyes and even of the whole body to the opposite side, can result from lesions in the frontal eye field anterior to the precentral gyrus. *Sensory epilepsy* will result from lesions near the sensory cortex, when paraesthesiae rather than jerking are the primary manifestation, though the latter may develop if spread to the motor cortex follows. When epileptic discharges begin in the occipital lobe, crude visual phenomena result (bright lines or flashes of light), while if visual association areas are involved the patient can experience formed visual hallucinations of people or of past events. Similarly a lesion near the speech areas may give transient aphasia and one near the auditory cortex auditory hallucinations, either crude or highly organised, depending upon whether the actual cortex or its association areas are primarily affected. Any of these manifestations can be the only epileptic experience that the patient has, but they may form the brief aura to an

episode of loss of consciousness which may be further complicated by a major tonic-clonic seizure. Focal epilepsy may appear clinically indistinguishable from generalised epilepsy (see below) if the focal disturbance is either too brief to be recognised or takes place in a relatively silent part of the cortex; thus loss of consciousness at the onset of an attack does not exclude focal epilepsy.

Many patients with both minor and major seizures have foci of epileptic discharge in one or other temporal lobe (temporal lobe epilepsy), a fact which may be indicated either by the content of the seizure or by the aura or sequelae of a major attack. The high incidence of this form of epilepsy is due to the frequency with which pathological changes occur in the anterior and medial parts of the temporal lobes (uncus, hippocampus, amygdaloid nucleus, Ammon's horn). These changes can result from birth injury, with 'moulding' of the head and herniation of the medial part of the temporal lobe through the tentorial hiatus, or from cerebral anoxia, however caused. Anoxic brain damage can indeed follow one or more 'febrile' convulsions in infancy. Transient anoxia occurring in repeated attacks of major epilepsy may increase such changes.

Although the lesions responsible are often present from birth, and some attacks of temporal lobe epilepsy begin in childhood, these seizures sometimes do not develop until adolescence or adult life, though acquired lesions (such as vascular malformations or neoplasms) are responsible in some older patients. The number of clinical manifestations which may be noted in such cases is legion and is clearly dependent upon the many important physiological functions which are subserved by the temporal lobes. Thus the attack may embrace intense *emotional experiences* (fear, depression, anxiety), feelings of unreality (*depersonalisation* or *jamais vu*) or a sensation of intense familiarity as if the patient were living through a vivid past experience (*déjà vu*). There may also be unpleasant hallucinations of smell or taste (*uncinate seizures*), *vasomotor manifestations* (sweating, salivation, palpitation and 'butterflies in the stomach'), or *vertigo*, while *irrational speech* or *behaviour* (automatism, such as undressing in public) or even episodes of *violent rage* can occur. It is, however, exceptional for crimes of violence to be committed in such attacks, although such a mechanism is sometimes postulated in epileptic patients charged with murder. *Gelastic epilepsy* (uncontrolled laughing during the attack) and *cursive epilepsy* (running or 'circling' as an epileptic phenomenon) are forms of automatism.

It is in occasional cases of this type that *permanent mental* changes of psychotic type may develop. The negativism and paranoid delusions which occur in some patients with severe and longstanding temporal lobe epilepsy can often be confused with schizophrenia. There is, however, no evidence that there is a specific 'epileptic personality'. Sometimes when there is spread of discharge to the lower end of the motor cortex, smacking of the lips or twitching of the corner of the mouth occurs, while if epileptic discharge spreads more posteriorly there may be distortion of visual images so that objects look smaller (*micropsia*) or larger (*macropsia*) or appear to be fading into the distance. Any such manifestations occurring episodically, without warning, either in isolation or in succession, should suggest a diagnosis of temporal lobe epilepsy, particularly if there is associated clouding of consciousness and certainly if they are followed by a major convulsion. Nevertheless, it may be difficult to distinguish between temporal lobe seizures on the one hand and episodes of phobic anxiety (with panic and depersonalisation) on the other, as fainting can result from the hyperventilation which often occurs in panic attacks. Any irritative focal lesion in the temporal lobe can produce the features described and while this may be a scar of long standing, it is sometimes an expanding lesion such as a tumour.

Powerful sensory stimuli can sometimes provoke focal epileptic discharges in patients who have foci in the appropriate area of the brain. Thus activation of epileptic seizures by music (*musicogenic epilepsy*) or intermittent light flashes (photic stimulation) has been observed and some children with '*self-induced*' *epilepsy* find that they can produce petit mal attacks by passing their open fingers rapidly between their eyes and a bright light. Other forms of '**reflex epilepsy**' include *television epilepsy* (attacks of minor or major type induced by watching television, particularly when the set is poorly adjusted), *reading epilepsy* (attacks induced by reading), and seizures (which are usually focal) precipitated by movement of the part of the body in which the fit begins (*kinesogenic epilepsy*). So-called 'drop' attacks (sudden falling without loss of consciousness) are rarely due to akinetic or inhibitory epilepsy; such episodes occurring in adolescents may be hysterical whereas in elderly patients they may be due to brain stem ischaemia but are more often unexplained. In contrast to reflex epilepsy, it is sometimes possible to abort an epileptic seizure by applying sensory stimuli which presumably compete for the occupancy of the fibre pathways along which the epileptic discharge is spreading. Some patients find that they can shorten minor attacks by means of powerful concentration; while others, for instance, who experience seizures with an aura of uncinate type (see above) can stop the attack by sniffing a substance with a powerful odour.

The rare condition of so-called **tonic epilepsy** is one in which one or more limbs suddenly become extended and rigid but there are no clonic movements; consciousness may or may not be lost. Usually such attacks result from organic brain disease. Focal tonic fits have been described in multiple sclerosis.

A type of attack which develops suddenly in infants and is characterised by momentary flexion of the head, neck and trunk with drawing up of the knees (salaam attacks) has been identified by the name of **infantile spasms**. The attacks may occur many times in the day and most affected infants eventually become spastic and severely retarded mentally even after the attacks cease, as they usually do after some months. The EEG usually shows hypsarrhythmia. The cause is unknown in many patients but some cases are due to tuberous sclerosis and the attacks rarely occur in patients with phenylketonuria. Anticonvulsants are relatively ineffective but steroid drugs may partially arrest the process.

While it is impossible to describe all the possible manifestations of partial epilepsy, the principles outlined indicate that almost any symptom of disordered cerebral function can occur as a manifestation of this condition.

Generalized seizures

Petit mal   Attacks of true petit mal (absence seizures) only begin in childhood between the ages of 5 and 15 years and occur in either sex with a slight female preponderance. The attacks nearly always cease in adolescence and only very rarely continue into adult life. There is a significantly increased history of epilepsy in first degree relatives. Petit mal itself is not symptomatic, but brain damage may act as a trigger factor in susceptible patients. The prognosis is relatively good for patients who only have absence seizures, particularly in those with a normal IQ and negative family history. Generalized tonic-clonic seizures occur in around 50% of patients with petit mal and these may coincide for a while in adolescence or may occur after the petit mal attacks have ceased.

An attack of petit mal is momentary, lasting from a few seconds up to about half a minute. Simple absence seizures form the minority, and the majority of attacks are more complex, associated with mild clonic components, tonic features, akinetic attacks or automatisms. The simplest form consists of a brief blank spell in which the child momentarily loses contact with his surroundings and, if it is brief, he may be able to continue to read aloud or carry on a conversation after an almost imperceptible pause; but if the attack lasts a little longer, the thread of conversation may be lost. A child's eyes often roll upwards and there may be a brief jerk of the limbs.

The diagnosis can usually be made without difficulty,

particularly if an attack is witnessed; they can sometimes be induced in the out-patient clinic by asking a child to hyperventilate. The EEG typically shows generalized bursts of 3 Hz spike-and-wave activity which may coincide with a clinically evident attack.

A 'petit mal variant' has been described in childhood associated with atypical absence as well as tonic seizures in association with mental retardation and an interictal EEG showing slow spike and slow wave discharges (the Lennox-Gastaut syndrome). This is a syndrome of multiple aetiology usually due to organic brain disease (including tuberous sclerosis as one example).

It is important to identify true petit mal because the drugs that are effective in this condition are not effective in other forms of epilepsy. Ethosuximide is still probably the drug of choice although some authorities prefer sodium valproate (see below). Treatment may be started with 250 mg a day or 15–25 mg/kg and the dose increased according to response. The therapeutic range of ethosuximide is 40–100 mg/l but higher levels are often tolerated. The drug is rapidly absorbed and is not protein bound. The long half-life of around 30 hours or more means that it can be given as a single daily dose, but a twice-daily regime is usually preferred because of the gastrointestinal discomfort that may result from taking too large a dose at any one time. Sodium valproate and clonazepam may also be effective in petit mal; these drugs are considered in more detail later.

Major seizures (clonic and tonic-clonic seizures)

A major convulsion or grand mal attack (Fig. 6.5) will result from a focal cerebral lesion, in the temporal lobe or elsewhere, if the spread of the epileptic discharge occurs rapidly throughout the cerebral hemispheres. It can also be a symptom of diffuse brain disease, but in many cases (though a diminishing number) no cause can be found and the attacks are presumed to be idiopathic or 'centrencephalic' in origin. The younger the patient, the more likely this is. Most patients with idiopathic major epilepsy first develop attacks in childhood or early adult life, whereas in middle age the number found to have cerebral tumours or vascular disease as a cause of the fits is much greater; however, even in late life no cause is demonstrable in many cases.

The typical major attack may begin with an aura or warning which indicates the situation of onset of the discharge but often this sensation is indefinable and little more than a 'sinking feeling' or an 'odd sensation in the head'. It is rare for an aura to last for more than a second or two and very often there is no warning at all. Consciousness is lost, the patient falls and may injure himself in the process, as when falling on to a fire. Cuts and bruises and falls downstairs are relatively common. The muscles then go rigid (the tonic phase), the teeth are clenched, the tongue is often bitten, the patient becomes cyanosed, and salivates at the mouth (frothing). Within a few seconds, the musculature relaxes and rhythmical repetitive jerking of the limbs and trunk occurs (the clonic phase). The patient is often incontinent of urine and occasionally of faeces. Sometimes the clonic phase is absent and the attack is so brief that the patient falls and then jumps up almost immediately (an akinetic attack). More frequently the jerking continues for a minute or two and is followed by relaxation. Often the patient falls into a deep sleep, but if roused he is briefly confused, or confusion may even last for several minutes or hours. In other cases he is lucid and co-operative almost at once. Often there is a headache and muscular aching which persists for some hours and vomiting occasionally occurs.

Death in a major convulsion is a very rare complication if the airway is kept clear, but if repeated convulsions

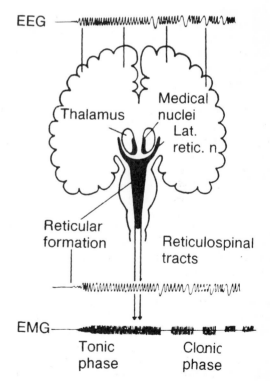

Fig. 6.5 Grand mal seizure. The high-frequency EEG discharge of the tonic phase is later interrupted by slow waves which inhibit cerebral activity and permit brief periods of muscular relaxation, responsible for the clonic phase of the seizure.
(Reproduced with permission from Lance & McLeod 1981.)

occur without recovery of consciousness between them (*status epilepticus*) there is some danger to life and treatment is an urgent matter.

It was once thought that mental disease might be a sequel of long-continued epileptic seizures. While some patients with temporal lobe epilepsy become psychotic, it is questionable whether it is the epilepsy itself or the primary pathological changes in the temporal lobe which are responsible. Similarly there is no evidence that epilepsy itself influences the mentality, but many diffuse cerebral disorders which give rise to dementia can produce symptomatic epileptic seizures. Diffuse brain damage resulting from anoxia occurring in repeated attacks of severe major epilepsy can, however, cause progressive dementia.

Myoclonic epilepsy   Myoclonus, a momentary shock-like contraction of a group of voluntary muscles, can accompany attacks of petit mal, but similar manifestations occur sporadically and repetitively in some cases without apparent impairment of consciousness, often occurring within the first hour of getting up in the morning. Sometimes repeated myoclonic jerks lead on to a major convulsive seizure and can be recognised as being likely to do so by the patient. Occasional myoclonic jerks occurring when falling asleep are physiological, but frequent nocturnal myoclonic jerks are often an epileptic manifestation and many such patients also have major seizures. Repeated myoclonic jerking can also be a symptom of diffuse progressive brain disease, in such conditions as various neuronal storage disorders (when it may occur particularly on startle), subacute sclerosing panencephalitis (when there is also progressive dementia) and the rare condition of progressive myoclonic epilepsy of Unverricht (in which the myoclonus becomes progressively more frequent and severe, dementia also occurs and the patient eventually dies from exhaustion and inanition). In such cases degenerative changes and intranuclear inclusions (Lafora bodies) may be found in the dentate nucleus of the cerebellum and abnormal mucopolysaccharides may be found in the serum.

Myoclonic jerking is also common in some cases of rapidly progressive degenerative brain disease (e.g. Creutzfeldt-Jakob disease) which give rise to progressive dementia and paralysis in middle or late life. Paramyoclonus multiplex is a name which has been given to a relatively benign disorder in which widespread myoclonic jerks of distressing frequency develop in adult life and involve facial and limb muscles to a variable extent but major fits and dementia do not occur. The condition may be familial (hereditary essential myoclonus) and is similar to another uncommon condition (hyperekplexia) in which severe sudden jerks resembling myoclonus occur only on startle (e.g. sudden noise).

Epilepsy and driving

Regulations concerning epilepsy and driving vary considerably throughout the world. In the United Kingdom a patient who has had epilepsy may drive after an attack-free period of two years whether or not the patient continues on anticonvulsant medication. However, if the patient, in consultation with his doctor, feels that he wishes to attempt withdrawal of medication after a prolonged attack-free period, many authorities believe that, because of the risk of withdrawal seizures, driving is not advisable for 12 months after withdrawal. The nature of the attack is irrelevant and even a minor temporal lobe aura is considered to be an attack of epilepsy for the purpose of this regulation. Patients who only suffer attacks while asleep (nocturnal epilepsy) may drive after a period of three years from the first attack even if the nocturnal attacks are continuing. A single epileptic attack is not usually considered sufficient to justify a diagnosis of epilepsy and these regulations do not therefore apply after a single episode. However, it is wise for such patients not to drive for a period of several months to make certain that further attacks do not occur as they would usually do within six months if the patient is to suffer from recurrent seizures. Similarly, isolated attacks which occur under exceptional circumstances which are not likely to be repeated may also be exempted. It is important to realize that physicians have no discretion in this matter and, once a diagnosis of epilepsy has been made, the patient is under an obligation to declare this to the licensing authorities who alone are empowered under the law to determine the patient's eligibility to hold a licence.

Epilepsy and pregnancy

It should be assumed that all female patients in the child-bearing age are likely to become pregnant during treatment with anti-convulsant medication which may extend from two or three years to the rest of their lives. Since carbamazepine is the drug of choice in pregnancy, this drug should be the first choice of anticonvulsants for a female patient in this age group. In common with phenytoin and phenobarbitone, carbamazepine is a powerful inducer of liver enzyme activity so that patients who wish to take the combined contraceptive pill should be given a preparation containing at least 50 μg of oestrogen; the more commonly used 30 μg preparations may not give adequate contraception, and good cycle control on a lower dose preparation does not necessarily indicate inhibition of ovulation.

Anticonvulsant medication should be continued throughout pregnancy. The adverse teratogenic effects of most drugs (which are in any event relatively slight—see below) occur in the first trimester so that by the time a patient seeks advice about the effects of her anticonvulsant medication on the fetus, it is often too late to make a worthwhile change, with the exception that it may be sensible to withdraw phenobarbitone, which has a depressant effect on the infant at term. The blood level of most anticonvulsants tends to decline during pregnancy and sometimes this results in an increase in the attack rate, but the dose of anticonvulsant medication should not be automatically increased during pregnancy unless this change occurs. Epilepsy seldom presents any difficulty at the time of delivery unless one or more doses is omitted and it is, of course, important to keep to a regular regime. The amount of anticonvulsant medication that is excreted in breast milk is very small and, with the exception of phenobarbitone, such treatment is not a contraindication to breast feeding.

There is a slightly increased but significant risk of congenital abnormalities in children born of women with epilepsy whether or not they are on anticonvulsant medication. This risk is further increased by some drugs, particularly phenytoin, which is associated with an increased risk of cleft lip and palate and congenital heart disease, and sodium valproate which is associated with an increased risk of neural tube defects.

The risk of a child born of a mother with epilepsy developing the same condition is critically dependent on whether there is any history of epilepsy on the father's side. If there is only a history of epilepsy in one parent, the risk of epilepsy developing in the child is only slightly greater than chance, but if there is a history of epilepsy in both parents, the risk of the child being affected becomes substantial.

Pseudoseizures

Hysterical fits can be extremely difficult to recognise and to treat. Patients may give a very plausible account of attacks and may even have witnessed attacks which are indistinguishable from the real thing, though incontinence, tongue biting or injury are rather rare in hysterical epilepsy unless the patient has been asked about these so often that he or she ultimately obliges. The situation is made more difficult by the fact that some patients with genuine epilepsy also have pseudoseizures. The problem may be compounded by the fact that some of these patients have slightly abnormal EEGs which turn out to be irrelevant. When pseudoseizures are suspected it is helpful to have a 24-hour tape or simultaneous video and EEG recordings (telemetry), though many patients with frequent pseudoseizures often stop having the attacks when these recordings are made.

An entirely normal EEG recorded during an apparently florid grand mal attack is almost certainly indicative of a pseudoseizure, but the surface EEG may be normal during some temporal lobe attacks, especially when these arise in the medial part of the temporal lobe.

Management of patients with epilepsy

Once the diagnosis has been made, it is well worth spending some time explaining to the patient what epilepsy is and how it is best managed so that they have as full an understanding as is possible about their condition. This is particularly important because they may need to accept the necessity of taking drugs for many years and there may well be serious consequences if they suddenly stop medication. With the exception of true petit mal (see above) all other forms of epilepsy respond to the standard drugs. The drugs of first choice are carbamazepine, phenytoin and valproate. Carbamazepine is to be preferred in all women of child-bearing age for reasons already given. Valproate is often very effective in patients with idiopathic grand mal epilepsy, particularly in those patients who have or have had petit mal or myoclonus. Other effective drugs include primidone, phenobarbitone and the benzodiazepines, particularly clobazam and clonazepam. Unfortunately, the benzodiazepines show 'drug fatigue' and may become less useful after a number of months, but may be particularly effective in myoclonus. Table 6.4 gives some basic data on the more commonly used anticonvulsant drugs.

Treatment should be started with a low dose of one drug. If this fails to control attacks, the blood level should be measured and the dose adjusted until either the attacks are under control or the blood level reaches the upper end of the therapeutic range. If attacks continue, then a second drug should be substituted for the first. It is desirable to keep to a single drug if at all possible and

Table 6.4 The commoner anticonvulsant drugs. Half-lives vary considerably from patient to patient with the duration of treatment and the concomitant use of other drugs. The therapeutic ranges should only be used as a guide; they are arbitrarily derived from clinical experience and patients may respond or show signs of intoxication at lower levels than indicated or tolerate higher blood levels.

Drugs	Daily dose range (mg)	Therapeutic range (mg/l)	T½ (hrs)
Phenytoin	200–400	7–17	12–36
Carbamazepine	200–1600	4–12	9–15
Valproate	600–3000	50–100	6–10
Clonazepam	1–6	10–70	25–30
Primidone	500–1500	<14	12–15
Phenobarbitone	30–120	10–30	80–110
Ethosuximide	250–1500	40–100	30–60

studies have shown that about 80% of all patients with epilepsy can achieve complete control on a single drug provided that the dose is properly adjusted. A second drug should only be added if monotherapy with all the principal drugs has failed despite monitoring blood levels after changes in medication. It is important to realise that many drugs take some time to equilibrate, notably phenytoin and primidone.

It is always very difficult to make a decision about stopping medication. There is some evidence that the chances of stopping medication and remaining attack-free increases with the attack-free period on treatment up to about three years and there may be some further gain up to five years, but after this it is likely that the patient will either need to take medication indefinitely or alternatively they may no longer need to be on it at all. This applies particularly to adults where the risk of recurrence is about 50%. In children the risk of recurrence is about 20%. There is some evidence that the longer the epilepsy took to control initially on medication, the less likely is the patient to be able to come off drugs even after a three to five year attack-free period. Unfortunately, the EEG is not a very good guide unless it is very abnormal. Some patients who have been receiving a small dose of an anticonvulsant drug for many years may be found to have subtherapeutic blood levels, in which case the chances of recurrence when the drug is stopped are less than if the drug level is fully therapeutic. It is clearly undesirable for a patient to continue with medication for the rest of his or her life unless this is necessary; but it is equally undesirable to stop treatment if the patient is going to have further fits, particularly as recurrent seizures may be more difficult to control than they were initially and they may not respond to the dose of drugs which had controlled them satisfactorily for the previous few years. The advantages and disadvantages must be discussed in full with the patient since they must accept the risk of having further attacks if the drugs are stopped. Of course any reduction in dosage must be very gradual and patients should be advised not to drive during the reduction in dose as they are at risk throughout this period and not just in the months after the drug has been stopped altogether.

Fortunately the complications of treatment with the standard anticonvulsant drugs, though common, are not usually serious. Overdosage, which can usually be identified by measurement of drug levels, is characterised by drowsiness, ataxia and dysarthria but usually resolves after reduction in dosage. Coarsening of the features, hirsutism and gum hypertrophy may result from phenytoin and its derivatives and very rarely a chronic cerebellar syndrome or polyneuropathy can develop. Anticonvulsant osteomalacia and macrocytic anaemia due to folate deficiency also occur from time to time, while hepatic failure is an occasional idiosyncratic reaction to valproate.

Status epilepticus

Repeated seizures without full recovery between are known as **status epilepticus**. Minor status is difficult to recognise and is often misdiagnosed, but can be readily identified on the EEG. Some authorities believe that minor status is rare in true petit mal and much commoner in the Lennox-Gastaut syndrome (see above). Major status has a significant mortality and should be treated as a neurological emergency. The initial treatment of choice is 10 mg of intravenous diazepam or 1–2 mg of intravenous clonazepam. These doses may be repeated once. Intramuscular diazepam should be avoided as it may produce prolonged sedation without controlling the seizures. If there is any doubt about the control of the attacks, the patient should be immediately transferred to a hospital where facilities for artificial ventilation exist. Chlormethiazole by intravenous infusion can be very effective and the patient's condition can be controlled from minute to minute by varying the drip rate. Intravenous infusions containing diazepam should be avoided as they are often ineffective. Chlormethiazole should not be used if there are no facilities for artificial ventilation since profound respiratory depression may occur, particularly if the patient is already taking phenobarbitone. If these measures fail, the patient should be paralysed with relaxant drugs and ventilated and an intravenous infusion of thiopentone begun. Under these circumstances it may be very helpful to have continuous EEG monitoring, and machines exist (known as cerebral function monitors) which have a very slow paper speed.

Status epilepticus occurs in two groups of patients. The first group is those who are already known to have epilepsy and in them status is often precipitated by the sudden withdrawal or reduction of drugs. It is important to re-establish the patient's normal anticonvulsant regime as soon as possible. Anticonvulsant blood levels taken on admission can be a useful guide to compliance. Sometimes status may be precipitated by alcohol. The second major group is of those patients with no previous history of epilepsy, in which case the development of status usually indicates some serious underlying organic cerebral lesion such as a cerebral abscess.

Conclusions

Epilepsy may thus be classified from the aetiological standpoint into idiopathic and symptomatic varieties and the idiopathic group is clearly one which is diminishing steadily, as newer techniques reveal more organic disorders of the brain which produce epilepsy as a symptom. Clinically true petit mal (absence seizures) is to be distinguished as a separate entity, at present of unknown aetiology; in many patients with major seizures, too, the condition must still be regarded as 'idiopathic'. Many patients with grand mal, however, and most of those with partial seizures, are suffering from focal organic brain disease, frequently affecting the temporal lobe. Accurate diagnosis is of great importance from the point of view of treatment.

Syncope and other brief disorders of consciousness

It is sometimes very difficult to differentiate clinically between simple faints or syncopal attacks and epileptic seizures. Syncope is most common in young patients, particularly adolescent girls, and is often produced by long periods of standing in one position (as in church, on parade or in morning school assembly), by an emotional shock ('the sight of blood') or by 'stuffy' atmospheres. It is particularly liable to occur in early pregnancy, can develop at any age in patients with uraemia or blood loss, or with heart block (**the Stoke–Adams syndrome**). In the latter condition, syncope with pallor occurs during a period of cardiac asystole, and when the circulation is restored, the patient's face flushes and there may even be convulsive movements. Indeed, syncope however caused can rarely result in transient epileptic manifestations, including transient twitching of the limbs and urinary incontinence, if cerebral anoxia is sufficiently prolonged. Cardiac lesions other than heart block, which diminish cardiac output (e.g. aortic stenosis, auricular fibrillation, paroxysmal tachycardia or other arrhythmias) can be associated with recurrent fainting. So too may be chronic bronchitis and emphysema, in that severe bouts of coughing with fixation of the chest wall in expansion may so impair venous return to the heart as to result in episodes of **cough syncope**. **Carotid sinus syncope** occurs in those in whom turning of the head or pressure upon the neck causes abnormal slowing of the heart rate or even asystole due to increased sensitivity of the carotid sinus. Rarely, fainting occurs in patients with stenotic lesions of the carotid and vertebral vessels which reduce cerebral blood flow. **Micturition syncope** is not uncommon, particularly in the elderly male patient who gets up during the night with a full bladder and loses his senses in the toilet.

In general terms, syncope is due to cerebral ischaemia, resulting usually from pooling of blood in the skin and viscera. Generally the patient feels a 'swimming in the head' and a sensation of heat; he then perspires and can

usually reach a place of safety before consciousness is lost (unless he is standing on parade). The loss of consciousness is usually brief, the patient's skin is deathly pale, cold and clammy, and his pulse is often thin and rapid, but occasionally slow. The aura of a syncopal attack is usually considerably longer than that of an epileptic seizure, there are often emotional or physical precipitants, and injury in attacks is uncommon, while convulsive movements and incontinence are rare. The attacks usually occur when standing and not when sitting or lying. Often they are brought on by standing up abruptly. These are the principal points upon which differential diagnosis is based. Syncope due to transient postural hypotension is particularly likely to occur after a hot bath, overindulgence in alcohol, after sympathectomy, in patients with spinal cord lesions impairing pressor reflexes (as in tabes dorsalis) and in those taking hypotensive drugs or some tranquillisers (especially phenothiazines).

In the uncommon condition of **chronic orthostatic hypotension** (the Shy-Drager syndrome), which is often familial and is due to degeneration in the autonomic nervous system, the blood pressure falls when the patient assumes the upright position and as the compensatory reflexes are impaired there is no pallor, sweating or tachycardia and consciousness is lost; recovery occurs as soon as the patient lies down. In many cases dysarthria and cerebellar ataxia eventually develop; at autopsy, degeneration of cells in the intermediolateral grey column of the spinal cord is usually found. Some patients develop progressive Parkinsonian features, dementia and impotence, even occasionally incontinence (so-called **progressive multi-system degeneration**).

Drop attacks are episodes in which the patient's legs give way until he falls but does not lose consciousness. They are commonest in elderly women and are either due to transient brain stem ischaemia or to an inhibitory mechanism of unknown cause involving the brain stem reticular substance.

Hysterical hyperventilation (rapid panting respiration) which is often accompanied by panic and which leads to paraesthesiae in the lips and tongue and even to tetany, may also cause syncope and is often misdiagnosed. The **tetany** which occurs as a result of hyperventilation is due to alkalosis resulting from loss of CO_2 in the expired air. Other disorders associated with tetany which reduce the serum ionised calcium (repeated vomiting, dietary alkalosis, rickets and osteomalacia, hypoparathyroidism and malabsorption) do not usually give rise to attacks of loss of consciousness. However, in idiopathic hypoparathyroidism attacks of epilepsy are common. The typical carpopedal spasms of tetany with other evidence of neuromuscular excitability (positive Cvostek's and Trousseau's signs) usually ensure that attacks of this nature are not confused with focal epilepsy and estimation of the serum calcium will be diagnostic.

Spontaneous hypoglycaemia can cause attacks of light-headedness, fatigue, sweating, paraesthesiae, giddiness and even confused and irrational behaviour. Rarely, major epileptic convulsions result, particularly in those patients who have a tumour of the islets of Langerhans, with excessive insulin production (organic hyperinsulinism). When reactive or functional hyperinsulinism is the cause, due to an excessive fall in blood sugar following the peak produced by a high carbohydrate meal, or after rapid gastric emptying (such as may follow gastrectomy or gastroenterostomy), the symptoms are as a rule less severe. Nevertheless this condition, too, must be considered in determining the cause of transient disturbances of consciousness.

REFERENCES

Adams R D, Victor M 1985 Principles of neurology, 3rd edn. McGraw Hill, New York

Cooper J R, Bloom F E 1986 The biochemical basis of neuropharmacology, 5th edn. Oxford University Press, Oxford

Eadie M J, Tyrer J H 1980 Anticonvulsant therapy, 2nd edn. Churchill Livingstone, Edinburgh

Jackson J H 1958 In: Taylor J (ed) Selected writings of John Hughlings Jackson, Vol 1. Staples, London

Johnson R H, Lambie D G, Spalding J M K 1984 Neurocardiology. Major problems in neurology, Vol 13 (Walton J, series ed). Saunders, London

Laidlaw J, Richens A 1982 A textbook of epilepsy, 2nd edn. Churchill Livingstone, Edinburgh

Lance J W, McLeod J G 1981 A physiological approach to clinical neurology, 3rd edn. Butterworth, London

Matthews W B 1975 Practical neurology, 3rd edn. Blackwell, Oxford, chs 3, 4

Parkes J D 1985 Sleep and its disorders. Major problems in neurology, Vol 14 (Walton J, series ed). Saunders, London

Patton H D, Sundsten J W, Crill W E, Swanson P D 1976 Introduction to basic neurology. Saunders, Philadelphia

Plum F, Posner J B 1980 Diagnosis of stupor and coma, 3rd edn. Davis, Philadelphia

Porter R 1984 Epilepsy: 100 elementary principles. Major problems in neurology, Vol 12 (Walton J, series ed). Saunders, London

Smythies J R 1970 Brain mechanisms and behaviour. Academic Press, New York

Sutherland J M, Eadie M J 1980 The epilepsies: modern diagnosis and treatment, 3rd edn. Churchill Livingstone, Edinburgh

Swash M, Kennard C (eds) 1985 Scientific basis of clinical neurology. Churchill Livingstone, Edinburgh

Teasdale C, Jennett W B 1974 Assessment of coma and impaired consciousness. Lancet ii: 81

Walton J N 1985 Brain's diseases of the nervous system, 9th edn. Oxford University Press, Oxford

Walton J N 1987 Introduction to clinical neuroscience, 2nd edn. Baillière Tindall, London

7. Behaviour, memory, intellect, personality and their disorders

The principal difference between the human and the subhuman brain consists in the great development of the cerebral cortex in man. The cortex is, in relation to perception, an end station at which are received nervous impulses derived from the eyes, the ears and other sensory organs. The corresponding regions of the cortex are linked by association paths through which the sensations which form the raw material of perception evoke memories and become enriched with meanings which can be communicated to others by means of speech, writing and gesture (see Ch. 5). The perceptual function of the cerebral cortex, therefore, is primarily discriminative, and its massive development in man compared with that in the lower animals is paralleled by the enhancement of his discriminative faculties. This has occurred in spite of there having been little improvement, and in some cases an actual retrogression, of man's sensory acuity.

By contrast there is far less difference between man and the lower animals with respect to the development of subcortical centres, in particular the thalamus and hypothalamus. These regions of the brain, basal alike in situation and in function, are intimately concerned with the affective element in feeling, with the emotional and instinctive life, with the regulation of the autonomic nervous system, and to some extent with metabolic and endocrine function. The brain, however, works as a whole and there is a constant interplay between cortical and subcortical activity. Perception evokes emotion and, conversely, emotion provides the interest which activates perception.

There is another aspect, however, of this relationship. Discrimination, the function of the cortex, implies inhibition as, if an organism is to react appropriately to a stimulus, inappropriate reactions must be simultaneously inhibited. This is true even at the level of a simple reflex arc. It is far more essential when the range both of potential stimuli and of potential reactions has been so enhanced by the development of the cortex. The cortex,

therefore, acquires inhibitory functions as the complement of its discriminative functions.

THE FUNCTION OF THE DIENCEPHALON

The thalamus plays a fundamental role in the organisation of animal behaviour. The dorsal thalamus is divided into an external portion and an internal core (Fig. 7.1). Each of these has nuclei that receive impulses from outside the thalamus (extrinsic nuclei) and other nuclei which, as far as is known, do not (intrinsic nuclei). The extrinsic nuclei of the external portion receive the somatic sensory tracts, the optic and auditory pathways; the intrinsic nucleus is the posterior nucleus. The extrinsic nuclei of the internal core receive impulses from the posterior hypothalamus and the central reticular formation; the intrinsic nucleus is the medial. The extrinsic nuclei of the external portion project to the primary sensory cortical areas concerned with somatic sensibility, hearing and vision in the parietal, temporal and occipital lobes, while the intrinsic, posterior nucleus projects to the rest of the parieto-temporo-occipital cortex. The extrinsic nuclei of the internal core project to the limbic areas of the medial aspect of the frontal and parietal lobes and to the anterior rhinencephalon and basal ganglia, and the medial (intrinsic) nucleus projects to the prefrontal cortex. There is an important corticofugal pathway (the medial fore-brain bundle) running from the medio-basal part of the frontal lobe to the thalamus and the hypothalamic nuclei, including the corpora mammillaria.

The projections from the extrinsic nuclei of the external part of the dorsal thalamus are the sensory afferent pathways, and interference with them causes sensory loss in the corresponding modalities. Damage to the parts of the cerebral cortex supplied by the projections from the intrinsic nuclei of the external part leads to a failure to differentiate and respond to patterns of sensory stimuli, a condition resembling agnosia (p. 66).

These nuclei, their projections, and the corresponding cortical areas therefore provide a higher level perceptual discriminative mechanism.

On the other hand ablations and stimulations of the anatomical systems represented by the nuclei of the internal core of the thalamus (and their projections through the medial and basal telencephalon) affect feeding (eating and drinking), fighting and aggression, fleeing and avoidance, mating, and maternal behaviour. They are therefore concerned with what may in the broadest sense be termed instinctive behaviour. All such activities are linked with emotion to a greater or a lesser extent.

The role of various hypothalamic nuclei in controlling the activity of the autonomic nervous system is now well documented. Emotional disorders and altered autonomic activity are closely interlinked. The hypothalamus, brain stem reticular system, parts of the thalamus, hippocampus, amygdala, fornix and cingulate gyrus are closely interlinked and play a fundamental integrating role in controlling emotion as well as memory and behaviour. Even though in anatomical terms parts of the hypothalamus and brain stem reticular substance are not strictly part of the limbic system, functionally they are so closely related that it is reasonable to regard all of these structures as forming the limbic brain (Figs. 7.2 and 7.3).

Some parts of the basal ganglia also possess behavioural functions. Thus the nucleus accumbens, anatomically related to the striatum, seems to act as a 'bridge', bringing limbic influences to bear on motor function. Various neurotransmitters and their respective functions were mentioned in Chapter 1; however, it is now well known that increased serotonin activity leads to psychomotor retardation, while serotonin antagonist drugs have a stimulant and antidepressant effect. Drugs which deduce catecholamine activity decrease spontaneous locomotion and inhibit conditioned responses and exploratory behaviour, while dopamine agonists can cause stereotyped behaviour. Both adrenergic and non-adrenergic activity are important in pleasure and reward responses and in hypothalamic activity. The mesolimbic dopamine system seems to be related to motivational arousal and that of the striatum to motor arousal, so that the proper functioning of these systems is needed for the integration of sensory inputs, memory, motivation and motor expression.

In the hypothalamus the anterior and posterior nuclei are concerned with temperature and cardiovascular control and with endocrine activity, and the supraoptic nucleus produces antidiuretic hormone (ADH) (p. 322). The perifornical nucleus, if stimulated, causes hunger, increased blood pressure and sometimes rage; the ventromedial nucleus, satiety; the lateral hypothalamic area, thirst and hunger; and the mammillary body, feeding reflexes. Many of these functions appear to be mediated through the reticular formation. A series of polypeptides containing between 17 and 21 amino acids, known as endorphins, may play a transmitter role in various parts of the limbic system, thus fulfilling a variety of behavioural functions. Their exact function has yet to be fully defined. Smaller polypeptides known as encephalins seem to act as intrinsic analgesic substances elaborated within the brain itself, as they combine with opiate receptors and are known as endogenous ligands.

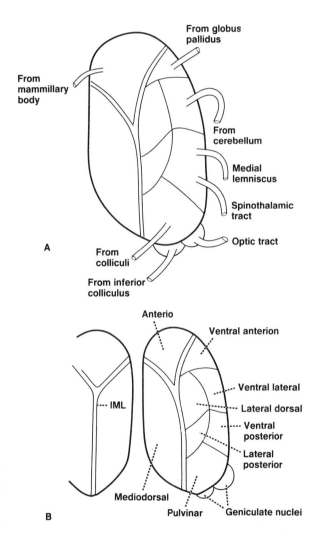

Fig. 7.1   A Thalamus from above, with nuclear subdivisions. IML = internal medullary lamina. **B** Diagram indicating sources of input to the specific thalamic nuclei. (Reproduced with permission from FitzGerald 1985.)

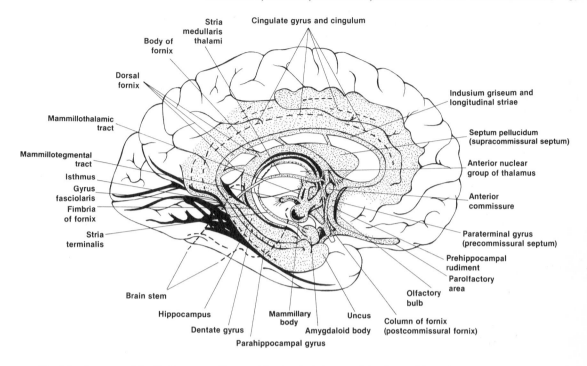

Fig. 7.2 Anatomy of the limbic system illustrated by the shaded areas of the figure. (Reproduced with permission from Warwick & Williams, *Gray's Anatomy*, 35th British edn., 1980.)

THE LIMBIC SYSTEM: BEHAVIOURAL FUNCTIONS

Many hypothalamic and other limbic centres are especially concerned with sensations that have an emotional content and are either pleasant (rewarding) or painful, probably in an emotional rather than a physical sense (punishment or aversion). Centres in the septum, hypothalamus, ventromedial nuclei, and medial forebrain bundle may produce such a feeling of reward or stimulation that if an indwelling electrode is inserted and an animal can then apply stimuli himself he will do so repeatedly. By contrast, stimulation of the perifornical nucleus of the hypothalamus and of the mesencephalic central grey matter may give manifestations suggestive of pain, displeasure and punishment, and will outweigh the effects of simultaneous stimulation of a reward centre. Physiologically, both habituation (diminishing response) and reinforcement have been shown with different stimulus patterns. Pharmacologically both reward and punishment can be suppressed by various tranquillising drugs. It seems probable that much human behaviour is dependent upon the balance of activity in reward and punishment centres.

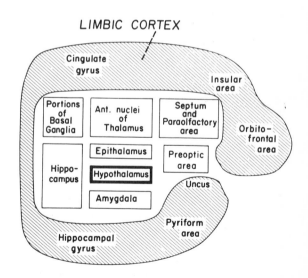

Fig. 7.3 The limbic system. (Reproduced with permission from Guyton 1981.)

Intense stimulation of the punishment centres (e.g. the periformical nucleus) of animals may produce a rage response, whereas stimulation more rostrally gives manifestations of fear and anxiety. By contrast, repeated stimulation of reward centres will result in docility and tranquillity. Stimulation dorsal to the mammillary bodies gives excessive wakefulness and excitement with evidence of sympathetic overactivity, while stimulation in parts of the septum, anterior hypothalamus, or some parts of the thalamic reticular nuclei causes somnolence and sometimes actual sleep.

THE LIMBIC SYSTEM AND EMOTION

Psychophysiologically, emotion involves a number of factors, including: (1) some external object which excites it, (2) specific feelings characteristic of particular emotions and, (3) the fact that the emotion tends to find expression in some characteristic action. Accompanying the feelings and the motor activities there are (4) certain other physiological manifestations in which the autonomic nervous system and endocrine activity play an important part. And, finally, there is often (5) a pre-existing physiological state which is necessary if the appetite or emotional need is to be fulfilled. This is most obvious in the case of hunger, thirst and the sexual impulse.

The limbic system controls not only the emotions but also memory and much of behaviour. However, the functions of many parts of the limbic system are still poorly understood and what little we know has been largely derived from experiments involving electrical stimulation.

Stimulation of the amygdala can cause changes in heart rate and blood pressure, defaecation and micturition, pupillary dilatation and an increased output of various anterior pituitary hormones. In other areas involuntary movements (tonic or circling movements, chewing or lip-smacking) may be elicited or, alternatively, an arrest reaction may be produced in which the animal 'freezes' in one posture. Yet other areas, if stimulated, give manifestations of rage, fear, reward or punishment as described above, while elsewhere stimuli produce sexual activity including erection, ejaculation, copulatory movements, ovulation or uterine contraction. Thus, many of the emotional and behavioural manifestations of temporal lobe epilepsy, including fear or hypersexuality, may be reproduced.

The hippocampus distributes many outgoing signals to the hypothalamus and other parts of the limbic system via the fornix. Its other major role appears to relate to memory (see below). Animal experiments suggest that the hippocampus also plays a part in 'gold-directed'

behaviour, but its principal function, in consort with the reticular formation and other parts of the limbic system, appears to lie in focusing attention and in acquiring and retaining new information in an orderly manner. Stimulation of other parts of the limbic cortex (the cingulate gyrus and orbitofrontal cortex) can give changes in respiratory and cardiac rate and blood pressure, facilitation of movements induced by cortical stimulation elsewhere, licking, swallowing, changes in gastrointestinal motility and secretion, and various affective reactions (e.g. rage or docility, increased or diminished awareness). Ablation of the cingulate gyri may give tameness in animals and suppression of previous rage reactions, while bilateral ablations of the orbitofrontal cortex may cause insomnia and motor restlessness. In man, cingulectomy and various other ablations of limbic cortex have been used as psychosurgical procedures for the treatment of obsessional states, hypersexuality and other behaviour disorders.

MEMORY

Types of memory and memory mechanisms

The recording and registration of information is a process known as memorising. In clinical practice, memory is usually divided into short-term and long-term memory as well as secondary and tertiary varieties. Short-term (or primary) memory is the ability to retain a few facts, words, numbers or letters (such as a telephone number or name and address) for a few seconds or minutes or more at a time. This information can be instantly recalled at will. Long-term memory is the storage in the brain of information which can be recalled minutes, hours, days, months or years later. Secondary memories are those long-term memories which are stored in the form of relatively weak memory traces so that some time may be needed to recall the information or else it can only be recalled for a few days after it has been recorded (recent memory). Tertiary memories, by contrast, are so deeply imprinted that they can be recalled at will throughout life (as in the case of the individual's own name, the letters of the alphabet, prime numerals, etc.).

The mechanism of short-term memory is still uncertain. The recall mechanism has been attributed to (a) activity in precisely defined reverberating neuronal circuits, (b) post-tetanic potentiation in appropriate neurones, and (c) prolonged depolarisation of neurones with the production of electrotonic dendritic potentials. Long-term memory is thought to depend upon physical changes in synapses, giving rise to permanent changes in excitability of postsynaptic neurones in appropriate neuronal circuits, thus leading to progressive synaptic facilitation. A role for RNA and for glial cell activity in this process has been postulated but remains unproven. The repetition of information (rehearsal) and the coding of sensory stimuli into different classes of information assist the consolidation of long-term memories and the transfer of short-term into long-term memory. It now appears that while short-term memory involves the modification of pre-existing proteins by second messenger systems, long-term memory requires the expression of additional genes.

The pathophysiology of memory

Clinical, behavioural and neuropathological evidence clearly indicates that the recording and registration of information occurs in the hippocampus and its connections, but that the storage of the memory trace (engram) plainly involves a considerable part of the limbic system. Severe loss of recent memory with inability to record and retain new impressions follows lesions of the mammillary bodies in the Wernicke-Korsakoff syndrome or after some surgical procedures. Remote memory is sometimes impaired in these subjects to a greater extent than is generally realised. Division of the fornix and extensive bilateral frontal lobe damage do not as a rule affect memory, while bilateral anterior cingulectomy produces only transient memory impairment. The effect of bilateral lesions of the thalamic dorsomedial nuclei in animals upon learning tasks may be more profound. In the 'split-brain' animal each hemisphere can be trained to store information so that the corpus callosum is not essential for information processing, storage and retrieval. However, after commissurotomy in man, some defects of memory have been found, suggesting that processes mediating the initial encoding of engrams and the retrieval and read-out of contralateral engram elements involve interhemispheric co-operation. Work carried out in flat-worms suggested that cellular RNA is involved in the memory process and that acquired information can be transferred to a worm that ingests RNA derived from one that has succeeded in learning a task. Much more work upon the transfer of memory by such chemical means has been done with results which have often been conflicting. As Cooper et al (1982) pointed out: 'There is evidence that protein and RNA synthesis may occur along with learning but the experiment has yet to be designed which explicitly relates these two events'.

In clinical practice, lesions of the anterior temporal lobe and particularly of the hippocampus have been the ones shown most often to impair memory. Investigations of temporal lobe epilepsy in man, involving electrical stimulation, have shown that memories can be evoked or temporary amnesia induced by hippocampal stimulation. Persistent, profound and generalised loss of recent mem-

ory has been reported in cases of bilateral hippocampal excision or infarction, the amnesia being unrelated to any deterioration of the intellect or personality of the subject. Cases of recent memory impairment have also been described after unilateral temporal lobe lesions, but it has been suggested that in such cases the corresponding area on the opposite side may previously have been damaged, and recent neuropathological studies have supported this hypothesis. The syndrome of transient global amnesia (see p. 96) is thought to result from bilateral temporal lobe ischaemia. The use of new and precise techniques of studying cognitive function, involving dichotic learning tasks and other methods of assessing auditory inattention, have shown that a unilateral defect of 'auditory memory' may follow unilateral anterior temporal lobectomy performed for temporal lobe epilepsy. Hence there is no doubt that bilateral hippocampal lesions are likely to cause permanent and continuing loss of memory for recent events. Such memory loss may be particularly prominent after recovery from herpes simplex encephalitis.

THE FUNCTIONS OF THE FRONTAL LOBE

In animals, experimental damage to the frontal cortex, which derives its thalamic input from the medial nuclear group, affects the ability of the animal to solve problems that depend upon the use of past experience. It has long been believed that the frontal lobes play a particularly important part in the control of intellect, initiative, personality and social consciousness. However, maximum amputation of the right or left frontal lobe produces little change except for some impairment of those processes necessary for planned initiative, sometimes with diminished inhibition of affective responses and a tendency to euphoria, less often with depression. Changes in psychomotor activity may take the form either of restlessness or lack of initiative and interest. The more automatic forms of intelligence are relatively well preserved, together with attention and memory, but the higher forms of reasoning, thinking in symbols and judgement may be impaired, especially after bilateral frontal lesions.

The operation of prefrontal leucotomy or lobotomy threw new light upon the functions of the frontal lobes, which have been summarised as follows:

According to Freeman and Watts, the prefrontal regions in man are concerned with foresight, imagination and the perception of the self. These psychological functions are invested with emotion by way of the association fibres that link the hippocampus and cingulate gyrus with the thalamus and hypothalamus. It would seem, then, that the functions of the prefrontal lobes are concerned with the adjustment of the personality as a whole to future contingencies. The imagination, therefore, in the pure sense of the term, may be said to reside in the prefrontal areas. Pure intellection in the sense of analysis, synthesis and selectivity does not appear to require the integrity of the frontal and prefrontal areas to the extent that was previously thought necessary.

Despite the virtual certainty that the frontal lobe is concerned with the storage and maintenance of certain social behaviour patterns, its exact functions are still poorly understood. Disturbances of micturition, including frequency, urgency and incontinence, are well recognised to occur in some patients with bifrontal lesions and less often as a consequence of a unilateral frontal tumour. The frontal lobes presumably possess a regulating function, shaping the development of intellectual resources and the pursuit of long-term goals. The effect upon personality of massive bifrontal lesions was well demonstrated by the celebrated case of Phineas Gage who in 1848 had a crowbar driven through the front of his skull. He was described as 'fitful, irreverent, indulging at times in the greatest profanity ... manifesting but little deference for his fellows, impatient of restraint or advice when it conflicts with his desires, at times pertinaciously obstinate, yet capricious and vacillatory'. Thus, a 'frontal lobe syndrome' has come to be recognised. An affected individual previously capable of judgement and sustained application and organisation of his life may thus become aimless and improvident, with loss of tact, sensitivity and self-control, and exhibiting impulsiveness and a failure to appreciate the consequences of reckless behaviour.

Destruction of the dorsomedial nuclei of the thalamus has been shown to produce effects similar to those of frontal leucotomy. The syndrome may follow stereotaxic surgery for parkinsonism. Since the efferent frontothalamic pathways are comparatively scanty, it has been suggested that leucotomy works by interrupting the afferent pathways from the dorsomedial nuclei to the frontal cortex and from the anteromedial nuclei to the cingulate gyri. Because the standard prefrontal operation all too often gave relief from stress at the cost of lethargy, social incompetence and other manifestations of the frontal lobe syndrome, it was replaced by more selective procedures such as undercutting of the orbital cortex, cingulectomy, frontal tractotomy and various stereotaxic techniques which aim at producing relief of emotional tension or behaviour disorder with minimal effects upon intellect and personality.

BRAIN, MIND AND INTELLECT

Although the formulation of thoughts and the correlation and analysis of thought processes are clearly functions of the brain, we still know comparatively little of the ultimate mechanisms by which these important activities are controlled. Memory, as discussed earlier, is clearly the ability to record and to recall thoughts and sensorimotor experiences, while learning is the ability of the brain to store these memories and to utilise them at will. Intellect is the ability to analyse complex sensory information and to formulate abstract thoughts and concepts. This requires:

a. the separation of complex sensory inputs into their constituent modalities, which may each be recorded in different areas of the cerebral cortex.
b. the analysis and interpretation of this information in relation to the content of the existing memory store.
c. the establishment of new memory engrams, and
d. the formulation of the appropriate abstract concept or thought, or alternatively of some physical activity which constitutes a response to the information received.

These processes may lead to modification of subsequent responses to similar inputs in the light of the past experience. There are many diseases of the brain which impair both intellect and memory, but these two qualities may be disordered independently, or one may be affected more severely than the other, as a consequence of selective and focal cerebral lesions. Subsequent parts of this chapter will deal with some of the mechanisms and disease processes through which they are disordered.

HALLUCINATIONS AND ALLIED DISORDERS OF PERCEPTION

Hallucinations may be defined as mental impressions of sensory vividness occurring without external stimulus, but appearing to be located or to possess a cause located outside the subject. An illusion is defined as a misinterpretation of an external stimulus, but some illusions are closely related to hallucinations and occur as symptoms of hallucinatory states. A delusion, by contrast, is an idea or thought (such as a false concept of persecution) which has no substance in fact. In contrast to visual and auditory hallucinations, it is a pure thought process with no sensory content. Hallucinations and delusions may occur together in various toxic/confusional states and in psychotic illnesses such as schizophrenia. Though hallucinations manifest themselves as changes in the content of consciousness, there is considerable evidence that they are often the result of disordered function of the reticulo-hypothalamic and associated pathways concerned with the state of consciousness as a whole.

The principal circumstances in which hallucinations may occur are:

1. in dreaming and the hypnagogic state (p. 71),
2. in disorders of sleep,
3. as a result of organic disease of the sense organs or of the central nervous system (including focal epilepsy),
4. in states of intoxication by alcohol and other drugs, and particularly after the administration of substances such as mescaline and lysergic acid or after withdrawal of alcohol, amphetamines or barbiturates, and
5. in certain psychoses (especially schizophrenia).

Visual hallucinations may occur in patients suffering from severe visual loss as a result of disease of the eyes, such as a detached retina, or may appear as the 'phosphenes' or sparks of light which can result from mechanical distortion of the globe. These are largely illusory, but probably depend upon entrophic images from retinal ganglion cells which exceptionally reach perception. They may also result from lesions in any part of the visual pathways as well as elsewhere in the nervous system. Visual hallucinations have been attributed in the past to lesions of the anterior part of the visual system (including the optic tracts and radiation). While lesions in these areas can cause brief flashes of light, these phenomena are uncommon, and certainly anterior lesions do not cause 'formed' images (see below). When a hemianopia is present, the hallucinations may be seen in the normal half fields or in the blind half fields.

Hallucinations arising in the occipital striate cortex take the form of stars and static lights, those from the parastriate area coloured flashes or rings or, less often, a grey or black 'fog'. Those which arise from visual association areas in the parietal and temporal cortex are more complex and often formed, sometimes involving the evocation of visual memories of people, places or things. Hallucinations arising in the parietal region may be associated with visual agnosia, defective localisation of images, perseveration of visual images, and errors in colour-naming or defective colour perception, while those of temporal lobe origin may be associated with auditory hallucinations. The latter, if originating in the primary auditory cortex, are crude and unformed sounds, but lesions of auditory association areas can reproduce auditory memories (music, well-recognised voices, etc.). Temporal lobe lesions not infrequently result in disorders of perception also in that objects look larger or smaller than normal and there may be similar alterations in auditory perception, feelings of unreality of the self and of the surroundings (depersonalisation or jamais vu) or conversely feelings of intense familiarity with actual recall of previous experiences (déjà vu). In temporal lobe epilepsy it is often impossible to remember after the attack the actual familiar experience which was recalled.

Visual hallucinations of the self have been described in which the individual feels that he is observing his own body from outside his physical self. This unusual phenomenon has some affinities with sensations of intense depersonalisation.

Some recent neuropharmacological studies

Hallucinogenic drugs such as lysergic acid diethylamide (LSD) may produce their effects through an action upon the serotonergic system of neurones and especially upon those in the median raphe of the midbrain. The activation of raphe cells by either noradrenaline or serotonin (5-HT) applied electrophoretically in experimental animals can be blocked by LSD, either by inhibiting 5-HT release or by acting at the 5-HT receptor site in the post synaptic membrane (Fig. 7.4). Mono-amine oxidase inhibitors and tryptophan, as well as tricyclic antidepressant agents (imipramine, amitriptyline and their derivatives), slow down the rate of discharge in median raphe neurones. They may elevate brain 5-HT levels locally through inhibiting its re-uptake. Patients with schizophrenia tend to have low mono-amine oxidase activity in their platelets. It has been postulated that this may allow the plasma level of tryptamine to rise, thus producing abnormal amounts of dimethyltryptamine, which is known to be a hallucinogenic agent. The possible sequence of events and the actions of various drugs upon a serotonergic synapse are summarised in Figure 7.4. Recently, evidence has accumulated to suggest that depression is associated with dysfunction of the hypothalamic-pituitary-adrenal axis and with a reduced availability of mono-amines, principally noradrenaline and serotonin at several cerebral receptor sites, while many of the physical accompaniments of anxiety are related to neurotransmitter release and can be relieved at least in part by β-adrenergic blockade. There are further complexities in that various dopaminergic drugs (except bromocriptine) which stimulate dopaminergic neurones have been shown to reproduce many of the symptoms of schizophrenia, in which disease increased numbers of cerebral dopamine receptors and reduced glutamic acid decarboxylase activity have also been reported. The role of hypothalamic endorphins as putative transmitters in the limbic system with their powerful potential influences upon behaviour and memory has already been mentioned.

ABNORMALITIES OF MEMORY, MOOD, INTELLECT AND PERSONALITY

A detailed survey of the classification and differential diagnosis of mental disorders would be inappropriate in a

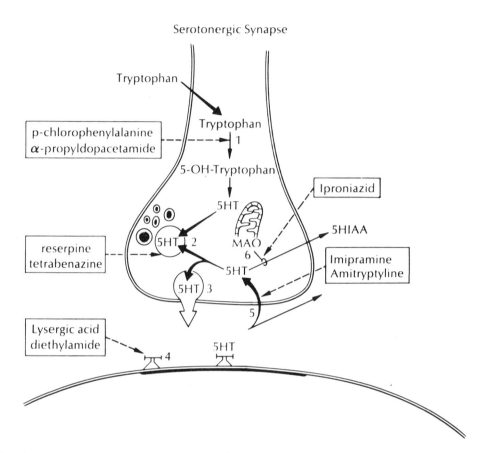

Fig. 7.4 Schematic model of a central serotonergic neurone indicating possible sites of drug action.

Site 1: Enzymatic synthesis. Tryptophan is taken up into the serotonin-containing neurone and converted to 5-OH-tryptophan by the enzyme tryptophan hydroxylase. This enzyme can be effectively inhibited by p-chloro-phenylalanine and α-propyldopacetamide. The next synthetic step involves the decarboxylation of 5-OH-tryptophan to form serotonin (5-HT).

Site 2: Storage. Reserpine and tetrabenazine interfere with the uptake-storage mechanism of the amine granules, causing a marked depletion of serotonin.

Site 3: Release. At present there is no drug available which selectively blocks the release of serotonin. However, lysergic acid diethylamide, owing to its ability to block or inhibit the firing of serotonin neurones, causes a reduction in the release of serotonin from the nerve terminals.

Site 4: Receptor interactions. Lysergic acid diethylamide acts as a partial agonist at serotonergic synapses in the CNS. A number of compounds have also been suggested to act as receptor-blocking agents at serotonergic synapses, but direct proof of these claims at present is lacking.

Site 5: Re-uptake. Considerable evidence now exists which suggests that serotonin may have its action terminated by being taken up into the presynaptic terminal. The tricyclic drugs with a tertiary nitrogen, such as imipramine and amitryptyline, appear to be potent inhibitors of this uptake mechanism.

Site 6: Mono-amine oxidase (MAO). Serotonin present in a free state within the presynaptic terminal can be degraded by the enzyme MAO, which appears to be located in the outer membrane of mitochondria. Iproniazid is an effective inhibitor of MAO.

(Reproduced with permission from Cooper et al 1982.)

commentary upon neurological pathophysiology. Nevertheless, so many mental symptoms can accompany or imitate organic brain disease that certain general principles must be set down against the background of the anatomical, physiological and pharmacological evidence discussed earlier in this chapter.

Some useful definitions

It was once thought that a **neurosis**, characterised by anxiety and related symptoms, resulting essentially from psychological causes, was different in both aetiology and prognosis from a psychosis, a term generally implying insanity and typified by a serious derangement of thought processes. It is now evident that the distinction between these two disorders is not absolute and that both neurotic and psychotic reactions can occur in response to organic disease. **Amnesia** implies loss of memory, while **mental retardation or handicap** (once called amentia, mental deficiency or oligophrenia) means defective development of intellectual function, and **dementia** disintegration of previously normal intellect resulting from organic brain disease. Abnormalities of personality and character are more difficult to define but include the shy and introverted or fanatical adherent of outlandish cults who is evidently different in personality from the norm, though not clearly abnormal, and who is often called **schizoid**, but more particularly the **psychopath** who, though not insane or mentally retarded, behaves in a socially abnormal manner. The term '**personality disorder**' is now generally preferred in modern psychiatric terminology to the more traditional 'psychopathy'.

Affective disorders are characterised by abnormalities of mood or affect of which the most prominent are **anxiety** and **depression**. Cyclothymic individuals show excessive mood swings from states of elation verging upon mania to periods of intense depression with psychomotor retardation. The **obsessive-compulsive** syndrome is a variant of neurosis largely determined by constitutional factors in which insistent thoughts so occupy the patient's mind that they may compel him to perform compulsive acts which he knows are foolish or unnecessary but which he cannot resist. **Hypochondriasis**, a state of intense introspection in which the patient is preoccupied with his own bodily symptoms, shows many affinities with obsessional neurosis. **Hysteria** is a common psychiatric reaction in which there are symptoms or signs often mimicking physical disease (loss of voice, blindness, or paralysis) which are not caused by organic pathological change but which are actuated by the desire to obtain real or imagined profit from the symptoms or to escape from stress.

The **schizophrenic** reaction is often characterized by introversion, severe distortion of thought processes, auditory hallucinations, and paranoid features commonly involving ideas of persecution. The disorder is constitutional and not usually a consequence of exogenous factors.

The assessment of mental changes in cerebral lesions

Many neuropsychological and psychometric tests are available for the assessment of memory, intellect, mood and personality and for the identification of specific defects of speech and perception. Some of these were mentioned in Chapter 1 and methods of identifying aphasia, apraxia and agnosia have been described previously (see p. 15). The Wechsler intelligence scale for children (WISC) is particularly useful in childhood for identifying through a discrepancy between verbal and performance intelligence quotients (IQ) defects in the acquisition of motor skills (developmental apraxia), and the measurement of Schonell's 'reading age' is valuable in cases of suspected dyslexia. The Wechsler adult intelligence scale (WAIS) is valuable in identifying early intellectual impairment in cases of presumed dementia and also gives a reasonable assessment of the patient's premorbid IQ. The ability to calculate can be tested by asking the patient to subtract serial 7's from 100.

In examining memory, the patient is asked to remember a series of numbers (normally one can recall at least seven digits forwards and five backwards) and recall a name, an address and the name of a flower. These are tests for short-term memory. In testing remote memory the patient is asked for details of his schooling, marriage, children, etc., and for the names of prime ministers or US presidents.

Disorders of personality, emotion and thought processes are more complex. Tests such as the Minnesota Personality Inventory (MMPI) or the Cattell are useful in assessing personality and emotional traits (extraversion, introversion, anxiety, depression, psychopathy). In psychotic states such as schizophrenia the patient sometimes gives concrete interpretations of proverbs, which are intended to be interpreted in an abstract manner. Interpretations of the Rorschach ink-blot test are of greater relevance to psychiatry than to neurology.

Amnesia

Bilateral temporal lobe disease or resection may seriously impair memory. Severe memory loss is characterised particularly by an inability to record, retain and recall recent impressions with comparative sparing of the memory for remote years. Very many metabolic, traumatic, neoplastic, inflammatory and degenerative diseases of the brain may be associated with memory loss. A few of the more specific syndromes are described below.

Transient global amnesia

This syndrome is usually due to transient ischaemia in one or both temporal lobes. It is generally of sudden onset in middle-aged or elderly individuals with evidence of cerebral atherosclerosis. It may be precipitated by emotional stress, sexual intercourse, intense pain or exposure to cold and has also been described as occurring in migraine, cerebral embolism and left temporal haemorrhage. It is rarely familial and recurrent attacks have been described. CT scanning sometimes shows unilateral, rarely bilateral, temporal lesions and is often negative. Memory loss for recent events develops rapidly. Despite their inability to register new impressions, the patients retain their personal identity, and show no abnormality of behaviour apart from anxiety and no evidence of impaired perception. Recovery is usually complete within a few hours, and retrograde amnesia shrinks rapidly, leaving the patient with no disability other than amnesia for the events occurring in the attack itself.

The Korsakoff syndrome

This disorder is sometimes called the 'amnestic syndrome' or the 'Wernicke-Korsakoff syndrome' because of its common association with Wernicke's encephalopathy. It is usually due to vitamin B_1 (thiamine) deficiency and is most commonly observed in alcoholic subjects. More rarely it can follow head injury, anoxia, encephalitis or subarachnoid haemorrhage or may be a manifestation of general paresis or other dementing disorders, intracranial neoplasm or granulomatous meningitis, including sarcoidosis. Malnutrition or malabsorption and the post-gastrectomy syndrome are other occasional causes. Loss of neurones and demyelination with gliosis, capillary proliferation and occasional haemorrhages are found predominantly in the thalamus, mammillary bodies and midbrain. There is characteristically a striking loss of the ability to record and retain new impressions. At one minute the patient appears alert and his conversation is lucid, but within a moment or two he will have forgotten the interview completely. The memory of his remote past may be intact. As a result he becomes disorientated, certainly in time and often in place, and in order to conceal this memory defect he confabulates. For instance, he will describe in detail fantastic activities which he claims to have carried out some few hours or days

earlier, though he may never have left his bed. Usually his descriptions have some basis in fact in the remote past, but he is utilising these previous experiences to fill in the recent period for which his memory is defective.

Hysterical amnesia

Psychological as well as physical causes can seriously impair memory. In hysterical amnesia the patient may have no recollection whatever of his identity, of his address, or of any other details concerning himself despite apparent alertness. The condition is presumably due to some process of psychological inhibition resulting in an inability to reopen voluntarily the pathways where memories are retained. Usually the condition develops acutely as a method of escape from undue stress. Hysterical amnesia may be feigned as a defence against a criminal charge and can then be difficult to distinguish from the genuine disorder. Other manifestations of hysteria will be considered below.

Disorders of mood

The neural basis of emotion and the integration of the accompanying bodily changes have already been discussed. It is to disorders of this mechanism and of its relationship with higher levels of the nervous system that we must look for the explanation of disorders of mood occurring as a result of organic nervous disease. For more detailed commentaries upon disorders of mood and emotion consequent upon affective and psychotic disorders the reader is referred to textbooks of psychiatry. Such conditions will be mentioned here only in so far as they enter into the differential diagnosis of those mood changes which occur in organic nervous disease.

Emotional instability

Emotional instability or lability is a common symptom of nervous diseases, especially of those in which the lesions are diffuse. The patient is easily moved by almost any form of emotion. He is quickly irritated or angered, easily becomes apprehensive, and is readily depressed or reduced to tears. Less often, he experiences pleasurable emotion with abnormal facility and is readily moved to laughter. Emotional instability of this kind is commonly encountered after head injury, after massive cerebral infarction, and in patients with diffuse cerebral arteriosclerosis. It is frequently present in the early stages of dementia, however produced, and is characteristic of the later stages of multiple sclerosis. This exaggerated emotional activity appears to result from impairment of the control which higher levels of the nervous system normally exercise over the thalamus and hypothalamus.

Impulsive disorders of conduct

The emotional instability described above does not usually lead to disorders of conduct, perhaps because conduct is normally more strongly inhibited than feeling. Exceptionally, however, impairment of higher control releases emotions which pass into action. This most often happens in children or adolescents in whom the control of impulsive action is as yet incomplete. Misdemeanours and acts of violence are sometimes committed by children and adolescents who have suffered disorders causing diffuse brain damage. Similar acts may be committed by aggressive psychopaths, and rarely by epileptics, either before an epileptic attack or in the phase of post-epileptic automatism, or even in the intervals between attacks. Such acts of aggression seem most likely to occur in patients with temporal lobe lesions.

Apathy

A general loss of emotional responsiveness without a proportionate intellectual deterioration was once most characteristically seen in association with parkinsonism due to encephalitis lethargica. In view of the known predilection of the virus of this disease for the diencephalic grey matter, it was reasonable to attribute the apathy to injury to the posterior hypothalamus. A similar picture is associated with mental deterioration in the later stages of dementia from any cause. Here it is probable that the apathy is in part, at least, secondary to the deterioration of thought and perception. However, apathy may also be observed in many forms of organic encephalopathy, degenerative brain diseases and some psychotic disorders, especially severe melancholia and schizophrenia. The apathetic patient loses all his former interests and affect and, lacking the drive of the instinctive life, becomes incapable of effort and sinks into a vegetative existence.

Euphoria

Euphoria is the term used to indicate a mood characterised by feelings of cheerfulness and happiness and a sense of mental well-being. Transitory euphoria is induced in many people by the consumption of alcohol. As a prevailing mood it is seen most characteristically, though uncommonly, in multiple sclerosis. Some sufferers from this disease remain persistently serene and happy in spite of their increasing physical disabilities. Euphoria is also encountered occasionally in patients with intracranial tumours, especially when the tumour is situated in the temporal lobe or, less frequently, in the frontal lobe or corpus callosum. Its psychophysiological basis is little understood.

Excitement

Excitement is a term somewhat loosely applied to several forms of mental overactivity, which may predominantly involve the intellectual, emotional or psychomotor spheres. All three may be affected together, as in acute mania, characterised by flight of ideas, elation and psychomotor restlessness. Disordered ideas may be linked with excitement in some delirious and confusional states, and in catatonic schizophrenia. Delirium has been defined as confusion with an overlay of excitement. Psychomotor restlessness is associated with anxiety in agitated depression, and the prevailing mood may be one of rage in the outbursts of aggressive psychopaths. There is some evidence that states of excitement can be caused by lesions of the anterior hypothalamus.

Depression

Depression may be regarded as the converse of euphoria. It is a mood of dejection and gloom for which frequently the patient can offer no explanation. It is encountered in a variety of states. It may be a reaction to an adequate external cause, such as failure or bereavement, or a neurotic reaction to personal difficulties (reactive depression). In sufferers from cyclothymia, depression is liable to occur as a recurrent disorder of mood, sometimes alternating with phases of excitement, though often these are no more than a mild general sense of elation. In cyclothymic individuals the depression is likely to be associated with psychomotor retardation, causing difficulty in concentrating, and with insomnia and loss of appetite. Such patients typically wake early and feel at their worst in the early part of the day. Depression also occurs as the predominant feature of endogenous depression or involutional melancholia, in which it may be associated with agitation. Patients suffering from psychotic depression in a severe form often have delusions of guilt or of a hypochondriacal nature. Individuals with endogenous depression frequently have physical symptoms including headache, fatigue and facial and/or limb or low back pain. Whereas it was once believed that reactive depression on the one hand and the endogenous disorder on the other were distinct disorders, it is now known that there is considerable overlap between the two, as a depressive illness with all of the features of the endogenous disorder is sometimes precipitated and is certainly accentuated by exogenous factors. Depression is also a mood which is common in patients suffering from organic disease of the brain, sometimes as a natural reaction to their disabilities. It is particularly common in individuals of a cyclothymic temperament in whom the nervous disease may be regarded as having released a pre-existing tendency to depression.

Anxiety

Fear is the emotional reaction to an imminent danger; anxiety is the reaction to a possible future danger—fear linked with anticipation. Anxiety may be produced in a variety of ways. It can be a normal emotional reaction. It may be the effect of certain toxins which appear to stimulate directly the nervous centres concerned. It can also be induced by drugs which have a stimulating effect upon the sympathetic nervous system, namely adrenaline, noradrenaline, ephedrine, amphetamine, nicotine and thyroxine. Anxiety may be the prevailing mood in patients suffering from organic disease of the brain, as after head injury, and it is then probably due in part to diminished control of emotional reactions by higher centres. Fear may be very evident in delirious states, when it appears as a reaction to terrifying hallucinations. It may also be linked with depression in involutional melancholia. In many cases, however, anxiety is neurotic—that is, it is the product of unconscious mental processes.

Anxiety is a common emotional disturbance which can be a normal reaction under stressful conditions. It is when the feeling of anxiety or apprehension is not clearly related to any specific object or thought that it becomes pathological and may then be thought to constitute an anxiety neurosis. Physical concomitants of anxiety are frequent and include sweating, feelings of suffocation or choking, sighing, restlessness, fatigue, 'dizzy bouts' and tension headaches. The anxious patient is often unable to rest or to relax. Whereas anxiety is common in many psychiatric syndromes and may accompany depression or even psychosis, it is those individuals who are constitutionally predisposed to developing severe anxiety symptoms as a result of minor stress who become neurotic. In such individuals episodes of anxiety may occur acutely as 'panic attacks', or may present with episodes of tension and with physical symptoms of the type outlined above, but with intervening periods when life is lived on a relatively even keel. In a chronic anxiety state, the patient exists in a state of continual worry and is irritable and unhappy. Often symptoms are focused upon one particular organ; for instance the patient with a cardiac neurosis or 'effort syndrome' complains of breathlessness, palpita-

tion and precordial pain. Reactive depression frequently co-exists with anxiety but self-reproach and suicidal ideas are much less common than in the endogenous variety, and patients with this type of depression have difficulty in getting to sleep but do not usually wake early in the morning.

Depersonalisation

Depersonalisation, or a feeling of unreality of the self, can co-exist with either depression or anxiety. Similar symptoms can be one feature of attacks of complex partial epilepsy from which differential diagnosis can at times be difficult. Patients can feel so intensely unreal or detached from the world about them that they feel themselves to be 'floating in air' and may even have delusional ideas that they are soon to die or that their bodies are shrinking. When depersonalisation is severe and combined with panic attacks and phobias (unreasoning fear of heights, of people, of enclosed places or of crossing the road) this syndrome has been called a 'phobic anxiety state'. Agoraphobia (fear of open spaces) is common in such cases and the patient is afraid of leaving the house alone ('the house-bound housewife'). A feeling of chronic instability, with associated lightheadedness and faintness, often confused with true vertigo unless the history is carefully taken, is often due to depersonalisation and is typically more troublesome out of doors than in the home.

Mental handicap (retardation)

Mental handicap implies an intellectual deficit which is present from birth and can be confirmed by psychometric testing, by means of which the intelligence quotient (IQ) and 'mental age' of the patient are assessed. It is customary now to talk of mental handicap rather than retardation and to classify cases into one of three groups, namely severe, moderate and mild handicap. The severely handicapped are incapable of guarding themselves against common dangers and must usually be confined in institutions. Moderately handicapped individuals are also incapable of managing themselves or their affairs, but are occasionally able to live satisfactorily in a protected domestic environment and may even be able to do work of a low-grade nature. The group which were once called high-grade mental defectives or morons, now known as cases of mild mental handicap, some of whom have IQs approaching the lower normal limit of 80, are common and mostly live outside institutions. Some can be educated in ordinary schools but others must attend schools for the educationally subnormal. The diagnosis of mild handicap can readily be overlooked and the patient is often regarded as being 'rather stupid', 'incapable of giving a resonable history', 'hypochondriacal'. Character defects are common in such individuals and many habitual petty criminals, prostitutes, sexual offenders and murderers fall into this group.

In many severely and moderately handicapped individuals, as well as in some of those less severely affected, there are associated congenital abnormalities involving other organs, while epilepsy or signs of 'cerebral palsy' may co-exist.

Among the many chromosomal anomalies which are usually associated with mental handicap are the 'cri du chat' syndrome due to partial deletion of the short arm of chromosome S, Klinefelter's syndrome (XXY or XXXY), Turner's syndrome (XO), trisomy E (17–18) and the fragile X syndrome. In **Down's syndrome**, formerly called mongolism, there is a characteristic facial appearance and disorders of skeletal development are also seen. The epicanthal folds are wide, the palpebral fissures oblique, the mouth is usually open with a protruding tongue, the bridge of the nose is broad, the ears are square, and the facial profile is flattened; muscular hypotonia and congenital heart disease are often present and mental handicap is moderate or mild. This condition usually results from a chromosomal disorder in that an extra chromosome may be attached to the 21st pair ('trisomy 21'). Occasionally it results from a chromosomal translocation or mosaic. The condition occurs in about 1 in 650 live births and shows a clear association with increasing maternal age. Accurate diagnosis of the nature of the chromosomal anomaly is important since the trisomy 21 defect would be likely to affect further children. Patients who survive beyond the age of 40 years usually show clinical and neuropathological evidence of Alzheimer's disease. Down's syndrome in the fetus and many inborn errors of metabolism can now be detected, when their presence is suspected, by examining amniotic cells (obtained by amniocentesis at about the 12th–14th week of pregnancy) in culture. Selective abortion of affected fetuses then becomes possible.

Very many endocrine and metabolic disorders, including innumerable inborn errors of metabolism, some common and some rare, have also been described in association with mental retardation. To quote but one example, in **phenylpyruvic oligophrenia (phenylketonuria)** the children, who are usually fair-haired and blue-eyed and may suffer from infantile convulsions, become severely handicapped if untreated. The diagnosis can be made in the first few days of life by detecting phenylpyruvic acid in the urine with the ferric chloride test. A simple paper-strip test is now used for routine screening of all newborn infants. Treatment with a diet low in phenylalanine may result in normal mental development. Of the many other enzyme defects causing retardation (including Tay-Sachs disease, Hartnup disease, oculo-cerebral dystrophy, maple-syrup urine disease, galactosaemia, fructosuria, and nephrogenic diabetes insipidus, to quote only a few) few can yet be controlled by dietary or other methods. Nevertheless, careful biochemical screening of infants with suspected mental handicap is paying increasing dividends, although approximately 50% of cases remain unexplained (non-specific mental handicap). The fact that non-specific handicap is commoner in males than in females led to the discovery that the fragile X syndrome (due to an X-linked gene with a secondary constriction or fragile site on the X-chromosome) is almost as common as Down's syndrome.

Dementia

Dementia, or progressive disintegration of the intellect, of memory and of the powers of abstract thought, results from organic disease and usually from physical or metabolic disturbances affecting the brain. The first sign of a dementing process may be an error of judgement incompatible with the patient's previous ability, or a failure to grasp all facets of a difficult situation. It may simply be felt that Mr X is 'losing his grip'. Subsequently, memory, particularly for recent events, often becomes impaired, so that the patient is forgetful, unable to concentrate and his attention wanders freely. Increasing emotional lability with inappropriate laughing or crying or with irritability and irrational impulsive acts may follow, with striking changes in mood, presenting as elation in some cases and apathy in others. By the time the patient becomes neglectful of his personal appearance and dirty in his habits, the diagnosis is usually obvious, but in the earlier stages it is much more difficult to make. Increasing unpunctuality, neglect of detail, and long periods spent in solitude, in contrast to the patient's customary previous behaviour, may be useful pointers. Aphasia, apraxia and/or agnosia occur in some cases. It is nevertheless remarkable how often patients with early dementia continue to hold responsible jobs, despite increasing 'eccentricity', until some major error of judgement or faux pas brings matters to a head. In the late stages, delusions occasionally occur, in the form of grandiose imaginings ('I am the King of Spain') or ideas of hostility or persecution towards relatives or business associates. Progressive dementing processes must be distinguished from reversible toxic confusional states, due to metabolic disorders or treatable intracranial lesions such as subdural haematoma, and from the pseudodementia (due to psychomotor retardation) which may be seen in severe endogenous depression or, rarely, in hysteria. Patients with benign senescent forgetfulness and without other cognitive deficits who readily forget, for example, proper names on some occasions but not on others, should be reassured that they are not suffering from dementia. In depressive pseudodementia there may be a family history of depression, the patient often complains bitterly of memory impairment but nevertheless does well on formal memory testing. Unlike the truly demented patient, he will often respond to a question by saying 'I can't remember' while the sufferer from dementia either offers a feeble excuse or an incorrect answer.

Many forms of organic brain disease give rise to progressive dementia. Some authorities differentiate between the so-called 'cortical' dementias such as Alzheimer's disease or general paresis in which focal symptoms or signs of cerebral cortical dysfunction may ultimately develop on the one hand and 'subcortical' forms (e.g. normal pressure hydrocephalus, Huntington's disease and parkinsonism) on the other, but this distinction is not universally accepted. Thus the common multi-infarct dementia (see below) can be associated with both cortical and subcortical lesions. Alzheimer's disease accounts for about 50% of all cases, multi-infarct dementia for about 20% and combined Alzheimer's disease and vascular disease for about 15–20% with all other causes producing about 10–15%. Most such disorders are progressive and incurable, but others are eminently treatable and may show no very specific clinical features so that remediable causes should always be borne in mind. One such is **neurosyphilis** (particularly general paresis), in which a fatuous euphoric dementia is common and there may also be Argyll Robertson pupils and rarely spastic paresis of the limbs. Diagnosis can be made by appropriate serological tests and cerebrospinal fluid examination. Another possible cause is **intracranial tumour**, either primary or secondary, and involving particularly the frontal lobes. In such cases memory and intellect are often severely affected when other aspects of behaviour and personality are reasonably well preserved, while there may be features (headache, vomiting and papilloedema) to indicate raised intracranial pressure. Recent evidence suggests that **communicating** (sometimes called 'low-pressure') **hydrocephalus** can sometimes cause a fluctuating confusional state and later progressive dementia, often associated with urinary incontinence, gait apraxia and increased unsteadiness in walking; diagnosis may be made by CT and/or MRI scanning, and in some cases improvement has followed continuous ventricular drainage through a valve inserted into a ventricle with drainage by catheter into the venous circulation (an atrioventricular 'shunt'). A number of **toxic and metabolic disorders** can also cause progressive dementia; **drug intoxication** and **alcoholism** are usually self-evident causes if the history is adequate, but are nevertheless often missed, while **pernicious anaemia** and **myxoedema** are other treatable conditions which are easily overlooked and in which the dementia may be reversible with appropriate treatment. When intellectual deterioration follows upon severe diffuse **head injury, anoxia, inflammatory disease**, such as encephalitis or meningitis, **multiple sclerosis, parkinsonism**, long-standing **temporal lobe epilepsy** or a **chronic psychosis**, the cause is generally apparent and little can usually be done. This also applies to cases of cerebral lipidosis, diffuse cerebral sclerosis and other **degenerative disorders** which cause dementia in childhood. The same is unfortunately true of cases of **cerebral atherosclerosis** in which, however, the dementia, though progressive, is usually step-like, rather than insidious in its advance, being accompanied by transient episodes of confusion, aphasia and/or motor or sensory disturbance, indicating minor 'strokes' due to focal cerebral ischaemia (**multi-infarct dementia**).

Alzheimer's disease

Alzheimer's disease is by far the commonest cause of progressive dementia, and the pathology is the same whether the patient is in the presenile (under 65 years) or senile (over 65) age group. No distinction is now made between presenile and senile dementia. The condition affects 10–15% of individuals over the age of 65 years and perhaps 20% over 80. Although a familial incidence is relatively uncommon and the condition has been described in one of a pair of monozygotic twins, there is increasing evidence of a significant genetic influence in its aetiology. The relentless downhill course usually results in death 5–15 years after the onset. In this condition, there is degeneration of cortical neurones and deposition of argyrophilic material in the form of plaques ('senile plaques') in the cerebral cortex. Granulo-vacuolar degeneration in hippocampal neurones is also found, along with neurofibrillary tangles within the cytoplasm of neurones. Senile plaques occur as a result of normal ageing processes but their number and density is greatly increased above the normal range in demented patients. Along with these changes there is macroscopic shrinkage of cortical gyri with dilatation of the cerebral ventricles, changes which are often readily demonstrable by CT scanning. Recent work has also demonstrated deposits of β-amyloid protein in the brain in such cases, as in older individuals with Down's syndrome. Recent genetic studies using DNA probes have indicated that the gene conferring susceptibility to this disease maps to a region of chromosome 21 which carries the amyloid protein gene, and raise the possibility that the latter may play a role in pathogenesis. In senile cases, the patient is usually in the seventh or eighth decade, the intellect and personality deteriorate hand in hand and very often there is characteristic nocturnal restlessness, so that the patient wanders about in the middle of the night. Alzheimer's disease may, however, cause progressive dementia in the 40 to 60 age group. Some workers differentiate between the form which develops insidiously in old age (AD-1) and that which begins in middle age and runs a more rapid course (AD-2). In the late stages, aphasia and spasticity of the limbs may develop, while epileptic seizures occasionally occur.

Recent research has demonstrated a deficiency of acetylcholine (ACh) and of choline acetyl transferase in the cerebral cortex of such patients and attempts have been made to treat the condition with choline or lecithin and with other acetylcholine precursors. Short-term benefit has been reliably demonstrated with such treatment and with neostigmine but is not sustained. And the discovery that the form of dementia which developed in some patients undergoing long-term renal dialysis, but only in certain centres (dialysis dementia), was due to brain damage produced by an abnormally high concentration of aluminium in the domestic water supply used in dialysis led to studies of trace elements in the brain in Alzheimer's disease. Undoubtedly some senile plaques contain aluminium and the role of this element in pathogenesis is still undecided.

Pick's disease

In Pick's disease, again a condition of late middle life, which is very much less common than Alzheimer's disease, there is often affection of more than one member of a family and the pathological changes are more circumscribed, often beginning in one or other frontal or temporal lobe. The upper three layers of the affected parts of the cerebral cortex are principally involved in this disease with chromatolysis and loss of ganglion cells. Senile plaques are relatively infrequent and neurofibrillary tangles are absent, but cortical neurones show numerous amphophilic and argentophilic Pick bodies which are the histological hallmark of the disease. As the changes are initially focal, epilepsy or neurological signs suggesting a localised brain lesion are occasionally seen, while aphasia and defective memory are common at a time when the personality remains reasonably well preserved; eventually, however, a global dementia supervenes. Psychomotor restlessness and inappropriate jocularity are somewhat commoner in this condition than in Alzheimer's disease. Females are affected slightly more often than males, the age of onset is usually between 50 and 60 years and the condition terminates fatally within 3–12 years of the onset. It is totally uninfluenced by treatment.

Other causes of dementia

Huntington's chorea must also be mentioned as a cause of dementia of relatively non-specific type. In such cases there is generally a clear-cut family history of the condition and the characteristic involuntary movements of the limbs and face are seen, though rarely dementia alone is the first manifestation. In the rare degenerative condition sometimes known as **cortico-striato-nigral degeneration**, a disorder which is sometimes familial and has sometimes been called erroneously Creutzfeldt-Jakob disease, a dementia is associated with signs of bilateral pyramidal tract dysfunction, with clinical features suggesting Parkinson's disease, and with weakness and wasting of peripheral limb muscles. This condition shows some resemblances to the so-called **parkinsonism-dementia complex** which has been endemic in the Chamorro people in the Mariana islands of the South Pacific. There is still uncertainty as to whether that condition is due to the accumulation of minor quantities of aluminium in the brain in an area where the soil and water are both deficient in calcium or whether a toxic factor related to the dietary consumption of the cycad nut is the principal cause. It is also well recognised that progressive dementia occurs more often in the later stages of idiopathic parkinsonism (**paralysis agitans**) than was once thought, and it is also a feature of **progressive multi-system degeneration** (the Shy-Drager syndrome, see p. 81 and of some of the hereditary ataxias. True **Creutzfeldt-Jakob disease** (often called also subacute spongiform encephalopathy) is a rapidly-progressive form of dementia accompanied by myoclonic jerking and progressive paralysis in most cases and by a characteristic irregular spike-and-wave discharge in the EEG; the condition is usually fatal in a few months. It is now known to be due to a transmissible agent (a 'slow virus') and has been transferred from one human subject to another by corneal transplantation. It shows several clinical and pathological resemblances to scrapie in sheep.

Hence many possible causes must be considered in any case of dementia; accurate diagnosis is of considerable importance, for in some conditions the prognosis is grave, while in others (neurosyphilis, intoxication, pernicious anaemia, myxoedema and benign intracranial neoplasms) the condition may be reversible with appropriate treatment. Of all the investigations available, apart from psychometric tests required to assess quantitatively the defects of intellect and cognition and those tests designed, for example, to exclude specific infective or metabolic causes, CT scanning is the most important. Ventricular dilatation is often proportional to the degree of dementia, evidence of cortical atrophy much less so, as some degree of the latter may be found in normal individuals.

Substantial ventricular dilatation with little CSF visible over the cortex favours low pressure hydrocephalus, while multiple small infarcts are often visualised in multi-infarct dementia and the scan is usually successful in revealing intracranial neoplasms or other space-occupying lesions (e g. subdural haematoma) which may be the cause.

Hysteria

The differential diagnosis between hysteria and organic disease is one of the most difficult in medicine. In clinical neurological practice this problem is particularly common and has been the graveyard of many a professional reputation; for although hysterical symptoms can simulate almost any physical disease, disorders of the nervous system are most often imitated. The most important point in the diagnosis of hysteria is that this condition must not be diagnosed by exclusion, as a label casually applied when clinical examination and ancillary tests fail to reveal organic disease. On the contrary, there must be positive evidence of hysteria, for hysterical symptoms are purposive (though unconsciously so, unlike malingering which is deliberate), arising in order to obtain for the patient some real or imagined gain, either to fulfil an ambition, to realise a fantasy, or to escape from stress. To lose a job or to fail an examination through illness is more respectable than to do so through inefficiency; whereas such motivations may not be wholly conscious, the end desired by the patient is usually revealed on careful enquiry.

Patients with hysterical symptoms often have characteristic personality traits. They commonly deceive themselves that they are more able or important than they really are, they are emotionally shallow, easily influenced and unreliable and often utilise hysterical symptoms in order to draw attention or sympathy upon themselves or to dominate relatives and friends. Hysteria may occur in both sexes but is commoner in females; as the basic abnormality is constitutional, symptoms usually appear first in adolescence or early adult life, though much depends upon the severity of the stress to which the individual is subjected. Unfortunately there is no objective test available to distinguish between hysteria (subconscious motivation) and malingering, in which motivation is wholly conscious. This problem in differential diagnosis often arises when manifestations suggestive of hysteria arise against a background of industrial injury or in any other situation where prospects of financial compensation are involved.

Anxiety symptoms are often prominent in hysterical reactions, but relatively few neurotic patients exhibit frankly hysterical manifestations. A typical group of mental symptoms due to hysteria results from an ability to dissociate one part of the personality from another. Thus, hysterical 'twilight states', trances, or simulation of insanity (Ganser states) may occur, but most common is the **hysterical amnesia** or **fugue**, in which the patient wanders away from home for hours or days, having lost all sense of his identity.

As a rule, hysterical symptoms are a result either of suggestion or of an idea or fantasy in the patient's mind. Suggestion is of particular importance; thus a hysteric may become paralysed because her mother had a stroke, or a symptom develops in response to a leading question asked by a doctor, which the patient then endeavours to justify. It is from discrepancies between the patient's idea of a physical illness and the signs of the organic disorder itself that most diagnostic assistance is obtained. Motivation is also important; thus a patient with 'stage-fright' loses her voice, while another who is dreading forthcoming examinations develops hysterical blindness and is then unable to study. In hysterical **aphonia** the patient is able to cough on demand, while the individual with **hysterical blindness** blinks on threat or avoids obstacles in his path. **Hysterical convulsions** are staged for their histrionic effect and invariably occur with an audience; the patient is careful not to injure himself and tongue-biting and incontinence do not occur unless the patient who has often been asked about these features decides to oblige by providing them. The convulsion is often preceded by **hyperventilation** and actual tetany may develop through respiratory alkalosis. In **hysterical paralysis**, a single limb is usually involved, though hemiplegia or paraplegia are seen. There are generally discrepancies between the clinical findings and those resulting from organic nervous disease. In particular, the reflexes are generally normal or show slight but symmetrical exaggeration and the plantar responses are flexor. Typically, when the patient tries to move the affected limb, there is a massive apparent expenditure of effort with little result, and palpation of the muscles involved reveals that agonists and antagonists contract simultaneously. Hysterical disorders of **gait** are seen in some patients who claim to have paresis of the lower limbs, but in others there is no abnormality at all on examining the patient in bed, although the gait is bizarre, and unlike that associated with any organic nervous disease. Falling may be frequent, but significantly without injury. One must be sure to exclude the broad-based gait of truncal ataxia due to a midline cerebellar lesion, in which, too, signs of cerebellar dysfunction are conspicuously absent in the recumbent patient. Hysterical **sensory loss** is common; it frequently occurs in 'glove and stocking' distribution, with a clear-cut upper margin (unlike polyneuropathy where the transition is gradual) or there may be a total hemianaesthesia affecting all forms of sensation. Loss of vibration sense over one half of the skull or sternum is invariably hysterical. Co-ordinated movements are also good in such patients despite apparent complete loss of position and joint sense. In a limb showing hysterical weakness or paralysis the sensory impairment often ends at the elbow, knee, groin or shoulder, giving a pattern of sensory impairment which could not be produced by an organic lesion. These patients are very suggestible and 'islands' of normal sensation can sometimes be induced by suggestion in anaesthetic areas. In any event, the sensory impairment never corresponds to the cutaneous distribution of any peripheral nerve, sensory root or tract. Other less common hysterical manifestations include **dermatitis artefacta**, produced by self-inflicted cutaneous trauma, and hysterical **pyrexia**, which is commonest in nurses and is usually an artefact produced by cups of tea, cigarettes or hot water bottles or by substituting thermometers. Some patients even produce subcutaneous or intra-articular abscesses by injecting themselves with bath water, in which case the infecting organism is generally *E. coli*. Related to hysteria, but psychiatrically more complex, is the condition often called '**Munchausen's syndrome**'; these patients become skilled at feigning organic disease and seek admission to one hospital after another. Some few are drug addicts but others simply demonstrate 'a desire to be ill'. Along with all the features described there is, in hysteria, a characteristic **belle indifférence** or seeming unconcern about what, if physically determined, would be a serious disability.

From this description it may be asked why the differential diagnosis from organic disease should sometimes be so difficult. Unfortunately the clinical picture is not always clear-cut. For example, the early manifestations of extrapyramidal disorders such as dystonia musculorum deformans can produce abnormalities of gait which initially look hysterical. Furthermore, hysterical manifestations arise in patients with organic disease and it may be difficult to determine how much is overlay and how much genuine. In multiple sclerosis, for instance, early manifestations of hysterical type are common even before distinctive physical signs have appeared. In many such patients the hysterical manifestations seem to develop as a means of impressing the doctor who may, inadvertently or deliberately, have given the impression to the patient that he does not understand the significance of the symptoms. Hysterical manifestations developing for the first time late in life can be the first symptoms of an endogenous depression or organic dementia. The most important principles to follow in establishing the diagnosis are first to seek assiduously for any motivation, unconscious or otherwise, which may be responsible for the symptoms and secondly to look for sources of suggestion which could be determining the pattern of the illness. Even when all clinical evidence suggests a diagnosis of hysteria the possibility of underlying organic disease or of more serious psychiatric illness should invariably be considered. It is in just this setting that such disorders are often overlooked when the hysterical overtones cloud the clinical picture.

Occupational neurosis

Of the many 'craft palsies' which have been described, writer's cramp is the commonest and is believed to be, like other disorders in this group, of emotional origin. It is typical that the affected hand can be used normally for all activities other than writing and it is difficult to see how this could be explained by an organic lesion in the basal ganglia or elsewhere. Nevertheless, some authorities believe that the condition represents a focal manifestation of dystonia. I remain firmly convinced that some such cases can only be psychogenic, while accepting that others in which movements other than writing are affected may well be dystonic. Typically, as the patient begins to write, the thumb and fingers grip the pen more and more tightly so that writing ceases and the pen may even be driven through the paper. If the patient learns to write with the other hand or to type, these activities may subsequently be affected. While tranquillising drugs and deconditioning techniques sometimes help, in many cases the prognosis is poor and the patient is eventually compelled to avoid writing. Similar problems affecting the specific movements involved in the craft concerned are well known to occur in typists, violinists, professional players of wind instruments, needleworkers and in many more occupations, making it difficult for the individual to continue in his or her normal employment.

REFERENCES

Agranoff B W 1975 Biochemical strategies in the study of memory formation. In: Tower D B (ed) Nervous system. Volume I in Brady R O (ed): The basic neurosciences. Raven Press, New York

Andrew J, Nathan P W 1964 Lesions of the anterior frontal lobes and disturbances of micturition and defaecation. Brain 87: 233

Anonymous 1987 Alzheimer's disease, Down's syndrome, and chromosome 21. Lancet i: 1011

Bloom F 1985 Neurotransmitter diversity and its functional significance. Journal of the Royal Society of Medicine 78: 189

Cooper J B, Bloom F E, Roth R H 1982 The biochemical basis of neuropharmacology, 4th edn. Oxford University Press, Oxford

FitzGerald M J T 1985 Neuroanatomy basic and applied. Bailliére Tindall, Eastbourne

Freeman W, Watts J W 1947 Psychosurgery during 1936–1946. Archives of Neurology and Psychiatry 58: 417

Gellis S S, Feingold M 1968 Atlas of mental retardation syndromes. US Department of Health, Washington DC

Goelet P, Castelluci V S, Schacher S, Kandel E R 1986 The long and the short of long-term memory—a molecular framework. Nature 322: 419

Guyton A C 1981 Textbook of medical physiology, 6th edn. Saunders, Philadelphia

Isaacson R L 1974 The limbic system. Plenum Press, New York

Menkes J L 1985 A textbook of child neurology, 3rd edn. Lea & Febiger, Philadelphia

Meyer A 1974 The frontal lobe syndrome, the aphasias and related conditions a contribution to the history of cortical localization. Brain 97: 565

Mulley G P 1986 Differential diagnosis of dementia. British Medical Journal 292: 1416

Penfield W, Mathieson G 1974 Memory. Autopsy findings and comments on the role of hippocampus in experimental recall. Archives of Neurology 31: 145

Smythies J R 1970 Brain mechanisms and behavior. Academic Press, New York

Strub R L, Black F W 1985 The mental status examination in neurology, 2nd edn. Davis, Philadelphia

Trimble M R 1981 Neuropsychiatry. Wiley, Chichester

van Praag H M 1982 Depression. Lancet ii: 1259

Walton J N 1985 Brain's Diseases of the nervous system, 9th edn. Oxford University Press, Oxford

Wells C E (ed) 1977 Dementia, 2nd edn. Contemporary neurology series, Vol 15. Davis, Philadelphia

Zaidel D, Sperry R W 1974 Memory impairment after commissurotomy in man. Brain 97: 263

8. The special senses

The special senses include the faculties of smell, vision, hearing and taste. Closely related to hearing, at least in an anatomical sense, is the maintenance of equilibrium (vestibular function). These functions are mediated by those cranial nerves which convey the sensory impulses concerned in appreciating these sensations to the appropriate areas of the cerebral cortex. Thus the first or olfactory nerve contains the peripheral pathway for the sense of smell, while the second or optic nerve carries visual impulses. The ability to see is closely related to mechanisms subserving binocular vision and ocular movement, so that in considering visual processes one must also discuss the functions of the third (oculomotor), fourth (trochlear) and sixth (abducens) cranial nerves which control external ocular movement. The third nerve, along with sympathetic fibres derived from the autonomic nervous system, also influences those intrinsic ocular muscles controlling the size of the pupils as well as the process of accommodation. Hearing and the control of bodily equilibrium are respectively mediated through the cochlear and labyrinthine divisions of the eighth or auditory nerve, while taste sensations from the anterior two-thirds of the tongue travel in the chorda tympani along with the seventh or facial nerve and those from the posterior one-third are conveyed by the ninth or glosso-pharyngeal nerve. Disorders of function of the special senses, produced by lesions of the primary sensory receptors, of the cranial nerves concerned, or of their central connections, are common in patients with neurological disease, and an adequate understanding of the means by which lesions produce their clinical effects is essential for accurate diagnosis.

SMELL

The olfactory receptors are bipolar nerve cells situated in the upper part of the mucous membrane on either side of the nasal cavity. Inhaled gases given off by all odorous materials become dissolved in the nasal secretions which continually bathe the surface of these sensitive cells.

Impulses so produced are conveyed by nerve fibres through the cribriform plate of the ethmoid bone into the cranial cavity to join the olfactory bulb which lies on the under-surface of the ipsilateral frontal lobe. Thence impulses travel posteriorly to the olfactory tracts to reach the prepyriform cortex and uncus in the parahippocampal gyrus of the temporal lobe which is the primary rhinencephalic (olfactory) area of the cerebral cortex. The anterior commissure unites the cortical olfactory regions of the two hemispheres, carrying fibres from each olfactory tract to the opposite side.

Disease of the nasal mucosa such as rhinitis, a severe coryza, or sometimes excessive smoking, can so impair the sensitivity of the olfactory nerve cells that the sensation of smell is lost or greatly impaired (**anosmia**). Bilateral loss does not, therefore, always indicate a neurological lesion, though it may follow a head injury with tearing of the olfactory nerve fibres as they traverse the ethmoid bone. Unilateral impairment of the sense of smell is, however, an important physical sign, since in the absence of a primary nasal abnormality it may indicate compression of one olfactory bulb or tract, possibly by a tumour underlying the ipsilateral frontal lobe. Total anosmia can also be hysterical or feigned and in such cases the patient may deny that he can appreciate concentrated ammonia which stimulates trigeminal rather than olfactory nerve endings. Olfactory hallucinations sometimes occur in schizophrenia and in patients with lesions in one or other temporal lobe, as in some cases of temporal lobe epilepsy (**uncinate seizures**), and are presumably due to abnormal discharges arising in the medial temporal cortex. **Parosmia** is an abnormal or perverted sense of smell, rarely due to organic lesions but more often occurring in mental illness (e.g. severe depression).

TASTE

Taste fibres from the anterior two-thirds of the tongue travel through the lingual nerve to the chorda tympani, joining the facial nerve at the geniculate ganglion and proceeding to the pons in the nervus intermedius with the seventh and eighth nerves. Taste sensations from the posterior one-third of the tongue are conveyed by the glossopharyngeal nerve. In the pons the fibres of these nerves enter the tractus solitarius, cross the midline and proceed in the gustatory fillet to the optic thalamus whence they are conveyed to the lower end of the post-central gyrus.

There is a very close relationship between the faculties of smell and taste, and these are often confused by patients. The sense of taste is concerned with the relatively crude sensations of sweet, salt, bitter and sour, whereas the sensation of flavour is mediated through the sense of smell. It is not uncommon for patients to complain of a complete loss of taste after a head injury but examination shows that it is the sense of smell which is lost and the primary taste sensations are found to be intact.

Loss of taste (**ageusia**) on the anterior two-thirds of the tongue can result from lesions of the geniculate ganglion. A facial paralysis due to a lesion at or proximal to this point is usually associated therefore with unilateral loss of taste, while one resulting from a more distally-situated lesion is not. A lesion of the glossopharyngeal nerve will result in loss of taste on the posterior third of the tongue on the same side, but taste sensation is so difficult to test with even a reasonable degree of accuracy, that disorders of this sense have little value in clinical neurological diagnosis. **Parageusia**, an abnormal or perverted sense of taste, is rarely the result of organic lesions and is more often due to depressive illness.

VISION

The visual pathways

Visual impulses recorded upon the retina are conveyed by the optic (second cranial) nerves through the optic chiasm and the optic tract to the lateral geniculate body and then via the optic radiation to the visual cortex.

The light-sensitive receptors in the retina itself are the rods which are found diffusely throughout the retina except in the fovea centralis or macular area, and the cones which are concentrated largely in the region of the fovea but are scanty elsewhere. The cones have a high stimulus threshold, function mainly in daylight or conditions of high illumination and are responsible for high-acuity vision and colour vision. The rods, by contrast, have very low thresholds of stimulation, are insensitive to colour and relatively to fine visual details, and subserve vision in conditions of poor illumination. For detailed

information about the physiology of vision, including the anatomy and electrophysiology of the retinal ganglion cells and the respective roles of light-sensitive pigments such as rhodopsin or visual purple in the rods and iodopsin and other pigments in the cones, the reader is referred to textbooks of physiology. Information recorded by the rods and cones passes to the retinal ganglion cells which lie in its superficial layers and whose axons form the fibres of the optic nerve and come together in the optic disc or nerve head.

In the optic chiasm, fibres from the nasal half of each retina decussate, whereas temporal fibres do not. Hence each optic tract carries fibres from the temporal half of the ipsilateral retina and from the nasal half of the contralateral one (Fig. 8.1). This means that impulses from the right half-field of both eyes are carried in the left optic tract and vice versa. The tract continues to the lateral geniculate body where its axons synapse with nerve cells which give origin to the optic radiation. The optic radiation then travels backwards through the temporal lobe, hooking around the tip of the temporal horn of the lateral ventricle, and onwards to that part of the cerebral cortex which lies in the lips and in the depth of the calcarine fissure of the occipital lobe. This is the primary visual receptive area and has profuse connexions with the surrounding association areas where visual sensations are recognised and interpreted.

In the optic nerve there also travel afferent fibres from the retina and from the muscles of accommodation, which influence pupil size; these synapse in the lateral geniculate body and in the superior corpora quadrigemina (colliculi) of the upper midbrain, whence fibres arise which travel to the third, fourth and sixth nerve nuclei and to a sympathetic centre in the hypothalamus. These pathways are responsible for constriction of the pupil in response to light or fixation on near objects, and dilatation when the visual field is darkened or when distant objects are observed. A similar reflex pathway, controlled by visual impulses from the retina, influences the ocular movements necessary for ocular convergence and fixation and for following objects with the eyes.

Visual acuity

The visual acuity in each eye can be measured independently by means of test-types of the Snellen and Jaeger type (see p. 16). The acuity is essentially a measurement of the efficiency of macular or central vision as it depends largely upon normal functioning of this part of the retina and of its nervous connexions, provided the mechanism for focusing light upon the retina is intact. Thus peripheral retinal lesions rarely influence acuity, but a small lesion of the macula or of optic nerve fibres which come from the macular area may seriously affect the ability to read or to distinguish small objects. This is seen particularly in retrobulbar neuropathy (see below) which often produces a central field defect or scotoma. Disorders of refraction (myopia, presbyopia, astigmatism) can seriously impair visual acuity as may other primary abnormalities of the eye (iridocyclitis, cataract, vitreous haemorrhages) which influence the passage of light to the retina, as well as disorders which damage retinal sensitivity (retinal detachment, glaucoma, etc.), but these local causes are usually self-evident and refractive errors can be corrected by the use of appropriate lenses.

Colour blindness

Colour blindness is an inherited defect which occurs in 8% of the male population and in less than 0.5% of females. It is generally inherited as a sex-linked (X-linked) recessive trait; the commonest type is red-green blindness, either partial or complete, in which the affected individual finds it difficult to distinguish reds from greens. Many complex defects of colour vision do, however, occur. **Trichromats** (three-colour vision) include normal individuals but also some with weak red vision (protanomaly) or weak green vision (deuteranomaly). **Dichromats** are those who cannot perceive red

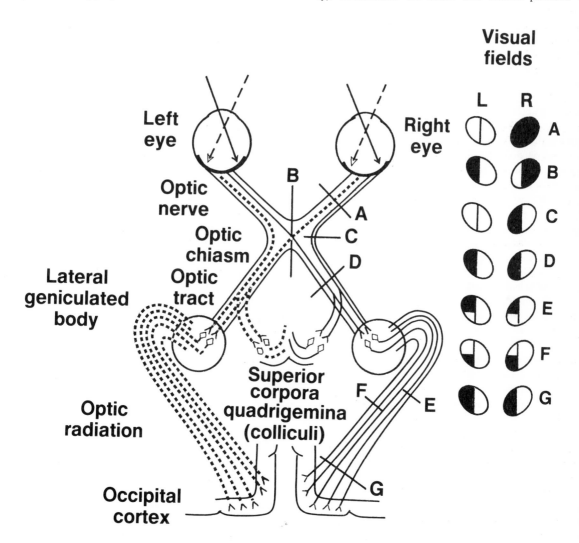

Fig. 8.1 A diagram of the visual pathways. On the right are examples of visual field defects produced by lesions interrupting these pathways at the points signified by the letters A to G.

(protanopia) or green (deuteranopia). **Monochromats** (with total colour blindness) are very rare and also have severe photophobia. Many patients with the less severe varieties are unaware of their colour blindness, as they recognise 'colours' by their brightness, but the diagnosis can be confirmed with the Ishihara charts. The defect is of no serious significance except in those occupations where the recognition of coloured lights or signals, say, is important. However in patients with minimal lesions of the visual pathways, field defects for coloured objects (red is commonly used) can be demonstrated at a time when the field for white objects is completed. The field for red is much smaller than that for white.

The visual fields

Defects in the visual fields can be assessed clinically by the technique of confrontation which depends on a comparison of the examiner's visual field with that of the patient. Hemianopic defects can be detected with great sensitivity by applying simultaneous small stimuli in both half-fields and looking for attention defects (see p. 23). These methods are of course qualitative. Charting the peripheral visual fields with a perimeter or of the central fields on the Bjerrum screen provides quantitative information. These two techniques have largely been superseded by the use of machines which can record both central and peripheral fields, such as the Goldmann or Topcon perimeters. From a knowledge of the anatomy of the visual pathways it is generally possible to localise with reasonable accuracy the site of the lesion which is responsible. Circumscribed defects of the central fields are referred to as scotomas. In each central field there is a normal 'scotoma', lateral to the fixation point; this is the caecum or 'blind spot, corresponding to the optic disc in which there are no visual receptors. A scotoma which surrounds the fixation point or macular area is called a **central scotoma**, and gives marked impairment of visual acuity. It is most commonly seen as a sequel of **optic or retrobulbar neuritis**, an inflammatory lesion of the optic nerve which is often due to multiple sclerosis. A central scotoma can rarely result from **compression of one optic nerve**, presumably because macular nerve fibres are more sensitive to pressure, in patients with a tumour (usually a meningioma) behind the orbit. It may also be found in **pernicious anaemia**, or in **neuromyelitis optica**, an acute demyelinating disorder related to multiple sclerosis, and in retrobulbar neuropathy due to many toxic and metabolic causes, of which **methyl alcohol poisoning** is a good example. **Tobacco amblyopia**, which is a cause of progressive visual failure in smokers of certain brands of pipe tobacco and which may be related to the effect of cyanide in the tobacco upon vitamin B_{12} utilisation,

usually gives a **centrocaecal scotoma**, joining the fixation point to the blind spot.

A severe lesion of one optic nerve gives, of course, complete blindness of the ipsilateral eye, while the peripheral field of the other eye is full. This may be seen, for instance, after severe head injury or occlusion of the central retinal artery due to embolism, atherosclerosis, cranial arteritis, or even severe papilloedema. Lesions of the optic chiasm can give a variety of field defects, depending upon the character and situation of the causal lesion. Compressive lesions are much the most common and these include parasellar neoplasms such as meningioma, chordoma and craniopharyngioma as well as aneurysms and tumours of the pituitary gland. The pattern of field defect depends on which part of the optic chiasm is compressed. Although pituitary tumours, as they protrude from the sella turcica, usually compress the centre of the chiasm and therefore damage the decussating fibres from the lower nasal portions of the retina, producing upper temporal field defects in both eyes and eventually a bitemporal hemianopia, if the chiasm is a little anterior then the posterior part of the chiasm may be affected first or even one optic tract, causing a hemianopia, perhaps with a temporal scotoma on the ipsilateral side. If the chiasm is a little posteriorly placed, then the presenting feature may be that of an optic nerve lesion, often with a temporal scotoma in the other eye. Chordomas and aneurysms usually compress the chiasm from the side, producing an initial defect in the ipsilateral nasal field. It can be seen, therefore, that many different types of defect can be found in chiasmal lesions in addition to the widely recognised bitemporal hemianopia.

A complete lesion of one **optic tract** produces a contralateral **homonymous hemianopia**, that is loss of the nasal field of the ipsilateral eye and of the temporal field of the contralateral eye. Thus in a lesion of the left optic tract, which can be produced by lesions like those which compress the chasm, the right half-field of both eyes is lost. However, since optic tract compression is frequently asymmetrical, a progressive increase in size of the defects in these half-fields may develop slowly and the defect may initially be larger in one field than in the other until the hemianopia is complete. When homonymous defects in the two fields are unequal in size and shape they are said to be **incongruous**.

Lesions of one **optic radiation**, whether in the internal capsule, temporal lobe, or occipital lobe, and whether of vascular (infarction, haemorrhage), neoplastic or inflammatory (encephalitis, diffuse sclerosis) aetiology, also cause homonymous defects. A large lesion will give a complete homonymous hemianopia, but a smaller one, say in the temporal lobe affecting the lower fibres of the radiation, may give a contralateral upper quadrantic homonymous defect. As the nerve fibres from the retina are closely intermixed in the radiation, so that those from homologous portions of the two retinae lie alongside one another, field defects due to radiation lesions are **congruous**, i.e. they are the same in both eyes. It has been suggested that there is bilateral representation of the macula in the two occipital lobes, so that in a homonymous hemianopia resulting from an occipital lobe lesion the macular area of the blind half-field is spared. This finding may be an artefact due to poor fixation during charting of the fields, and in such a case the macular field is actually split, but in vascular lesions it may be due to the fact that the macular area can receive some blood supply from both the posterior and middle cerebral arteries and may thus be spared in patients with a dense hemianopia due to middle cerebral artery occlusion. Visual acuity is unimpaired in a patient with a complete homonymous hemianopia, but reading is difficult, as in normal reading words are read in groups of two or three and in a patient with a hemianopia ability to see only half the words in the group can cause great difficulty. Patients with a right homonymous hemianopia read slowly because they are unable to scan ahead of the word they are reading, whereas patients with a left homonymous hemianopia have difficulty in finding the start of the next line. Some representative visual field defects are illustrated in Figure 8.2.

Abnormalities of the visual fields can also result from local ocular conditions such as glaucoma and retinal detachment, but these disorders are generally apparent on examining the eye and rarely give diagnostic difficulty. Some **concentric diminution** of the fields with enlargement of the blind spot is seen in severe papilloedema and less often in optic atrophy due to syphilis or constriction of the optic nerve due to arachnoiditis. Loss of the peripheral field with retention of only a small central area (**tubular vision**) is usually an hysterical phenomenon but can occur in retinitis pigmentosa.

The optic fundus and its abnormalities

Ophthalmoscopic examination of the optic disc, of the retinal vessels, and of the retina itself is an essential and often revealing part of a neurological examination. The optic disc is normally slightly pink in colour, but its temporal half is generally paler than the nasal, while some lack of definition of its nasal margin is common. In the centre of the disc, or slightly more towards its temporal margin, is the physiological cup into which the vessels dip; this cup is often much paler than the rest of the disc and its appearance must not be confused with that of optic atrophy. Excessive cupping is, of course,

seen in glaucoma. Sometimes a leash of pale fibres is seen spreading for a short distance across the retina, in fan-like manner, from one part of the edge of the disc; these **medullated nerve fibres** are common' and have no pathological significance.

The two most frequent abnormalities of the optic disc are swelling (papilloedema) and excessive pallor (optic atrophy).

Papilloedema (Fig. 8.3) generally results from obstruction to the venous return from the retina, so that the first sign may be distension of the retinal veins, which look unusually tumid and lose pulsation. This is followed by obliteration of the physiological cup and later the centre of the disc becomes raised above the level of the surrounding retina, while its margins become progressively more blurred and indistinct. When swelling is severe, haemorrhages and sometimes patches of white exudate develop around the disc margins in a radial manner. A star-shaped patch, of white exudate ('macular star') may also develop in the macular area, which is normally a relatively avascular area of the retina, lying about two disc-breadths lateral to the disc. The principal cause of papilloedema is **increased intracranial pressure**, transmitted to the optic nerve sheath and so compressing the veins, as in cases of intracranial tumour, abscess, haemorrhage, hydrocephalus or meningitis. Severe papilloedema due to increased intracranial pressure is often present without loss of visual acuity, though there may be some concentric diminution of the fields with enlargement of the blind spot, and the patient sees flashes of light or 'haloes' around lights, symptoms which may presage impending visual failure. These symptoms indicate that urgent measures to reduce the intracranial pressure are needed, since if visual loss occurs as a result of papilloedema it is due to compression of the central retinal artery and is usually complete and irreversible. Transient episodes of visual loss in patients with papilloedema, provoked often by stooping, are due to retinal ischaemia and give warning of impending occlusion. Papilloedema can also be due to severe arterial disease, as in **chronic nephritis** and **malignant hypertension**, to local lesions giving venous obstruction in the orbit or elsewhere (**central retinal vein thrombosis, cavernous sinus thrombosis, cor pulmonale**), or to **polycythaemia vera**.

The other principal cause of disc swelling is papillitis which occurs when the lesion of optic or retrobulbar neuritis lies close to the nerve head. This is an 'inflammatory' neuritis of the optic nerve, due most often to a demyelinating lesion of multiple sclerosis or the related neuromyelitis optica, but rarely resulting from syphilis or from toxic, nutritional and metabolic disorders. These two causes of disc swelling can generally be distinguished by the fact that visual acuity is seriously impaired at an

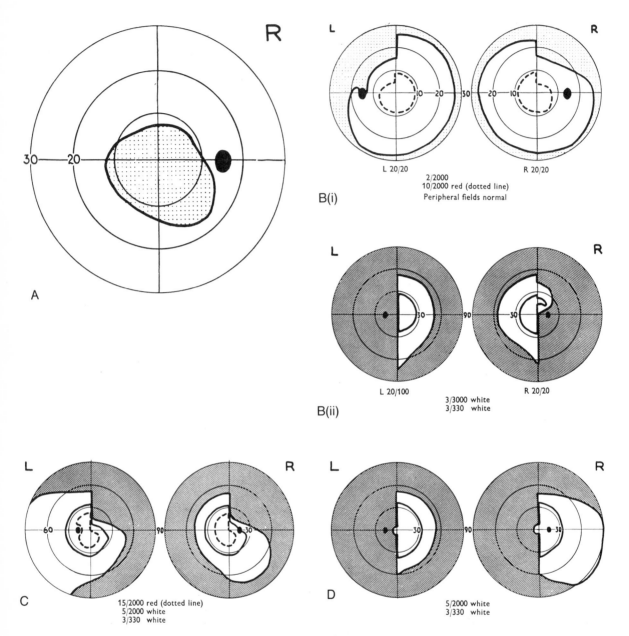

Fig. 8.2 A   A central scotoma due to retrobulbar neuritis. **B**   (i) Visual fields of a patient with a chromophobe adenoma of the pituitary, showing early changes in the upper temporal quadrants. (ii) Field changes in a patient with a chromophobe adenoma of the pituitary. There is an almost complete bitemporal hemianopia. **C**   Fields of a patient with a glioma in the left temporo-occipital region. **D**   Fields of a patient with a metastasis from a breast carcinoma involving the right geniculocalcarine pathway. (Reproduced with permission from Walton 1985.)

early stage in retrobulbar neuritis. Furthermore, disc swelling is rarely as great in retrobulbar neuritis as in papilloedema, while haemorrhages and exudates are uncommon; indeed the disc may look surprisingly normal even in the acute stage when visual acuity is severely impaired unless the plaque of demyelination is very close to the disc. The typical history is one of progressive failure of vision in one eye, often associated with local pain, and usually leading to partial or total monocular blindness within a few hours or days. There is often complete recovery from this condition after several weeks or months, although a central scotoma may persist. Nowadays the condition is presumed to be due to multiple sclerosis unless some other cause is clearly apparent; however it may be many months or years before other neurological manifestations develop, and in some cases they never do so. Occasionally, congenital hyaline bodies ('drüsen') lying on or in relation to the optic disc can give sufficient blurring of its margins (**pseudopapilloedema**) to make diagnosis from true papilloedema

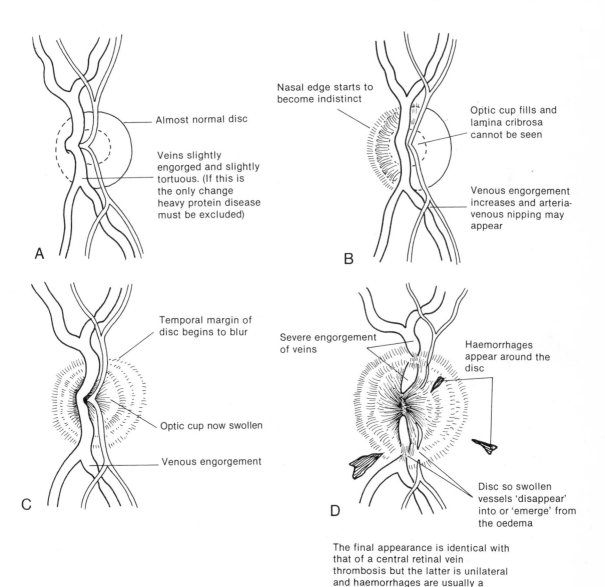

Fig. 8.3 The sequence in developing papilloedema. (Reproduced with permission from Patten 1977.)

difficult. Fluorescein retinal angiography may then be diagnostic, and calcification may be seen in the disc on the CT scan.

The optic disc in patients with **optic atrophy** is chalky-white or grey in colour, its pallor contrasting with the surrounding retina. The edges of the disc are clear-cut and often irregular. The form of optic atrophy seen in **multiple sclerosis** which typically follows an attack of retrobulbar neuritis, although no history of such an episode may be obtained, affects the temporal half of the disc much more than the nasal, as the fibres from the macular area of the retina enter this part of the disc. This so-called **temporal pallor**, which may be difficult to distinguish from the normal comparative pallor of the temporal part of the disc, except through experience, is almost diagnostic of multiple sclerosis. Optic atrophy may also be inherited; it is a feature of **cerebral lipidosis** of the Tay-Sachs type (cerebromacular degeneration), in which case there may also be a cherry-red spot at the macula; it is a common accompaniment of diseases in the **hereditary ataxia** group (see pp. 188–189). It also occurs in **retinitis pigmentosa**, a genetically-determined disorder which causes progressive bilateral visual failure, usually in early adult life, and in which there is also spidery pigmentation of the periphery of the retina and narrowing of the retinal vessels.

Leber's optic atrophy is another inherited condition (usually due to a sex-linked (X-linked) recessive gene) in which bilateral optic atrophy develops comparatively rapidly in young adult males. The history is often reminiscent of that of retrobulbar neuritis but vision recovers only temporarily, if at all. The condition may be due to an inherited defect of cyanide metabolism and in occasional cases hydroxocobalamin seems to have produced temporary improvement. **Syphilis** is also an important cause of optic atrophy; up to 15% of patients with tabes dorsalis, particularly of the congenital type, have pale discs and the visual fields show peripheral constriction with enlargement of the blind spot. Of more immediate consequence as a cause is **compression of the optic nerve**, whether by a tumour of the nerve itself or of its sheath, or by a meningioma, pituitary neoplasm or aneurysm which lies in relation to the nerve in its intracranial course. Less commonly a **head injury** will injure one optic nerve with a similar result, while severe papilloedema, glaucoma, choroidoretinitis, occlusion of the central retinal artery or central retinal venous thrombosis may all in time give rise to optic atrophy. When this occurs as a sequel of long-standing papilloedema, it is referred to as **secondary** or **consecutive optic atrophy**. Various **metabolic, toxic and nutritional disorders** may also damage the optic nerves. Thus, blindness can result from methyl alcohol poisoning while quinine, arsenical

drugs and chloroquine have all been known to produce such an effect, as may the dietary ingestion of cyanide in cassava root in cases of tropical ataxic neuropathy with amblyopia. Cyanide has also been implicated as the cause of tobacco amblyopia. It is uncertain whether nutritional amblyopia (as observed in some prisoners of war) is due to vitamin B_1 deficiency or to lack of other B vitamins, while pyridoxine deficiency (as in patients taking isoniazid) rarely, and B_{12} deficiency (pernicious anaemia or dietary deficiency in vegans) more commonly, can cause optic atrophy.

Changes in **retinal vessels** are also of considerable diagnostic value. The venous engorgement of papilloedema has already been mentioned. In subarachnoid haemorrhage, the rapid inflow of blood into the optic nerve sheath can give such severe venous obstruction that a large brick-red **subhyaloid haemorrhage** may be seen extending from the edge of the optic disk. Early changes of **atherosclerosis** and **hypertension** may take the form of slight 'silver-wiring' of retinal arteries (Grade I retinopathy) with subsequent narrowing of veins where the arteries cross them (Grade II); when the changes are more severe, flame-shaped haemorrhages and patches of hard white exudate appear in the retina (Grade III) and eventually papilloedema develops (Grade IV). In **diabetic** patients, small micro-aneurysms are sometimes found on peripheral retinal arteries. **Occlusion of the central retinal artery** may give sudden unilateral blindness; the arteries are seen to be reduced in calibre and optic atrophy follows. While this syndrome can result from atherosclerosis, in elderly patients it is often due to **cranial arteritis**, and thickening of the temporal arteries with other features of this disease are generally found. Transient unilateral blindness is often due to embolism of the artery, and occurs most commonly in patients with internal carotid artery stenosis: emboli of platelets or cholesterol may be seen in retinal arteries during attacks ('amaurosis fugax').

Among other retinal abnormalities of diagnostic value are **retinal angiomas** (tangles of abnormal blood vessels) found in patients with haemangioblastoma of the cerebellum (Lindau-von Hippel disease) **retinal tubercles** (yellowish nodules, often about half the size of the optic disk) which help to confirm a diagnosis of tuberculous meningitis or miliary tuberculosis, and flat yellow plaques or **phakomas** which may be seen in tuberous sclerosis or neurofibromatosis.

The cornea and lens

A cloudy 'ground-glass' opacity of the cornea, due to interstitial keratitis consequent upon congenital syphilis, may help to confirm that a patient's neurological symptoms are due to neurosyphilis. Arcus senilis may occur prematurely in patients with hypercholesterolaemia and atherosclerosis, but a paler white rim around the periphery of the cornea (marginal keratitis) is usually indicative of hypercalcaemia. Of even greater diagnostic value, though rare, is the golden-brown peripheral rim of pigmentation (the Kayser-Fleischer ring) of Wilson's disease, which may only be visible on examination with a slit-lamp. The latter instrument may also be needed to detect the early cataract of dystrophia myotonica and the lens opacities seen in some rare storage disorders (such as the mucopolysaccharidoses) of childhood.

The pupils

The parasympathetic nerve fibres which innervate the constrictor of the pupil travel in the third cranial (oculomotor) nerve, while sympathetic fibres responsible for pupillary dilatation arise in the hypothalamus and traverse the tegmentum of the brain stem and the cervical cord to the lateral horn of grey matter in the eighth cervical and first and second dorsal segments. They leave the cord in the anterior roots to reach the superior cervical ganglion, from which postganglionic fibres arise which enter the skull in the plexus in the wall of the internal carotid artery. Some then pass to the ophthalmic division of the fifth (trigeminal) nerve and enter the orbit with its branches, while others go from the carotid plexus directly to the ciliary ganglion in the orbit, giving rise to the short ciliary nerves.

Both pupils normally constrict when a light is shone upon one retina; the reaction in the illuminated eye is called the direct reaction, that in the opposite eye the consensual one. The afferent pathway for the light reflex travels in the optic nerve to the lateral geniculate body and superior corpora quadrigemina (colliculi) and thence to the third nerve nuclei, whence efferent constrictor fibres arise. Hence a lesion on the afferent side of the pathway (e.g. optic atrophy) impairs both the direct and the consensual reaction to light, while a lesion in the efferent pathway (e.g. third-nerve paralysis) to the eye being stimulated will affect the direct but not the consensual reaction. Constriction of the pupil also occurs when vision is focused upon a near object, a procedure which involves both accommodation (through contraction of the ciliary muscle) and convergence, and which is subserved by a series of reflexes involving the oculomotor nuclei. Both the light and accommodation reactions are impaired by a lesion of the third nerve. Paralysis of the pupillary reaction to accommodation with preservation of the light reflex is rare, though it can occur occasionally in lesions of the midbrain and may seem to be present when ocular convergence is impaired, as may be seen with ageing or in post-encephalitic-parkinsonism. Loss of

the light reflex with retention of that to accommodation-convergence is, however, one feature of the **Argyll Robertson pupil** of tabes dorsalis, which is also sometimes present in general paresis. Additional features are that the pupils are small, irregular and unequal; there is atrophy of the iris, and loss of the ciliospinal reflex (pupillary dilatation on pinching the skin of the neck). There is some controversy about the location of the lesion responsible for the Argyll Robertson pupil; some believe it to be in the periaqueductal region of the midbrain, others in the ciliary ganglion. In congenital syphilis, the light reflex may be lost, but the pupils are often large and are not therefore of typical Argyll Robertson type.

A lesion of the **third-nerve nucleus** or of the nerve in its intracranial course can paralyse the pupillo-constrictor muscles, so that the pupil becomes dilated and fixed. As the parasympathetic fibres lie relatively superficially in the nerve trunk, along with those innervating the levator palpebrae superioris, this pupillary change may be the first sign of a third-nerve lesion, being followed by ptosis and later by external ophthalmoplegia. Pressure upon the nerve by an aneurysm or pituitary neoplasm, and ischaemia or infarction of the nerve in diabetes mellitus, are common causes of a unilateral third-nerve palsy. A similar effect can result from herniation of the temporal lobe through the tentorial hiatus so that a unilateral fixed dilated pupil may be an early sign of a space-occupying lesion in or overlying one cerebral hemisphere (such as an extradural or subdural haematoma).

A lesion of the sympathetic pathway gives a constricted pupil (myosis) and usually the other features of **Horner's syndrome** (myosis, ptosis, enophthalmos and loss of sweating on the affected side of the face). The lesion responsible may lie in the descending pathway in the brain stem (as in certain cases of brain stem infarction, e.g. posterior inferior cerebellar artery thrombosis), in the neck, involving one of the cervical sympathetic ganglia, or in the internal carotid artery, damaging sympathetic fibres which run in the wall of the vessel (e.g. aneurysm). In the latter case, facial sweating, mediated by fibres in the coat of the external carotid artery, is unimpaired (**Raeder's paratrigeminal syndrome**). Sympathetic overactivity, due for instance to fright, dilates the pupils. Lesions in the brain stem often affect the size and reactivity of the pupils; changes of localising value in comatose patients and in identifying the site of brain stem lesions are described on page 73.

Drugs have a profound influence upon pupillary size and activity. Myotics, which cause pupillary constriction, include morphine, pilocarpine, neostigmine and eserine, while mydriatics or dilators include the long-acting atropine, homatropine which is used to dilate the pupil for ophthalmoscopy, and cocaine. When examining the pupils it should also be remembered that **local ocular conditions** can influence their shape and size. Iridocyclitis, for instance, often gives irregularities of the iris and adhesions to the lens (synechiae), which may restrict the range of pupillary movement. **Hippus** is a phenomenon of intermittent rhythmical pupillary contraction and dilatation; though sometimes observed in patients with neurological disease it has no diagnostic value. The detection of an afferent pupillary defect is strong evidence of an optic nerve lesion and is nearly always found in patients with retrobulbar neuritis. There is loss of the direct light reaction in the affected eye but a brisk consensual reaction in the affected eye when the other eye is stimulated. If a light is shone alternately into both eyes, the pupil in the affected eye follows that of the unaffected eye and the pupil therefore dilates as the light is shone into the affected eye, in striking contrast to the normal reflex. These signs are collectively known as the retrobulbar pupil reaction.

Another interesting pupillary abnormality is that known as the **myotonic** or **Adie's pupil** (Fig. 8.4). When this pupillary abnormality is associated with sluggishness or absence of the tendon reflexes, the condition is referred to as the **Holmes-Adie syndrome**. Characteristically it occurs in young women, though it is occasionally seen in males. The patient may notice a sudden onset of blurring of vision in one eye or alternatively she observes on looking into the mirror that one pupil is dilated. On examination the pupil is widely dilated and shows a sluggish, delayed reaction to light. The reaction to accommodation is usually better but this too may be impaired and indeed it may be impossible to produce pupillary constriction with either stimulus. The condition is benign but its aetiology is unknown and it is

uninfluenced by treatment. The lesion responsible is a loss of cells in the ciliary ganglion.

The eyelids and orbital muscles

That part of the levator palpebrae superioris consisting of voluntary muscle is innervated by the third cranial nerve but there is also a smooth muscle component (Muller's muscle) innervated by the sympathetic. Hence paresis of the third nerve or of the sympathetic can cause **ptosis**. Ptosis can also be congenital and is then either unilateral or bilateral; it also occurs in myasthenia gravis when it typically worsens as the day wears on, in tabes dorsalis, and in myopathic degeneration of the external ocular muscles (ocular myopathy). **Blepharospasm**, a prolonged or intermittent spasm of the orbicularis oculi, causing eye closure, is often due to habit spasm or hysteria but is sometimes seen in parkinsonism and other extrapyramidal disorders. When persistent blepharospasm is associated with oromandibular dyskinesia this combination of signs, usually due to a degenerative process of unknown aetiology in the extrapyramidal system, is often called **Meige's** or **Brueghel's** syndrome.

Lid retraction, or a failure of the upper lid to follow the globe on downward movement of the eye, is typically seen in thyrotoxicosis in which **exophthalmos**, or protrusion of the eye, is also common. The term **proptosis** is sometimes used to identify a unilateral exophthalmos, particularly when asymmetrical. Severe exophthalmos, sometimes unilateral, but more often bilateral, can result from excessive output of the exophthalmos-producing substance, which is neither LATS nor thyrotropic hormone, by the anterior pituitary. Some recent evidence (the discovery of circulating antibodies against ocular muscle and improvement resulting from steroids in high

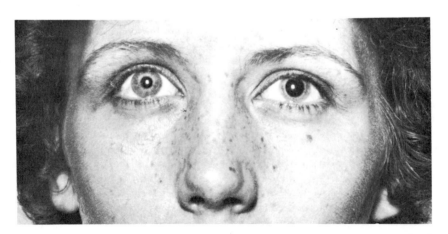

Fig. 8.4   The myotonic pupil. (Reproduced with permission from Spillane & Spillane 1982.)

dosage) has raised the alternative possiblitity of an autoimmune pathogenesis. In this condition there is swelling of the external ocular muscles and orbital tissues, and ophthalmoplegia is common (**exophthalmic ophthalmoplegia, ophthalmic Graves' disease** or **Graves' ophthalmopathy**). Sometimes the condition begins with minimal exophthalmos on one side only and often with weakness limited to one superior rectus muscle. By contrast, severe painful exophthalmos with total paralysis of all ocular movement and severe conjunctival chemosis can develop in acute cases within a few days and papilloedema may ensue, so that urgent surgical decompression may be needed. Other conditions which may cause exophthalmos include orbital tumour, 'pseudotumour' (see below) other inflammatory lesions in the orbit or paranasal sinuses, retro-orbital intracranial tumours (meningiomas in particular) and thrombosis of, or arteriovenous aneurysm in, the cavernous sinus. Intermittent exophthalmos, occurring particularly on coughing or stooping, may be due to an orbital venous angioma; that due to an arteriovenous fistula in the cavernous sinus may pulsate and a systolic bruit will be heard over the globe of the eye. A painless exophthalmos, often unilateral, is rarely due to an orbital pseudotumour resulting from autoimmune orbital myositis in which the histology of the ocular muscles resembles that of polyarteritis nodosa or polymyositis. This condition, too, may require surgical decompression but in many cases there is a good response to treatment with steroid drugs. A mucocele of the ethmoid sinus, by contrast, usually gives unilateral proptosis with lateral deviation and protrusion of the globe of the eye.

External ocular movement and its abnormalities

The nature and control of ocular movements

The ocular movements include horizontal movement outwards (abduction); horizontal movement inwards (adduction); vertical movement upwards (elevation); vertical movement downwards (depression). The eye is capable of diagonal movements at any intermediate angle. The term 'rotation' should be reserved for wheel-like movements around an imaginary pivot passing through the centre of the pupil; such movements of rotation are not normal but only occur as a result of the unbalanced action of certain muscles. Inward rotation is a movement like that of a wheel rolling towards the nose, outward rotation the opposite. Normally the movements of the two eyes are harmoniously symmetrical constituting conjugate ocular movement, whether horizontal or lateral, upward or downward. Conjugate adduction of the two eyes is known as convergence. Other varieties of ocular movement will be considered below.

The nuclei of the ocular muscles The lower motor neurones which innervate the ocular muscles originate in the nuclei of the third, fourth and sixth cranial nerves. The first two lie in the midbrain just anterior to the cerebral aqueduct at the level of the superior and inferior colliculi. The nuclei of the sixth nerve lie in the pons beneath the floor of the fourth ventricle and partly encircled by the fibres of the seventh nerve (Fig. 8.5). Immediately below the third nerve nucleus lies that of the fourth nerve which innervates the opposite superior oblique. This nucleus and the adjacent lowest part of the third nerve nucleus innervate the two muscles concerned in depression of the eye, and the two elevating muscles are innervated by mutually adjacent portions of the upper half of the nucleus of the third nerve.

The extrinsic ocular muscles The extrinsic ocular muscles are the four recti, superior and inferior, lateral and medial, and the two obliques, superior and inferior. The action of each of these muscles is shown in Figure 8.6. Only the lateral and medial recti act in a single plane.

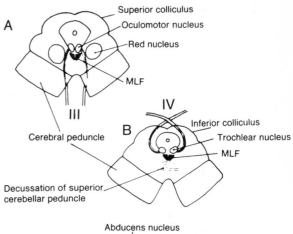

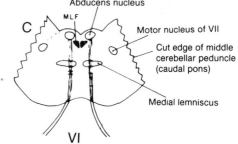

Fig. 8.5 Diagrammatic cross sections at the levels of the nuclei for the (**A**) oculomotor nerve (III), (**B**) trochlear nerve (IV), and (**C**) abducens nerve (VI). MLF locates the medial longitudinal fasciculus. (Reproduced from Patton et al 1976, by kind permission of the authors and publisher.)

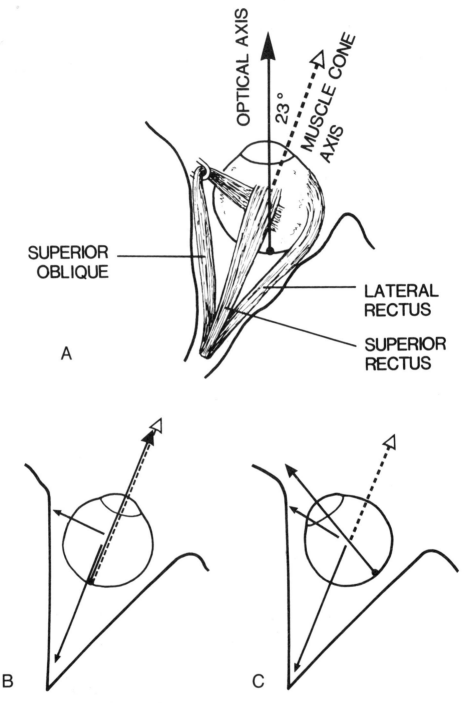

Fig. 8.6 **A** Diagram of the right eye viewed from above to show the superior oblique, lateral rectus and superior rectus muscles and the optical and muscle cone axes. **B** With the eye 23° abducted, the muscle cone axis and the optical axes are in line; in this position the superior rectus is a pure elevator and the superior oblique can only rotate the eye. **C** With the eye adducted, the superior oblique causes depression of the eye, while the action of the superior rectus is largely one of rotation.

The other muscles always act in concert; thus when the two obliques aid the lateral rectus in abduction their vertical and rotatory forces cancel out; and when the superior rectus and inferior and inferior oblique contract together to elevate the eye their horizontal and rotatory components also cancel. But owing to the anatomy of the superior and inferior recti and the obliques, their actions are influenced by the position of the eye in the orbit. When it is rotated outwards 23° the superior rectus is a pure elevator and the inferior rectus a pure depressor. The more it is turned inwards the more they act as internal and external rotators. The converse is true of the obliques. In conjugate deviation there is a harmonious contraction of the appropriate muscles of the two eyes. In lateral conjugate deviation the lateral rectus of one eye and the medial rectus of the other are associated; in conjugate deviation upwards and downwards, the elevators and depressors of the two eyes respectively; and in convergence, the medial recti. Graded contraction and relaxation of their antagonists play an important part in orderly movement.

Paralysis of individual ocular muscles The more important results of paralysis of an ocular muscle are:

1. defective ocular movement
2. squint
3. erroneous projection of the visual field and
4. diplopia.

Defective ocular movement is demonstrated by asking the patient to fix his gaze on an object, such as the observer's finger, which is then moved upwards and downwards and to either side, convergence being tested by bringing it towards the patient. The movement is defective in the direction in which the eye is normally moved by the muscle which is paralysed.

Squint, or **strabismus**, is the term applied to a failure of the normal coordination of the ocular axes. Paralytic squint must be distinguished from concomitant squint. Paralytic squint may be present when the eyes are at rest, due to the unbalanced action of the normal antagonist of the paralysed muscle; for example, the affected eye may be slightly adducted when the lateral rectus is paralysed. More often it is seen only when the eyes move in the direction in which the eye should be pulled by the paralysed muscle, or squint present at rest is increased by this movement. Concomitant squint, however, is present at rest and is equal for all positions of the eyes; if the fixing eye is covered, the movements of the squinting eye are full. Concomitant squint is not usually associated with diplopia; paralytic squint, at least in the early stages, usually is. However, when there is long-standing ocular muscle imbalance (latent concomitant squint or hetero-

phoria) the patient may be able for many years to contract the ocular muscles so as to fuse the images from the two eyes; as he becomes older the effort is no longer possible so that the latent squint breaks down and diplopia may result. Similarly, in long-standing paralytic squint, one image may ultimately be suppressed so that diplopia disappears; suppression of this type often results in one eye becoming amblyopic as a result of untreated concomitant squint in early childhood. When the lateral rectus is paralysed the ocular axes converge and the squint is said to be convergent. Paralysis of the medial rectus causes divergent squint.

Erroneous projection of the visual field If we look directly at an object in any position of the eyes, the image of the object falls upon the macula. When the right lateral rectus is paralysed, on conjugate deviation to the right the left eye moves normally but the right eye remains directed forwards. The image of the object falls in the left eye upon the macula, in the right eye upon the nasal half of the retina. The patient is accustomed to regard an object, the image of which falls upon the nasal half of the right retina, as being situated to the right of one of which the image falls upon the macula. Consequently he sees two images and projects the false image perceived by his affected eye to the right of the true image perceived by his normal eye. If now his normal eye is covered and he is asked to touch the object, he will direct his finger to the right of its true position. The erroneous projection is always in the normal direction of action of the affected muscle. Hess's screen can be used to record the position of the false image. Erroneous projection of the visual field of the affected eye is thus responsible for **double vision** or **diplopia**. When both eyes are used, two images are seen, one correctly and one erroneously projected, the true and the false image. From the facts outlined, three simple rules about diplopia can be deduced:

1. The separation of the images increases the further the eyes are moved in the normal direction of pull of the paralysed muscle.
2. The false image is displaced in the direction of the plane of action of the paralysed muscle.
3. In vertical diplopia the double vision is due to an oblique palsy if it is maximal with the affected eye adducted, and due to a rectus palsy if the separation of the images is maximal with the affected eye abducted. The true and false images can readily be identified by placing coloured glasses over each eye.

From these facts it is a relatively easy matter to deduce which muscle or muscles are involved in a patient with paralytic squint.

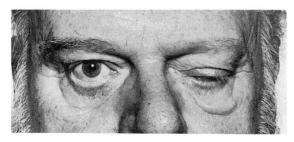
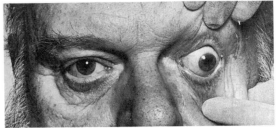

Fig. 8.7 A left third-nerve palsy in a diabetic subject who also had a carcinoma of the left ethmoid sinus (Fig. kindly supplied by Dr J.D. Spillane). Note the ptosis and the abduction of the eye due to the unopposed action of the lateral rectus. (Reproduced with permission from Walton 1985.)

Nuclear and infranuclear lesions which affect ocular movement Having confirmed which muscle or muscles are affected and hence which nerve is diseased, it is then necessary to decide the nature of the lesion responsible. A lesion of one third nerve gives ptosis, a fixed dilated pupil, lateral and downward deviation of the globe (due to unopposed action of the lateral (sixth nerve) and superior oblique (fourth nerve) muscles) with loss of all movements except lateral and downward and outward movement (Fig. 8.7). A sixth nerve lesion causes loss of lateral deviation of the affected eye (Fig. 8.8). Rarely, an isolated paralysis of abduction of one eye simulating a sixth nerve lesion is congenital and often familial (Duane's syndrome) and is due to fibrosis of the lateral rectus muscle. Many traumatic, inflammatory, neoplastic and degenerative disorders arising in the brain stem or in the basal cisterns or orbital foramina can cause lesions of one or more of the oculomotor nerves. In the brain stem itself, **infarcts**, **gliomas** and **Wernicke's disease** are the most common, while in the basal cisterns, the third, fourth or sixth nerve lesion is congenital and often familial (Duane's syndrome) and is due to fibrosis of the lateral rectus **tumour**. A third or sixth nerve palsy of sudden onset in an

elderly person may result from compression of the trunk of the nerve by an **atherosclerotic artery**, or from actual infarction of the nerve trunk itself, and these palsies generally clear up spontaneously in from three to six months. They are particularly common in patients with **diabetes mellitus**. The third nerve in particular is also vulnerable in patients with basal **arterial aneurysms** or **pituitary tumours**, while it can be paralysed as a result of a cerebral hemisphere lesion giving **tentorial herniation**. When complete third, fourth and sixth nerve palsies develop and are associated with sensory loss in the upper face, then an **aneurysm in the cavernous sinus**, compressing also the first and second divisions of the trigeminal nerve, which accompany these nerves within the sinus, may be present. A similar syndrome results from lesions in the neighbourhood of the **superior orbital fissure**; one such is so-called orbital apicitis or 'painful ophthalmoplegia' (the Tolosa-Hunt syndrome) resulting from a steroid-responsive inflammatory process of unknown aetiology at the apex of the orbit. Pain behind the eye often precedes the ophthalmoplegia in such cases.

Lesions of the myoneural junction and of the ocular muscles themselves can also produce ptosis, strabismus

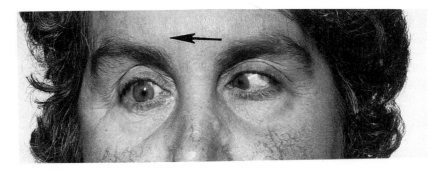

Fig. 8.8 A right sixth-nerve palsy, evident on right lateral gaze. (Reproduced with permission from Spillane & Spillane 1982.)

and diplopia. In **myasthenia gravis**, for instance, drooping of the eyelids towards the end of the day and
intermittent or fluctuant squint and diplopia are common. An uncommon condition in which there is slowly
progressive bilateral ptosis, with, eventually, impairment
of ocular movement in all directions, is **ocular myopathy**.
Most cases of this type were previously referred to as
progressive nuclear ophthalmoplegia on the assumption
that the disease was one of the oculomotor nuclei, but it is
now recognised that the process responsible is only
occasionally nuclear and is more often a progressive
dystrophy or mitochondrial myopathy of the external
ocular muscles. In some such cases there is associated
retinal pigmentation and cerebellar degeneration with
abnormal mitochondria not only in the ocular muscles
but also in the cerebellum (the Kearns-Sayre syndrome).

*The supranuclear and internuclear control of
ocular movement*

During **conjugate** or **version** movements of the eyes the
visual axes remain parallel, while during **disconjugate** or
vergence movements the axes intersect. Version movements are of two types: in one (**saccades** or **saccadic
movements**) the eyes jump rapidly and successively from
one point of fixation to another, while in the other
(**smooth-pursuit movements**) the eyes follow smoothly a
moving object. All voluntary eye movements (except
when viewing a moving object) take the form of fast
saccades; thus in reading a line of print the eyes read one
to four words in the course of a single fixation and then
jump to the next series of words. Speed and efficiency of
reading depend upon the number of words read during
each fixation. Smooth pursuit movements, used to track
moving objects, are much slower than saccades and
cannot be performed at will without the stimulus of a
moving target. By contrast, vergence movements, which
are slow, track approaching (convergence) or receding
(divergence) objects, and during these the eyes move in
opposite directions.

Supranuclear and internuclear pathways   The supranuclear pathway concerned with voluntary conjugate
eye movement (saccades) in a lateral direction originates
in the frontal eye field in the contralateral middle frontal
gyrus (Brodmann's area 8). Stimulation in this area gives
contralateral saccades, while destructive lesions give
difficulty in carrying out voluntary version movements of
the eyes to the opposite side. The pathway from this
cortical area descends through the corona radiata, internal capsule and cerebral peduncle, subsequently decussating in the midbrain and descending in the pons to join
the medial longitudinal fasciculus at about the level of
the sixth nerve nucleus. Thus stimulation in the pons,
below the decussation of this pathway, causes conjugate

deviation of the eyes towards the lesion or point of
stimulation, while a unilateral lesion of the ponto-
mesencephalic reticular formation may cause paralysis of
conjugate gaze towards the affected side. Another important cortical centre controlling ocular movements lies in
or near the visual cortex in the occipital lobe and is
probably concerned especially with smooth pursuit
movements and with vergence.

Because coordination of the movement of the two eyes
is essential for binocular vision, the nuclei of the
individual third, fourth and sixth cranial nerves are
linked together in the medial longitudinal bundle or
fasciculus which is the principal internuclear pathway
involved in the control of ocular movement. Supranuclear pathways as described above all feed into this
fasciculus. Cerebellar lesions often cause over- or under-
shoot of saccadic movements and/or the breaking down
of smooth-pursuit movements into saccades. In Huntington's chorea saccadic movements often become slow,
jerky and irregular.

Reflex ocular movement   In voluntary conjugate
deviation of the eyes the patient may turn his eyes
spontaneously or on command, but some ocular movements are reflexly induced. Visual stimuli usually result
in movement of the head or eyes in order to keep the
image upon the macula. Continuous movement of a
series of objects or lines in one direction evokes optokinetic nystagmus (see below). Similarly, auditory stimulation may give deviation of the eyes towards the origin of
the sound, while caloric or electrical excitation of one
labyrinth evokes conjugate ocular deviation and nystagmus (see below). If the patient fixes his gaze upon an
object and the head is then flexed, rotated or extended at
the neck, reflex ocular deviation occurs in an attempt to
keep the image of the object upon the macula. This
oculocephalic reflex (the doll's head manoeuvre) is
dependent upon the integrity of the medial longitudinal
fasciculus and of its connections with the vestibular
system, and is thus valuable in determining whether
pontine vestibulo-ocular connections are intact in
patients in coma.

Supranuclear and internuclear lesions   **Spasmodic
conjugate lateral movement** of the eyes may occur in
focal attacks of epilepsy due to lesions involving the
contralateral frontal eye field. **Paralysis of conjugate
lateral movement** may occur as the result of a lesion at
any point in the supranuclear pathway, but this effect is
always transient in lesions situated above the pons,
though one involving the decussation of the pathways at
the ponto-mesencephalic junction can give paralysis of
conjugate gaze to both sides. However, a unilateral
pontine lesion can cause long-lasting paralysis of both
voluntary and reflex conjugate gaze to the affected side.

This can result from encephalomyelitis or Wernicke's disease but is more often due to brain stem infarction. **Dissociation of conjugate lateral movement** is usually a consequence of a lesion of the medial longitudinal fasciculus (an internuclear lesion). Much the commonest effect is the so-called **anterior internuclear ophthalmoplegia** (Harris' sign or **'ataxic nystagmus'**) in which there is phasic nystagmus confined to the abducting eye associated with failure of medial movement of the adducting eye. While this sign can rarely be a consequence of brain stem tumour or infarction, it is much more often due to multiple sclerosis and can be unilateral or bilateral.

Skew deviation of the eyes, in which one eye is deviated upwards and outwards, the other downwards and out, is a rare consequence of an acute cerebellar or pontine lesion. **Spasmodic conjugate vertical movement** of the eyes upwards is a rare phenomenon, occasionally occurring in an attack of epilepsy, especially petit mal, but it is also seen in the oculogyric crises of post-encephalitic parkinsonism. **Paralysis of conjugate vertical deviation** in an upward direction is not uncommon, but paralysis of downward movement is excessively rare. In midbrain lesions involving the region of the superior colliculus, voluntary upward deviation can be lost even though the movement can still be excited reflexly. The term 'Parinaud's syndrome' is often applied to isolated defects of upward conjugate gaze, which can rarely be congenital, but in the fully-developed syndrome due to lesions of the midbrain tectum there is often loss of the pupillary light reflexes and paralysis of convergence in addition. This may result from encephalitis, front tumours of the third ventricle, midbrain or pineal body, from Wernicke's disease or from infarction. **Paralysis of convergence** is occasionally seen in post-encephalitic parkinsonism, as a result of head injury or midbrain infarction, and rarely results from ageing. Loss of convergence is occasionally, and spasm of convergence invariably, hysterical.

Progressive supranuclear degeneration (the Steele-Richardson-Olszewski syndrome) is a rare degenerative disorder characterised by progressive ophthalmoplegia affecting vertical and especially downward gaze with early loss of saccadic movements. The ophthalmoplegia is associated clinically with variable parkinsonian and dystonic features, with dysarthria, pseudo-bulbar palsy, inconstant cerebellar and pyramidal signs and sometimes dementia; pathologically there is neurofibrillary and granulovacuolar degeneration of neurones with gliosis and demyelination in the brain stem (sometimes involving the oculomotor nuclei), basal ganglia and cerebellum. The disease is progressive and uninfluenced by treatment.

Nystagmus

Nystagmus is an oscillatory movement of the eyes which is often rhythmical and repetitive; it is sometimes present with the eyes at rest, but may only appear when they are moved conjugately, or, if present at rest, it may be accentuated by ocular movement. It can be rotary in type (occurring in more than one plane) or may occur only in a lateral or vertical direction. Occasionally both phases of the to-and-fro oscillation are of equal duration but more often there is a quick phase in one direction succeeded by a slower recoil (**phasic nystagmus**); in this case the nystagmus is said to occur in the direction of the quick phase. This phenomenon is a disorder of the posture of the eyes and can be produced by disease of the reflex pathways which influence ocular posture. Stimuli from the retina and labyrinths are important in the maintenance of posture of the eyes as of other parts of the body, as is cerebellar activity, so that lesions of any of these structures can cause nystagmus.

Nystagmus must be distinguished from other rare spontaneous ocular movements such as **opsoclonus**, a repetitive shock-like myoclonic jerking of the eyes, seen in subacute myoclonic encephalopathy of infancy and childhood, and **ocular bobbing**, in which the eyes bob rhythmically upwards and downwards as a very rare and often transient manifestation of a pontine lesion.

Congenital nystagmus, which may be familial, is a benign disorder of unknown aetiology in which a continuous pendular movement of the eyes occurs at rest and is often accentuated by movement of the head and eyes in any direction. It is usually asymptomatic. **Optokinetic nystagmus** is a physiological phenomenon which occurs when the eyes are fixed upon a moving object such as a rotating drum or the landscape observed from a moving vehicle. The slow phase occurs in the direction in which the object moves and is followed by a quick recoil. Optokinetic nystagmus to one side may be lost as a result of lesions of the contralateral frontal or parietal cortex or of the upper brain stem and this has been used as a diagnostic test. Absent, sluggish or irregular optokinetic responses usually indicate a pontine lesion; contralateral parieto-occipital lesions impair the slow phase of optokinetic nystagmus, frontal lesions the fast. **Nystagmus of peripheral origin** may be seen in any local ocular condition (such as amblyopia or optic atrophy) which impairs visual fixation; it may then be monocular, involving only the affected eye, and is generally pendular in type. Impairment of ocular fixation resulting from ocular muscle weakness, as in polyneuropathy or myasthenia gravis, can rarely give similar nystagmus. **Miner's nystagmus**, which was generally gross and pendular in type, was due to impaired macular vision and visual fixation resulting from prolonged work in poor illumination, but there were many associated symptoms (headaches, giddiness) and neurosis was an important complicating factor; the condition is now rare since lighting in mines has been improved.

Nystagmus of labyrinthine origin can be evoked by caloric stimulation of the semicircular canals; if only the horizontal canals are stimulated it is lateral in type, but involvement of the vertical canals gives a rotary type which is therefore more common in disease of the internal ear, and the quick phase of the nystagmus takes place in a direction away from the affected ear. This is seen in acute labyrinthine vertigo (see below); the amplitude of the nystagmus is increased on looking to the side away from the lesion. Sometimes nystagmus is produced only by sudden movement of the head in a particular direction (positional nystagmus); this occurs in benign positional nystagmus (see below), but is occasionally seen in brain-stem lesions or in patients with neoplasms in the region of the fourth ventricle.

The commonest causes of nystagmus in neurological practice are **lesions of the cerebellum or of cerebellar and vestibular connexions in the brain stem**. However, phasic nystagmus on lateral gaze may be due to many drugs including alcohol, barbiturates and anticonvulsants (**toxic nystagmus**). In a unilateral cerebellar lesion the nystagmus is increased on lateral deviation of the eyes towards the side of the lesion. So profuse are the structures in the brain stem which are concerned with cerebellar, vestibular and oculomotor function (the medial longitudinal bundle is one of the most important) that virtually any lesion in this situation, whether inflammatory, neoplastic, degenerative or metabolic, can produce this physical sign; it is almost impossible to attribute to it any specific localising or diagnostic value under these circumstances, except in the case of the **ataxic nystagmus** previously mentioned (see p. 119). Often the nystagmus due to a brain-stem lesion occurs particularly on lateral ocular movement, the quick phase occurring towards the direction of gaze, but many other varieties occur and **vertical nystagmus** is particularly common in cases of the Chiari malformation or in other lesions at or near the foramen magnum. Statistically, multiple sclerosis is the commonest cause, but encephalitis, vascular lesions, syringobulbia, Wernicke's encephalopathy and tumours can also produce this sign. An uncommon variant, called **primary position upbeat nystagmus**, associated with lesions of the vermis or of cerebellar connections in the lower brain stem, is characterised by upward nystagmus occurring during ocular fixation, increased by looking upwards, but decreased by downward gaze. There is no convincing evidence that lesions in the cervical spinal cord, or indeed at any level lower

than the medulla oblongata and cerebellar tonsils, ever produce nystagmus. **Rebound nystagmus** is an uncommon phenomenon, usually due to cerebellar degeneration, in which phasic nystagmus which appears on looking laterally quickly fatigues but recurs to the opposite side when the eyes return to the midline. Uncommonly, in patients with multiple sclerosis, cerebellar degeneration or posterior fossa malformations, another variant, **periodic alternating nystagmus**, occurs, giving nystagmus occurring now in one direction and later in the opposite direction. In the rare **see-saw nystagmus** one eye moves up as the other moves down; this is usually due to a third ventricular tumour or less often to a pontine lesion. **Pseudonystagmus** is sometimes seen in hysteria; crude and disorganised ocular movements superficially resembling nystagmus are seen during voluntary ocular movement but disappear during conscious ocular fixation and are often accompanied by blepharospasm.

THE AUDITORY NERVE

Auditory impulses are received by the cells of the organ of Corti, travel along the peripheral processes of the

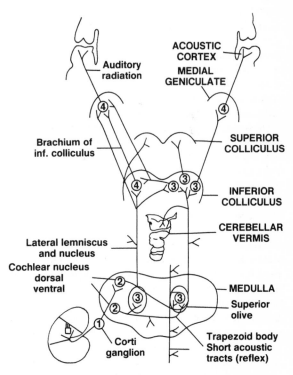

Fig. 8.9 Central auditory pathways. Numbers label first-, second- , third- and fourth-order neurones. (Reproduced with permission from Patton et al 1976.)

bipolar cells of the spiral ganglion of the cochlea and thence in the central processes of these cells in the auditory nerve to the cochlear nucleus in the pons; they then cross the midline and travel upwards in the lateral field to the inferior corpora quadrigemina and medial geniculate body; from this relay station they pass to the cortical centre for hearing in the middle and superior temporal gyri (Fig. 8.9). The principal symptoms of disease of the auditory system are deafness and tinnitus. **Conductive or 'middle-ear' deafness** due to inflammation or otosclerosis can generally be distinguished by tuning-fork tests, but audiometry is needed for accurate assessment (see Ch. 2, and p. 47).

Nerve deafness can result from damage to Corti's organ as in Ménières disease (see below) or occupational deafness. Spread of inflammation from the middle ear will sometimes damage the cochlea, as may syphilis. Nerve deafness can be congenital (deaf mutism), when it is usually due to an atresia of the cochlea and labyrinth. In childhood it can also be due to head injury, perinatal anaemia, maternal rubella or kernicterus. The auditory nerve in its intracranial course may be damaged by head injury, by inflammatory lesions (meningitis, meningovascular syphilis), by drugs or toxins (streptomycin) or by tumours, of which acoustic neuroma is the commonest. Nerve deafness resulting from a lesion of Corti's organ can often be distinguished from that due to an acoustic nerve tumour by the recruitment test (see p. 47). Deafness due to lesions of the cochlear nucleus in the brain stem is rare (but can be seen unilaterally in pontine infarction or, less often, multiple sclerosis); it is not produced by cortical lesions unless they are bilateral and extensive.

Tinnitus, or noise in the ears, is an important symptom of disease of the auditory nerve, though it can result from wax, from Eustachian catarrh or middle-ear disease. Typically it is a hissing or machinery-like noise which may be unilateral or bilateral, continuous or intermittent. It is often severe in elderly people and can be so distressing as to interfere seriously with sleep and hearing, so that some become almost suicidal; it may be due to atherosclerotic ischaemia of the inner ear, though it can also be a manifestation of severe depression. Drugs such as quinine, salicylates and streptomycin will also produce it. When unilateral, however, it may be an important symptom of disease of the labyrinth (e.g. Ménière's disease) or of the auditory nerve (e.g. acoustic neuroma).

THE VESTIBULAR NERVE

The end-organs which subserve vestibular function are the semicircular canals, which are concerned with the appreciation of movements of the head in any direction, and the utricle and saccule which convey information concerning the position of the head in relation to gravity. In the ampullae of the semicircular canals and in the utricle and saccule, where they lie in contact with the crystalline otoliths, are hair cells which transmit impulses to the cells of the vestibular ganglion of Scarpa. Thence they are conveyed by the vestibular nerve to the vestibular nuclei of the pons (Fig. 8.10) which have profuse connexions with the cerebellum, with the oculomotor nuclei via the medial longitudinal bundle, and with the spinal cord via the vestibulospinal tract.

The most important symptom produced by disorders of the vestibular system is **vertigo**. This term implies a disorder of equilibrium characterised by a sensation of rotation of the self or of one's surroundings. Often it is the objects around the patient which seem to be moving, either continuously in one direction or in a to-and-fro manner, but sometimes the patient feels that it is he himself that is twisting or spinning. Commonly vertigo is accompanied by staggering or even by actual falling, with clumsiness of the limbs, vomiting, depression and pallor. Nystagmus is generally present and in severe cases the vision is blurred or momentarily lost while rarely transient fainting may occur. It is important to distinguish true vertigo from mild 'giddiness' or 'swimming in the head' which are commonly psychogenic, or else may be due to syncope or presyncope.

In considering the aetiology and diagnostic significance of vertigo one must remember the many organs and mechanisms concerned in the normal maintenance of posture, as disorders of many different nervous pathways may cause this symptom. Firstly, visual impulses from the retina and from proprioceptive receptors in the external ocular muscles convey information concerning the relationship between the individual and his surroundings. Thus we can experience transient vertigo when looking down from heights or when observing a rapidly-moving object. Secondly, the labyrinth is very important; the commonest forms of vertigo are of aural origin and will be discussed below. Thirdly, and closely related to labyrinthine function, are the proprioceptive impulses derived from neck muscles, while similar stimuli from the muscles of the trunk and limbs give information concerning the position of the body. Whereas lesions of these proprioceptive pathways do not usually cause vertigo it can, however, result from disorders of the central co-ordinating mechanisms in the brain stem and of the cerebellum; the latter is important in the efferent mechanisms controlling posture. Lesions of the cerebral cortex rarely cause vertigo, although it has been described as the aura of an epileptic seizure and can occasionally result from tumours of the temporal lobe.

Even though the cerebellum is so important in the control of posture, it is comparatively uncommon for cerebellar hemisphere lesions, however massive, to give rise to vertigo. An exception is primary intracerebral haemorrhage in which intense vertigo and vomiting often occur at the outset. Brain-stem lesions involving central cerebellar connexions, however, often cause severe vertigo. Whereas it may result from **encephalitis**, **pontine tumours** or **syringobulbia**, the two most common brain-stem causes are **multiple sclerosis** and **infarction** or transient ischaemia. Occasionally the first symptom of multiple sclerosis is a sudden attack of severe vertigo, often lasting for hours or days, and associated with severe nystagmus and usually with other signs of a brain-stem lesion. The lateral medullary infarct pro-

duced by posterior inferior cerebellar artery thrombosis typically produces sudden vertigo, vomiting and prostration at the outset, while less severe attacks can occur in the recurrent ischaemic episodes of vertebro-basilar insufficiency.

Lesions of the labyrinth itself are, however, the most frequent cause of vertigo. Whereas some patients with compression or irritation of the eighth nerve, say, by an acoustic neuroma, suffer from it intermittently, disease of the internal ear is more often responsible. Sudden vertigo may result from an extension of a middle-ear infection to the labyrinth, but an **acute vestibular neuronitis**, often erroneously but conveniently called labyrinthitis, can occur without a preceding middle-ear infection. In such a case vertigo develops suddenly and is generally associated

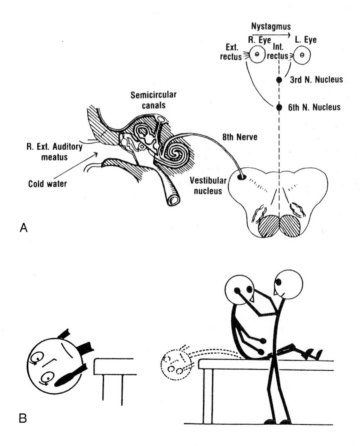

Fig. 8.10 A Diagram of mechanism of caloric nystagmus. Cooling of the right horizontal semicircular canal by irrigating the ear with cold water. This sets up currents in the endolymph, the labyrinth is stimulated and the resulting nystagmus is horizontal with the quick phase to the left. (Reproduced with permission from Spillane & Spillane 1982.) **B** Diagram to illustrate method of inducing positional nystagmus. The vertigo and nystagmus usually cease within a minute or so, but may recur transiently when the patient sits up. (Reproduced with permission from Hallpike 1955.)

with severe vomiting and prostration, some ataxia, and a rotary nystagmus which can be unilateral and to the opposite side if the lesion is unilateral but is more often bilateral. The patient is often pyrexial and the illness may last for hours, days or weeks. The condition can occur in epidemic form and is then believed to be due to an acute virus infection of the brain stem, involving vestibular nuclei, rather than a labyrinthitis, as diplopia and a lymphocytic pleocytosis in the CSF may be found. Hence the title 'epidemic vertigo' is often preferred, even for sporadic cases. A similar clinical picture, usually with a shorter time course, and generally identified by the accompanying unilateral deafness, can result from atherosclerotic **occlusion of the internal auditory artery**. The distinction between epidemic vertigo and a first episode of multiple sclerosis due to a plaque in the brain stem can be difficult and may depend solely upon the subsequent course, as acute vestibular neuronitis generally recovers completely, whereas in multiple sclerosis subsequent manifestations of neurological disease are to be expected. Furthermore, other signs of brain stem dysfunction (e.g. diplopia) often accompany the vertiginous presentation of multiple sclerosis. Even in the benign labyrinthine disorder, however, one or more relapses may occur within the first few months.

Ménière's disease (recurrent aural vertigo) is a condition characterised by recurrent attacks of vertigo, often with vomiting and prostration, and accompanied by unilateral tinnitus and progressive nerve deafness. The condition can occur at any age, but is rare in children; it is commonest in middle life and somewhat more frequent in males. It seems to be due to a hydrops of the membranous labyrinth, of unknown aetiology, resulting in dilatation of the endolymph system with consequent pressure atrophy of the organ of Corti. Sometimes deafness and tinnitus are present for some time before the attacks of vertigo develop but more often the latter are the presenting feature. Attacks may initially be mild and brief, increasing in severity and frequency, but the manifestations are very variable. Typically a sudden attack of vertigo occurs with unsteadiness, vomiting and prostration and can be so violent that the patient is literally thrown to the ground. Pallor, perspiration, depression and tachycardia are common accompaniments and rotary nystagmus is present. Occasionally transient loss of consciousness due to syncope occurs in a severe attack. The attack may last only a few minutes or several hours but the patient is often lethargic, unsteady and depressed for several days afterwards. The episodes can occur at intervals of a few days, weeks or even months, but tend to become less frequent and eventually to disappear completely when deafness is complete in the affected ear. Unfortunately the contralateral ear is occasionally affected, sometimes concurrently but more often subsequently. To be distinguished from Ménière's disease is the syndrome of **benign recurrent vertigo**, a disorder of unknown aetiology in which patients suffer repeated attacks of acute vertigo lasting from minutes to hours, and these are followed by a period in which positional nystagmus is present. The condition is often familial, deafness and tinnitus do not occur and audiometry and caloric test are normal. There is a weak association with migraine and prophylactic propranolol or pizotifen may control the episodes. A form of self-limiting **benign paroxysmal vertigo of childhood** is also recognised which gives recurrent attacks of vertigo, without deafness, in children under the age of three years; it usually resolves spontaneously after a few months and its cause is unknown.

During acute attacks of vertigo, an intramuscular injection of chlorpromazine 50 mg may give symptomatic relief but vestibular sedatives such as dimenhydrinate, promethazine, thiethylperazine maleate or prochlorperazine are more often used and are also given prophylactically in patients with recurrent attacks. In intractable cases of Ménière's disease, surgical section of the vestibular nerve is effective and spares hearing but is a major neurosurgical operation. Ultrasonic destruction of the labyrinth is also effective but reduces hearing in about one-third of cases. Endolymphatic subarachnoid shunt or decompression and cannulation of the endolymphatic sac are now preferred by many otological surgeons.

A somewhat similar condition giving episodic attacks of vertigo is **benign positional nystagmus**, which results from a degenerative lesion, again of unknown aetiology, in the otolith of the utricle and saccule. In this condition, however, the attacks occur only on certain specific movements of the head (e.g. stooping or lying down on one side) and can be reproduced at will by carrying out this movement. Most patients learn to avoid the offending position which evokes the attacks (Fig. 8.10) and often the condition improves spontaneously after months or years.

It is important to note, however, that vertigo elicited by change in posture (bending or stooping or any movement of the head, rather than the single specific movement of the benign positional syndrome) is seen in cases of epidemic vertigo and can also be a manifestation of organic lesions (such as an ependymoma or metastasis) in the region of the fourth ventricle.

Motion-sickness is also a closely related disorder, and is due to the stereotyped repetitive stimulation of the semicircular canals produced by movement of a motor car, ship, train or aeroplane. There is a wide variation in individual susceptibility. Commonly lassitude, vague depression and drowsiness are early symptoms and are followed by vomiting and vertigo, though the latter is not usually severe. Considerable adaptation usually occurs in the habitual traveller.

REFERENCES

Adams R D, Victor M 1985 Principles of neurology, 3rd edn. McGraw-Hill, New York

Ashworth B, Sherwood I 1981 Clinical neuro-ophthalmology. Blackwell, Oxford

Baloh R W, Honrubia V 1979 The clinical neurophysiology of the vestibular system. In: Plum F, McDowell F (eds) Contemporary Neurology Series. F A Davis , Philadelphia

Cogan D G 1977 Neurology of the visual system, 2nd edn. Thomas, Springfield, Ill.

Dix M R, Hood J D (eds) 1984 Vertigo. John Wiley, Chichester

Hallpike C S 1955 Ménière's disease. Postgraduate Medical Journal 31: 330

Kandel E R, Schwartz J H 1985 Principles of neural science, 2nd edn. Arnold, London

Leigh R J, Zee D S 1983 The neurology of eye movements. F A Davis, Philadelphia

Mayo Clinic, Section of Neurology 1976 The cranial nerves, and neuro-ophthalmology. In: Clinical examinations in neurology, 4th edn. Saunders, Philadelphia

Newman P P 1980 Neurophysiology. SP Medical and Scientific Books, New York

Patten J 1977 Neurological differential diagnosis. Harold Starke, London

Patton H D, Sundsten J W, Crill W E, Swanson P D 1976 Introduction to basic neurology. Saunders, Philadelphia

Spillane J D, Spillane J A 1982 An atlas of clinical neurology, 3rd edn. Oxford University Press, London

Walton J N 1985 Brain's Diseases of the nervous system, 9th edn. Oxford University Press, Oxford

Walton J N 1987 Introduction to clinical neuroscience, 2nd edn. Baillière Tindall, London

9. The motor system

Disorders of movement of the parts of the body produce some of the commoner symptoms described by patients with nervous disease or dysfunction. Sometimes the ability to move a part voluntarily is impaired (weakness or paresis) and sometimes it is lost completely (paralysis). Alternatively, willed movements may be clumsy, ill-directed or uncontrolled (ataxia or inco-ordination), or else the part moves spontaneously or independently of the will (involuntary movements). On examination the examiner can readily elicit these abnormalities but may also discover abnormalities of tone in which the normal response to passive stretching of a muscle is altered; it can be reduced (hypotonia) or increased in two ways (spasticity, rigidity). Abnormalities of this type, and particularly weakness or paralysis are sometimes emotionally determined (hysteria); or else they can be apraxic, resulting from a cortical lesion impairing the ability to recall and utilise acquired motor skills (see p. 66). More often, however, they are due to a disorder of function of that motor pathway which begins in the motor area of the cerebral cortex and ends in the voluntary musculature. There are many important physical signs which help to localise lesions within this motor apparatus, but to appreciate their significance a working knowledge of the organisation and pathophysiology of movement is essential.

The human motor system consists first of the descending pathways derived from the cerebral cortex and brain stem (the corticospinal and corticobulbar (pyramidal) system) which are concerned with the suprasegmental control of movement, secondly of the basal ganglia and cerebellum, thirdly of the continuation of these pathways within the spinal cord, and fourthly of the neuromuscular system which is made up of the nuclei of the motor cranial nerves and the muscles which they innervate, as well as the spinal cord anterior horn cells along with the segmentally organised voluntary musculature of the trunk and limbs. Both at higher and at segmental levels major afferent pathways project to these motor structures, providing information about the relative positions of different parts of the body and about muscle length; the latter is provided through the fusimotor spindle system of the muscles, which fulfils an important role in the control of movement. The basal ganglia and cerebellum do not project directly to the segmental motor structures of the brain stem and spinal cord but process information from other parts of the nervous system and project backwards on to the cortical and brain-stem structures from which the suprasegmental pathways arise.

ANATOMY AND PHYSIOLOGY

The **upper motor neurones**, which constitute the pyramidal or corticospinal tracts, arise in part from nerve cells in the motor cortex of the cerebrum. This area of cortex lies anterior to the Rolandic fissure, in the precentral convolution. Whereas some of these neurones arise from the giant Betz cells which are common in this area, there are far more fibres in the pyramidal tracts than could be accounted for by the axons of all the Betz cells, so that many other upper motor neurones must arise from nerve cells in or near this area which are not structurally distinctive. Stimulation experiments have shown that activation of cells in the lower end of the precentral gyrus causes bilateral movement of the pharynx and larynx, while just above are others which, if stimulated, give movement of the contralateral half of the tongue (Figs. 9.1, 9.2 and 9.3). Facial movement can be elicited at a point slightly higher still and it is of interest that stimulation gives bilateral movement of the upper face but unilateral movement only of the lower face. Movement of the contralateral hand, arm, trunk, leg and foot is then produced in turn as one ascends the gyrus, and in each case 'representation' is strictly unilateral. The leg and foot 'area' lies partly on the medial surface of the hemisphere and partly on its superior aspect. Nerve fibres arising from the cells in this cortical area then come together in the corona radiata and converge upon the internal capsule which lies deep in the hemisphere between the thalamus and caudate nucleus medially and

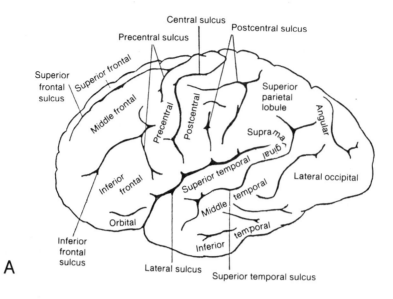

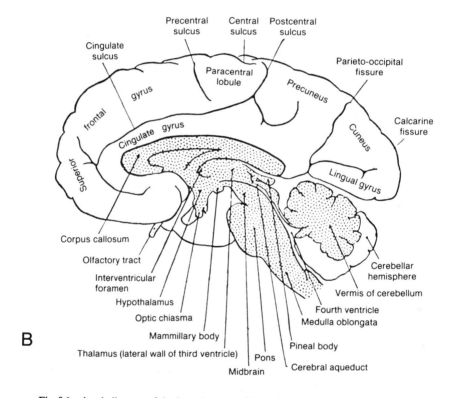

Fig. 9.1 A A diagram of the lateral aspect of the left cerebral hemisphere.
B A diagram of the medial aspect of the right cerebral hemisphere. (From
Fundamentals of Neurology, by E. Gardner, 4th edition, Saunders, Philadelphia
and London, 1963)

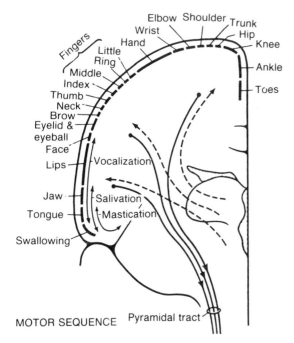

Fig. 9.2 Corticospinal motor pathway (pyramidal tract). Cross-section through right hemisphere along the plane of the precentral gyrus. The sequence of responses to electrical stimulation of the surface of the cortex (from above down, along the motor strip from toes through arm and face to swallowing) is unvaried from one individual to another. The broken arrows represent afferent thalamocortical pathways. (Reproduced with permission from Walton 1985.)

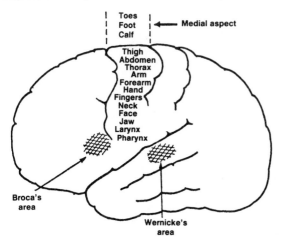

Fig. 9.3 A diagram of the lateral aspect of the left cerebral hemisphere indicating the situation of the motor and sensory speech areas and also the 'representation' of the parts of the body in the motor area (precentral gyrus) of the cerebral hemisphere. The areas of the motor cortex concerned with movement of the lower limb lie on the medial aspect of the hemisphere in the paracentral lobule. 'Representation' in the sensory area (postcentral gyrus) is similar.

the lenticular nucleus laterally (Fig. 9.4). The pyramidal tract occupies the posterior one-third of the anterior limb, the genu, and the anterior two-thirds of the posterior limb of the capsule. Behind it lie sensory fibres travelling to the postcentral sensory cortex and others forming the optic radiation, while anteriorly are fronto-pontine fibres. From the internal capsule the tract passes down in the middle three-fifths of the cerebral peduncle to enter the midbrain; in the pons it is broken into bundles by transverse pontine fibres, but in the medulla it is again a compact tract, the pyramid, which forms an anterior prominence. Throughout the brain stem the tract gives off fibres to the contralateral motor nuclei of the cranial nerves. In the lower medulla, most of the fibres in the pyramidal tract decussate to form the crossed pyramidal tract which travels down in the lateral column of the spinal cord on the opposite side, but a small proportion continue downwards in the anterior column of the cord, forming the direct or uncrossed pyramidal tract (Figs. 9.5 and 9.6). Fibres of the pyramidal tract do not as a rule synapse directly with the anterior horn cells from which the lower motor neurones arise, but rather with internuncial (propriospinal) neurones in the grey matter of the spinal cord, which in turn pass on to synapse in the anterior horns. The organisation and function of the neuromuscular system will be described later.

The anatomical schema laid out above outlines the basic functional units through which a movement is initiated and performed. However, the organisation of movement is much more complex than this simple schema would suggest. For instance, no single cell in the motor area of the cerebral cortex can be said to innervate any single muscle. Stimulation experiments have shown that it is not single muscle twitches, but organised movements, which are initiated in the motor cortex. These movements involve several muscles or muscle groups, of which only some act as prime movers or agonists. Others, the antagonists, must be enabled to relax smoothly as the agonists contract, while yet others must fix a limb proximally, say, in order to allow a movement occurring distally to be efficient. Other muscles, or synergists, may also be used to counteract unwanted effects which would be produced by the unmodified action of the agonists. The many internuncial neurones in the spinal cord, which receive impulses from many pyramidal axons and may influence many anterior horn cells, are clearly important in this organisation. However, incoming sensory impulses from stretch receptors (muscle spindles) in the muscles themselves, as well as other proprioceptive impulses giving information about the position of the part which is being moved, can also modify this activity through a series of spinal reflexes. Additional modifying influences are exerted through sensory impulses from the eyes and labyrinths which

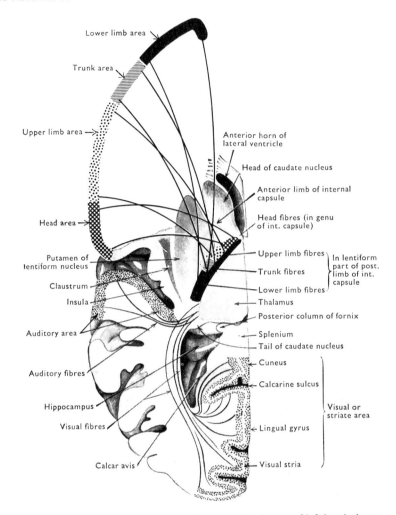

Fig. 9.4   A   Diagram of motor, auditory and visual areas of left hemisphere and their relation to the internal capsule. (Reproduced with permission from Walton 1985.)

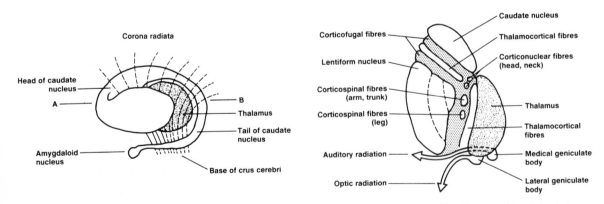

Fig. 9.4   B   Left, a lateral view of the internal capsule showing its relationship to the caudate and lentiform nuclei and the thalamus; right, an axial view through A–B.

Fig. 9.5   The motor pathways. The corticospinal (pyramidal) tract arises in the cerebral cortex from the precentral gyrus and the region immediately anterior to it; it also arises in part from the postcentral gyrus (the 'sensory area'). The tract then traverses the internal capsule and brain stem and largely decussates in the medulla. The main crossed corticospinal tract then runs in the lateral white column of the spinal cord to terminate in the ventral grey column (the anterior horn) around the motor cells. The axons of these motor cells leave the cord by the anterior roots and supply the voluntary muscles.

The so-called extrapyramidal tracts are derived from neurones in the caudate and lentiform nuclei (the corpus striatum) and are relayed in the substantia nigra, the red nucleus and the reticular formation in the mid-brain. The rubrospinal tract immediately decussates and passes down the spinal cord in the lateral white column immediately anterior to the lateral corticospinal (pyramidal) tract; its fibres connect with ventral grey column (anterior horn) cells. The vestibular and reticular nuclei also project to the ventral grey columns (anterior horn) cells via the vestibulospinal and reticulospinal tracts. A schematic spinal reflex arc is also shown. (Reproduced with permission from Mann 1975.)

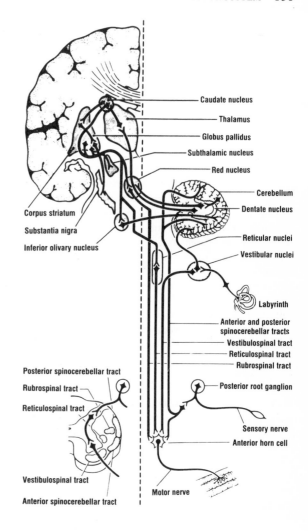

Fig. 9.6   Diagrammatic representation of the motor reflex arc and of the principal fibre tracts of the spinal cord. **A**, a simple two-neurone reflex arc. **B**, a three neurone reflex arc with an internuncial neurone between the sensory and motor neurones. **C**, a corticospinal fibre influencing the activity of the reflex arc.

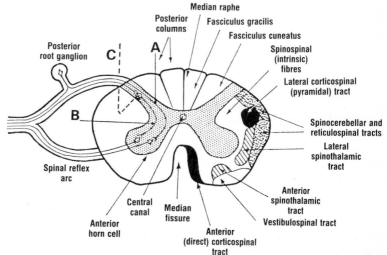

enter the brain stem and initiate activity in the vestibulo-spinal tracts.

Not only can sensory impulses influence movement in this way, but other important effects are exerted by the **extrapyramidal motor system**. Several nuclear masses in the basal ganglia and upper brain stem, and particularly the lenticular and caudate nuclei, the thalamus, the subthalamic nuclei, the substantia nigra, the brain-stem reticular formation and the olivary nuclei, exercise profound controlling influences upon movement. The basal ganglia influence movement largely through thalamic relays which project to the motor cortex, by integrating their output with cerebellar input to the ventrolateral nucleus of the thalamus and by descending impulses conveyed by the rubrospinal and reticulospinal tracts. It is now evident that the corpus striatum (consisting of the caudate nucleus, the globus pallidus and putamen, the latter two of which together form the lenticular nucleus) plays an important role in controlling posture and that the globus pallidus is the final efferent cell station; lesions of this nucleus can give akinesia (inability to initiate movement) or bradykinesia (excessively slow movement). The basal ganglia also control the balance between alpha and gamma motor neurone activity so that when disease distorts this balance, abnormalities of muscle tone or tremor result. The concerted activity of the nuclei of the basal ganglia gives smooth integration of voluntary movement; lesions of individual components of the system may allow the release, due to removal of inhibitory mechanisms, of typical involuntary movements (chorea, athetosis, dystonia, hemiballismus) which will be described below. It is now known, too, that many neurones of the substantia nigra, especially in the nigrostriatal pathway, are dopaminergic, while others in the striatonigral system employ GABA as a neurotransmitter and many neurones in the corpus striatum are cholinergic. Reserpine or phenothiazines may deplete dopamine stores giving drug-induced parkinsonism, but may also produce troublesome facial dyskinesia; there is loss of dopamine in the substantia nigra in idiopathic parkinsonism, but this can be restored with clinical improvement by levodopa, a dopamine precursor which, however, may cause involuntary movements like those of athetosis; and cholinergic activation can accentuate the features of parkinsonism. It thus appears that many of the clinical features of disease or dysfunction of the basal ganglia are due to an imbalance in the relative activities of cholinergic and dopaminergic neurones and their receptors.

The **cerebellum** is made up of the archicerebellum, palaeocerebellum and neocerebellum. The archicerebellum, consisting of the flocculonodular lobe and uvula, is concerned with the control of eye movements, with postural neck and axial reflexes and thus with the maintenance of equilibrium. The palaeocerebellum, consisting of the vermis and contiguous parts of the cerebellar hemispheres, exercises a modulating influence upon muscle tone through the spindle system. Lesions of these central cerebellar structures often cause severe dysequilibrium without vertigo (truncal ataxia) with a broad-based unsteady gait and sometimes postural nystagmus. The neocerebellum, which is made up of the major part of the two cerebellar hemispheres, is especially concerned with the regulation and smooth coordination of limb movements, fulfilling a graduating and harmonising role (see Fig. 9.7).

We presume that a movement is initiated when the concept of it is first invoked in the 'association' areas of the cortex. The appropriate cells of the precentral cortex are then activated and impulses travel down the pyramidal tracts, in order to activate the appropriate anterior horn cells and their motor units. Simultaneously the movement is influenced and controlled by the activity of the cerebellum and of the extrapyramidal motor system; at the same time as agonists are being stimulated to contract, synergists to assist and fixators to fix, an inhibitory mechanism is invoked to produce controlled relaxation of antagonists. Once the movement has begun it is then subject to continued modification through sensory impulses arriving from the proprioceptors or from the eyes and labyrinths. Clearly, therefore, movement can be disorganised by lesions of many different nervous pathways, and principles which aid in deciding which pathway or pathways are diseased will be considered later.

The neuromuscular system

The lower motor neurones

The cell bodies of the lower motor neurones are situated in the motor nuclei of the brain stem and in the anterior horns of grey matter of the spinal cord. The cell bodies or perikarya of the alpha neurones which innervate voluntary muscle are remarkably consistent in total number and distribution throughout the various segments of the spinal cord. Various groups of cells lying in specific locations constantly supply certain muscle groups and even individual muscles. The gamma neurones supply the intrafusal fibres of the muscle spindles. Each motor neurone is influenced by impulses concerned with both excitation and inhibition. Spinal interneurones constitute an important set of networks for processing both peripheral sensory inputs (feedback) and commands descending from centres in the brain. The axons of the motor neurones leave the central nervous system via the cranial nerves or the spinal ventral roots. From the latter the axons enter the peripheral nerves, those destined for the limbs being organised into brachial and lumbosacral plexuses.

The structure and function of voluntary muscle

A voluntary muscle is composed of muscle fibres, each of which is a multinucleate cell, consisting of myofibrils, sarcoplasm and a number of discrete intracellular organelles including mitochondria, ribosomes and the sarcotubular system. Each fibre is enclosed within a sarcolemmal sheath (with an outer basement membrane and an inner plasma membrane), deep to which the muscle nuclei are situated, and each has a motor end-plate in which the nerve fibre terminates. Under normal conditions muscle fibres never contract singly. The functional unit of muscle activity is known as the motor unit, being that group of muscle fibres supplied by a single alpha neurone and its axon. Discharge of such a single anterior horn cell results in the simultaneous contraction of all of the muscle fibres which it innervates. In most human limb muscles each motor unit contains between 500 and 2000 muscle fibres.

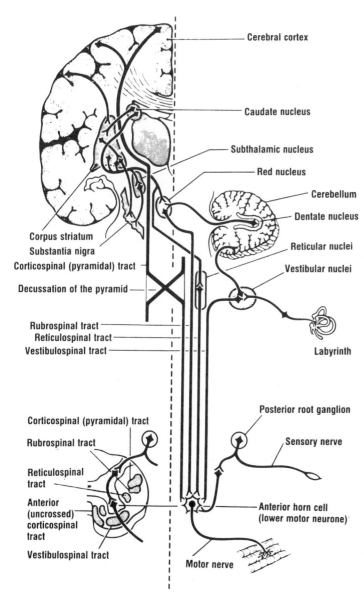

Fig. 9.7 The pathways concerned in muscular co-ordination and tone. Information is received from sensory nerve endings in muscle, tendon and joints. The central processes of the primary sensory neurones (with cell-bodies in the dorsal root ganglia) terminate in the thoracic nucleus of the dorsal grey column, connecting with interneurones which give rise to the largely crossed anterior spinocerebellar tract and the uncrossed posterior spinocerebellar tract. The cerebellum also receives fibres from the vestibular nuclei and the labyrinth. Efferents from the cerebellum reach the red nucleus and the thalamus. The red nucleus also receives fibres from the corpus striatum.

From the red nucleus, the rubrospinal tract conveys impulses to the anterior horn cells, as also do the vestibulospinal and reticulospinal tracts. The corpus striatum has 'feed-back' connections via the inferior olivary nucleus to the cerebellum.

Note that the corpus striatum, the red nucleus and olivary nuclei subserve the *opposite* side of the body; the cerebellum, the vestibular and reticular nuclei subserve the *same* side of the body.

Proprioceptive fibres giving conscious indication of sense of position run in the posterior white columns and these are shown in Figure 10.2. (Reproduced with permission from Mann 1975.)

The motor unit

The fibres of a single motor unit are usually widely scattered throughout a muscle rather than being gathered into groups or fasciculi. Only after denervation and subsequent re-innervation by regenerating neurones are fibres innervated by a single anterior horn cell gathered together into groups. Contraction of the muscle fibres which make up a motor unit is preceded by electrical excitation of the fibre membranes. The appearance of this electrical activity in the electromyogram (EMC) depends on physical factors such as the dimensions of the electrode used, as well as on the muscle chosen for examination. For example, in the biceps brachii of a healthy young adult, the electrical activity of a single motor unit usually appears as a di- or triphasic wave with a duration of 5–10 ms and an amplitude of 250–500 μV. The variation in form, amplitude and duration of the motor unit action potential is considerable, however.

Neuromuscular transmission

The release of acetylcholine (ACh) is responsible for transmission of the nerve impulse at the neuromuscular or myoneural junction (Fig. 9.8). The synaptic vesicles in the motor nerve terminal are actually packets of ACh. Single packets of ACh are continually being released spontaneously and give rise to small depolarisations (miniature end-plate potentials) which can be recorded electrically with a microelectrode in the region of the end-plate. ACh so released combines with ACh receptors (AChR) on the postjunctional membrane. The arrival of a nerve impulse at the motor end-plate results in the synchronous release of many packets or quanta of ACh, which produces a localised depolarisation of the muscle fibre membrane in the region of the end-plate. This is the end-plate potential. When the end-plate potential reaches a certain critical size it triggers off an excitatory wave, the action potential, which then travels away from the end-

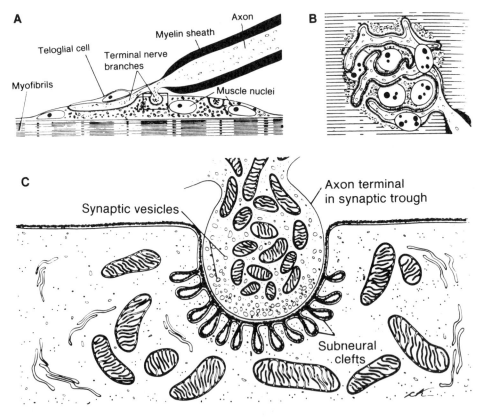

Fig. 9.8 Schematic drawings of motor end-plates. **A** and **B**: Views from the side and from above, respectively. **C**: Enlarged view (as seen in electron micrographs) of the region outlined by the rectangle in **A**. (Reproduced with permission from Bloom & Fawcett 1970.)

plate along the surface membrane of the fibre. There is evidence that the wave of excitation spreads inwards into the substance of the muscle fibre along the transverse system of tubules—the 'T' system—and that the consequent mobilisation of calcium ions in the sarcoplasmic reticulum initiates contraction of the myofibrils. Among the many biochemical reactions which follow, creatine phosphate, in the presence of calcium, is broken down into creatine and phosphate, and adenosine triphosphate (ATP) to adenosine diphosphate (ADP), also releasing phosphate. This release of high-energy phosphate bonds provides much of the energy required for muscular contraction.

Muscle ultrastructure

The unit of structure of the individual myofibril of skeletal muscle is the sarcomere (Fig. 9.9) extending from one Z line (situated in the midst of the I band) to the next. Attached to each Z line is a series of thin filaments of actin. There is also a second thicker type of filament composed of myosin. These filaments correspond to the dark (birefringent) A bands of the myofibrils. Each filament of myosin is surrounded by a hexagonal array of actin filaments and, in addition, molecular cross-bridges reach out from the myosin to the actin filaments. During contraction, the cross-bridges repeatedly disengage and

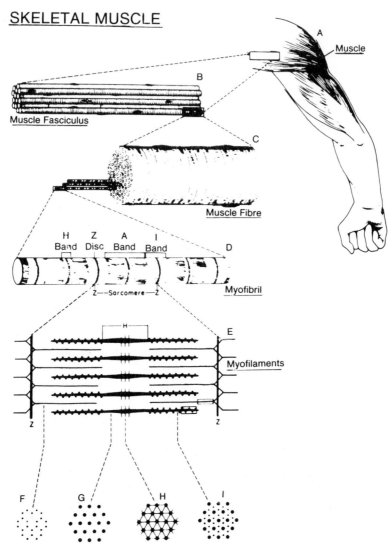

SKELETAL MUSCLE

Fig. 9.9 Histological and molecular structure of skeletal muscle. (Reproduced with permission from Bloom & Fawcett 1970.)

re-engage at successive sites on the actin filaments. The propulsion imparted to the actin filaments causes them to slide over the myosin filaments so as to interdigitate more fully with the latter. In this way the whole myofibril, and consequently its parent fibre, shortens.

Types of muscle fibre

Skeletal muscles are not homogenous. In man they contain at least two main types of muscle fibre which are morphologically and histochemically distinct. The so-called type I fibre has a high concentration of mitochondria and enzymes such as succinic dehydrogenase and NADH diaphorase which are concerned with aerobic metabolism. The larger type II fibres contain fewer mitochondria but a higher concentration of glycogen and enzymes such as phosphorylase and myofibrillar adenosine triphosphatase, which are concerned with anaerobic metabolism. In man, all skeletal muscles contain an admixture of type I and type II fibres so that in transverse sections stained histochemically, a characteristic checker-board pattern is observed. These fibres are functionally different, and histochemical techniques have shown that the type II fibres can be further subdivided into subtypes IIa and IIb. In mammals other than man there are certain muscles (such as soleus) which are made up predominantly of type I fibres (so-called red muscles). These muscles are concerned largely with the maintenance of posture, and upon stimulation contract and relax relatively slowly (slow 'twitch' muscles). By contrast, other muscles concerned more directly with phasic motor activity, such as the flexor digitorum longus, are made up predominantly of type II fibres (white muscle) and contract more rapidly (fast 'twitch' muscles). The motor nerve not only controls the physiological behaviour but also largely determines the histochemical structure of the muscle fibres. Transposition of the motor nerve supply from a fast muscle to a slow muscle, and vice versa, may thus alter the physiological and histochemical characteristics of the muscle fibres. The neurones control the behaviour of the muscle fibres which make up their motor units, so that one can speak of type I and type II alpha neurones. When a group of muscle fibres which have lost their nerve supply are re-innervated by a sprouting neurone they become of uniform histochemical type (so-called 'type grouping').

The effect of drugs

A number of drugs may act upon the neuromuscular junction. When ACh is released at the neuromuscular junction, it is broken down by cholinesterase, which is normally present in the subneural apparatus. Curare acts on the postjunctional membrane, where it reduces or prevents the depolarising effect of the transmitter excited by the nerve impulse. Botulinum toxin blocks ACh release. Drugs such as physostigmine and neostigmine inhibit cholinesterase and allow ACh liberated at the myoneural junction to accumulate. Guanidine hydrochloride increases the output of ACh at the nerve endings and may thus be helpful in botulism. If ACh accumulates in excess, as in overdosage with neostigmine or guanidine, depolarisation of the muscle fibre membrane persists and may result in blockage of the muscle action potential (depolarisation block). Tubocurarine and gallamine compete with ACh for the end-plate chemical receptors and are therefore competitive inhibitors. Decamethonium and suxamethonium first produce muscle paralysis as a result of depolarisation block but subsequently also produce competitive block, so that they are said to have a 'dual' action. In myasthenia gravis ACh receptors become coated with circulating anti-AChR antibodies, preventing ACh from having its full normal effect.

The muscle spindles (the fusimotor system) and other muscle and tendon receptors

The stretch detectors of muscle and tendon are the Golgi tendon organs and the muscle spindles. Strictly, the Golgi organs are tension receptors and the muscle spindles are length detectors. The Golgi neurotendinous endings lie most often on tendons and are thus excited by stretch, as in tension applied to the tendon during muscular contraction. These stimuli produce a tonic generator potential and repetitive spike discharge in the afferent fibres. The effect of such discharge is to activate inhibitory motor neurones which inhibit alpha neurone activity.

The muscle spindles (Fig. 9.10) are present in all voluntary muscles and contain on the average seven or eight muscle fibres, called intrafusal because they are enclosed in a fluid-containing connective tissue capsule. These fibres are of two types: nuclear bag fibres, which are few, relatively large in diameter and show a collection of nuclei at their equator, and the narrower and often more numerous nuclear chain fibres, each of which contains a single row of nuclei. Axons of gamma (effector) neurones enter the striated poles of these fibres. At the equatorial region of the fibres there are two types of sensory endings (a) annulospiral endings giving rise to group I myelinated axons, and (b) secondary or flower-spray endings, which give origin to group II myelinated axons. Both types of receptors are tonic receptors which are depolarised by stretch. Gamma-neurone discharge increases the sensitivity of the muscle to tension through contraction of the intrafusal fibres and stretching of the sensory receptors in the equatorial region.

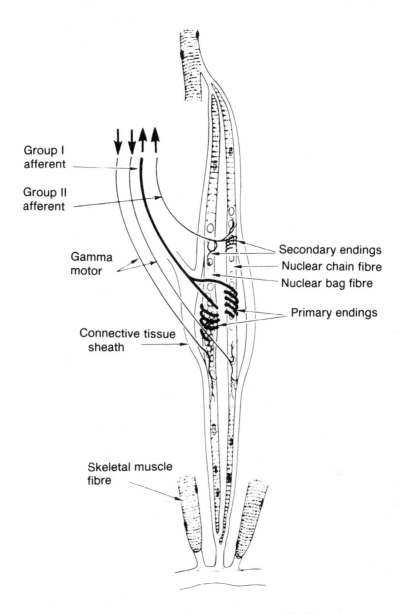

Group I afferent

Group II afferent

Gamma motor

Connective tissue sheath

Skeletal muscle fibre

Secondary endings

Nuclear chain fibre

Nuclear bag fibre

Primary endings

Fig. 9.10 Schematic representation of a neuromuscular spindle. Parts of three skeletal muscle fibres are shown (cross-striated, nuclei at edge). Inside the connective tissue sheath of the spindle are two muscle fibres (thinner than regular skeletal muscle fibres, with central nuclei, and striations minimal or absent in region of sensory endings). Sensory nerve fibres form primary (annulospiral) and secondary (flower-spray) endings, the primary arising from the large fibres. (The form of primary and secondary endings varies according to species. In some, such as rabbit and man, the primary endings of the large fibre may be flower-spray in type, not winding around the muscle fibre.) Small nerve fibres (gamma efferents) form motor endings at each end of the spindle muscle fibres. Motor discharges over gamma efferents cause the muscle spindle fibres to contract at each end, thus stretching the intervening, non-contractile sensory region and activating the sensory endings. Arrows indicate direction of conduction. (Reproduced with permission from Gardner 1975.)

Passive stretching of a muscle gives rise to afferent impulses which reach the spinal cord, stimulating the alpha neurones which then discharge, causing the muscle to contract and regain its former length. This process is responsible for monosynaptic spinal reflex activity as in the tendon jerks (see below). Sensory impulses from the spindles also reach the brain stem, cerebellum and cerebral cortex by a number of ascending pathways. In turn the descending pathways from these structures influence the excitability of gamma neurones, thus exercising important controlling influences over muscle tone. Sudden and transient stretching of a muscle, as in the tendon jerks, causes selective discharge in group I afferents, thus eliciting a monosynaptic reflex. Steady stretch or vibration applied to the muscle, by contrast, excites group I and group II afferents from all of the receptors in the muscle, eliciting stretch reflexes which are more complex, often polysynaptic, and which are modulated by activity in the many descending pathways concerned in the control of posture and of muscle tone. Essentially the response consists of tonic or continuous muscle contraction (the tonic stretch reflex).

Segmental and peripheral organisation of the neuromuscular system

In the adult the anatomical organisation of motor nuclei in the brain stem retains some semblance of segmental organisation, but this is much less clear than is the segmental arrangement of the spinal cord. Corresponding to each spinal segment is one pair of spinal nerves composed of the ventral and dorsal roots derived from that segment. The sensory neurones in the dorsal root ganglia are completely separated in each segment from those of the contiguous segments. The organisation of the alpha motor neurones is less clearly segmental in that their cell bodies are arranged in longitudinal columns and those innervating a single muscle often extend over more than one segment. Several muscles may be represented in one segment. A lesion of the anterior horn of a single segment gives weakness of all muscles innervated by that segment but paralyses completely only those which have no nerve supply from adjacent segments.

WEAKNESS, PARALYSIS, HYPERTROPHY AND ATROPHY

Weakness (paresis) of a muscle group implies that the power produced by voluntary contraction of the affected muscles is reduced, whereas paralysis indicates that the power to move the part concerned is totally lost. Weakness of one limb is called a **monoparesis**, total paralysis a **monoplegia**. **Hemiplegia** is the term used to identify paralysis afflicting one side of the body, and particularly the arm and leg, while **paraplegia** signifies a paralysis of both lower limbs. When all four limbs are paralysed, the terms **quadriplegia** or **tetraplegia** are used; a symmetrical weakness of all four limbs, affecting the lower more markedly than the upper, and occurring in children with cerebral palsy, is often called a **diplegia**. The term palsy can be used interchangeably with 'paralysis', but is more often utilised in practice to identify paralysis of individual muscles or muscle groups resulting from peripheral nerve lesions.

Paralysis may be due to a lesion of the upper or lower motor neurone, and under certain circumstances it can be due to a defect in conduction at the neuromuscular junction or to a biochemical or structural abnormality of the muscle itself. Clinical methods of differentiating these causes of paralysis will be discussed below.

Hypertrophy simply means enlargement, **atrophy** wasting. In neurology these terms are used almost exclusively to describe changes in skeletal muscle. Hypertrophy can result from repeated work as in body-builders, weight-lifters and some athletes, and can also be a consequence of prolonged medication with anabolic steroids. As a manifestation of disease it may occur in some neuromuscular disorders (see Ch. 18). Atrophy can be due to disuse as in muscles paralysed as a result of upper motor neurone lesions (see below) but is not then as a rule severe, as long as the reflex arc is intact. But in lower motor neurone lesions or primary diseases of muscle, atrophy may be severe.

THE MOTOR CRANIAL NERVES

The pathophysiology of the third, fourth and sixth cranial nerves, which innervate the external ocular muscles, is described in Chapter 8. The motor root of the **fifth or trigeminal nerve** leaves the lateral aspect of the inferior surface of the pons, passes forward beneath the gasserian ganglion, leaves the skull via the foramen ovale, and unites with the third sensory division to form a single trunk in the infratemporal fossa. Its branches then innervate the temporalis, masseter and pterygoid muscles as well as the anterior belly of the digastric, the mylohyoid muscle, the tensor tympani and the tensor palatini. Lesions of this root therefore give weakness of the masticatory muscles, and when the mouth is opened the mandible deviates to the side opposite to the lesion.

The **seventh or facial nerve** (*see* p. 288) is primarily motor, but it also contains fibres which excite salivary secretion and others carrying taste impulses from the anterior two-thirds of the tongue. The nerve emerges from the lateral aspect of the pons, enters the internal auditory meatus with the eighth nerve, and then travels through the middle ear in the facial canal (Fig. 9.11) to emerge from the skull via the stylomastoid foramen. In the middle ear it gives a branch which innervates the stapedius. After leaving the skull it gives branches to the stylohyoid muscle, the posterior belly of the digastric, and the posterior part of the occipitofrontalis before entering the parotid gland, where it divides into several branches which then innervate the facial musculature or muscles of expression, including the frontalis, orbicularis oculi, orbicularis oris, buccinator and platysma.

Facial weakness due to supranuclear lesions of the contralateral corticospinal tract affects movements of the lower part of the face much more severely than those of the upper part. Voluntary retraction of the corner of the mouth is impaired, whereas eye closure remains relatively normal, as do emotional movements of the face as in smiling. Such emotional movements may, however, be reduced (mimetic paralysis) a result of lesions of the opposite frontal lobe anterior to the precentral gyrus, or less often as a result of lesions in the region of the thalamus where there may be a centre for emotional expression. Lesions of the facial nerve itself may involve the nucleus in the pons, as in pontine tumour or infarction, for example. The nerve can also be involved in

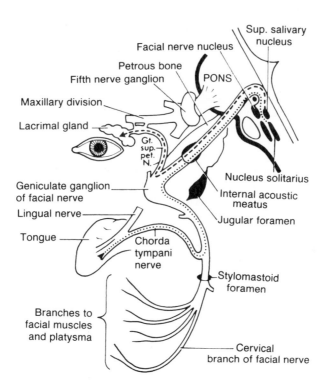

Fig. 9.11 The facial nerve. Lesions involving the facial nerve trunk above the geniculate ganglion will cause loss of lacrimation (greater petrosal nerve), and loss of taste in the anterior two-thirds of the tongue (chorda tympani nerve), as well as paralysis of both upper and lower facial muscles. Lesions between the geniculate ganglion and the point where the chorda tympani nerve leaves the facial nerve (6 mm above the stylomastoid foramen) will cause loss of taste sensation in the anterior two-thirds of the tongue, as well as paralysis of the facial muscles, but lacrimation will still be present. Lesions below the point where the chorda tympani leaves the facial nerve will cause paralysis of the facial muscles, but both taste and lacrimation will be present. (Reproduced with permission from Walton 1985, and redrawn from an original drawing by Charles Keogh.)

its intracranial course in the posterior fossa (e.g. by acoustic neuroma), or within the petrous temporal bone (e.g. by otitis media or cholesteatoma). Herpes zoster of the geniculate ganglion (the Ramsay Hunt syndrome) often gives facial paralysis and loss of taste on the anterior two-thirds of the tongue, sometimes with ipsilateral deafness and facial sensory loss due to involvement of the fifth and eighth nerves. Vesicles are usually seen in the external auditory meatus and on the soft palate. Perineural and interstitial oedema of undetermined cause of the nerve in its canal above the stylomastoid foramen appears to be the mechanism usually responsible for idiopathic facial paralysis (Bell's palsy). Fibrosis and irritation of the nerve in a similar location has been thought to be the usual cause of clonic facial spasm (hemifacial spasm), a benign but embarrassing condition which gives rise to irregular intermittent twitching or spasm of the muscles of one side of the face, but it has become apparent that compression of the intracranial trunk of the nerve in the subarachnoid space, caused by an aberrant artery (a condition readily relieved by surgery) is a commoner cause. Aberrant re-innervation of regenerating facial nerve fibres after facial paralysis can result in various patterns of paradoxical facial movement and/or in gustatory sweating (facial sweating during meals). After leaving the skull the fibres of the nerve may also be damaged in the parotid gland. Facial muscle weakness is seen in various forms of myopathy but here it is the muscles themselves rather than the facial nerve which are affected.

The **ninth or glossopharyngeal** nerve is principally sensory, carrying taste from the posterior one-third of the tongue. Its few motor fibres, arising from the nucleus ambiguus, supply the stylopharyngeus muscle. The motor function of this nerve can for practical purposes be ignored in clinical neurology.

The motor fibres of the **tenth or vagus nerve** originate in the nucleus ambiguus and leave the medulla oblongata in a series of radicles at the anterior margin of the inferior cerebellar peduncle in line with the roots of the glossopharyngeal nerve above and the accessory below. These radicles combine into a single trunk which leaves the skull through the jugular foramen with the accessory nerve and then comes to lie in the carotid sheath behind the carotid arteries and the internal jugular vein. In the thorax the course of the two vagus nerves differs on the two sides. That on the right passes downwards behind the trachea and superior vena cava to reach the right lung root, while that on the left passes between the left common carotid and subclavian arteries and then crosses the aortic arch to reach the root of the left lung. In the posterior mediastinum both nerves contribute parasympathetic fibres to the pulmonary and oesophageal plex-

uses and enter the abdomen at the oesophageal opening in the diaphragm, the left in front, the right behind the oesophagus, going on in a purely parasympathetic capacity to supply the stomach and other abdominal organs. The principal motor branches of the vagus are:

a. the pharyngeal branch, which leaves the inferior ganglion of the nerve just below the jugular foramen and which innervates the muscles of the soft palate,
b. the external laryngeal division of the superior laryngeal branch, which innervates the cricothyroid muscle (the remainder of the superior laryngeal nerve is sensory), and
c. the recurrent laryngeal branch, which innervates most of the intrinsic muscles of the larynx as well as the cricopharyngeus, which is the principal muscle of the inferior pharyngeal sphincter. The right recurrent laryngeal nerve arises in the root of the neck and loops backwards and upwards behind the subclavian artery. The left nerve loops similarly around the arch of the aorta, where it is especially vulnerable to damage by aortic aneurysm but more particularly by other lesions in the mediastinum such as metastases in lymph nodes.

A unilateral lesion of the vagus gives ipsilateral paralysis of the muscles of the soft palate, the three pharyngeal constrictors, the intrinsic and extrinsic laryngeal muscles, and the lower pharyngeal sphincter. This results in difficulty in swallowing food and saliva, hoarseness of the voice, and sometimes a nasal intonation as well as impaired coughing. With unilateral palatal paralysis there may be few if any symptoms, but when the patient opens his mouth and says 'ah' the soft palate and uvula deviate to the opposite side. Bilateral palatal paralysis gives a nasal quality to the voice, mouth breathing, and loud snoring and regurgitation of ingested fluids through the nose. Palatal myoclonus is a rare rhythmical and repetitive movement of the soft palate due to a degenerative lesion of unknown cause in the inferior olivary nucleus.

Unilateral pharyngeal paralysis causes delay in pharyngeal emptying with the accumulation of mucus overflowing into the larynx. On attempting to swallow there is a 'curtain' movement of the posterior pharyngeal wall towards the normal side. In bilateral lesions dysphagia is more complete.

In the normal larynx the cricothyroid muscles (external laryngeal nerve) tense the vocal cords, while the abductors and adductors of the cord are supplied by the recurrent laryngeal. Abduction of the cords occurs during inspiration, and the cords are adducted during phonation and coughing. A unilateral lesion of one vocal cord and of the cricopharyngeus muscle on the same side

(Fig. 9.12) results in hoarseness of the voice (dysphonia) and some accumulation of mucus with dysphagia. If the external laryngeal nerve is also damaged or if the lesion affects the vagus between the nucleus ambiguus and its inferior ganglion, these symptoms are more severe. In the latter instance, the palate and pharynx are paralysed on the same side. Bilateral paralysis of the larynx usually gives inspiratory stridor and a weak but clear voice, a very poor cough, and difficulty in expelling mucus from the larynx.

The **eleventh or accessory nerve** arises in part from the most caudal portion of the nucleus ambiguus and in part from the anterior horn cells of the first to the fifth cervical segments of the spinal cord. At the jugular foramen the medullary fibres join the vagus; the spinal fibres form a single trunk which lies between the internal carotid artery and the internal jugular vein, descending to supply the sternomastoid muscles and the upper part of the trapezius in conjunction with branches of the second, third and fourth cervical nerves. A unilateral lesion of this nerve gives paralysis of the sternomastoid, which results in difficulty in rotating the head to the opposite side and (owing to weakness of the trapezius) in elevating the shoulder on the same side, while the affected shoulder also droops at rest. Lesions damaging this nerve are much the same as those which damage the vagus except that isolated lesions of this nerve rarely result from inflammation (in cervical lymph nodes) or from penetrating injuries or surgical operations on the neck.

The **twelfth or hypoglossal nerve** originates in the hypoglossal nucleus of the medulla, this nucleus being an upward extension of the anterior horn of the cervical cord. It emerges from the medulla between the inferior olive and the pyramid and leaves the skull via the hypoglossal canal. Near the hyoid bone it turns medially over the two carotid arteries and between the mylohyoid and hypoglossus muscles to reach the tongue, where it innervates all the intrinsic tongue muscles. Other branches supply the infrahyoid and thyrohyoid muscles. Lesions of this nerve cause weakness and wasting of the affected half of the tongue, in which fasciculation can often be seen. The tongue deviates to the paralysed side when protruded. Unilateral lesions do not cause impairment of articulation (dysarthria), but when paralysis is

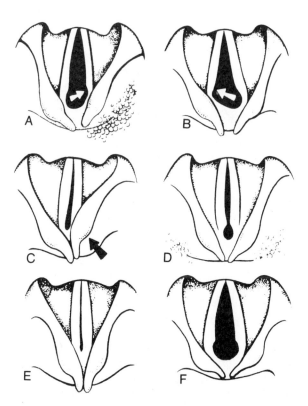

Fig. 9.12 Paralysis of the larynx (as seen through a laryngeal mirror). **A:** Paralysis of the left recurrent laryngeal nerve (neurofibroma). The paralysed arytenoid always lies slightly in front of the non-paralysed right arytenoid. Froth tends to collect around the opening of the oesophagus, owing to paralysis of the left cricopharyngeus muscle (lower sphincter of the pharynx, supplied by the same recurrent laryngeal nerve). On adduction, the non-paralysed right vocal cord moves across to meet the paralysed left cord. **B:** Paralysis of the right recurrent laryngeal nerve (thyroidectomy). There is no collected froth at the opening of the oesophagus, because compensation is so good by the intact left paired cricopharyngeus muscle that it has been able to overcome the delay due to the paralysis of the right cricopharyngeus muscle. **C:** The same case as B, showing closure of the larynx on adduction. The left non-paralysed cord now moves up to the paralysed cord, and the non-paralysed arytenoid now lies in front of the paralysed arytenoid. **D:** Paralysis of both vocal cords at the same time (thyroidectomy). The cords are held in adduction because their muscles are all paralysed except for the chief tensors of the cords, the cricothyroid muscles (supplied by the external branch of the superior laryngeal nerve). **E:** Normal closure of the vocal cords as seen in a laryngeal mirror. **F:** Normal abduction of the vocal cords as seen in a laryngeal mirror. (Reproduced with permission from Walton 1985, and redrawn from an original drawing by Charles Keogh.)

bilateral (as in advanced progressive bulbar palsy—motor neurone disease), speech is markedly impaired. Spasticity of the tongue giving dysarthria without atrophy can result from bilateral corticospinal tract lesions in the cerebral hemispheres or upper brain stem, as in progressive bulbar palsy (motor neurone disease), pseudo-bulbar palsy due to bilateral infarction, and brain-stem tumour.

The innervation and organisation of the voluntary muscles of the trunk and limbs

The axons derived from the alpha and gamma motor neurones in each spinal cord segment leave that segment in the anterior or ventral root which joins with the posterior root in the spinal nerve of that segment. After leaving the spinal column via the intervertebral foramina, each spinal nerve divides into dorsal and ventral rami. The dorsal rami largely supply the muscles of the trunk, the larger ventral rami those of the limbs. But in the brachial and lumbosacral plexuses the axons are redistributed and enter into new groupings in the peripheral nerves. Hence the fibres from a single spinal segment may reach several peripheral nerves, and con-

versely a single peripheral nerve often receives fibres from several spinal segments. In addition many peripheral nerves divide into several branches, each supplying one or more voluntary muscles. In clinical neurology a working knowledge of anatomy of the peripheral neuromuscular system is necessary in order to be able to distinguish between lesions involving:

a. a spinal cord segment or anterior horn or one ventral root,
b. a spinal nerve, in which case somatic sensory afferent fibres are also involved,
c. one or more components (e.g. cords) of the brachial or lumbosacral plexus,
d. a single peripheral nerve or one of its branches, and
e. the voluntary muscles themselves.

To assist the reader in this differential diagnostic process, the brachial plexus is illustrated in Figure 9.13 and the distribution to the musculature of various peripheral nerves in Figure 9.14; the root and nerve supply of the muscles commonly examined in clinical practice are listed in Table 9.1. The principles governing the examination of the individual skeletal muscles were described earlier.

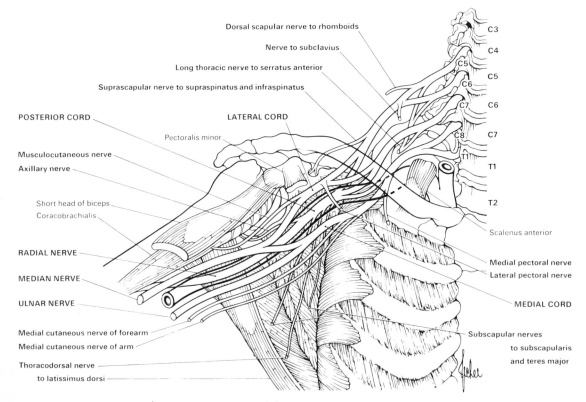

Fig. 9.13 Diagram of the brachial plexus, its branches and the muscles which they supply. (Reproduced with permission from Guarantors of Brain 1986.)

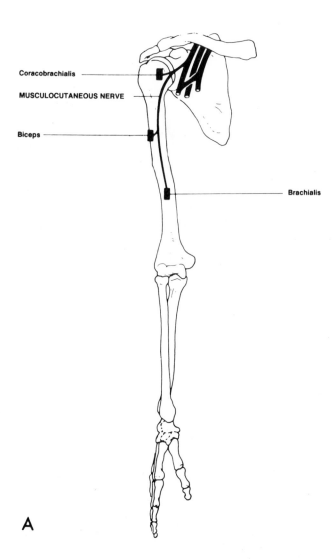

Coracobrachialis

MUSCULOCUTANEOUS NERVE

Biceps

Brachialis

A

Fig. 9.14 A Diagram of the musculocutaneous nerve and the muscles which it supplies.

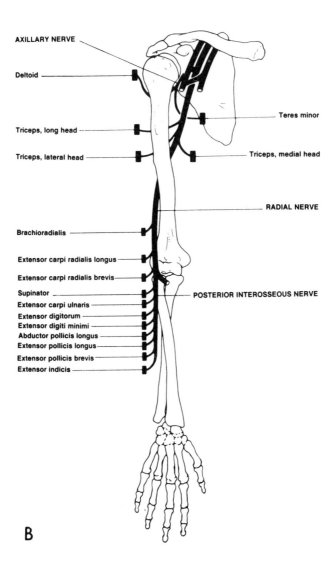

AXILLARY NERVE

Deltoid

Teres minor

Triceps, long head

Triceps, lateral head

Triceps, medial head

RADIAL NERVE

Brachioradialis

Extensor carpi radialis longus

Extensor carpi radialis brevis

Supinator

POSTERIOR INTEROSSEOUS NERVE

Extensor carpi ulnaris

Extensor digitorum

Extensor digiti minimi

Abductor pollicis longus

Extensor pollicis longus

Extensor pollicis brevis

Extensor indicis

B

Fig. 9.14 B Diagram of the axillary and radial nerves and the muscles which they supply.

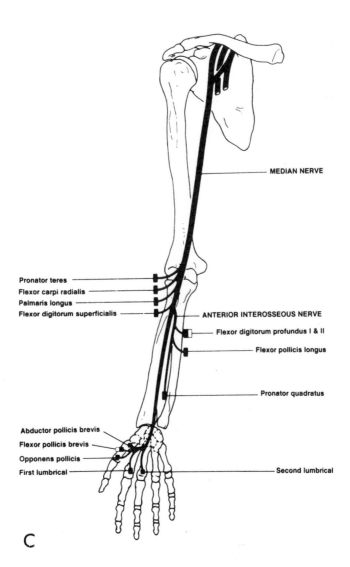

Pronator teres

Flexor carpi radialis

Palmaris longus

Flexor digitorum superficialis

MEDIAN NERVE

ANTERIOR INTEROSSEOUS NERVE

Flexor digitorum profundus I & II

Flexor pollicis longus

Pronator quadratus

Abductor pollicis brevis

Flexor pollicis brevis

Opponens pollicis

First lumbrical

Second lumbrical

C

Fig. 9.14 C Diagram of the median nerve and the muscles which it supplies.

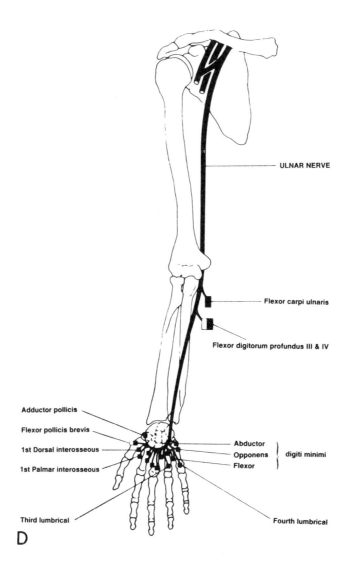

ULNAR NERVE

Flexor carpi ulnaris

Flexor digitorum profundus III & IV

Adductor pollicis

Flexor pollicis brevis

1st Dorsal interosseous

1st Palmar interosseous

Abductor
Opponens   } digiti minimi
Flexor

Third lumbrical

Fourth lumbrical

D

Fig. 9.14 D   Diagram of the ulnar nerve and the muscles which it supplies.

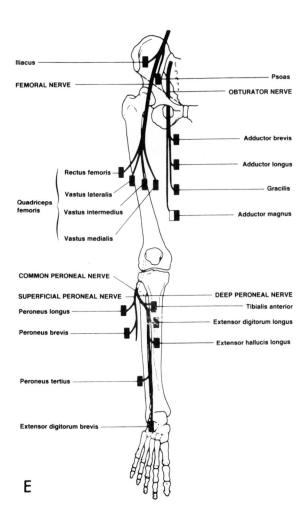

Iliacus

FEMORAL NERVE

Psoas

OBTURATOR NERVE

Adductor brevis

Adductor longus

Rectus femoris

Vastus lateralis

Gracilis

Quadriceps
femoris

Vastus intermedius

Adductor magnus

Vastus medialis

COMMON PERONEAL NERVE

SUPERFICIAL PERONEAL NERVE

DEEP PERONEAL NERVE

Tibialis anterior

Peroneus longus

Extensor digitorum longus

Peroneus brevis

Extensor hallucis longus

Peroneus tertius

Extensor digitorum brevis

E

Fig. 9.14 E Diagram of the nerves on the anterior aspect of the lower limb, and the muscles which they supply.

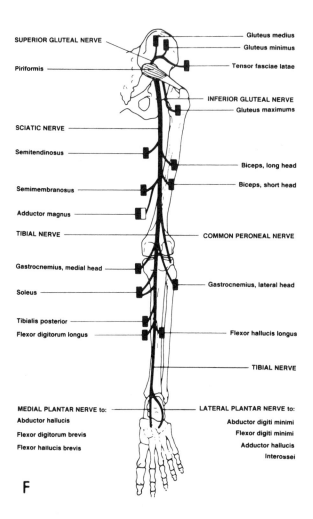

Fig. 9.14 F   Diagram of the nerves on the posterior aspect of the lower limb, and the muscles which they supply. (Fig. 19.4 A–F reproduced with permission from Guarantors of Brain 1986.)

Table 9.1 Nerve and main root supply of muscles. The list given below does not include all the muscles innervated by these nerves, but only those more commonly tested, either clinically or electrically, and shows the order of innervation. (Reproduced from Guarantors of Brain, 1986 with the permission of the authors and publishers.)

Upper limb	Spinal roots
Spinal accessory nerve	
Trapezius	C3, C4
Brachial plexus	
Rhomboids	C4, C5
Serratus anterior	C5, C6, C7
Pectoralis major	
Clavicular	**C5**, C6
Sternal	C6, **C7**, C8
Supraspinatus	**C5**, C6
Infraspinatus	**C5**, C6
Latissimus dorsi	C6, **C7**, C8
Teres major	C5, C6, C7
Axillary nerve	
Deltoid	**C5**, C6
Musculocutaneous nerve	
Biceps	C5, C6
Brachialis	C5, C6
Radial nerve	
Triceps { Long head / Lateral head / Medial head }	C6, **C7**, C8
Brachioradialis	C5, **C6**
Extensor carpi radialis longus	C5, **C6**
Posterior interosseous nerve	
Supinator	C6, C7
Extensor carpi ulnaris	**C7**, C8
Extensor digitorum	**C7**, C8
Abductor pollicis longus	**C7**, C8
Extensor pollicis longus	**C7**, C8
Extensor pollicis brevis	**C7**, C8
Extensor indicis	**C7**, C8
Median nerve	
Pronator teres	C6, C7
Flexor carpi radialis	C6, C7
Flexor digitorum superficialis	C7, **C8**, T1
Abductor pollicis brevis	C8, **T1**
Flexor pollicis brevis*	C8, **T1**
Opponens pollicis	C8, **T1**
Lumbricals I & II	C8, **T1**
Anterior interosseous nerve	
Pronator quadratus	C7, **C8**
Flexor digitorum profundus I & II	C7, **C8**
Flexor pollicis longus	C7, **C8**

Upper limb	Spinal roots
Ulnar nerve	
Flexor carpi ulnaris	C7, **C8**, T1
Flexor digitorum profundus III & IV	C7, **C8**
Hypothenar muscles	C8, **T1**
Adductor pollicis	C8, **T1**
Flexor pollicis brevis	C8, **T1**
Palmar interossei	C8, **T1**
Dorsal interossei	C8, **T1**
Lumbricals III & IV	C8, **T1**

Lower limb	Spinal roots
Femoral nerve	
Iliopsoas	L1, **L2**, L3
Rectus femoris }	
Vastus lateralis } Quadriceps	
Vastus intermedius } femoris	L2, **L3**, **L4**
Vastus medialis }	
Obturator nerve	
Adductor longus }	
Adductor magnus }	**L2**, **L3**, L4
Superior gluteal nerve	
Gluteus medius and minimus }	
Tensor fasciae latae }	**L4**, **L5**, S1
Inferior gluteal nerve	
Gluteus maximus	**L5**, **S1**, S2
Sciatic and tibial nerves	
Semitendinosus	L5, **S1**, S2
Biceps	L5, **S1**, S2
Semimembranosus	L5, **S1**, S2
Gastrocnemius and soleus	S1, S2
Tibialis posterior	L4, L5
Flexor digitorum longus	L5, **S1**, **S2**
Abductor hallucis }	
Abductor digiti minimi } Small muscles	
Interossei } of foot	S1, S2
Sciatic and common peroneal nerves	
Tibialis anterior	**L4**, L5
Extensor digitorum longus	**L5**, S1
Extensor hallucis longus	**L5**, S1
Extensor digitorum brevis	L5, S1
Peroneus longus	L5, S1
Peroneus brevis	L5, S1

*Flexor pollicis brevis is often supplied wholly or partially by the ulnar nerve.

DISORDERS OF TONE

The tone of a muscle is the response it shows to passive stretching. A relaxed and resting muscle is not in a state of continuous partial contraction; it has elasticity, but no tone. Tone can only therefore be assessed when the muscle is moved or when it is concerned with maintaining a posture against an applied force such as that of gravity. **Postural tone** is thus that state of partial contraction of certain muscles which is needed to maintain the posture of the parts of the body; clearly the muscles involved and the force of muscular contraction required will depend upon the position of the parts concerned at any one time.

In neurological practice, tone is usually assessed by moving a limb or some other part passively and by observing the reaction which occurs in the muscles which are being stretched. As this stretching begins, stretch receptors in the muscle concerned, and particularly the muscle spindles, give out afferent stimuli and reflex partial contraction of the muscle results. Variations in the sensitivity of this reflex, which is also responsible for the tendon reflexes, account for the alterations in tone which result from nervous disease. Forceful continued contraction of a muscle group (e.g. clenching one hand or pulling firmly with the flexed fingers of both hands opposed to one another) temporarily causes an increased flow of afferent impulses in the sensory fibres from the spindles. This in turn gives increased gamma neurone activity with contraction of intrafusal fibres. This leads to a generalised slight increase in tone, and the tendon reflexes become more brisk due to a secondary increase in alpha neurone discharge as the 'set' of the spindle (the state of contraction of its intrafusal fibres) is altered, with resultant increased sensitivity to stretch. This phenomenon, often known as reinforcement, or Jendrassik's manoeuvre, is often used to bring out tendon reflexes which at first seem absent. In spasticity and extrapyramidal rigidity the 'set' of the spindles is continuously abnormal.

On stretching, the tone of the muscle may be increased (spasticity or rigidity or hypertonia) or it may be reduced (flaccidity or hypotonia) and these changes are very helpful in neurological diagnosis.

Muscle tone is normally regulated by reticulospinal fibres which accompany the pyramidal tract throughout its course and which have an inhibitory effect upon the stretch reflex. This inhibition balances the background facilitatory impulses conveyed by the pontine reticulospinal and vestibulospinal pathways; these influences are in turn modified by multisynaptic arcs traversing the cerebellum, basal ganglia and brain stem. When lesions of the pyramidal and reticulospinal tract release stretch reflexes from inhibition, the increased tone and exaggerated tendon reflexes which result are initially associated with hyperactivity in dynamic fusimotor neurones, but if such increased tone (**spasticity**) persists, increased alpha neurone discharge develops so that spasticity in man at different stages may be associated with both increased gamma (dynamic fusimotor) and alpha neurone activity. If the dorsal reticulospinal system, closely related anatomically in the spinal cord, is also damaged, afferent flexor reflex pathways are also released from inhibition giving flexor spasms in the lower limbs in response to stimulation of the legs; the 'extensor' plantar response, or Babinski reflex, one component of the flexor withdrawal reflex, is similarly released. In spasticity the affected limb or limbs show an increase in resistance to passive stretching; this resistance is particularly severe initially, but then 'gives' suddenly as the movement is continued. Hence this sign, seen particularly well in the legs of a patient with a spastic paraplegia due to bilateral pyramidal tract disease, is known as 'clasp-knife' rigidity. In individuals with spastic weakness movement is impaired owing to defective conduction of motor impulses by the pyramidal tracts while there is also 'clasp-knife' rigidity on passive movement.

Rigidity of extrapyramidal type, in patients with disease of the basal ganglia or substantia nigra, is different. It is seen characteristically in parkinsonism. In such cases the rigidity is either uniform in degree throughout the entire range of passive movement, when it is known as 'plastic' or 'lead-pipe rigidity, or else it intermittently 'gives' and returns throughout the movement, being then described as 'cog-wheel' in type. In extrapyramidal rigidity, unlike spasticity, alpha neurone rather than gamma neurone discharge predominates from the beginning. In **dystonia** there is simultaneous contraction of agonists, antagonists and synergists, reciprocal inhibition of antagonists is seriously deranged and alpha neurone discharge is greatly increased. A particular form of muscular rigidity, known as **decerebrate rigidity**, develops as a result of severe transverse lesions of the upper mid-brain at the level of the superior colliculus or red nucleus. Excitatory mechanisms cause increased tone in extensor muscles, inhibitory mechanisms reduce tone in flexor muscles. These mechanisms are mediated by reticulospinal and vestibulospinal pathways, and tonic as distinct from phasic stretch reflexes are increased, while there is increased gamma efferent discharge to extensor muscles, involving especially static fusimotor fibres. In such a case all four limbs are rigidly extended, the back is arched and there may be neck retraction, so that the patient, if lying supine, is virtually supported by the back of the head and the heels. This posture is known as **opisthotonos**; the arching of the back is increased by any sensory stimulus and there is striking resistance to any attempt at flexing the limbs passively.

Flaccidity, or **hypotonia**, is a reduction in tone. When this is severe, as in patients with total flaccid paralysis, all resistance to passive stretch is lost and the limbs are limp and flail-like. Less severe hypotonia in the upper limbs, for instance, can be elicited by asking the patient to hold out his arms horizontally. The forearms are then tapped briskly; when tone is increased (spasticity) the recoil is sharp, immediate and exaggerated. When one limb is hypotonic the recoil is slower and the arm swings through a wider range. If the patient is asked to contract the biceps brachii against resistance, by bending the arm towards his face, and the examiner's restraining hand is suddenly removed, the patient's hand may strike his face if the limb is hypotonic, whereas if the tone is normal he will stop the movement before it does so. Furthermore, if the subject is asked to raise his arms above his head with the palms facing forwards, the palm of a hypotonic limb is externally rotated and facing more laterally than the other. In the lower limbs it is useful to place a hand beneath the knee and to lift the leg from the bed, then to allow it to fall back quickly; with experience it is soon possible to judge from the resistance of the limb to this movement, whether tone is increased or reduced.

ATAXIA AND INCO-ORDINATION

Ataxia is clumsiness of motor activity, resulting from inability to control accurately the range and precision of movement. It can result from a defect in the sensory pathways carrying proprioceptive information from sensory receptors in the periphery. Appreciation of the position of the parts of the body in space is then impaired, and since controlled movement requires continuous and accurate information of this type for its continued performance it may be seriously deranged. This phenomenon known as sensory ataxia, will be considered in Chapter 10. In such a case, the cause of the unsteadiness is revealed by sensory examination. Similarly, afferent stimuli from the labyrinths are important in the maintenance of posture and if, as a result of disease of the labyrinths, of the vestibular nerves or of their central connexions, distorted information about the position of the head is received, the patient's gait will become grossly unsteady and the movements of his limbs clumsy and poorly controlled. Thus ataxia can also be due to **labyrinthine dysfunction**.

The commonest cause of ataxia is **disease of the cerebellum** or of its central connexions in the brain stem. The controlling activity of the cerebellum upon the motor system is concerned particularly with the fine co-ordination of movement and with the judgement of

distance; these faculties are selectively impaired by cerebellar disease. Much depends upon which part of the cerebellum or its connexions is diseased, and there are several general principles which help in deciding that the function of the cerebellum or of cerebellar pathways is impaired. The archicerebellum and palaeocerebellum as defined above have important vestibular connexions and are concerned particularly with equilibration. Lesions in this situation produce an ataxia which involves central structures of the body and is thus particularly apparent when the patient walks. He is unsteady and staggers in a drunken manner, walks on a wide base and has considerable difficulty in stopping suddenly or in turning. Lesser degrees of ataxia can be brought out by asking the patient to walk 'heel-to-toe'; even in mildly ataxic individuals this is usually impossible. In such a case the tests of cerebellar function to be described below, which are concerned with demonstrating ataxia in lateral structures such as the limbs, may be singularly uninformative. When the tests are negative it is a common pitfall to regard such patients as hysterical, particularly if the doctor fails to recognise that a central cerebellar lesion gives this particular type of so-called **truncal or central ataxia**. This sign is particularly common in children with medulloblastomas.

Lesions of the lateral cerebellar hemispheres, affecting the neocerebellum, give physical signs which are more readily identifiable. If the lesion is predominantly unilateral, these signs appear in the limbs on the same side as the lesion. There may also be **ocular signs**; thus in an acute cerebellar lesion *skew deviation* is occasionally seen, in which the eye on the affected side is deviated downwards and inwards, while the contralateral eye is turned upwards and out; but this rare manifestation is more common in upper brain stem lesions. *Nystagmus* is commoner and usually prominent, being of greatest amplitude on looking to the side of the lesion. **Hypotonia** is often present in the ipsilateral limbs, and **ataxia** causes a striking clumsiness and inco-ordination of movement. The patient is unable to fasten buttons with the affected hand and his hand-writing may be scrawling and illegible. Judgement of distance is also impaired, a phenomenon known as **dysmetria**, and the hand or digit performing a movement may wildly overshoot the mark (**past-pointing**). Tremor of the limbs may be apparent at rest but is greatly accentuated by movement, being worse towards the end of an action (**intention-tremor**). The latter sign is, however, much more common in disease of central cerebellar connections than of the cerebellar hemispheres and in fact is rarely seen in any condition other than multiple sclerosis. These 'neocerebellar' signs are particularly apparent on carrying out the 'finger-nose' and 'heel-knee' tests and there is also an irregularity of movement if the patient is asked to tap quickly and repetitively upon a smooth surface, or to make dots within a small circle with a pencil. Rapid alternating movements of the limbs, such as pronation and supination of the hands and forearms, are poorly and jerkily performed (**dysdiadochokinesis**). The patient with a unilateral cerebellar lesion also tends to stagger and to deviate towards the affected side when walking. A minimal cerebellar lesion on one side is sometimes easily identified by asking the patient to walk a few paces with his eyes closed, when he turns or walks to the affected side. Alternatively, if asked to walk in a circle around the examiner, first clockwise then anticlockwise, there is deviation away from the examiner in one direction and towards him in the other.

THE REFLEXES

The simplest reflex arc consists of an afferent or sensory neurone and an efferent or motor neurone with whose parent cell the terminal fibres of the afferent neurone synapse (Fig. 9.6). Stimulation of the sensory neurone then produces a motor response mediated by the motor neurone. Very few reflexes are as simple as this, then being called monosynaptic, though the spinal reflex arc through which withdrawal of a limb follows a painful stimulus cannot be much more complex. In many pathways concerned with reflex activity, however, the sensory and motor neurones are separated by connecting or internuncial neurones, most of which lie in the spinal grey matter; they receive impulses from ascending and descending fibre pathways which exercise important controlling influences upon reflex activity. Unquestionably some long reflex pathways run a course involving brain stem as well as spinal structures, while some may even traverse the cerebral cortex. There are many reflexes concerned with autonomic and visceromotor activity, and even endocrine secretion, but in clinical neurology we are largely concerned with the simpler reflexes which, when activated, result in somatic motor activity.

Clearly reflex activity is lost or impaired if a lesion is present at any point in the reflex arc. Thus a break in the afferent or efferent pathway will abolish that particular reflex. For instance, the **corneal reflex** (the contraction of the orbicularis oculi which follows stimulation of the cornea) is lost if the cornea is anaesthetic due to a lesion of the trigeminal nerve or if the face is paralysed due to a lesion of the seventh nerve. Similarly, the **palatal and pharyngeal reflexes** which give contraction of muscles of the soft palate or pharynx on tactile stimulation may be impaired unilaterally. This occurs if one trigeminal (palate) or glossopharyngeal (pharyngeal) nerve is diseased (the afferent pathway), or if there is a lesion of the vagus (the efferent pathway).

There is also a facial reflex which is useful in clinical neurology. A brisk tap on the glabella above the bridge of the nose causes bilateral blinking. In the normal individual, on repeated tapping the blinking ceases after two or three taps, but in patients with parkinsonism it may continue in time with the taps (the 'glabellar tap' sign). Electrophysiological recordings from the orbicularis oculi have shown that there is an initial monosynaptic reflex response of low amplitude, followed by a larger response of longer latency which is clearly polysynaptic and which habituates in normal individuals but not in parkinsonism.

The most informative reflexes in the physical examination of patients with nervous disease are the stretch and cutaneous reflexes.

The first of the **stretch reflexes** to be regularly tested is the *jaw jerk*, elicited by means of a sharp downward tap on the chin with the mouth held partly open. A positive response consists in contraction of the masseters with elevation of the lower jaw; if this reflex is exaggerated it usually indicates a bilateral pyramidal tract lesion in or above the upper brain stem. The **'snout' reflex** (see p. 22) occurs under similar circumstances, while if there is bilateral frontal lobe destruction or degeneration as in certain varieties of dementia, a **'sucking' reflex**, like the normal sucking response of the young infant, may be present.

The stretch reflexes normally sought on examining the limbs are the tendon reflexes or 'jerks'. These consist of a reflex contraction of the relevant muscle, produced in practice by a sharp blow upon its tendon near its point of insertion. Those commonly elicited were described in Chapter 2. In the upper limb they are the biceps and radial jerks which obtain their motor innervation from the fifth and sixth roots, the triceps jerk which is mainly innervated by the seventh, and the finger jerk which receives its supply from the seventh and eighth roots. In the lower limbs, the knee jerk is innervated by the second, third and fourth lumbar roots, the ankle jerk by the first and second sacral. Any tendon reflex can be diminished or lost if there is a lesion of the sensory pathway which carries different impulses from the muscle to the spinal cord, or at any point in the lower motor neurones supplying the muscle concerned, or even when a primary disorder of the muscle itself, a myopathy, has impaired its ability to contract. These reflexes are also lost temporarily during the stage of so-called 'shock' which follows an acute and severe lesion of the brain or spinal cord, even when there is no break in the reflex arc. All the tendon reflexes may be symmetrically exaggerated by tension and anxiety or by increased neuromuscular excitability due to metabolic or other causes, but they are most strikingly increased when there is a lesion of the pyramidal tract. A unilateral lesion is easier to identify, as the reflexes are exaggerated on one side of the body and not on the other. The finger jerk, for instance, is normally present in some patients and not in others; it is only of real significance if present unilaterally. The phenomenon of *clonus* often accompanies exaggeration of stretch reflexes. It consists of an intermittent muscular contraction and relaxation evoked by sustained stretching of a muscle; it can occur apparently spontaneously in spastic limbs, but is best elicited as a physical sign in the lower limbs by sudden pressure applied in a distal direction to the upper margin of the patella (*patellar clonus*), or by sharp dorsiflexion of the foot carried out with the leg extended (*ankle clonus*).

Inversion of upper-limb reflexes is an important physical sign of spinal cord disease. Thus if there is a lesion of the C5 or C6 segments of the spinal cord, this can break the reflex arc for reflexes innervated by these segments, namely the biceps and radial jerks, which are therefore lost or diminished. If, however, the same lesion is compressing the spinal cord and causing pyramidal tract dysfunction, reflexes innervated by lower segments (triceps, finger jerks) are exaggerated and are obtained by stimuli applied over a wide field. Thus tapping the biceps tendon may produce contraction of triceps, while on attempting to elicit the radial jerk, finger flexion, but no radial jerk, is obtained. This so-called inversion of either reflex is diagnostic of a cervical cord lesion.

The **cutaneous or superficial reflexes** commonly utilised in neurological diagnosis are the abdominal reflexes, the cremasteric, anal and plantar reflexes. The *abdominal reflexes* are elicited by stroking the skin of the abdomen (the point of a pin is a suitable instrument), when movement of the umbilicus towards the stimulus should follow. The level of a segmental lesion in the dorsal spinal cord can sometimes be identified by loss of the lower abdominal reflexes and preservation of the upper. Even more useful is the fact that the abdominal reflexes are unilaterally diminished in amplitude or lost, or may simply fatigue rapidly on repetitive stimulation, when there is a lesion of the pyramidal tract on the same side of the body. There are some conditions (e.g. multiple sclerosis) in which the abdominal reflexes are lost at a comparatively early stage of the disease, whereas in others (e.g. motor neurone disease), in which there may also be other evidence of pyramidal tract disease, they often survive much longer. Total absence of the abdominal reflexes is usually a finding of pathological significance, except in the very obese, in multipara with lax abdominal muscles, and in the elderly. The *cremasteric reflex* (contraction of the cremaster on stroking the medial side of the thigh) is also impaired or lost in pyramidal tract lesions. The *anal reflex* (contraction of the external sphincter on scratching the perianal skin) is particularly likely to be lost when there is a lesion of the

cauda equina involving the fourth and fifth sacral roots.

Probably the most important reflex in clinical neurology is the **plantar response**. On stroking the lateral aspect of the sole of the foot from the heel towards the fifth toe, plantar-flexion of all five toes (the flexor response) normally occurs. The abnormal response which consists of dorsiflexion of the great toe and a simultaneous downward and 'fanning-out' movement of the remaining toes, is known as an extensor response or the Babinski response. The Babinski response refers only to the abnormal extensor reflex and it is semantically inaccurate to say that 'the Babinski was negative or positive'. It is better to avoid the eponymous term and to refer to the plantar response as being 'flexor' or 'extensor'. An extensor plantar reflex is virtually diagnostic of a lesion of the pyramidal tract at any point in its course from the contralateral motor cortex down through the brain stem and the ipsilateral lateral column of the spinal cord. It is part of a primitive withdrawal response 'uncovered' or 'released' by a pyramidal tract lesion; often it is accompanied by contraction of the hamstrings. Indeed, if the spinal cord lesion is severe and complete, stroking the sole will also evoke flexion at the hip and knee and even evacuation of the bladder and bowels (a 'mass' reflex). In such a case the extensor plantar response is readily elicited by a variety of stimuli applied over a wide area (e.g. pressure upon the shin, pricking the leg with a pin, etc.).

Among the many other reflexes which are altered by nervous disease there are few which are of sufficient practical importance to be mentioned here. However, in decerebrate patients, as in neonates, the **tonic neck reflexes** may be greatly exaggerated so that on forcibly turning the head to one side the limbs on that side extend while the contralateral limbs flex (Magnus-de Klejn reflex). Persistence of this reflex after the first three months of life, and of the Moro reflex (flexion of all four limbs on sharply tapping the bed upon which the baby lies) indicates a serious disorder of cerebral development. Similarly, the activity of the frontal lobes in man is sufficient after the first year or two of life to inhibit the reflex grasping and groping which results from stroking the palm of the hand. This grasp reflex may, however, return unilaterally due to a lesion of the contralateral frontal lobe.

THE CLINICAL FEATURES OF UPPER AND LOWER MOTOR NEURONE LESIONS

An illustrative example of the effects of an **upper motor neurone lesion** is the hemiplegia produced by an extensive lesion of the contralateral motor area of the cerebral cortex, or of the internal capsule. If the lesion is acute, say, a massive haemorrhage, the paralysed limbs are at first flaccid, immobile and without tone, owing to the phenomenon of 'shock', through which a sudden and extensive lesion causes abrupt depression of reflexes subserved by relatively remote areas of the nervous system, even though the reflex arcs concerned remain intact. All reflexes are lost at this stage on the affected side. Gradually over the course of days or weeks flaccidity lessens and the affected limbs become spastic, though there are a few cases in which, particularly if there is also an extensive parietal lobe lesion, the hemiplegia remains permanently flaccid. Whereas the affected arm and leg are completely paralysed, those parts of the body which are bilaterally 'represented' in the cerebral cortex can still be moved voluntarily, even on the paralysed side. Thus facial weakness affects mainly the lower part of the face and the upper part slightly or not at all, and there is no defect of palatal movement. And since emotional movement of the face, as in smiling, seems to be controlled not by the cerebral cortex but by thalamic mechanisms, a patient who cannot move the lower half of one side of the face at will may yet smile symmetrically.

As flaccidity passes off in the paralysed limbs and spasticity appears, so the tendon reflexes return, become greatly exaggerated and may be accompanied by clonus. The abdominal and cremasteric reflexes on the affected side remain absent and the plantar response extensor. Spasticity is often greatest in the flexor muscles of the upper limbs and in the extensor muscles of the lower, so that in a patient with a long-standing hemiplegia, the arm is flexed at the elbow and at the wrist and fingers while the leg remains extended.

When the lesion of the pyramidal tract is not sufficiently severe to cause total paralysis, but only relatively slight weakness, it is the finer and more skilful movements, those most recently acquired by man in the process of evolution, which are most severely impaired (Hughlings Jackson's law). Thus independent finger and toe movements are poor, though the strength of movement at proximal joints such as the elbow and knee remains good. A useful sign of early pyramidal tract dysfunction is to observe the hands and arms outstretched in front of the patient when the eyes are closed; a downward 'drift' is an early sign of upper motor neurone weakness. Furthermore, while difficulty in opposing the thumb and individual fingers may be an early sign, objective testing of muscle power often shows that 'pyramidal' weakness is first apparent on abduction of the shoulder and in hand-grip in the upper limbs and in hip flexion and foot dorsiflexion in the lower. And during the process of recovery from a pyramidal tract lesion, movement usually returns first at the proximal joints; the cruder movements are first regained, while the more delicate and precise activity of the fingers and toes is the

last to return. A patient recovering from a hemiplegia resulting from, say, cerebral thrombosis, may be able to use his hand to grip or to lift objects, but is often unable to write or to fasten buttons or shoelaces. He walks with his arm flexed across his chest and with stiffness, dragging and circumduction of the affected leg.

Similar physical signs are found in patients with bilateral pyramidal tract lesions causing spastic paraplegia. If the lesion responsible is an acute transverse lesion of the cord, say, from infection or injury, there is total flaccid paralysis of the limbs below the affected segment during the initial stage of spinal shock; subsequently spasticity, increased tendon reflexes and extensor plantar responses appear. As the lower motor neurone and the spinal reflex arc are intact, severe wasting of muscles does not occur, although when paralysis has been present for some time, disuse atrophy, affecting all muscles of the limb or limbs, appears. When the spinal cord lesion is incomplete the tone of the spastic lower limbs may be particularly increased in the extensor muscles (paraplegia-in-extension) but when both pyramidal tracts are severely diseased and there are lesions of reticulospinal and vestibulospinal pathways, the legs become progressively flexed at the knees and hips and stimulation will provoke painful flexor spasms (paraplegia-in-flexion).

Much depends, in an individual case, upon the rate of evolution of any upper motor neurone lesion. Whereas an acute lesion, e.g. cerebral haemorrhage or cord transection, gives a total flaccid paralysis initially with spasticity evolving slowly over subsequent days or weeks, a chronic or slowly progressive lesion such as a tumour may give little more initially than a slight impairment of fine finger movement in one hand, or else a minimal increase in tendon reflexes in the affected arm; subsequently however a spastic monoparesis or hemiparesis slowly develops.

The pathological causes of upper motor neurone lesions are many and varied—too many for their differential diagnosis to be considered in detail here. Once the lesion has been localised by means of the physical signs, the clinical history should again be analysed to see if any clue can be obtained as to the nature of the pathological process. The scheme of pathological classification given in Chapter 2 is often useful. Thus if we take the cerebral causes of spastic weakness, these may include traumatic (cerebral contusion, extradural haematoma), developmental (cerebral palsy) inflammatory (cerebral abscess, encephalomyelitis) neoplastic (meningioma, glioma metastases), and degenerative (cerebral infarction or haemorrhage) disorders.

The natural history of these and of the many other conditions which may affect the pyramidal tract differ considerably, and associated signs indicating involvement of other nervous structures or other systems may be invaluable. Similarly, there are many possible causes of spinal cord disease giving rise to spastic paraplegia. These include developmental causes (basilar impression, Chiari malformation), trauma (fracture dislocation of spine, haematomyelia) inflammation, either extradural (abscess) or intramedullary (transverse myelitis), neoplasia (meningioma, neurofibroma, glioma, metastases, reticulosis) and a group of common degenerative, demyelinating and metabolic disorders. Of these, multiple sclerosis is characterised by a remittent course and often by involvement of brain-stem structures; it sometimes gives temporal pallor of the optic discs, nystagmus or diplopia and cerebellar signs as well as signs of a spastic paraplegia with impaired appreciation of 'posterior column' type sensation in the lower limbs. Some few cases, however, run a progressive course with only a spastic paraplegia and no signs of involvement of brain-stem structures, although even in these, visual evoked potential measurement may demonstrate unsuspected lesions of the optic nerves or pathways. In these cases the condition may be difficult to distinguish from amyotrophic lateral sclerosis or cervical cord compression due to tumour or cervical spondylosis. In the latter disorder, however, particularly if the long-standing disc protrusions extend laterally, spinal roots are often compressed as well as the cord, and there may be muscle wasting and weakness in the arms or inversion of upper limb reflexes as well as a spastic paraplegia. Patients with motor neurone disease usually demonstrate some wasting, weakness and fasciculation of muscles in the limbs, as well as signs of a spastic paraparesis, and in this condition there is no sensory impairment, but in early cases presenting with the clinical syndrome of amyotrophic lateral sclerosis, as distinct from progressive muscular atrophy, the signs may simply be those of spastic paraparesis. In syringomyelia, on the other hand, dissociated anaesthesia to pain and temperature sensation with retention of touch is often found in one upper limb, combined with some wasting and weakness of muscles due to lower motor neurone involvement, while in the lower limbs there are usually signs of a spastic paraparesis. Spastic weakness of the legs is also present in some cases of subacute combined degeneration of the cord, but here sensory symptoms and signs indicating dysfunction of the posterior columns of the cord usually predominate; there may be tenderness of the calves and absent ankle jerks owing to a neuropathy interrupting the sensory side of the reflex arc, while signs of pyramidal tract disease, though present, are often relatively unobtrusive. In spinal cord infarction, if the cord is infarcted over several segments, due to occlusion of the anterior spinal artery resulting from thrombosis, embolism or compression, the paraplegia may be permanently flaccid, but the plantars, if not absent, are extensor.

The features of a **lower motor neurone lesion** are very different. As the final common path of all forms of motor activity is interrupted, the muscle or muscle groups involved become totally paralysed and flaccid, and remain so. Any reflex movement for which the paralysed muscles are necessary is lost. Another invariable feature is that all muscles deprived of their motor nerve supply undergo rapid atrophy; they may shrink to half normal size within about six weeks and eventually disappear almost completely, being virtually replaced by fibrous connective tissue. Before this stage of total atrophy is reached, and particularly if the lesion responsible lies in the anterior horn cells of the spinal cord (e.g. motor neurone disease), **fasciculation** is common. The latter is a phenomenon, visible through the intact skin unless the subject is very obese, in which individual muscle fasciculi contract spontaneously, and random, repetitive flickering of these fibre bundles is seen to be occurring in a muscle which is apparently at rest. Fasciculation, though most often seen in motor neurone disease, is not diagnostic of that condition, as it may occur after old poliomyelitis, and is also seen occasionally in polyneuropathy and in other conditions involving anterior horn cells and peripheral nerves. Furthermore, it may be benign and of no pathological significance; it is often noticed by doctors in their calf and small hand muscles. A benign condition in which widespread and coarse fasciculation occurs along with profuse sweating and muscular cramps is known as one variety of **myokymia**. Benign myokymia of the lower eyelid is a flickering in that lid often experienced by normal individuals when fatigued. Another rare and obscure form of myokymia is characterised by fasciculation, myotonia, distal muscular wasting and contracture and by continuous muscle fibre activity in the EMG (Isaacs' syndrome or neuromyotonia). Yet another (facial myokymia) is a repetitive rippling or wave–like movement of the muscles of one side of the face, sometimes seen in multiple sclerosis, sometimes of unknown cause.

Fibrillation, or spontaneous contraction of single muscle fibres, also follows a lesion of the lower motor neurone, but cannot be seen through the skin, though it can be recorded in the EMG (p. 36). Hence the clinical features of an acute lower motor neurone lesion are flaccid paralysis, absent reflexes, and rapid atrophy of the affected muscle or group of muscles. In a slowly progressive lesion weakness and atrophy increase gradually, and eventually the reflexes are lost. In such a case it can be difficult to decide whether the lesion involves a single peripheral nerve, multiple peripheral nerves, spinal anterior roots, or the anterior horn cells of the cord. All-important in making this distinction is a knowledge of the anatomy and innervation of muscles. If more muscles are affected than could be supplied by one peripheral nerve, it must then be asked whether lesions of one or several spinal roots could be responsible, in which case there may be other evidence of spinal cord dysfunction. If the muscular weakness and wasting is more widespread still, and particularly if it occurs symmetrically in the periphery of the limbs, the two most likely diagnoses are polyneuropathy and motor neurone disease (progressive muscular atrophy). The presence of sensory loss, particularly if present symmetrically and distally, will support the former diagnosis, while if there is widespread fasciculation, no sensory loss, and some evidence of pyramidal tract disease, motor neurone disease can be diagnosed with reasonable confidence.

Muscular weakness and wasting which can mimic that due to a lower motor neurone lesion may result from disease of the muscles themselves, a myopathy. Here too there is flaccid weakness with atrophy and absence of tendon reflexes. Even in disorders of conduction at the motor end-plate, such as myasthenia gravis, the muscles may be weak and hypotonic, though atrophy is uncommon. In general, however, myopathic as distinct from neuropathic disorders (see Ch. 18) tend to affect the proximal rather than the distal muscles of the limbs; fasciculation is rare. Considerable help in differential diagnosis is obtained from electromyography, since in polyneuropathy and motor neurone disease the motor unit potentials, though reduced in number, are often normal or larger than normal, whereas in myopathy, owing to patchy degeneration of individual muscle fibres, they are broken-up and polyphasic or of short duration. Measurement of motor and sensory conduction velocity in peripheral nerves can be of particular value in identifying lesions of such nerves and in helping to distinguish the different varieties of polyneuropathy.

INVOLUNTARY MOVEMENTS

Movements which do not occur in response to the will and are thus involuntary can be of great importance in neurological diagnosis.

The first type of movement commonly classified in this group, though not strictly involuntary, is the so-called **tic** or **habit spasm**. This term embraces many twitching or jerking movements which occur irregularly and involve particularly the muscles around the eyes, the remainder of the face and the shoulders. The subject is aware of the movement, and on close questioning it is clearly performed voluntarily since from it the patient obtains relief of tension which would otherwise become intolerable. This affliction is clearly related to anxiety. Though initially under the control of the will the movements become so habitual as to be almost involuntary. However,

there is evidence that multiple tics can result from organic disease as these are the principal manifestations of Gilles de la Tourette's syndrome in which coprolalia (recurrent compulsive utterances, often of an obscene nature) also occur.

The epileptic fit or convulsion, whether focal or general, clearly involves involuntary movement, but is considered in Chapter 6. A closely related phenomenon is **myoclonus**, a sudden shock-like muscular contraction which can involve a small group of muscles, several muscle groups or even the greater part of the voluntary musculature, either simultaneously or successively. Myoclonic jerks may occur while falling asleep and are not then pathological, though when they occur repeatedly throughout the night they probably represent an epileptic manifestation and many affected individuals have occasional major seizures. A brief myoclonic jerk of the limbs is a common accompaniment of an attack of petit mal. Myoclonus in response to startle (say, by noise) is a feature of cerebral lipidosis, but in some individuals it is a benign but troublesome disorder unaccompanied by other evidence of disease (hyperekplexia, or the 'essential startle disease'), while myoclonic jerks also occur in several cerebral degenerative diseases such as subacute sclerosing panencephalitis and Creutzfeldt-Jakob disease (see pp. 226 and 101). When myoclonus involves many parts of the body and occurs repetitively or at times almost rhythmically, this clinical syndrome has been called paramyoclonus multiplex; sometimes the condition is familial and the patients show no other features of epilepsy (hereditary essential myoclonus). However there are some patients developing severe myoclonus in childhood who go on to develop major epilepsy and dementia with progressive degenerative changes in the cerebrum and cerebellum. This fatal condition is known as progressive **myoclonic epilepsy** (or Lafora body disease, since the affected nerve cells, especially in the dentate nuclei of the cerebellum, show cytoplasmic acidophilic inclusions consisting of abnormal polysaccharides, known as Lafora bodies). Occasionally in elderly persons a repetitive myoclonus of plate and throat muscles develops. This condition, **palatal myoclonus**, also interferes with respiration and speech which then occur in a series of staccato jerks. Though distressing, the condition, which is due to degenerative changes in the olivary nuclei and the central tegmental tract of facial midbrain is not progressive.

Repetitive irregular twitching (not the wave-like ripple of facial myokymia) in one half of the face must not be confused with either habit spasm or myoclonus, as this condition, **hemifacial spasm** (see p. 140) is probably due to an irritative lesion of the facial nerve.

Tremor is a rapid, rhythmically repetitive movement which tends to be consistent in pattern, amplitude and frequency, and usually consists of intermittent contraction of a muscle group and then of its antagonists. It may be *static* (present at rest), *action* (present throughout the range of movement), or *intention* (accentuated towards the end of movement) in type. A *static tremor* of the head and hands, rapid in frequency and small in range, and not generally abolished by movement, is typical of the *senile tremor* seen in some elderly persons. A more coarse rhythmical nodding of the head occurs in some patients with cerebellar disease. Senile tremor is closely related to, if not identical with, benign familial tremor (see below), but develops in later life. The most typical form of static tremor, however, is the 'pill-rolling' movement of the fingers and hands, often with associated tremor of the arms and legs and sometimes the lips and tongue, which is seen in Parkinson's disease. Though accentuated by embarrassment and attention, this tremor is generally abolished by movement, though occasionally in parkinsonism an action tremor is present as well. The lesion responsible for this tremor appears to lie in the substantia nigra. Rarely, a similar tremor (often called, perhaps erroneously, 'striatal' tremor) is seen in other degenerative diseases of the nervous system (e.g. olivo-ponto-cerebellar degeneration).

Many different diseases can cause an *action tremor* which is readily observed in the actions of writing, of taking hold of an object, or in holding the arms outstretched. The fine tremor of the outstretched hands of thyrotoxicosis is usually easy to recognise, while much coarser movements occur in individuals with many toxic and metabolic disorders including delirium tremens (alcoholism), mercury poisoning and chronic liver disease; in the latter condition there is 'flapping' movement of the outstretched hands, like the beating of wings ('asterixis'). In Wilson's disease (hepatolenticular degeneration), a similar movement of the hands is seen if the liver disease is severe, but facial grimacing, rigidity and tremor of the limbs are also present as a result of the pathological changes which occur in the lenticular nuclei. In general paresis, tremor not only affects the hands but often also the lips and tongue. So-called *benign familial* or *essential tremor* is also accentuated by movement. Remarkably this tremor, though sometimes gross, does not often interfere with fine movements such as threading a needle, which would at first sight seem impossible. Curiously, this condition, which often develops first in early adult life but occasionally not until middle life, is often relieved considerably by alcohol. However, B$_2$-adrenoreceptor antagonists such as propranolol (120–240 mg daily) are also effective and some patients are helped by primidone (up to 750 mg daily). Some patients also develop tremor of the head, as in senile tremor. The most bizarre and gross form of tremor is often that of hysteria, and is produced for histrionic effect; it is coarse, irregular and variable and diminishes when the patient's attention is distracted.

Intention tremor is diagnostic of disease of the cerebellum or more often of its brain-stem connections. When unilateral it indicates a lesion on the affected side. Whereas the lesion, if severe, may also cause static tremor, this invariably becomes much worse towards the end of movement, which cannot therefore be accurately controlled, and activities such as writing and feeding are grossly disorganised. The patient may spill a cup whenever he brings it towards his mouth.

Many types of involuntary movement result from lesions of the extrapyramidal system, in addition to the parkinsonian tremor already described. The movements of **chorea**, for instance, though involuntary, may seem at first sight to be semipurposive and to show a high degree of organisation. Facial grimacing, raising of the eyebrows and rolling of the eyes, curling of the lips and protrusion and withdrawal of the tongue are common. In the limbs the movements are largely peripheral with intermittent 'wriggling' or 'squirming' of the fingers and toes. Often, too, there is striking limb hypotonia, and the reflexes may be 'pendular' in type in that a single blow on the quadriceps tendon causes the dependent leg to swing forwards and backwards several times like a pendulum. The limb movements cease during sleep. The exact situation of the causal pathological change is not known, though the caudate and lenticular nuclei have been implicated. The condition occurs in two main forms, namely rheumatic or Sydenham's chorea, and Huntington's chorea, a degenerative disease of late adult life, which is inherited as an autosomal dominant trait, and in which progressive dementia also occurs. A choreiform syndrome can also occur in chronic liver disease. Chorea, particularly the rheumatic form, is often accompanied by emotional lability and movement is often uncontrolled and ill-directed with undue expenditure of effort in performing simple actions. In other words, 'associated' movements are increased in chorea, in contrast to parkinsonism in which they are diminished.

Athetosis involves the more proximal limb muscles to give movements which are writhing in character, slower in their execution and of greater amplitude than those of chorea. Often choreiform and athetotic movements occur together in the same patient, when the condition is called choreo-athetosis. Athetosis can be bilateral and congenital due to degenerative changes (*état marbré*) in the corpus striatum. It is sometimes a sequel of birth injury, occurring particularly in those children with cerebral palsy who initially have a flaccid diplegia, and it rarely follows kernicterus due to Rh-factor incompatibility. It may also occur unilaterally in children with infantile hemiplegia in whom the lesion responsible has extended to involve the basal ganglia.

Another type of involuntary movement with an ill-defined pathological basis is **dystonia musculorum deformans** once called torsion spasm but more often called in modern parlance simply dystonia (Fig. 9.15). In this condition there is a striking increase in tone with irregular spasmodic contraction of the muscles of the neck, back and abdomen, and also of the limbs, giving

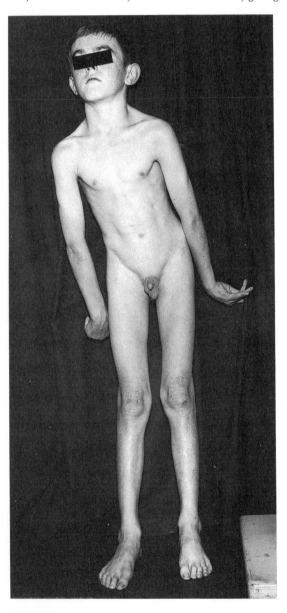

Fig. 9.15 A case of torsion dystonia; note the abnormal posture of the head, neck, trunk and upper limbs. (Reproduced with permission from Spillane & Spillane 1982.)

bizarre alterations in posture. These postural changes are often constant over long periods with superimposed painful spasms and the affected muscles often show marked hypertrophy. The condition often begins in childhood with an abnormal posture of a limb (e.g. inversion of one foot) resulting in a gait which is so remarkable that it may at first be thought hysterical. It is unfortunately progressive, depending upon degenerative changes of unknown aetiology which occur in the basal ganglia and is sometimes inherited as a dominant trait. Dystonic posturing and movement can also develop in paretic limbs following cerebral haemorrhage or infarction. Some authorities believe that occupational 'neuroses' such as writer's cramp (p. 103) represent fractional forms of dystonia. Many believe that **spasmodic torticollis**, a condition of frequent spasm of the sternomastoid and of other neck muscles, which results in a spasmodic turning of the head and neck to one side, is also a fractional variety of dystonia; there is often a constant increase in the tone of neck and shoulder muscles, and in some cases the condition progresses to involve other parts of the body, although in others it remains localised. Spasmodic retrocollis (backward movement of the head) is similar. The inadequacy of present histopathological methods is revealed by the fact that the situation and nature of the lesion responsible for this condition too, are not yet clearly defined.

That biochemical rather than structural abnormalities often account for involuntary movements is evident from recent work in neuropharmacology. Drugs of the phenothiazine group, given over long periods, can cause irreversible **facial** or **'tardive' dyskinesias** (involuntary grimacing and protrusion of the tongue), while athetosis, foot-tapping and paddling movements are among the many side-effects of treatment of parkinsonism with levodopa. However, the cause of blepharospasm-oromandibular dystonia (Meige's or Brueghel's syndrome), which is characterised by severe and almost continuous blepharospasm and by repetitive spasms of the facial, mandibular and lingual musculature, is quite unknown and the condition is almost totally uninfluenced by treatment.

One final but characteristic form of involuntary movement which can result from extrapyramidal disease is **hemiballismus**, a wild, purposeless, 'flinging' movement of one arm and leg which may occur in elderly patients as a result of a lesion, generally an infarct, which involves particularly the subthalamic nucleus of Luys on the opposite side (Fig. 9.16). The movements can be so violent and distressing that if untreated they result in death from exhaustion. The condition resembles in many respects a very violent form of unilateral chorea and similar but less severe movements occurring in the elderly, often unilaterally but occasionally bilaterally, are often called **senile chorea**.

CONCLUSIONS

Although the organisation of voluntary movement is complex and still incompletely understood, a careful analysis, based upon anatomical and physiological knowledge, of the ways in which it is disorganised in any single case, whether through weakness or paralysis, ataxia or involuntary movements, can be of the greatest value in localising the situation of the lesion responsible; observed changes in muscle tone and in the reflexes may give invaluable aid. Once localised, reconsideration of the mode of evolution of the lesion will often indicate its nature.

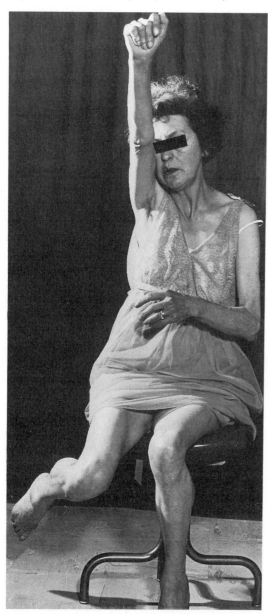

Fig. 9.16 Hemiballismus. (Reproduced with permission from Walton 1985; photograph kindly supplied by Dr J.D. Spillane.)

REFERENCES

Adams R D, Victor M 1985 Principles of neurology, 3rd edn. McGraw Hill, New York

Bloom W, Fawcett D W 1970 A textbook of histology. Saunders, Philadelphia

Denny-Brown D 1962 The basal ganglia and their relation to disorders of movement. Oxford University Press, London

FitzGerald M J T 1985 Neuroanatomy basic and applied. Baillière Tindall, Eastbourne

Ford F R 1973 Diseases of the nervous system in infancy, childhood and adolescence, 6th edn. Thomas, Springfield, Ill.

Gardner E 1975 Fundamentals of neurology, 6th edn. Saunders, Philadelphia

Gilman S, Bloedel J R, Lechtenberg R 1981 Disorders of the cerebellum. Contemporary Neurology Series, Vol. 21. F A Davis, Philadelphia

Gordon N 1976 Paediatric neurology for the clinician. Spastics International Medical Publications, Heinemann, London

Guarantors of Brain 1986 Aids to the examination of the peripheral nervous system. Baillière Tindall, London

Holmes G 1968 An introduction to clinical neurology, revised by Matthews W B. Livingstone, Edinburgh

Kandel E R, Schwartz J H 1985 Principles of neural science, 2nd edn. Arnold, London

Lance J W, McLeod J G 1981 A physiological approach to clinical neurology, 3rd edn. Butterworth, London

Mann W N (ed) 1975 Conybeare's textbook of medicine, 16th edn. Churchill Livingstone, Edinburgh

Marsden C D 1985 The basal ganglia, In: Swash M, Kennard C (eds) Scientific basis of clinical neurology. Churchill Livingstone, Edinburgh

Martin J P 1967 The basal ganglia and posture. Pitman, London

Matthews W B 1975 Practical neurology, 3rd edn, Blackwell, Oxford

Patton H D, Sundsten J W, Crill W E, Swanson P D 1976 Introduction to basic neurology. Saunders, Philadelphia

Pearlman A L, Collins R C 1985 Neurological pathosphysiology, 3rd edn. Oxford University Press, Oxford

Spillane J D, Spillane J A 1982 An atlas of clinical neurology, 3rd edn. Oxford University Press, London

Walton J N 1985 Brain's Diseases of the nervous system, 9th edn. Oxford University Press, Oxford.

Walton J N 1987 Introduction to clinical neuroscience, 2nd edn. Baillière Tindall, London

Wartenberg R 1945 The examination of the reflexes. Year Book Publishers, Chicago

10. The sensory system

Somatic sensory input is of two principal types: first, there are impulses which lead to motor responses through the segmental reflex systems (discussed earlier) and secondly there are impulses which ascend to reach those centres in which sensory experiences are recorded and enter perception. The latter are known as sensory responses. These two processes are not totally independent as a single primary afferent nerve fibre can initiate reflex responses, while its long ascending collateral branches may also convey sensory information which reaches consciousness (sensory awareness). Generally the term 'sensory' relates only to those neurones and pathways that convey impulses to levels of the nervous system (thalamus and cortex) at which the sensation conveyed evokes conscious awareness, and not to the segmental reflex system. The distinction is not always useful in clinical practice, since proprioceptive sensory information, relating to the position and interrelationship of the parts of the body, does not as a rule enter consciousness, yet defects of this sense produce striking clinical manifestations. Sensory mechanisms in the strict sense outlined above will be considered below as well as some of the pathophysiological consequences of impaired reflex responses due to dysfunction of afferent pathways.

The examination of sensory function and the interpretation of abnormalities of sensory perception present considerable difficulties, as in no part of the neurological examination is the patient's co-operation more important. Objective assessment can thus be difficult and it is often necessary to make allowances for the patient's state of co-operation and intellectual capacity. Areas of cutaneous sensory impairment, particularly to light touch and pinprick, subsequently shown to be spurious, are commonly elicited even by the most skilled observers. Indeed sensory examination is sometimes easier in children and in adults of less than average intellect, as it is virtually impossible to achieve uniformity of sensory stimulation in clinical practice. Intelligent patients often perceive and remark upon relatively slight variations which prove in the end to be of no pathological

significance, but which nevertheless can cause confusion during the examination. Furthermore, individuals vary greatly in their reaction to sensory stimuli, a sensation which appears acutely painful to one being well tolerated by another. And while it is conventional to examine sensory function and to record the results of this examination independently of those obtained on examining the motor system, motor and sensory functions are intimately connected, the one being largely dependent upon the other. Thus motor activity is grossly impaired if there is a defect in proprioception: a limb from which no afferent stimuli are received (deafferentation) is virtually immobile even though its motor pathways are intact. A serious disorder of movement can therefore be entirely due to a defect of sensation in the affected part.

THE ANATOMICAL AND PHYSIOLOGICAL ORGANISATION OF SOMATIC SENSATION

The sensory apparatus consists of (a) a series of sensory receptors in the skin and other organs, (b) the first sensory neurone, whose unipolar cells are located in the posterior root ganglia, and (c) secondary sensory neurones which are responsible for the conduction of impulses through the spinal cord and brain stem to the thalamus; further neurones then relay certain forms of sensation to the cerebral cortex. Cells in the substantia gelatinosa of the spinal cord and the network of internuncial neurones to which they relate clearly play a major role in modulating sensory input. Visceral sensation, which is conveyed initially alongside fibres of the autonomic nervous system, enters the spinal cord along with somatic sensory impulses and is conveyed centrally in a similar manner.

Receptors

Sensory receptors can be divided into **exteroceptors**, which are largely situated in the skin and are concerned with recording information about the external environment of the body, and **proprioceptors** and **interoceptors**,

161

which are situated in muscles , tendons, joints and viscera and which inform us of the position and condition of these deeper structures. For many years controversy abounded over the question as to whether there were specific cutaneous sensory receptors responding to specific stimuli or whether different forms of sensation were related to patterns of stimulation of relatively undifferentiated networks of fine nerve endings terminating in the skin. This dispute has now been settled in favour of the specificity theory which accepts that individual cutaneous sensory receptors are most sensitive to a particular form of natural stimulation but that this specificity is not absolute and other types of stimuli may also excite the ending. Three broad classes of receptors can be distinguished in mammals, namely **mechanoreceptors**, which respond to mechanical displacement of the skin, **thermoreceptors**, which respond to temperature changes, and **nociceptors**, which are insensitive to stimuli that excite the other two varieties, but which are excited by higher intensity, potentially damaging stimuli.

Of the **mechanoreceptors**, some are rapidly-adapting. These include the large subcutaneous Pacinian corpuscles which respond to vibration or tickle, the Meissner corpuscles and hair follicle receptors which respond to tapping, and the Krause end-bulbs whose function is still not entirely clear though they probably respond to similar stimuli. There are also slowly-adapting receptors, including Merkel cells and Ruffini endings that also respond to touch and to pressure which indents the skin, but which continue to discharge during continuing indentation. The Merkel discs and cells are specifically pressure receptors, but no specific perceived sensation is associated with stimulation of Ruffini endings. Most mechanoreceptors are supplied by large myelinated axons, whereas the smaller myelinated (Aδ) and non-myelinated (C) axons innervate thermoreceptors, nociceptors and (a few) mechanoreceptors, which are known as C-mechanoreceptors and which are excited by lightly moving hairs or light pressure on the skin.

Thermoreceptors are relatively or absolutely insensitive to mechanical stimuli but respond to changes in skin temperature. Cold receptors are excited by a fall in temperature, warm receptors by a rise, and these receptors can discharge continuously and more or less indefinitely at a constant temperature within their range of sensitivity, the rate of discharge depending upon the actual temperature. Most cold units have myelinated fibres, while warm units have non-myelinated fibres, and each have spot-like receptive fields corresponding to the warm and cold spots on the skin which can be identified clinically with fine thermal stimulators.

Nociceptors, which are innervated either by small myelinated (Aδ) or non-myelinated (C) afferent fibres, have small receptive fields. Some are mechanical and are excited by firm pressure or by penetrating the skin with a sharp object; those responsible for pain sensation are often called fine C-terminals. Others are thermal or mechanothermal receptors, innervated by C-fibres; they can be excited by severe mechanical stimuli but are principally responsive to high skin temperatures (i.e. 42°C or above), well above the normal threshold (about 40°C) that stimulates warm thermoreceptors. Algogenic chemicals such as bradykinin, 5-HT and prostaglandins E_1 and E_2 produced in the skin during inflammation either excite or enhance the excitability of C-nociceptors.

Proprioceptive sensory input comes from the muscle spindles, the muscles themselves, the joint capsules and Golgi tendon organs. This information is conveyed by fibres of group Ia afferents (carrying impulses from muscle spindle primary afferents), group Ib afferents (from Golgi tendon organs) and group II afferents (from spindle secondary afferents). Some information also comes via somatosensory afferents from joint capsules and via slowly conducting afferents originating in muscle (the flexor reflex afferents). Comparatively few proprioceptive stimuli reach consciousness; most are concerned with reflex activity mediated through the spinal cord and cerebellum by means of which posture and movement are controlled.

Somatic sensation: its nature, coding and measurement

Sensory parameters

Somatic sensation is not a uniform sensory experience. It is a fusion of several qualities which cannot be consciously dissociated but which may be differentially affected by disease or dysfunction. Each sensory experience has a quality or modality (touch, pain, heat and cold, etc.); the various sensory modalities will be considered below. Different receptors respond to different modalities. Similarly some secondary sensory neurones in the posterior horn of spinal cord grey matter, some fibres in the ascending sensory tracts, some thalamic neurones, and, to a lesser extent, neurones in the cortex are modality-specific. Thus, for example, in the dorsal horn of grey matter there are mechanoreceptive neurones, multireceptive neurones (receiving stimuli from both mechanoreceptors and nociceptors) and nociceptive neurones (excited only by afferent input from nociceptors); but as yet neurones responding to thermoreceptors have not been identified. The substantia gelatinosa of the dorsal horn contains a very large number of small neurones, and most non-myelinated cutaneous axons end within it. The cells of this area clearly receive an excitatory input from many synapses and there is an interplay of excitation and inhibition from mechanoreceptors and nociceptors. Several neuropeptides, notably substance P (which is important in relation to pain sensation) have been identified in this region. Clearly, therefore, the dorsal horn provides a site of excitation and inhibition of activity in dorsal horn neurones, thus modulating sensory input before it enters ascending tracts leading to higher levels of the neuraxis.

Intensity is another important parameter enabling us to distinguish between a light pinprick and a fierce jab. Intensity discrimination is pattern-coded, i.e. it depends upon frequency of firing in sensory receptors and in neurones and afferent fibres at all levels of the nervous system. Phasic (on-off) receptors, such as those concerned with light touch, are more complex, intensity being little if at all related to frequency. The normal human subject is also skilled in localising sensory stimuli. This faculty is related to the segmental organisation of cutaneous sensory input. Localisation of visceral sensation is less accurate, though even this may be aided by the interpretation, for instance, of referred pain. Specific groups of neurones can be excited by specific sensory stimuli applied to specific areas of the body surface. There is a clear, consistent and precise somatotopic localisation in the posterior roots of the spinal cord and their ganglia, in the posterior horns of grey matter, in the ascending pathways in the spinal cord, in the principal sensory nuclei of the brain stem, in the thalamus and in the sensory cortex. The density of sensory receptors differs in different areas of skin. This variability of distribution accounts for the striking differences observed in the ability to discriminate between two points applied at set distances apart (two-point discrimination—see Fig. 10.1). The receptive fields of somatosensory cortical neurones show an inverse relationship to sensory acuity in that these fields are small, for instance, in respect to sensory input from the tips of the fingers, and large for many areas of the trunk.

The nervous system can also recognise the duration and temporal pattern of sensory stimuli. The onset and the termination of a stimulus and its reaction time (the time taken for its conscious perception) can be recognised, as can recurring stimuli such as the perception of vibration. Different fibres in peripheral nerves conduct at different rates, depending upon their diameter and upon whether or not they are myelinated, and different modalities of sensation are therefore conducted at different rates. Reaction time is directly related to conduction velocity in both the peripheral and the central nervous systems. The mechanism of perception of vibration is more complex. Such recurrent stimuli specifically excite phasic (on-off) mechanoreceptors (especially Pacinian corpuscles), each oscillation exciting a single spike, but different thalamic and cortical neurones may respond to different frequencies so that both place and pattern coding are involved.

Most somatic sensations evoke affective responses which determine whether the sensation perceived is pleasant (warmth), unpleasant (pain, excessive heat or cold) or neutral (touch, light pressure, change of position, etc). Cerebral and hypothalamic centres concerned with pleasure, reward and punishment also influence the response to somatic sensory experiences. Sedative drugs such as barbiturates and phenothiazines, for example, and surgical procedures such as prefrontal leucotomy or lesions which interrupt connexions between the prefrontal cortex and subcortical centres may all diminish or even abolish affect, while leaving intact the ability to recognise sensory modalities. The patient continues to feel and to recognise pain but it no longer disturbs him.

The coding of sensory information allows the subject to recognise the nature of the somatic stimulus which he perceives, its intensity, where it is situated, how long it lasts and whether it is repetitive, and its character and emotional connotations.

The simpler sensory modalities

Several clearly definable forms of somatic sensation can be recognised whose integrity is customarily assessed during a neurological examination. **Touch** is commonly tested with a light application to the skin of a pledget of cotton wool. It can be assessed quantitatively by using von Frey hairs, so graduated that differing pressures are needed to bend them. The threshold for the appreciation of touch varies considerably on different parts of the body surface, depending upon such variables as the thickness of the epidermis and the number of hair follicles present. **Pain** sensation is generally assessed by pin-prick, which can also be of graduated severity if an algesiometer is used. The patient must be asked to assess the painful quality of this stimulus and not the sensations of pressure or touch which may be simultaneously evoked. Squeezing the tendo Achilles or other deep tendons will determine whether the appreciation of **deep pressure** is intact, but this sensation can also be painful. **Thermal sensation** is generally tested by applying metal test tubes to the skin, one filled with ice, the other with water at 45°C. Again the patient must be told that it is the feeling of heat or cold he is being asked to note and not those of touch or pressure. The assessment of **position and joint sense** is generally carried out by moving the terminal phalanx of the forefinger or the great toe in a vertical plane and by asking the patient, whose eyes are closed, to describe the direction of movement each time the digit is moved. After making an initial movement of substantial amplitude it must then be decided whether the patient can appreciate movements through a very small range (about 1 mm). Another test of position and joint sense is to ask the patient, with his eyes closed, to point towards a part of his body, when the position of the part in space has been altered by the examiner. **Vibration sense**, as tested with a tuning fork of 128 frequency applied to bony prominences, is not a physiological sensation, being compounded of both touch and pressure, but nevertheless its absence is of considerable significance in clinical neurology. **Tactile discrimination** is assessed by recording the threshold distance at which the two blunt points of a compass, simultaneously applied, are independently perceived (Fig. 10.1). The normal threshold for two-point discrimination on the tip of the tongue is 1 mm, on the tips of the fingers 2–3 mm, on the palm of the hand or sole of the foot 1.5–3 cm, and in the centre of the back 6–7 cm. Appreciation of the texture, weight, size and shape of objects can also be assessed, somewhat crudely, by asking the patient, with his eyes closed, to identify objects placed in the hand, while tactile localisation is tested by asking him to identify on a diagram of model, or on the examiner, the point or points on his body which were stimulated. He may also be asked to identify figures or letters traced with a blunt point on his skin (graphaesthesia). There is considerable individual variation in the ability to perceive and interpret these more complex sensations, but retention of such functions on one side of the body and their absence on the other is always a finding of pathological significance.

The sensory pathways

The cells of the first sensory neurone are situated in the posterior root ganglia and are bipolar in type, having peripheral axons which convey afferent impulses from the sensory receptors, and central axons which enter the spinal cord in the posterior nerve roots. Sensory fibres in the **peripheral nerves** vary in diameter and in their rate of conduction; the large, heavily-myelinated rapidly-conducting A fibres are primarily concerned with the conduction of impulses subserving touch, pressure and proprioceptive sensation, but some (the Aδ fibres) undoubtedly transmit painful and thermal sensations. The most slowly-conducting unmyelinated C fibres seem capable of carrying touch, temperature, and pain sensation so that there is no exact relationship between the size and myelination of sensory axons on the one hand and their function on the other. Since some peripheral nerve disorders, and especially peripheral neuropathy, can have a selective effect upon fibres of one particular size or degree of myelination, there are some cases in which the appreciation of painful stimulation is more severely affected than that of touch or vice versa. And while cutaneous and pressure sensations travel in pure sensory (cutaneous) and later in mixed sensory and motor nerves,

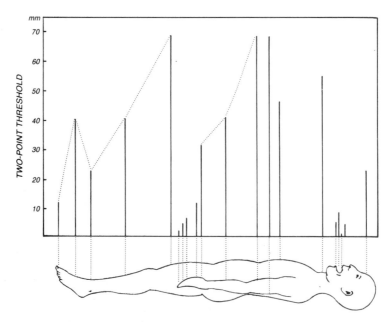

Fig. 10.1 Regional variation in tactile two-point threshold in man. (Reproduced with permission from Patton et al 1976.)

proprioceptive stimuli, particularly from the muscle spindles, travel centrally first of all in motor nerves.

As the central axons of the first sensory neurone enter the spinal cord, some regrouping of fibres occurs, according to their function. Initially most enter the posterior column, lying just medially to the posterior horn of grey matter. At this point internuncial neurones arising from cells in the substantia gelatinosa exert a modifying or 'gating' influence (see p. 49), especially upon painful sensations. Fibres concerned wih proprioception, position and joint sense, vibration sense and tactile discrimination, and some conveying touch, turn immediately upwards in the **posterior columns** and travel to the nuclei gracilis and cuneatus in the medulla. Since entering fibres continually displace medially those which entered the cord at a lower level, it follows that fibres from the lower limbs lie medially in the posterior column (the fasciculus gracilis or column of Goll), while those from the upper limbs lie more laterally (the fasciculus cuneatus or column of Burdach) (Fig. 10.2).

A second group of entering fibres, concerned with the appreciation of touch, also enters the lateral part of the posterior column where they ascend for several segments, then entering the posterior horn of grey matter to synapse with cells in this area. The axons of these cells then cross the midline close to the central canal to join the **ventral spinothalamic tract**. Fibres subserving pain and temperature sensation run a similar course, but only ascend in the posterior column for a few segments before crossing the midline to end in the more **lateral portion of the spinothalamic tract** in the opposite lateral column of the cord (Fig. 10.2). As in the posterior columns, there is some lamination of fibres in the spinothalamic tracts, those from the lower limbs lying nearest the cord surface and those from the upper limbs being situated more centrally. This probably explains why a lesion causing spinal cord compression may impair pain sensation first in the lower limbs; the sensory 'level' then ascends steadily but finally becomes arrested on the trunk at the level of a dermatome corresponding to a cord segment several segments below the actual point of compression; presumably fibres situated nearest to the surface of the cord are the first to be affected by pressure.

When the sensory fibres of the spinal cord reach the medulla oblongata, the spinothalamic fibres enter it laterally and pass upwards through the pons and midbrain to the thalamus. The fibres of the posterior columns, however, end in synapses in the nucleus gracilis and nucleus cuneatus. From the cells of these nuclei new axons arise which immediately cross the midline and then travel upwards as the **medial fillet** or **lemniscus**, again to enter the thalamus.

The pathway followed by sensory impulses from the face deserves special mention. The fibres of the trigeminal nerve which carry touch and tactile discrimination enter the main trigeminal nucleus and then, in the **quintothalamic tract**, cross the midline to join the medial fillet. Those subserving pain and thermal sensation enter the pons but then travel downwards in the **descending root of the trigeminal nerve** to end in a nuclear mass which extends downwards as far as the second cervical segment of the cord; then they, too, forming another part of the quintothalamic tract, cross the midline and travel upwards in the spinothalamic tract. 'Representation' of the parts of the face in the descending root is inverted; thus a lesion of its lower end in the upper cervical cord gives loss of pain and temperature sensation only, but not of touch, over the area supplied by the ophthalmic division on the same side of the face. It should also be noted that proprioceptive stimuli from the face travel centrally in the facial nerve, so that sense of position in the facial muscles (a difficult faculty to test) is not abolished by a lesion of the trigeminus.

Thus all sensory pathways which ascend as far as the brain stem terminate in the thalamus. Throughout their course in the spinal cord and brain stem many of these fibres give off collaterals or synapse with internuncial neurones. These connexions complete the sensory side of the arcs concerned with those spinal and brain-stem reflexes which are necessary for the maintenance of posture and other functions. There are, for instance, many sensory fibres, some of which synapse in Clarke's columns of the posterior horn of grey matter, which ascend the spinal cord in the dorsal and ventral spinocerebellar tracts and which are concerned with supplying information through which the cerebellum exerts control over posture and movement. The **thalamus** is, however, the first important sensory relay station. The sensory relay nuclei which are concerned with somatic and visceral sensation are the nucleus ventralis posterolateralis (VPL), which receives afferent stimuli from the trunk and limbs, and the ventralis posteromedialis (VPM), which is similarly concerned with input from the face. Both nuclei send thalamocortical neuronal projections to the somatosensory and parietal association areas of the cortex and receive corticothalamic projections from the same areas. The lateral and medial geniculate bodies are concerned with vision and hearing respectively, the ventralis lateralis (VL) with cerebellar and extrapyramidal function, the ventralis anterior (VA) with activity of the basal ganglia, and the nucleus anterior (A) with hypothalamic function. The dorsomedial nucleus (DM), which projects to the prefrontal cortex, is not primarily concerned with the awareness of somatic sensations but appears to have a role relating to the affective response to sensory input, especially of pain. There is a clear

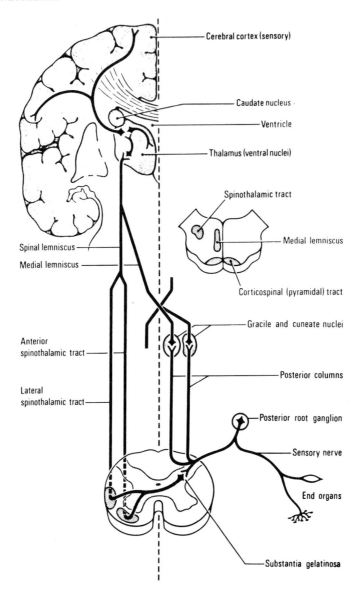

Fig. 10.2 The sensory pathways. The central fibres of the sensory nerves enter the cord through the posterior roots. The ascending branches of those mediating fine touch, vibration and kinaesthetic sensation run in the posterior white columns to the gracile and cuneate nuclei. Here they relay and cross to form the medial lemniscus which traverses the medulla and pons and midbrain. The fibres mediating pain and temperature and gross touch enter the dorsal grey column and relay in the substantia gelatinosa. The second order neurones cross the cord and form two tracts, the anterior and lateral spinothalamic tracts. These come together in the medulla and then join the medial lemniscus. This large sensory bundle of fibres (the lemniscus) which carries all forms of sensation from the opposite side of the body terminates in the ventral nuclei of the thalamus. From the thalamus, tertiary neurones pass to the sensory cortex. (The small drawing to the right shows the relative positions of the medial lemniscus and the spinothalamic tract in the medulla.) (Reproduced with permission from Mann 1975.)

somatotopic representation of parts of the body in the sensory relay nuclei of the thalamus, with caudal areas projecting to the lateral parts of the VPL, rostral segments more medially, and the face most medially in the VPM.

The **primary somatosensory area of the cerebral cortex** is concerned with the appreciation of most of those stimuli which enter consciousness. The integrity of the sensory cortex is particularly important if we are to recognise form, texture, size, weight and consistency of objects, or changes in position of parts of the body. It is also essential for the accurate localisation and recognition of the nature of stimuli applied to the body, for discrimination between two simultaneously applied stimuli, and even more for the ability to relate sensory experiences to others experienced previously, or to sense data perceived through the special senses. Clearly, numerous association pathways are concerned in the interpretation and recognition of these more complex sensory experiences, which may nevertheless be grossly deranged if there is a lesion of the primary sensory cortex, an important cell-station in

all sensory association mechanisms. As with the motor cortex, stimulation experiments have shown that specific portions of the post-central gyrus are concerned with the appreciation of sensations from particular areas of the opposite side of the body (Fig. 10.3). 'Representation' in the sensory cortex corresponds topographically with that in the motor area; thus a lesion of the lower end of the postcentral gyrus will impair sensory perception in the contralateral face and hand, while one involving the superior and medial aspects of the hemisphere will result in a failure to appreciate 'cortical' forms of sensation in the opposite leg.

However, cortical or subcortical lesions, even if they divide all thalamocortical fibres, do not destroy completely the ability to perceive sensory experiences in the opposite half of the body. In the presence of such a lesion, sensitivity to pain and temperature is affected comparatively little, while crude touch is still felt, though finer forms of sensory experience are greatly impaired. Hence the cruder varieties of sensation can be recorded in consciousness at a thalamic level.

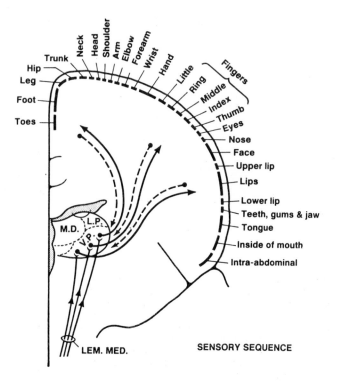

Fig. 10.3 Somatic sensation. Cross-section of the left hemisphere along the plane of the postcentral gyrus. The afferent pathway for tactile and kinaesthetic sensation is indicated by the unbroken lines coming up, through the medial lemniscus and the posterolateral ventral nucleus of the thalamus, to the postcentral gyrus. (Reproduced with permission from Walton 1985.)

Cutaneous sensory segmentation

Early in its development the human fetus demonstrates metameric segmentation, and each somatic segment, or metamere, is linked to the corresponding segment of the neuraxis by a pair of spinal nerves. In the course of evolution with specialisation of the anterior end of the human organism to form the head and with the growth of the complicated motor and sensory functions of the limbs, this metameric segmentation of the nervous system has been disrupted, persisting only in the dorsal region. After the fusion of ventral and dorsal roots to form a spinal nerve, the dorsal primary division conveys motor fibres to the spinal muscles and sensory fibres to the overlying cutaneous area. In the mid-dorsal region the ventral primary division supplies motor fibres to the intercostal muscles and sensory fibres to a narrow zone extending more or less horizontally around the thorax on one side as far as the midline. In the cervical and lumbosacral regions the arrangement is complicated by the formation of the limb plexuses in which several ventral primary divisions unite and subsequently subdivide to form the peripheral nerves supplying the limbs. Through the intervention of the plexuses a single spinal nerve may send both motor and sensory contributions to several peripheral nerves, and, conversely, a single peripheral nerve may receive contributions from several spinal nerves. It follows that the sensory loss resulting from interruption of a peripheral nerve differs in its distribution from that produced by interruption of a posterior root or spinal nerve. A segmental or radicular cutaneous area—a dermatome—is an area of skin which receives its sensory supply from a single dorsal root and spinal nerve. In the trunk these segmental areas still exhibit a metameric arrangement. In the limbs this has been modified, but as a rule the segmental areas occupy elongated zones in the long axis of the limb (Fig. 10.4). Owing to the specialisation of the ventral primary divisions of the lower cervical and first thoracic spinal nerves in the innervation of the upper limb, these have lost their cutaneous supply to the trunk anteriorly. At the level of the second rib the fourth cervical segmental cutaneous area is contiguous with the second thoracic. The lower six thoracic spinal nerves supply the abdominal wall as low as the inguinal ligament. The dorsal primary divisions of the spinal nerves take no part in the formation of the limb plexuses, so that all spinal segments appear to be represented in the cutaneous supply of the back.

There is considerable overlapping of contiguous segmental cutaneous areas. The division of a single dorsal root does not cause any sensory loss detectable by ordinary clinical methods. Each root supplies fibres for pain, heat and cold to a larger area than that to which it supplies fibres for light touch.

In the sensory innervation of the head the trigeminal nerve represents a fusion of the sensory supply of several segments, though the seventh, ninth and tenth cranial nerves still possess rudimentary sensory branches distributed to the neighbourhood of the auricle. The posterior and inferior boundaries of the trigeminal cutaneous area are contiguous with those of the first and second cervical segments respectively.

SOME COMMON ABNORMALITIES OF SENSATION

In considering the disorders of sensation commonly noted in clinical neurological practice, it is first necessary to understand the meaning of several terms often utilised to describe sensory disorders. The word **numbness** can have many meanings; when a patient says that a part of the body is numb he may mean that sensation in the part is abnormal, but sometimes the term is used to denote weakness or clumsiness. Hence careful enquiry is needed in order to determine the significance of this symptom. Many other sensory abnormalities, occurring apparently spontaneously, can be found in patients with neurological disease. Of these, one of the commonest is **pain**, which has been discussed fully in Chapter 4. Pain may result from disease of any pain-sensitive structure; if, for instance, it is due to irritation of a sensory nerve or root, the distribution of the pain will be in the cutaneous area supplied by the nerve or root concerned. Pain can alternatively be felt in the organ or organs which are diseased, while if arising in a viscus or in a muscle, it can be referred to an area of skin which sometimes overlies the viscus but may be anatomically remote. Referred pain seems to be due to a spread of impulses to contiguous sensory neurones within the cord (see p. 51). Spontaneous pain in the limbs or trunk can result from thalamic lesions, when it has a peculiarly unpleasant burning character, often with additional 'grinding' or 'tearing' qualities. This so-called **thalamic pain** is most often felt in the face, around one angle of the mouth and in the hand and foot on the affected side. A closely-related sensation of continuous burning, of pricking, of warmth or even cold, may result from a spinothalamic tract lesion, but tends to be more diffusely felt in the area of altered cutaneous sensation. Disordered sensations of this type, occurring spontaneously, are called **dysaesthesiae**. In addition, patients who have lesions of the spinothalamic tract often note that they cannot feel pain or temperature in the affected part. They have perhaps injured or burned a limb without discomfort or may admit that they cannot assess the temperature of bath water.

Other abnormal sensations which the patient may feel are called **paraesthesiae**. These include feelings of tingling, pins and needles, of swelling of a limb, sensations suggesting that tight strings or bands are tied around a part of the body, or as if water were trickling over the skin. These sensory experiences result from disordered function in the pathways conducting the finer and discriminative aspects of sensibility. Thus tingling or pins and needles can result from ischaemia of peripheral nerves, from polyneuropathy, from transient ischaemia of the sensory cortex, or from sensory Jacksonian epilepsy due to a cortical lesion. Similar symptoms are described by patients with lesions of the posterior columns of the cord and it is usually in such individuals that the 'tight, constricting band' or the 'trickling' type of sensation is felt. Often the affected part feels swollen, although inspection shows that this is not the case, or the patient may feel, for instance, as if the limb is encased in a firm glove or plaster cast. If there is a lesion of the posterior columns in the cervical region, sudden flexion or extension of the neck may give an 'electric shock' sensation which travels rapidly down the trunk and sometimes into the hands and feet; this sign (Lhermitte's sign) is most often due to multiple sclerosis or cervical spondylotic myelopathy. Similarly, tapping over the trunk of an ischaemic nerve (as in patients with median nerve compression in the carpal tunnel) or over a sensory nerve which has been injured in some other way, often gives paraesthesiae which shoot along the cutaneous distribution of the nerve concerned. A comparable sign produced by tapping a nerve in which regeneration is occurring is known as Tinel's sign.

As well as experiencing paraesthesiae, patients with dysfunction of the spinal posterior columns or of the sensory cortex often find that the affected part has become clumsy or even useless. If a hand is affected, they may be unable to use it except under direct vision and cannot recognise objects felt in a pocket or handbag, unless they can be taken out and examined visually. Fine movements such as fastening buttons or threading needles are grossly impaired. If both lower limbs are affected the patient is unsteady; he feels as if he were walking on cotton wool, and is worse in the dark. When the eyes are covered while washing the face, he tends to fall forwards into the washbasin.

Turning to sensory abnormalities found on physical examination, **anaesthesia** is generally used to describe a cutaneous area in which the sensation of touch is totally lost, while **hypaesthesia** implies impaired touch appreciation. Similarly, **analgesia** is absence of and **hypalgesia** diminution of the appreciation of pain. When thermal sensations cannot be appreciated, the term **thermoanaesthesia** is sometimes utilised, but this is rarely found unless hypalgesia is also present. **Hyperalgesia** is allegedly an increased sensitivity to painful stimuli and **hyperaesthesia** a heightened perception of touch. In fact, however, careful examination will usually show that in the one case the pain threshold, and in the other that for touch, is actually raised above normal, owing to a disorder of the pain or touch pathways. The apparent overreaction is due to an abnormal and often unpleasant additional quality added to the primary sensation which is in itself impaired; for this reason the term **hyperpathia** (Head's protopathic pain) is preferred to hyperalgesia which is semantically incorrect.

Romberg's sign is an important (if relatively crude and insensitive) sign of impaired position and joint sense in the lower limbs. Preservation of the upright posture depends upon labyrinthine, cerebellar and visual postural reflexes as well as upon those reflexes whose afferent pathway is from lower limb proprioceptors. So long as the eyes are open, even if the conduction of proprioceptive stimuli from the lower limbs is grossly impaired, the patient can maintain his position, but once the eyes are closed he will sway or fall. Cerebellar or labyrinthine disease can also cause excessive swaying, but severe instability and a tendency to fall results only from severe impairment of position and joint sense in the lower limbs. The same patient will show **sensory ataxia** when he walks; being unsure of the position of his feet in relation to the ground, he lifts them unusually high and then bangs them down heavily (the steppage gait). Owing to loss of visual control of posture, he is much more unsteady in the dark.

Ataxia of sensory type is also found in the upper limbs if affected by similar lesions. The hands are clumsy, and fine movements are impossible, particularly when the hands are out of sight (e.g. tying a necktie). If the affected arm is held outstretched with the eyes closed, it 'wanders' in space, upwards or sideways or indeed in any direction, unlike the downward drift of the limb showing motor weakness from pyramidal tract disease. There are also purposeless movements of the outstretched fingers, of which the patient is unaware, and these may have a 'writhing' character (**pseudoathetosis**).

Abnormalities of the finer and discriminative aspects of sensibility are more difficult to assess, although in a patient with a lesion of the sensory cortex, the threshold for two-point discrimination is much greater on the abnormal than on the normal side, and there may be total inability to recognise figures or letters drawn on the skin. Sensory stimuli are also incorrectly localised. Lesions of the parietal lobe of less severity may be demonstrated by the phenomenon of **sensory inattention**. The patient is well able to appreciate stimuli applied independently to the two sides of the body, but when two similar stimuli

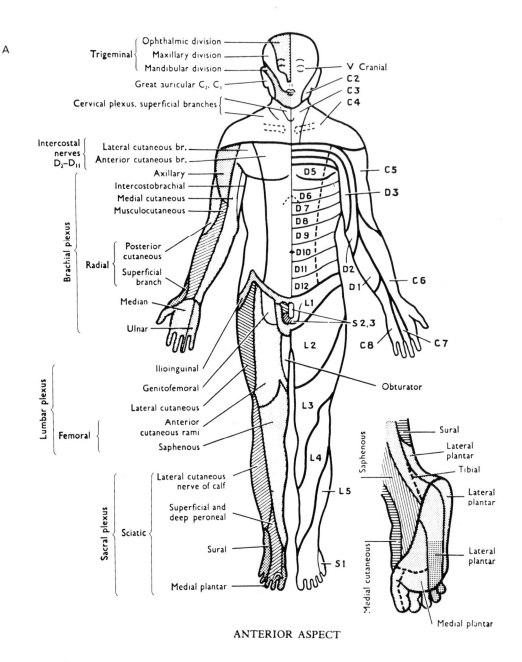

Fig. 10.4 Cutaneous areas of distribution of spinal segments and of the sensory fibres of the peripheral nerves. **A**: anterior aspect. **B**: posterior aspect. (Reproduced with permission from Walton 1985.)

B

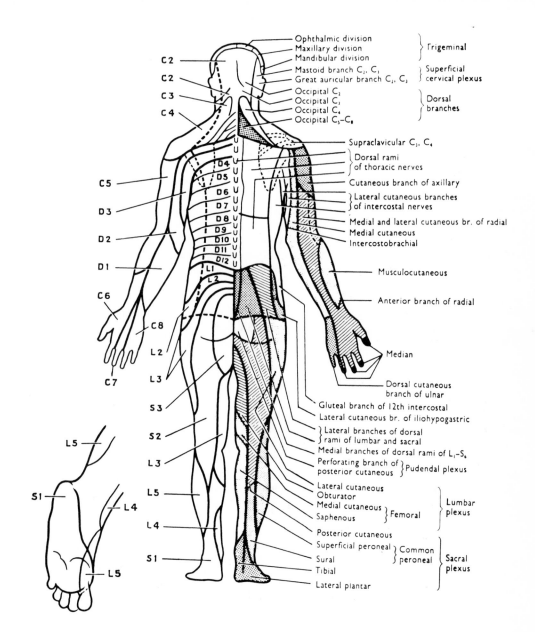

POSTERIOR ASPECT

are applied simultaneously to homologous points on the skin of the two sides, one is ignored, a finding which implies dysfunction of a contralateral sensory association area of the cerebral cortex. After amputation of a limb or of another member, it takes time, in a sense, for the brain to realise that the limb is no longer there, and there is often a clear-cut 'phantom' sensation as if the amputated part were still present and were able to move; sometimes the phantom is painful. A phantom limb can be abolished by a lesion of the contralateral sensory cortex.

Another defect observed in some patients with lesions of the arm area of the opposite sensory cortex is an inability to appreciate the form and texture of objects placed in the hand. Correctly this abnormality is entitled **stereoanaesthesia**, but the term **astereognosis** is more often used. Strictly speaking the latter term should be reserved for a failure to recognise the nature of objects when the primary sensory modalities are intact. That is an agnosic defect, due to a disorder of sensory association and akin to the other more complex disorders of parietal lobe function which were described in Chapter 5 (p. 67).

THE CLINICAL SIGNIFICANCE OF SENSORY ABNORMALITIES

In localising the lesion causing an abnormality of sensation, it must be asked whether the sensory changes found could be due to a lesion of one or several peripheral nerves, to one of sensory roots, of the spinal cord, of the brain stem, of the thalamus, or of the sensory cortex.

Identification of the sensory abnormalities which result from **peripheral nerve lesions** or from lesions of the brachial and lumbosacral plexuses can only stem from a knowledge of the cutaneous distribution of the various peripheral nerves and of the components of the plexuses (see Fig. 10.4). If a nerve is divided, and it is one with an extensive cutaneous distribution, there is a central area of sensory loss to all forms of sensation and a surrounding zone in which tactile loss is more extensive than that for pain and temperature sensation. There is considerable overlap in the cutaneous supply of individual peripheral nerves so that section of a small cutaneous nerve may produce no definable sensory abnormality. This is even more true of the dermatomes innervated by individual **sensory roots**; these have a strictly segmental distribution (see Fig. 10.4) but if a single root is divided it may be impossible to find an area of sensory loss, in view of the overlap in the supply of neighbouring roots. When more than one root is interrupted, however, there is generally some cutaneous sensory loss and its distribution clearly indicates the roots involved. A working knowledge of the dermatome distri-

bution of the individual sensory roots is essential in clinical neurology. This makes it relatively easy to distinguish on clinical grounds the sensory loss resulting from a root lesion from that due to one of a peripheral nerve. Associated signs of a lower motor neurone lesion also help greatly in this respect.

In clinical practice, for instance, the sensory loss due to an ulnar nerve lesion affects mainly the little finger and the ulnar half of the ring finger, while that due to a disorder of the median nerve involves chiefly the thumb, the first two fingers and the radial half of the ring finger. An ulnar nerve lesion also gives wasting of most of the small hand muscles, while median nerve damage, for practical purposes, affects only those in the lateral part of the thenar eminence. In contradistinction compression of the inner cord of the brachial plexus, which can also cause wasting and weakness of small hand muscles, gives sensory impairment in the medial aspect of the arm and forearm and only occasionally in the little finger.

When multiple peripheral nerves are symmetrically involved, as in **polyneuropathy**, it is the longest sensory fibres which tend to be most severely affected. Hence sensory impairment, which usually involves all forms of sensation, but may affect one more severely than the others, is most severe in the periphery of the limbs. Although this type of sensory loss is often described as of 'glove and stocking' distribution, the borderline between normal and abnormal areas of sensory perception is not usually abrupt, but there is a gradual transition between the two. When there is widespread disease of posterior spinal roots (as occasionally occurs in the Guillain-Barré syndrome) there may be ascending sensory loss which eventually involves the entire trunk and all four limbs, but the disease can cease to progress at any stage. The condition may mimic a transverse lesion of the spinal cord, as motor paralysis is generally even more severe. Indeed in most cases motor weakness predominates and sensory impairment is slight or absent. A rare variety of hereditary sensory neuropathy exists in which pain fibres are affected almost exclusively and there is peripheral insensitivity to pain, often giving perforating ulcers of the feet and extensive destruction of bones and joints (Morvan's syndrome).

Sensory abnormalities resulting from **spinal cord disease** depend upon which sensory pathways are principally affected. Total transection of the cord gives total loss of all forms of sensation below the dermatome level on the trunk corresponding to the segment at which the cord transection took place. Often there is a zone of 'hyperaesthesia' (see p. 169) in the skin area supplied by the segment immediately above the lesion. In hemisection of the spinal cord (**the Brown-Séquard syndrome**) there is loss of tactile discrimination, impaired touch perception and loss of position and joint sense on the same side of the body as that on which the cord has been divided, and these sensory faculties are impaired on the trunk up to the dermatome of the cord segment where the lesion lies. There are also signs of pyramidal tract dysfunction on the same side. On the opposite side of the body there is loss of pain and temperature sensation, but the sensory level for these modalities is a few segments lower, since pain fibres ascend in the posterior horn for a few segments before crossing to join the contralateral spinothalamic tract. A Brown-Séquard syndrome can result from trauma or from asymmetrical cord compression and is occasionally the initial manifestation of multiple sclerosis.·

The principal lesion of **tabes dorsalis** is in the root entry zone of the posterior roots; there is ascending degeneration of the posterior columns and to a lesser extent of the spinothalamic tracts. Hence patients with this disease have severe sensory ataxia and there is often pain loss, with impairment of deep pressure sensation, over the bridge of the nose, centre of sternum, perineum and Achilles' tendons, while position and joint sense and vibration sense are greatly impaired in the lower limbs. The tendon reflexes are lost owing to a break on the sensory side of the reflex arc. Similar impairment of lower limb tendon reflexes may be seen in **subacute combined degeneration of the cord**, in which disease sensory ataxia is also usual and vibration and position sense are commonly lost in the lower limbs; signs of pyramidal tract disease are also present as a rule. The cavity of **syringomyelia** usually damages the central grey matter of the cervical spinal cord; hence decussating pain and temperature fibres are interrupted, resulting in dissociated anaesthesia, i.e. loss of pain and temperature sensation but preservation of touch and of position and joint sense. Commonly, but not invariably, this sensory loss is unilateral, affecting the whole of one upper limb and shoulder and ending on the trunk at the midline and with a sharp lower level like the edge of a cape. As the cavity generally extends into the anterior horns, there is loss of tendon reflexes and muscular atrophy in the affected upper limb or limbs, while compression of the pyramidal tracts gives spastic weakness of the legs. The sensory changes of **multiple sclerosis** are usually due to lesions of the posterior columns, giving impaired tactile discrimination, vibration sense and sense of position, sometimes in one arm, in both lower limbs, or even in all four limbs. Occasionally, however, a plaque of demyelination affects one trigeminal nucleus to give facial hemianaesthesia and sometimes, though rarely, a unilateral lesion of the cord involves the spinothalamic tract and gives loss of pain and temperature sensation in one lower limb.

Lesions of the brain stem cause sensory abnormalities which can easily be interpreted anatomically. Dissociated sensory loss in the face can result from syringobulbia, due to involvement of the descending root of the trigeminus, while lesions of the pons and medulla can give unilateral facial sensory loss (due to a lesion of the trigeminal nucleus) with hemianaesthesia and/or hemianalgesia of the trunk and limbs on the opposite side due to involvement of ascending sensory tracts. A lesion of the upper pons or midbrain, however, can give a complete contralateral hemianaesthesia. More often such unilateral sensory loss is dissociated, involving only pain and temperature sensation, owing to selective involvement of the spinothalamic tract.

Patchy contralateral hemianaesthesia and hemianalgesia can also be due to a **thalamic lesion** and there is often in addition spontaneous pain of a peculiarly unpleasant and disturbing nature on the partially anaesthetic side. Fortunately this **thalamic syndrome**, which usually results from cerebral infarction, is rare. The pain is often most severe in the face, hand and foot.

Lesions of the **sensory cortex**, if irritative in type, give sensory Jacksonian epilepsy, often in the form of spreading paraesthesiae whose 'march' corresponds closely to the anatomical 'representation' of the parts of the body in the postcentral gyrus. This symptom is easy to confuse with the paraesthesiae which often occur during the aura of migraine, or during transient cerebral ischaemic attacks. When there is destruction of a part of the gyrus, then in the corresponding part of the opposite half of the body there is no impairment of pain sensibility and comparatively little of touch, but the appreciation of position, of tactile discrimination and localisation and of form and texture is profoundly impaired. Figures written upon the skin cannot be recognised, and the threshold for two-point discrimination is raised. In a less severe cortical lesion, there may simply be tactile inattention on the affected side. Defects of recognition and interpretation of sensory data found in parietal lobe lesions were discussed in Chapter 5.

One final diagnosis which must be considered as a possible cause of sensory abnormalities found on clinical examination is **hysteria**. In a suggestible patient it is only too easy to discover areas of spurious sensory loss. A total hemianaesthesia affecting all modalities of sensation, even including vibration sense over one half of the skull or sternum, is a common hysterical manifestation, as is anaesthesia of the palate or of the limbs in 'glove and stocking' distribution. Alternatively such sensory loss may be found in one limb only, particularly after minor injury in a compensation setting, when there is usually associated hysterical weakness and the sensory impairment ends at the level of a joint (e.g. the elbow, shoulder, knee or hip). In such cases, in contradistinction to polyneuropathy, there is an abrupt line of demarcation between the area of complete sensory loss and that where all sensation is normal. In a patient with hysterical sensory loss it may be possible to 'find' (with suggestion) an area within the anaesthetic region (impossible to explain on an anatomical basis) where pin-prick is felt acutely. Another useful pointer is that the patient, though claiming that all forms of sensation are impaired in the affected part, is yet able to localise accurately in space one finger or toe, say, with his eyes closed, indicating that the sense of position is in fact well preserved.

Sensory examination is a technique which can only be learned by experience and which even so is full of pitfalls, particularly with an anxious and suggestible patient. Nevertheless consistent and clear-cut sensory abnormalities are of great value in localising accurately a lesion within the nervous system, while the precise nature of the changes may give invaluable help in determining its character.

REFERENCES

Adams R D, Victor M 1985 Principles of neurology, 3rd edn. McGraw-Hill, New York

Bickerstaff E R 1980 Neurological examination in clinical practice, 4th edn. Blackwell, Oxford

FitzGerald M J T 1985 Neuroanatomy basic and applied. Baillière Tindall, Eastbourne

Gardner E 1975 Fundamentals of neurology, 6th edn. Saunders, Philadelphia

Guarantors of Brain 1986 Aids to the examination of the peripheral nervous system. Baillière Tindall, London

Iggo A 1985a Cutaneous sensation. In: Swash M, Kennard C (eds) Scientific basis of clinical neurology. Churchill Livingstone, Edinburgh

Iggo A 1985b Sensory receptors in the skin of mammals and their sensory functions. Revue Neurologique (Paris) 10: 599

Kandel E R, Schwartz J H 1985 Principles of neural science, 2nd edn. Arnold, London

Lance J W, McLeod J G 1981 A physiological approach to clinical neurology, 3rd edn. Butterworth, London

Mann W N (ed) 1975 Conybeare's Textbook of medicine, 16th edn. Churchill Livingstone, London

Matthews W B 1975 Practical neurology, 3rd edn. Blackwell, Oxford

Mayo Clinic, Section of Neurology 1981 Clinical examinations in neurology, 5th edn. Saunders, New York

Patton H D, Sundsten J W, Crill W E, Swanson P D 1976 Introduction to basic neurology. Saunders, Philadelphia

Sunderland S 1978 Nerves and nerve injuries, 2nd edn. Churchill Livingstone, Edinburgh

Wall P D 1985 Future trends in pain research. In: Iggo A, Iversen L L, Cervero F (eds) Nociception and pain. Philosophical Transactions of the Royal Society B308: 217

Walton J N 1985 Brain's Diseases of the nervous system, 9th edn. Oxford University Press, Oxford

Walton J N 1987 Introduction to clinical neuroscience, 2nd edn. Baillière Tindall, London

11. The autonomic nervous system

The autonomic nervous system is largely concerned with the control of visceral activity; its influences are widespread, affecting the cardiac rhythm and output, respiration, blood-vessel tone and the behaviour of the hollow viscera of the alimentary and urogenital systems, as well as the secretion of the ducted and ductless glands. It is probably as well that these activities are in a sense automatic and reflexly controlled, and that they are but little influenced by the will, for many of them are too vital to allow of any interference from the capricious behaviour of the mind. The combined activities of the autonomic nerves and of the endocrine glands are concerned in maintaining the constant internal thermal and biochemical environment of the body, a function which Cannon entitled homeostasis. Although many of the visceral functions of the autonomic nervous system and particularly its control of the heart, lungs and abdominal viscera are beyond the scope of this volume, there are many ways in which disease of the central or peripheral nervous system can affect autonomic activity, and accurate interpretation of the abnormalities so produced may be invaluable in diagnosis. Owing to the complex arrangement of the autonomic pathways it is easy to overlook some of the general principles upon which interpretation of autonomic disorders depends. However, a basic knowledge of their anatomy and pathophysiology is necessary for these principles to be rationally applied.

ANATOMY AND PHYSIOLOGY

The autonomic nervous system can be divided into two principal components, namely the **sympathetic** and the **parasympathetic** systems (Fig. 11.1). These two systems are in a sense antagonistic in their effects for where one excites the other inhibits. Thus activity of the sympathetic system produces dilatation of the pupil and slight protrusion of the eye, increased cardiac output with tachycardia, dilatation of the bronchioles, vasoconstriction of skin vessels but dilatation of the coronary and intramuscular arteries, sweating, inhibition of intestinal movement, closure of the internal anal sphincter, and erection of hairs (the pilomotor effect) on the skin. In other words the animal is prepared for action in response to an emergency. Activity of the parasympathetic system gives constriction of the pupil, slowing of the heart and diminished cardiac output, constriction of the bronchioles, increased intestinal peristalsis, increased intravesical pressure during micturition through contraction of the detrusor muscle, and increased secretory activity of the salivary and lacrimal glands. The parasympathetic system also plays a principal role in sexual activity, including penile erection and ejaculation in the male, and orgasm in the female.

There are areas of the **cerebral cortex** which exercise a controlling influence upon autonomic activity, but the exact areas of the cerebrum concerned and the mechanisms by which they produce their influence are not yet fully defined. However it is known that stimulation of the prefrontal cortex provokes sweating in the opposite arm and leg. Furthermore, the voluntary act of evacuation of the bladder and bowels seems to be initiated in the paracentral lobule; probably motor impulses from this area, destined to activate the appropriate parasympathetic nerves, travel downwards with the pyramidal tract. It is also evident that certain areas of cortex in the temporal lobe and insula, and particularly the hippocampal gyrus, may, with the amygdaloid nucleus, exercise important control over visceral as well as emotional activity.

Although the cerebrum influences autonomic activity, the most important cell stations from which visceral and other autonomic activity are finally controlled lie in the **hypothalamus**. Nuclei in this area receive fibres from the 'visceral' areas of cerebral cortex mentioned above and in turn they give rise to descending pathways which enter the brain stem and spinal cord. The anterior hypothalamic nuclei are particularly concerned with parasympathetic activity and with controlling the pituitary gland, while posterior nuclei, by contrast, influence sympathetic activity. Lesions of this area give rise to

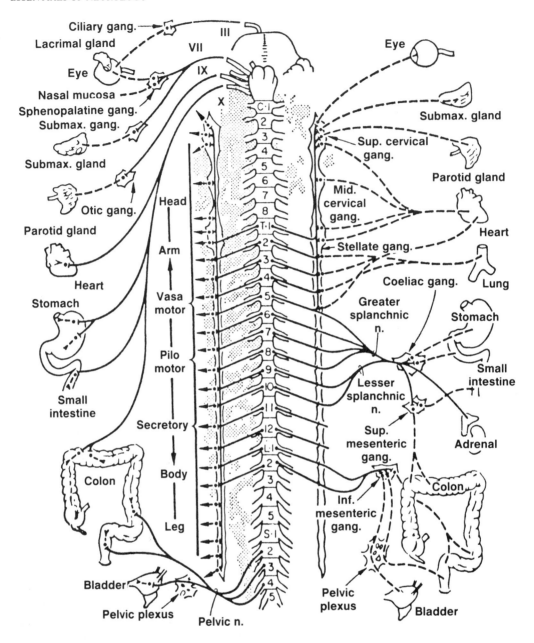

Fig. 11.1 A diagram of the spinal cord and brain stem showing thoracolumbar or sympathetic nerves and ganglia on the right, and craniosacral or parasympathetic nerves and ganglia on the left. The dual autonomic supply of the viscera is demonstrated. (By courtesy of the late Dr. Eaton and W. B. Saunders Co.)

emotional disturbances such as 'sham rage' in animals or to lethargy and hypersomnia. Temperature regulation, control of the emotions and of sleep are also mediated through hypothalamic nuclei. The corpora mammillaria, too, which form a part of the hypothalamic system, are clearly important in memory regulation, as lesions in this area may prevent the patient from recording new impressions, a feature seen typically in the Korsakoff syndrome (see Ch. 6, p. 96). The endocrine functions of the hypothalamus are considered in Chapter 19.

Descending pathways from the hypothalamus control both sympathetic and parasympathetic activity. These travel downwards, in the case of the sympathetic fibres, to the dorsal portion of the spinal cord to end in relation to the cells in the lateral horn of grey matter, while the parasympathetic fibres end in the nuclei of the oculomotor, facial, glossopharyngeal and vagus nerves, or in the sacral region of the spinal cord. No central autonomic fibres travel directly to any viscus, but in each case a ganglion lying outside the central nervous system is interposed, so that there are always preganglionic fibres arising within the central nervous system and postganglionic fibres arising in the ganglia. The sympathetic ganglia lie lateral to the vertebral bodies and with connecting fibres form the sympathetic chain; the postganglionic fibres to the effector organs are therefore long. Many of the parasympathetic ganglia are situated close to the effector organ so that in this case the preganglionic fibres are long.

Autonomic neurotransmitters

Acetylcholine or noradrenaline are released at autonomic nerve endings; all preganglionic fibres, both sympathetic and parasympathetic, are cholinergic. Circulating biogenic amines such as noradrenaline and adrenaline, secreted by the adrenal medulla, which influence sympathetic activity, as well as acetylcholine, produce their effects upon target organs by combining with receptor sites which lie in close relationship to the nerve endings.

Acetylcholine receptors are of two types, namely the muscarinic receptors which are found in all effector cells stimulated by postganglionic parasympathetic neurones and in cholinergic endings of the sympathetic system, and nicotinic receptors, found especially in the neuromuscular junctions of skeletal muscle but also at synapses in sympathetic and parasympathetic ganglia themselves. Adrenergic receptors are also of two types; alpha-receptors are stimulated mainly by noradrenaline and are concerned especially with vasoconstriction, dilatation of the iris, intestinal relaxation and pilomotor contraction in the skin, while beta-receptors are stimulated mainly by

adrenaline and to a lesser extent by noradrenaline; the latter account for an increased heart rate, vasodilatation of intramuscular blood vessels, intestinal and uterine relaxation and bronchodilatation. The rational use of many drugs depends upon receptor specificity. Thus parasympathomimetic drugs like pilocarpine and methacholine have a muscarinic effect and neostigmine is essentially nicotinic; atropine blocks the muscarinic but not the nicotinic effect of such drugs. Similarly the activities of sympathomimetic drugs depend upon their relative affinities for alpha- and beta- receptors.

Beta-receptors can be further divided into beta-1 receptors, which are found mainly in the heart, and beta-2 receptors which are present on all vascular smooth muscle and also on the smooth muscle in the bronchi. Some beta-blocking agents such as atenolol and metoprolol have a greater effect on beta-1 receptors and these are called cardioselective beta-blockers. The non-cardioselective beta blockers, such as propranolol, affect both beta-1 and beta-2 receptors and should therefore be avoided in patients prone to bronchospasm. Labetalol blocks both alpha- and beta-receptors and may thus be useful in the treatment of hypertension, while phenoxybenzamine only blocks alpha-receptors.

The sympathetic nervous system

Preganglionic medullated sympathetic fibres (white rami) arise from the lateral horn of grey matter in each segment of the spinal cord from the first thoracic to the second lumbar. They then pass laterally to the sympathetic chain in which there are ganglia corresponding to each of those segments of the cord from which sympathetic fibres arise; from these ganglia non-medullated postganglionic fibres (grey rami) join the corresponding somatic spinal nerve, to be distributed to the blood vessels and skin of the appropriate dermatome. However, fibres also run up and down in the chain to three cervical ganglia (superior, middle and inferior or stellate) and to four lumbar ganglia; these are necessary since there is no sympathetic outflow from the spinal cord in these regions. The thoracic and abdominal viscera receive a sympathetic supply through postganglionic fibres of the thoracic ganglia; these fibres form the splanchnic nerves and the coeliac, mesenteric and hypogastric plexuses. The sympathetic innervation of the cranium and of the upper limbs comes from the cervical ganglia and that of the lower limbs from the lumbar ganglia. Fibres travelling to the cranium traverse the inferior and middle cervical ganglia to synapse with nerve cells in the superior cervical ganglion, whence postganglionic fibres arise which enter or overlie the cranium in the coats of the internal and external carotid arteries and are then distributed to the blood vessels, smooth muscle, sweat glands, lacrimal and salivary glands.

Whether there are afferent sympathetic fibres concerned with the transmission of visceral sensation is controversial. Some regard the autonomic nervous system as entirely motor and suggest that afferent fibres accompanying sympathetic efferents are not themselves sympathetic. Whatever their nature, these fibres enter the posterior nerve roots, and visceral sensation is thereafter conveyed centrally along with somatic sensation.

The parasympathetic nervous system

This part of the autonomic system is often called the craniosacral outflow as its function is motor and its fibres only leave the central nervous system in the cranial nerves and in the sacral region. Fibres arising in the oculomotor nucleus supply the eye (see below). The superior salivary nucleus in the brain stem gives origin to fibres which travel with the facial nerve; in the geniculate ganglion some of these leave to form the greater superficial petrosal nerve. This nerve enters the sphenopalatine ganglion from which arise secretomotor fibres to the lacrimal gland. Other fibres from the superior salivary nucleus are conveyed by the chorda tympani to the submaxillary ganglion from which come fibres which innervate the submaxillary and sublingual glands. The axons of the inferior salivary nucleus, on the other hand, travel with the glossopharyngeal nerve; they form the lesser superficial petrosal nerve, enter the otic ganglion, and its postganglionic fibres promote secretion by the parotid gland. Finally, so far as the cranial outflow is concerned, the preganglionic fibres which arise in the dorsal nucleus of the vagus nerve end in many ganglia which lie in the walls of the numerous viscera innervated by this nerve.

The sacral outflow of the parasympathetic system leaves the spinal cord in the second, third and fourth sacral nerves, the so-called nervi erigentes. These preganglionic fibres pass to the vesical plexus and to numerous ganglia in the walls of the bladder, rectum and other pelvic organs, and from these ganglia postganglionic fibres arise.

The eye

The parasympathetic nerves supplying the pupil and ciliary muscle arise in the Edinger-Westphal nucleus in the midbrain and run with the third nerve to the orbit where they relay in the ciliary ganglion and then pass to the ciliary muscle and to the pupil via the short ciliary nerves. The sympathetic supply to the eye arises in the superior cervical ganglion and travels in the wall of the internal carotid artery to the cavernous sinus and then with the first division of the trigeminal nerve to the orbit and eventually to the pupillary muscle via the long ciliary nerves. Lesions of the parasympathetic supply to the eye may accompany third nerve palsies (see p. 113) when the pupil is dilated due to the unopposed action of the sympathetic system. Lesions anywhere in the sympathetic pathway will cause a Horner's syndrome (see p. 180) when the pupil is found to be constricted due to the unopposed action of the parasympathetic.

The bladder and bowel

The wall of the bladder consists of unstriped muscle, which forms the detrusor; it and the internal sphincter are both supplied by parasympathetic nerves arising from the nervi erigentes. Stimulation of these fibres gives contraction of the detrusor and relaxation of the internal sphincter. Evacuation of the bladder cannot, however, occur until the external sphincter relaxes; this consists of striped muscle, being supplied by the pudendal nerve and being thus under voluntary control. Normally the tone of the detrusor keeps the bladder contracted upon its contents, but when the intravesical pressure rises to a certain level rhythmical contractions of the bladder wall develop and after a time there is reflex relaxation of the internal sphincter; evacuation is then resisted only by voluntary contraction of the external sphincter. When the latter is relaxed and micturition occurs, the abdominal muscles also contract.

Sympathetic fibres from the hypogastric nerves also supply the bladder wall and, if stimulated, may inhibit contraction. In fact, however, section of these nerves has little practical effect upon bladder function. Some of the afferent fibres concerned in the vesical reflexes travel with these fibres but others travel with the pelvic nerves.

The physiological stimulus for bladder evacuation is an increase in the intravesical pressure which gives the desire to micturate. If this desire is unfulfilled, repeated contractions eventually follow. As previously mentioned there are also higher centres in the paracentral lobule of the cerebral cortex and probably also in the midbrain which exercise control over micturition; these produce their influence through fibres which descend with the pyramidal tracts. Hence disease of the spinal cord, as will be seen below, can profoundly influence bladder function. Disordered function is assessed by measuring the changes in intravesical pressure following the introduction of increasing volumes of fluid into the bladder via a catheter. Normally this cystometrogram shows a rise in pressure as the fluid is introduced, followed by a gradual fall; this response follows the introduction of each volume increment and eventually rhythmical contractions of the bladder wall occur. The point at which the patient is aware of a 'full bladder' sensation can be recorded, as can the volume and pressure at which voiding becomes inevitable. If radio-opaque fluid is used, a video camera coupled to an X-ray screening device can be used to visualise the bladder contractions and eventually the process of micturition; it is therefore possible to visualise the function of both the bladder wall and the urethral sphincters.

In many respects the innervation of the rectum resembles that of the bladder. Stimulation of the parasympathetic nerves gives contraction of the rectal musculature but relaxation of the internal sphincter, as both consist of smooth muscle. The striated external sphincter of the anus, however, is supplied by the pudendal nerve and enables evacuation to be resisted voluntarily. As with the bladder, distension with faeces gives reflex rectal contraction and the desire to defaecate.

Sexual activity

Sexual function in the male can be divided into first, desire or libido which is essentially an emotional function; secondly, erection of the penis due to tumescence of the corpora cavernosa, and thirdly, ejaculation of semen. The second and third functions are mediated through the activity of parasympathetic nerves, while closure of the internal sphincter through sympathetic action is also necessary during ejaculation. Loss of libido may be due to disease of the mind or of the endocrine glands, while impotence (retention of desire but inability to achieve an effective penile erection) can also be psychologically determined. However, impotence can also result from disease of the sacral cord or cauda equina, and is then due to a lesion of the parasympathetic motor pathway or of the afferent sensory pathways; in such a case the ability to ejaculate is also absent. However, since the sexual act is a function which, once initiated, is largely controlled reflexly, erection and ejaculation can occur despite a severe transverse lesion of the cord above the sacral segments. Indeed in some cases of spinal cord injury persistent erection of the penis (priapism) is seen. Disorders of sexual function in the female are less well understood. Lack of desire (frigidity) is relatively common in otherwise normal females and is usually psychogenic. Disease of the cauda equina or of the lower spinal cord may abolish the ability to achieve orgasm, but the effects of nervous disease upon female sexuality are much less apparent than in the male.

Precocious sexual development is generally due to overactivity of the adrenals or ovaries but is occasionally seen in patients with hypothalamic or midbrain neoplasms or in male patients with pinealomas. Excessive sexuality is generally a constitutional disorder, of psychic rather than physical origin, and often shows some affinities with psychopathy (personality disorder).

Some autonomic and related sensory reflexes

In addition to the visceral reflexes mentioned above, certain cutaneous reflexes dependent upon autonomic pathways assist in neurological diagnosis. Thus local warming of a limb initially gives vasodilatation and flushing of the skin, followed by sweating in the part that is warmed. Subsequently general vasodilatation and sweating occur in other parts of the body; this occurs even when all nervous connexions between the stimulated limb and the remainder of the body have been divided and must therefore depend upon stimulation of the hypothalamus by the warmed blood. Converse effects (vasoconstriction, pilomotor responses) follow cooling of a limb. Sweating and pilomotor activity are, however, lost in a part of the body which has lost its sympathetic nerve supply, whether the postganglionic or preganglionic fibres have been divided. Absence of cutaneous sweating can be demonstrated by dusting the skin with either quinizarin powder or a starch and iodine mixture; sweat turns quinizarin purple and starch and iodine blue.

The 'flare' reaction is another important reflex. It is an axon reflex; in other words the afferent stimulus travels centrally along a fibre, but then spreads to other branches of the same fibre, in which stimuli travelling peripherally are evoked; these produce a peripheral effect. If the skin is scratched firmly there is temporary blanching along the scratch-line due to local capillary injury, but this is soon followed by a spreading vasodilatation or 'flare', resulting from the axon reflex. A central weal also occurs due to local histamine release, but the 'flare', and the pilomotor response which may also occur in the same area, are reflexly determined. Since this axon reflex does not traverse the spinal cord it remains intact in spinal cord lesions and in lesions lying central to the posterior root ganglia; it is only impaired when the afferent sensory fibres or the ganglia themselves are diseased. Hence absence of the 'flare' can be a valuable physical sign of a lesion of somatic sensory nerves. Another useful test is the cold vasodilatation response; if normal fingers are immersed in water at 5°C they cool rapidly but 5 or 10 minutes later there is vasodilatation. This does not happen if the finger is denervated; like the flare, this is not strictly an autonomic reflex as it depends upon the integrity of sensory axons. Thus in disease of the efferent sympathetic pathways, whether preganglionic or postganglionic, reflex vasodilatation (flushing of the skin) and sweating are abolished but a 'flare' will develop.

When the sensory nerves from an area of skin are diseased, sweating may occur, but the 'flare' and cold vasodilatation are abolished.

SOME COMMON DISORDERS OF THE AUTONOMIC NERVOUS SYSTEM

Horner's syndrome

A lesion of the cervical sympathetic chain or ganglia causes constriction of the pupil on the same side due to unopposed action of the parasympathetic; drooping of the eyelid, due to paralysis of that part of the levator palpebrae superioris which is composed of smooth muscle and is innervated by sympathetic nerves; slight retraction of the globe of the eye into the orbit because of paralysis of smooth orbital muscle which is similarly innervated; and loss of sweating on the affected side of the head and neck. Hence the features of Horner's syndrome are myosis, ptosis, enophthalmos and anhidrosis of head and neck. A Horner's syndrome is a very good lateralising sign as it is always on the same side as the lesion, but it is a poor localising sign as the condition can result from a lesion anywhere in the sympathetic pathway from the midbrain to the internal carotid artery. Horner's syndrome may, therefore, be found in brain stem infarction and often accompanies the lateral medullary syndrome due to thrombosis of one posterior inferior cerebellar or vertebral artery. The sympathetic fibres may also be involved in the brain stem or cervical spinal cord in syringobulbia or syringomyelia. Lesions affecting the lower brachial plexus such as Pancoast's tumour or metastases in cervical lymph nodes from carcinoma of the breast may also affect the cervical sympathetic chain. Horner's syndrome can also occur in lesions of the internal carotid artery such as aneurysm or thrombosis, although facial sweating is usually then preserved as fibres responsible for this travel in the unaffected external carotid artery and its branches. This clinical picture of a Horner's syndrome with normal facial sweating on the affected side is seen in Raeder's paratrigeminal syndrome. Although the appearance of a Horner's syndrome demands investigation and the exclusion of the more obvious causes, in a number of patients even the most thorough investigation fails to reveal the cause.

Cranial nerve syndromes

A lesion of one oculomotor nerve usually gives a fixed dilated pupil on the affected side, owing to paralysis of parasympathetic fibres and unopposed action of the sympathetic. Diseases of the glossopharyngeal and vagus nerves rarely produce any clinical evidence of autonomic disturbance, but after a facial palsy misdirection of regenerating parasympathetic fibres can result in fibres intended for the salivary glands reaching the lacrimal gland so that lacrimation occurs when the patient eats (the syndrome of crocodile tears). Facial sweating during meals (gustatory sweating) is another reflex phenomenon which is occasionally seen in apparently normal individuals and can often be controlled by atropine and related drugs. The myotonic pupil (Adie's syndrome), due to a lesion of the ciliary ganglion of undetermined cause, is described on p. 114.

Lesions of the cauda equina and spinal cord

A severe lesion of the cauda equina can have profound effects upon bladder and bowel function because of damage to the sacral parasympathetic outflow. The bladder becomes toneless and reflex contraction can no longer occur as it distends, so that urinary retention develops. As distension increases, so the elasticity of the bladder wall forces urine into the urethra, and as the external sphincter is usually paralysed as well, dribbling incontinence or retention with overflow occurs. If the cauda equina lesion is permanent, reflex bladder activity cannot be re-established and these patients may require permanent catheterisation, although it is sometimes possible to avoid this by the use of external drainage devices such as Paul's tubing or intermittent catheterisation which has proved very successful in many patients, particularly in children with spina bifida. Sometimes it is possible to achieve evacuation by manual compression but many of these techniques leave some residual urine and patients are prone to repeated urinary tract infections. Proper management can usually avoid the long-term consequences of repeated infection, and urinary diversion by surgical means is only very rarely required. Similarly, faecal retention often occurs, with incontinence, and regular enemas may be required to empty the bowel.

The initial effects of an acute transverse lesion of the spinal cord are similar; there is retention of urine with overflow and also faecal retention. However, as spinal shock wears off, reflex bladder and bowel evacuation are gradually established, occurring solely in response to increasing intravesical and intrarectal pressure and independently of the will. Thus automatic bladder and bowel activity develop; micturition and defaecation can be evoked by anything which increases intravesical pressure, including pressure upon the abdomen, or straining. They can also occur as a result of stimuli applied to the lower limbs, as part of the 'mass reflex' which includes flexor withdrawal of the limbs. The patient with a total transverse cord lesion may become aware that his bladder is full through sensations of headache, sweating or abdominal fullness and may then be able to initiate micturition by pressure upon the abdomen.

Retention of urine can also result from parasagittal lesions affecting both cerebral paracentral lobules, while incomplete lesions of the spinal cord affecting the pyramidal tracts, in relation to which descending fibres controlling micturition are believed to travel, can also affect bladder function. Sometimes, in such a case, there is delay in the initiation of micturition and even incomplete retention with overflow. More often, in a patient with spastic paraplegia, say, as a result of multiple sclerosis, there is heightened reflex activity of the bladder and precipitancy or urgency of micturition results. The patient cannot resist the desire to micturate and precipitate bladder evacuation occurs. Incontinence of urine also occurs in some patients with bilateral lesions of the medial aspect of the frontal lobes, as may occur in falx meningiomas, medial frontal gliomas (particularly if they extend across the midline in the corpus callosum) and in patients with communicating hydrocephalus (see p. 185). Bilateral frontal lobe infarction in patients with anterior cerebral or anterior communicating artery aneurysms is another cause, as are the dementias.

Apart from their effect upon bladder and bowel function, lesions of the spinal cord influence other autonomic activities. Thus after an acute transverse lesion, and during the stage of spinal shock (diaschisis) the skin of the body below the level of the lesion is dry, pale and cool, but subsequently when reflex activity is established, profuse sweating in the affected area is common and can be provoked by many cutaneous or other stimuli. It should also be remembered that local disease of the dorsal spinal cord may damage the lateral horn of grey matter and will give sympathetic denervation of the affected segments with signs corresponding to those produced by division of preganglionic fibres.

Referred pain

The afferent pathway for visceral sensation is initially along afferent fibres which accompany autonomic nerves, and particularly the sympathetic. These fibres enter posterior nerve roots and travel centrally with somatic afferents. Visceral pain is often felt in skin areas which are not at first sight anatomically related to the viscus concerned; thus cardiac pain may be referred to the substernal region, but also to the left arm, to both arms or to the jaw. The mechanism of referred pain is discussed on p. 51.

Degenerative disorders of the autonomic nervous system

A progressive failure of autonomic function may occur in isolation without any evidence of degeneration of any other part of the nervous system. This is known as **progressive autonomic failure** or **idiopathic orthostatic hypertension** (the Shy-Drager syndrome). It is caused by a progressive fall-out of the preganglionic autonomic cells in the brain stem and the intermediolateral columns of the spinal cord. It presents in middle life with symptoms of postural hypotension eventually leading to such profound orthostatic hypertension that it may be impossible to maintain adequate cerebral perfusion when upright; this is associated with urinary and rectal incontinence, loss of sweating, iris atrophy and impotence. It is not known whether this is a specific clinical entity on its own or a forme fruste of multisystem atrophy since many of these patients also show signs of degeneration in other systems. Parkinson's disease is the most common associated degenerative disease but there may be clinical evidence of more widespread striatonigral or olivopontocerebellar involvement.

Familial dysautonomia (the Riley-Day syndrome) is an autosomal recessive disease which is usually found in Ashkenazi Jews. In addition to the involvement of the sympathetic nervous system giving rise to the features of progressive autonomic failure, the sense of taste is always profoundly affected and so is the peripheral sensory system with profound reduction in the size of the dorsal root ganglia and severe depletion of axons distally.

The autonomic nervous system may be affected in a number of other conditions including diabetes, amyloidosis and tabes dorsalis, and autonomic abnormalities occur in some paraneoplastic syndromes, including the Lambert-Eaton syndrome.

Acute autonomic neuropathy is a rare disorder of unknown cause presenting in childhood or adult life with the rapid onset of postural hypotension, paralysis of ocular accommodation, anhidrosis and urinary and faecal retention. Spontaneous recovery usually occurs within a few months, so that the condition is also known as 'pure pan-dysautonomia with recovery'.

Peripheral nerve lesions

Whereas section of a sensory nerve peripheral to its posterior root ganglion usually abolishes the 'flare' response in the cutaneous anaesthetic area, a lesion of the lower motor neurone usually produces no recognisable autonomic effects. However, as a result of disuse the skin of the affected part may become smooth, shiny and inelastic while subcutaneous tissue and even bone, as well as denervated muscle, will atrophy. Owing to loss of the 'pumping' action of muscles upon the veins, the affected part, especially a hand or foot, is often cyanosed and oedematous. These so-called trophic changes are due to disuse and not to a lesion of autonomic nerves; the autonomic reflexes are intact. The sequelae of a sensory nerve lesion are often more serious, particularly if pain fibres are involved as, if the part is analgesic, injury to the insensitive skin and joints readily occurs, giving indolent or perforating ulcers and gross disorganisation of joints (Charcot's arthropathy). Other trophic changes, such as loss of sweating and of the pilomotor response, only follow a lesion of preganglionic or postganglionic sympathetic efferents and hence do not always result from lesions of somatic peripheral nerves, unless these contain sympathetic fibres.

After an incomplete lesion of a peripheral nerve, particularly in the region of the forearm and wrist, a curiously unpleasant burning pain may develop in the affected hand, with excessive sweating and excessive sensitivity to touch and pain. This syndrome is called **causalgia**; it seems that stimuli responsible for the pain travel with autonomic nerves and not along somatic afferents, as block or division of somatic sensory nerves fails to relieve the pain, while sympathectomy does so. The pathogenesis of causalgia is poorly understood (p. 59). Similarly, the mechanism by which painful swelling of the hand, often giving eventually atrophy of muscles and even of bone (Sudeck's atrophy), develops in some cases of pericapsulitis of the shoulder joint or 'frozen' shoulder (**the 'shoulder-hand' syndrome** or **reflex sympathetic dystrophy of the upper extremity**) is obscure, but this condition, too, is often relieved by cervical sympathectomy.

Hyperhidrosis

Though excessive sweating, particularly of the hands and feet, can be due to emotional disturbances or to endocrine disorders such as thyrotoxicosis, it may also be congenital and, if intolerable, can be alleviated by sympathectomy. It is also seen sometimes in Parkinson's disease. Localised cutaneous areas of increased sweating can occur following peripheral nerve lesions, as in causalgia, while excessive perspiration in response to any peripheral

stimulus is seen below the level of a transverse lesion of the spinal cord.

THE ASSESSMENT OF AUTONOMIC FUNCTION

In clinical practice there are a number of useful bedside tests which can be used to assess autonomic function; the following have been found particularly helpful:

1. Measure the blood pressure lying down and then again immediately on standing, to record the effect of posture.

2. Measurement of the variation in R-R interval in the electrocardiogram (ECG) at rest and with forced respiration.

3. Estimation of cutaneous sweating following external heating sufficient to raise the body temperature by 1°C. Quinazarin or starch and iodine powder can be used to assess sweating on the legs but facial sweating is usually obvious.

4. Analysis of the effect of the Valsalva manoeuvre on the R-R interval in the ECG.

Many other tests are available but those listed above can easily be carried out at the bedside and some of them can be quantified, which may be useful for serial testing. It should be recognised that these are tests of the integrity of specific autonomic reflexes concerned with the postural control of blood pressure, changes in heart rate and blood pressure and in the ECG R-R interval elicited either by changes in respiratory rate or by increased intrathoracic pressure or reduced venous return to the heart (in the Valsalva manoeuvre), and with the control of sweating. The tests cannot, however, invariably be used to determine which part of the reflex arc is defective; this may be dependent upon other evidence.

REFERENCES

Appenzeller 0 1976 The autonomic nervous system, 2nd edn. North-Holland, Amsterdam
Bannister R 1988 Autonomic failure, 2nd edn. Oxford University Press, Oxford
Johnson R H, Spalding J M K 1974 Disorders of the autonomic nervous system. Blackwell, Oxford
Patton H D, Sundsten J W, Crill W E, Swanson, P D 1976 Introduction to basic neurology. Saunders, Philadelphia
Walton J N 1985 Brain's diseases of the nervous system, 9th edn. Oxford University Press, Oxford

12. Developmental, hereditary and degenerative disorders

Among the many nervous disorders considered in this volume there is a group of syndromes or diseases which are difficult to classify according to rational criteria. Some are clearly inherited but we do not know how the gene or genes responsible for them produce their effects upon the nervous system. Nor do we know in the case of many of them whether they are separate diseases or are merely variants of a single disease process. Others are clearly due to an abnormality which has afflicted the developing nervous system of the affected individual in utero, while others which are normally grouped together for convenience on account of clinical similarities are probably due to a variety of causes, some well-recognised and others obscure. And in yet another group of conditions there is evidence of a pathological process involving part of the central or peripheral nervous system, a process so inexplicable in our present state of knowledge that we can only classify it as being degenerative. This chapter outlines some of the commoner nervous disorders in these categories and considers their interrelationship. It should be noted that many hereditary and degenerative disorders are also considered in other chapters; for example, the dementias in Chapter 7 and the neuromuscular disorders in Chapter 18. And many uncommon developmental defects, such as the microcephalies, macrocephalies and ageneses of portions of the brain will not be discussed here, in view of their rarity. These are described in larger textbooks to which reference is made at the end of the chapter.

CEREBRAL PALSY

The term cerebral palsy is used to identify a group of nervous disorders which are apparent from birth, which are very variable in their clinical manifestations and severity, and probably also in their aetiology. Although abnormalities of movement are generally the most prominent clinical features in such cases there are often associated defects of intellect, of emotional development, of speech in the broadest sense, and of sensation. Between one and two in every thousand children are victims of some form of cerebral palsy. In most of the affected children the limbs are stiff and spastic and this is why these cases are often referred to, particularly by the lay public, as spastic children. In fact, in as many as 10% of cases it is involuntary movements of athetoid type and not spasticity which constitute the principal disability, while in about 5% the limbs are actually hypotonic and the child is ataxic rather than spastic.

The aetiology of cerebral palsy has been a fertile source of dispute. Some claimed that virtually all cases were due to **birth injury** with meningeal haemorrhage, a view now clearly untenable, while others suggested that an encephalitis or some degenerative cerebral process of known aetiology, occurring in utero, was the cause. The truth appears to be that the pathological changes seen in such cases are so diverse that no single cause can be implicated. A **genetic factor** may be responsible for the condition in up to 10% of cases, as other members of the family, particularly sibs, are afflicted, either with cerebral palsy or with mental defect or epilepsy. Probably in some cases, **intra-uterine cerebral anoxia** due to placental insufficiency is responsible, and there is certainly a high incidence of threatened abortion or accidental haemorrhage in pregnancies resulting in the birth of spastic children. Possibly, too, the anoxia resulting from a prolonged convulsion in early infancy can give rise to similar changes, as may anoxia or direct trauma to the brain during a breech or forceps delivery or any prolonged labour. Certainly 50% of spastic children have abnormal deliveries and many are born prematurely. There is increasing evidence that prenatal or perinatal anoxia is the predominant aetiological factor, but complex neonatal metabolic abnormalities, including hypoglycaemia, as well as disorders of cerebral perfusion resulting from cerebral oedema and hypotension all play a part. Pathologically the principal changes are those of periventricular encephalomalacia, but multiple areas of cortical scarring are found in some cases, porencephalic cysts communicating with the ventricles in others and spongiform changes in the basal ganglia in yet others. **Kernicterus**, the degeneration and bilirubin-staining of the basal ganglia which may occur in untreated Rh-incompatibility (icterus gravis neonatorum) can cause a type of cerebral palsy in which mental defect, deafness and athetosis are prominent features.

Although all forms of cerebral palsy usually reveal themselves through delay in development, and failure to pass intellectual and physical milestones at a normal age, most cases fall into one of several distinctive clinical syndromes. The age at which the parents realise that their child is abnormal varies depending upon severity, but it is usually within the first 12 to 18 months of life; in some, delay and difficulty in walking are not apparent until late in the second year.

The condition can simply cause **mental retardation**, but more often there is clumsiness and spasticity of the limbs as well. The diagnosis of mental defect in early life, depending as it does upon failure to achieve new milestones of intellectual development (smiling, following lights, groping for objects, forming syllables and words, etc.) at the normal age, is a matter which requires great skill and experience in assessing the infant's behaviour against a background of known developmental variations. Certain children with cerebral palsy have specific defects of motor function (**apraxia**), of sensory function (**agnosia**), of the special senses (**nerve deafness**) or of speech (**aphasia, articulatory apraxia, dyslexia**) which can give a false impression of mental retardation if the clinical appraisal is too superficial. In some cases developmental disorders of execution and cognition (learning defects) occur in isolation without accompanying manifestations of spasticity or ataxia. Congenital reading defect (developmental dyslexia) is a good example, but apraxic and agnosic disorders ('clumsy children') also occur (see p. 67) and are difficult to recognise in the early stages, though a discrepancy between high verbal and low performance scores in an IQ test may be a useful pointer. These and other forms of so-called minimal cerebral dysfunction are often overlooked or may only become apparent when school performance falls short of expectation.

The commonest form of cerebral palsy is **spastic diplegia** (Little's disease) which may or may not be associated with mental defect. In its mildest form it presents with little more than a delay of a few months in learning to walk, with some clumsiness and unsteadiness of gait, symmetrical exaggeration of the lower limb reflexes and extensor plantar responses. In a severe case, walking is never possible, all four limbs are spastic and there is also severe spastic dysarthria and/or dysphagia. More often the patient cannot walk until the fifth or sixth year and then does so with the characteristic 'scissors gait', and contractures develop in the Achilles tendons and hamstrings.

In patients with **athetosis** (see p. 157) which is usually bilateral and symmetrical, there may also be facial grimacing and an intermittently explosive dysarthria. Voluntary movements of the limbs sometimes override the abnormal movements but are slowly and clumsily performed. Often the athetotic movements are not seen until the second year of life or later, and at an earlier stage the limbs are hypotonic and movement is inco-ordinate while the plantar responses are flexor. Some cases, however, show associated spasticity. More rarely patients with a hypotonic or flaccid variety of diplegia do not develop involuntary movements but have nystagmus and asymmetrical **ataxia** of all four limbs, usually due to cerebellar dysfunction (**cerebellar diplegia**).

The prognosis of cerebral palsy varies, depending upon the severity of the intellectual and motor deficit. When mental retardation is severe, little can be done and this is unfortunately true of some cases in which the motor abnormality is gross. Sometimes abnormal movements can be modified or partially alleviated by stereotaxic surgery, while many patients, with appropriate training and appropriate techniques of physiotherapy and rehabilitation, can be helped to lead useful lives. Children with specific disorders of language and reading, though requiring patient individual training, are particularly profitable subjects.

Infantile hemiplegia is another condition commonly classified as a form of cerebral palsy, although it clearly differs considerably from the diffuse and symmetrical cerebral disorders mentioned above. It can occur bilaterally (double hemiplegia) and is then distinguished from cerebral diplegia through the fact that the upper limbs are more severely affected than the lower. The condition can be present from birth (congenital hemiplegia), when it may be due to a congenital cystic deformity of one cerebral hemisphere (porencephaly), to the Sturge-Weber syndrome (see p. 280), or possibly to infarction occurring in utero. More commonly it develops acutely in infancy or early childhood, often during an acute illness such as whooping cough or an exanthem, or after a so-called 'febrile convulsion'. Probably the commonest pathological cause is infarction due to either arterial or venous occlusion, resulting in scarring and atrophy of the hemisphere and localised dilatation of the lateral ventricle (secondary porencephaly). It may in some cases be due to an inflammatory process of unknown cause involving the wall of the internal carotid artery. Characteristically the arm on the affected side is severely paralysed, finger and hand movement being virtually abolished, and the hand and forearm assume a typically flexed posture, lying across the front of the chest. The leg, though spastic with exaggerated deep reflexes and an extensor plantar response, is less severely affected, and all patients eventually walk, often with surprisingly little difficulty. If the dominant hemisphere is involved, aphasia occurs; the earlier the age at which the hemiplegia develops, the more complete and rapid is the recovery of speech function. Indeed if the patient is a young infant, the development of speech is not perceptibly delayed and this function becomes established in the contralateral hemisphere. The residual neurological deficit can be of all grades of severity and occasionally the resulting disability is trivial. In more severe cases, however, epilepsy is a common complication, as the scar in the affected hemisphere acts as a focus of epileptic discharge. Particularly in those cases in which epileptic seizures are frequent and severe, intellectual impairment and behaviour disorders are common. In some such cases, and especially if the epileptic seizures fail to respond to appropriate anticonvulsant therapy, the operation of hemispherectomy is very successful in abolishing or alleviating the attacks and in improving behaviour.

HYDROCEPHALUS

Hydrocephalus can be defined as an increase in the volume of CSF within the cranial cavity. This may occur as a compensatory phenomenon when the brain or any part of it is atrophic through disease (hydrocephalus ex vacuo), but no symptoms then result from the presence of excess fluid. It is when the increase in fluid is accompanied by a rise in the intracranial pressure that clinical effects become apparent. This variety of hydrocephalus results from obstruction to the circulation of the fluid, or from impaired absorption. Any increase in CSF production without obstruction is matched by increased absorption.

When hydrocephalus is due to an obstruction to the flow of fluid through a part of the ventricular system (lateral ventricle, third ventricle, aqueduct, fourth ventricle), it is known as **obstructive hydrocephalus** and there is enlargement of those ventricles which lie between the choroid plexuses and the block. An obstruction to the flow of fluid through the subarachnoid space, usually in the basal cisterns at the tentorial hiatus or in the region of the superior longitudinal sinus (with impaired absorption), gives **communicating hydrocephalus** and there is then dilatation of all the cerebral ventricles.

Obstructive hydrocephalus can be **congenital** or **acquired**. The commonest congenital cause is stenosis or malformation of the aqueduct of Sylvius (aqueduct

stenosis, in which the third and lateral ventricles are dilated but the posterior fossa is small), but less often there is membranous occlusion of the foramina of Magendie and Luschka (the so-called Dandy-Walker syndrome, in which the fourth ventricle is also dilated and the posterior fossa is large). Another cause is the Arnold-Chiari malformation which is a congenital abnormality in the region of the craniocervical junction. There are several different types according to the degree of abnormality. In type I there is ectopia of the cerebellar tonsils which lie in the upper cervical canal and there may be some descent of the medulla. In type II there is sufficient downward displacement of the medulla for the lower part of the fourth ventricle to lie in the upper cervical canal and this is associated with spina bifida. Both of these types can be associated with syringomyelia, syringobulbia and hydrocephalus. In most cases of congenital hydrocephalus there is conspicuous enlargement of the head, present sometimes at birth, but usually developing subsequently. The head is excessively translucent, it yields a typical 'cracked-pot' note on percussion, there is separation of the sutures and the eyes tend to be pushed forwards and downwards (the rising-sun sign). Convulsions, mental impairment, optic atrophy and spastic weakness of the limbs often develop. Without treatment some patients die within the first four years of life, but the condition becomes arrested in many others, who then survive with a variable degree of disability. These patients may subsequently decompensate following quite minor head injuries and then show again all the features of raised intracranial pressure associated with obstructive hydrocephalus. **Acquired** obstructive hydrocephalus can result from any lesion, whether inflammatory or neoplastic, which distorts intracranial hydrodynamics in such a way as to cause an obstruction to CSF flow in a cerebral ventricle or in the aqueduct. Space-occupying lesions in the posterior fossa often present with the features of hydrocephalus because of the small volume of the posterior fossa and the ease with which the CSF pathways can become obstructed.

Communicating hydrocephalus presents with the more insidious onset of a triad comprising dementia, gait apraxia and incontinence of 'frontal lobe' type. It may occur without any obvious or detectable cause but can be a complication of meningitis, particularly the basal granulomatous meningitides such as those due to tuberculosis, syphilis and sarcoidosis, but it may also follow subarachnoid haemorrhage which causes adhesions in the subarachnoid space and so occludes the arachnoid villi. It may also follow head injury. This condition was at one time known as low pressure or normal pressure hydrocephalus because the CSF pressure at lumbar puncture was usually normal. However, continuous monitoring of intracranial pressure has shown that these patients have intermittent periods of raised intracranial pressure (plateau waves). The diagnosis should be suspected in patients with the typical clinical features or may be suggested by the appearance of the CT scan in patients with dementia, which shows gross enlargement of the ventricles and obliteration of the cortical sulci, though the Sylvian fissures are sometimes quite prominent (Fig. 12. 1). The response to ventriculo-atrial or ventriculo-peritoneal shunting can be dramatic, but the selection of suitable patients to shunt is difficult as many of these patients are elderly and also have some degree of cerebral atrophy. There is a significant risk of causing subdural haematomas from shunting patients with atrophic brains. The patients who respond best to this procedure are those with the typical clinical picture and a readily identifiable cause, particularly if plateau waves can be demonstrated on 24-hour intracranial pressure monitoring.

The syndrome of **otitic hydrocephalus** is one of headache and severe papilloedema which may complicate middle-ear disease and is generally due to aseptic thrombosis of the lateral and/or superior longitudinal sinuses, giving impaired absorption of CSF. This condition is self-limiting, and complete recovery usually occurs provided there is no associated venous cortical infarction (see p. 277) and vision is preserved.

HUNTINGTON'S CHOREA

This genetically-determined degenerative disorder, in which pathological changes are most striking in the frontal and temporal cortex and caudate nuclei, is inherited as an autosomal dominant trait with complete penetrance and is usually first apparent in late middle-life. The characteristic features are progressive dementia, facial grimacing and uncontrollable choreiform movements of the limbs. Rarely, dementia develops before the choreiform movements; more often the latter are evident for some years before intellect declines. Some subjects become very depressed when they realise that they have inherited the family disease and the resulting emotional and intellectual retardation may be mistaken for dementia, but is of course amenable to treatment. Very occasionally the condition presents in childhood or early adult life, with generalised rigidity of the limbs (the 'rigid' form of the disease). The CT scan in such cases often demonstrates atrophy of the caudate nuclei. Neuropharmacologists are attempting, so far without success, to define the fundamental biochemical defect in such cases. A specific diagnostic test, applicable in the preclinical phase of the illness, is urgently required since each child

of an affected individual has a 50:50 chance of developing the disease and most sufferers have passed through their active reproductive phase before manifestations of the condition are first recognisable. The discovery of a cloned DNA sequence closely linked to the Huntington gene on chromosome 4 has raised the hope that a gene-specific marker may soon be identified, thus providing a reliable test.

STORAGE DISEASES

This is a very heterogenous group of genetically determined conditions in which there is a partial or complete interruption in a metabolic pathway, usually because of the deficiency of a particular enzyme, which results in the abnormal accumulation or storage in the tissues of the substance upon which the defective enzyme would normally act. The enzyme concerned and the accumulating substance have been identified in many of these conditions, while in others only the location of the deficiency is known, such as that it lies in the lysosomes or mitochondria. This has resulted in a much more logical classification than that formerly based on clinical features, although eponyms are still used for the more common conditions.

The most commonly accumulated substances include the sphingolipids (cerebrosides, galactosides, sphingomyelin and sulphatides), glycogen, mucopolysaccharides and mucolipids, glycoproteins, cholesterol and phytanic acid.

Most of these conditions present in the first few years of life, but in a number of cases the progression is sufficiently slow for the condition to present in adolescence or early adult life. The more important of these include GM1 gangliosidosis and GM2 gangliosidosis (adult **Tay-Sachs disease**) due to a deficiency of galactosidase and hexosaminidase A respectively. These conditions present with a progressive cerebellar syndrome with some involvement of motor pathways and also with seizures. **Metachromatic leucodystrophy** is due to the deposition of sulphatide because of a deficiency of aryl-sulphatase A. It presents with intellectual impairment and sometimes with psychosis and impairment of gait, and with both cerebellar and corticospinal involvement, and most patients also have a peripheral neuropathy. The diagnosis can be made by peripheral nerve biopsy and estimation of urinary and leucocyte aryl-sulphatase. **Krabbe's disease** is due to a deficiency of galactocerebrosidase with the deposition of galactocerebroside. There are cerebellar and corticospinal abnormalities associated with a peripheral neuropathy, and bulbar involvement is often a prominent feature. In **Pompe's disease** there is storage of glycogen and patients present with a slowly progressive

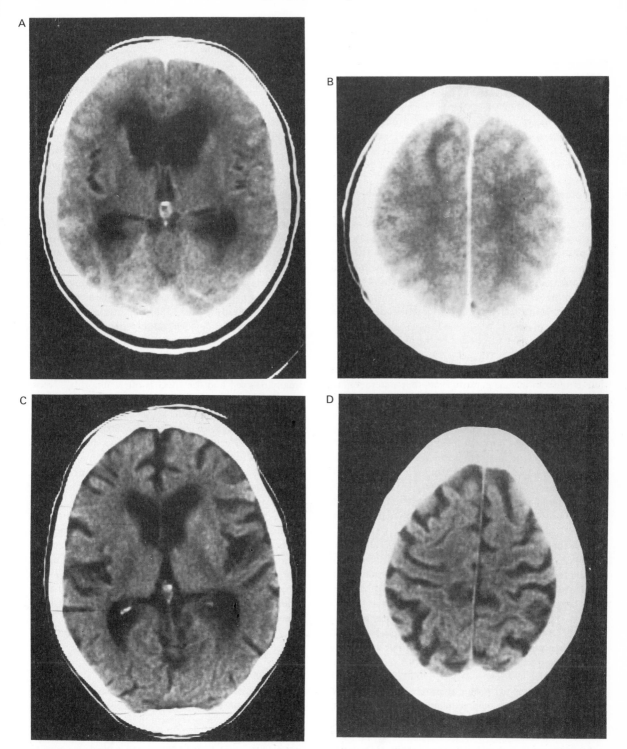

Fig. 12.1 **A** and **B**. Communicating hydrocephalus, axial CT scans. Note the dilated ventricles with periventricular lucencies and the absence of sulci. **C** and **D** (for comparison). Cerebral atrophy in a case of Alzheimer's disease, axial CT scans. Note the dilated ventricles and dilated Sylvian fissures and cortical sulci.

limb girdle weakness. **Fabry's disease** is due to a deficiency of galactosidase and the prominent feature is involvement of small blood vessels involving the brain, the heart and the kidneys. **Refsum's disease** is associated with the deposition of phytanic acid because of a deficiency of phytanic acid hydroxylase. These patients have retinitis pigmentosa, nerve deafness, cerebellar ataxia and polyneuropathy with hypertrophy of peripheral nerves; they may be helped considerably if the diagnosis is made early and the patients are given an appropriate diet low in dietary precursors of phytanic acid.

In **progressive myoclonic epilepsy**, a familial disorder, first described by Unverricht, repeated myoclonic jerking of the face, trunk and limbs of increasing and uncontrollable severity is associated with progressive dementia; this disease, too, is eventually fatal. Pathologically there is degeneration of the dentate nuclei of the cerebellum. In many such cases abnormal mucopolysaccharides can be found in the serum and inclusion bodies (Lafora bodies) may be found in affected cells in the cerebellum and even in voluntary muscle.

THE HEREDITARY ATAXIAS

The hereditary ataxias constitute another heterogenous group of hereditary degenerative conditions in which the predominant characteristic is cerebellar ataxia. Harding (1984) has suggested a clinically useful classification based on a combination of clinical features, particularly the age of onset, the underlying abnormality (particularly in those with a known metabolic cause) and the mode of inheritance.

The **congenital cerebellar ataxias** present in infancy and are usually not progressive. They are due to dysgenesis of parts of the cerebellar system.

Hereditary ataxia associated with metabolic disorders may be intermittent or progressive. The intermittent syndrome may be associated with hyperammonaemia, aminoaciduria (e.g. Hartnup disease) or disorders of pyruvate and lactate metabolism such as occur in Leigh's disease. There is a variety of defects associated with progressive ataxic syndromes and these include abetalipoproteinaemia. There are also a number of ataxic syndromes associated with defective DNA repair such as ataxia telangiectasia (see p. 191).

The other principal group of **progressive ataxic disorders** is those of unknown aetiology and it is likely that in time some of these syndromes will be reclassified as the nature of the underlying abnormality becomes apparent. This group can be divided into those in whom the onset occurs before the age of 20 years (these are usually inherited as an autosomal recessive trait) and those in whom the syndrome presents later in life (these are usually inherited as an autosomal dominant trait).

Friedreich's ataxia is the most common of the early-onset autosomal recessive progressive ataxic disorders. The onset of symptoms is usually in the second decade of life, but may occur earlier. It commonly presents with disequilibrium producing a disturbance of gait followed by limb ataxia and dysarthria. In addition to the signs of cerebellar dysfunction, these patients have pyramidal tract involvement as shown in the early stages by extensor plantar responses and later there may be weakness of corticospinal type in the legs. They also have a peripheral neuropathy with resulting loss of reflexes in the early stages and later there is impairment of joint position and vibration sense, particularly in the legs. Many patients develop nystagmus, optic atrophy and pes cavus. If the condition presents in early childhood, scoliosis is common. About 10% of patients have diabetes mellitus and in most of these it is insulin-dependent. Most patients have ECG abnormalities due to an associated cardiomyopathy, which may lead to heart failure; this is one of the common causes of death in these patients. The responsible gene has now been located on chromosome 9.

The diagnosis of Friedreich's ataxia is usually evident on clinical grounds. The visual evoked responses are usually delayed and the ECG is often abnormal. Nerve conduction studies show marked slowing of the motor conduction velocity and the sensory action potentials are usually undetectable. Friedreich's ataxia is a steadily progressive disorder and most patients depend on a wheelchair in their thirties, but survival may be quite prolonged, early deaths occurring in patients with marked chest deformity, cardiomyopathy and diabetes.

The **autosomal dominant late-onset cerebellar ataxias** (ADCA) may be divided into two types, both of which usually show the pathological features of olivopontocerebellar atrophy at autopsy. ADCA type 1 is associated with dementia, supranuclear ophthalmoplegia, optic atrophy or extrapyramidal features. ADCA type 2 is associated with retinitis pigmentosa, and some of these patients may later develop supranuclear ophthalmoplegia and extrapyramidal features.

HEREDITARY SPASTIC PARAPARESIS (USUALLY CALLED PARAPLEGIA)

On clinical grounds, hereditary spastic paraplegia can be divided into those patients with a pure spastic paraplegia and those in whom the spastic paraplegia is associated with other features; the latter are also a heterogeneous group. The pure hereditary spastic paraplegia may be either autosomal dominant or autosomal recessive. The age of onset is very variable but often runs true within families. The development of symptoms is insidious with the gradual onset of increasing spasticity with relative preservation of power, which is always a sign of chronicity. The upper limbs are usually spared. In the early stages, antispasmodic drugs such as baclofen or dantrolene may be very effective and even in the late stages of the disease these drugs can be useful in reducing flexion spasms.

HEREDITARY NEUROPATHIES

The hereditary neuropathies may also be classified according to the clinical features and method of inheritance.

Hereditary motor and sensory neuropathy type 1 (HMSN-1, peroneal muscular atrophy or Charcot-Marie-Tooth disease)

This is an autosomal dominantly inherited demyelinating neuropathy which usually presents in the late teens or early twenties and presents with weakness of the ankles associated with wasting of the muscles of the lower leg and foot; these patients usually have pes cavus. The small hand muscles are affected early. The condition is slowly progressive but seldom involves the proximal limb muscles, so that patients develop striking wasting and weakness of both lower limbs and of the forearms and hands. Nerve conduction studies show marked slowing of motor conduction and reduced or absent sensory action potentials. The condition usually runs a very benign course; the so-called 'inverted champagne bottle leg' is characteristic and many patients are able to continue walking, despite profound distal weakness and wasting of lower limb muscles, until late life. Appropriate appliances (plastic moulded splints or below knee calipers and toesprings) can be very helpful.

Hereditary motor and sensory neuropathy type 2 (HMSN-2, peroneal muscular atrophy or Charcot-Marie-Tooth disease)

This second form of Charcot-Marie-Tooth disease is also inherited as an autosomal dominant trait but is due to an axonal neuropathy. The age of onset is later, often as late as the fourth or fifth decade, and the rate of progression usually slower. However, muscular wasting and weakness sometimes spread more proximally than in the hypertrophic type. Apart from these clinical features, the two types of Charcot-Marie-Tooth disease can be differentiated on nerve conduction studies, since one is a demyelinating and the other an axonal neuropathy.

Hereditary motor and sensory neuropathy type 3 (HMSN-3, progressive hypertrophic interstitial polyneuropathy or Dejerine-Sottas disease)

This is an autosomal recessively inherited dysmyelinating neuropathy which presents in childhood with distal motor and sensory involvement. The peripheral nerves are usually markedly thickened and this is most easily appreciated in the ulnar nerve and common peroneal nerve. This enlargement is due to proliferation of Schwann cells which form concentric layers around nerve fibres. The condition is steadily progressive but at widely differing rates. Those affected early in childhood often have marked chest deformity and are usually quite severely disabled by late adolescence.

Hereditary sensory neuropathy types 1 and 2 (HSN1 and HSN2)

These two conditions are clinically identical and present in young adults. HSN1 is dominantly inherited and HSN2 is recessive. The condition is due to a neuropathy with degeneration of the dorsal root ganglia and this results in severe sensory impairment distally, particularly in the feet. Perforating neuropathic ulcers are very common and most patients develop Charcot joints. The peripheral nerves are involved in very many genetically determined degenerative conditions including Refsum's disease, ataxia telangiectasia, abetalipoproteinaemia, metachromatic leucodystrophy, Friedreich's ataxia and Fabry's disease. In these conditions, the peripheral neuropathy is one part of a much more extensive clinical picture and these diseases are described elsewhere.

THE NEUROCUTANEOUS DISORDERS (PHAKOMATOSES)

Neurofibromatosis

The two major forms of neurofibromatosis are NF1 (**von Recklinghausen's disease**) and NF2 (**bilateral acoustic neurofibromatosis**). These conditions are clinically and genetically distinct, but both are inherited as autosomal dominant traits.

NF1 has an estimated frequency of 1:4000; there is virtually 100% penetrance and a spontaneous mutation rate of about 50%. The predominant diagnostic features of NF1 are café-au-lait spots on the skin, peripheral neurofibromas, axillary and groin freckling and Lisch nodules (iris hamartomas). Phakomata (round yellow patches about half the size of the optic disc) are sometimes seen in the retina. Macrocephaly frequently accompanies NF1 and short stature is well recognised. The complications of NF1 are legion and occur at random even within families. They range from plexiform subcutaneous neurofibromas sometimes so large as to give the appearance of 'elephantiasis', orthopaedic problems including scoliosis and pseudoarthrosis, to malignancy. Neurological abnormalities include intracranial tumours, particularly gliomas of the optic nerve or elsewhere (see p. 254) and intellectual impairment is found in about 30% of patients. Hamartomatous lesions have been reported in the form of glial heterotopias, intramedullary schwannosis, meningiomatosis and angiomatosis. NF1 is associated with developmental abnormalities including syringomyelia, lateral thoracic meningocele, aqueductal stenosis and grey matter heterotopia which is usually associated with developmental delay. Epileptic seizures occur more commonly than in the general population. Multiple tumours of the peripheral nerves are pathognomonic of the disorder and are usually neurofibromas, although schwannomas can occur. Spinal neurofibromas may cause cord or cauda equina compression (Fig. 12.2), and phaeochromocytomas are a rare complication. Even in the absence of evidence of spinal cord compression, a characteristic concave 'scalloping' of the posterior borders of the vertebral bodies can be seen in spinal radiographs. The gene for NF1 has been located on the long arm of chromosome 17 by genetic linkage analysis.

NF2 is also inherited as an autosomal dominant trait with over 95% penetrance. The hallmark of the disorder is bilateral acoustic neuromas; symptoms, usually loss of hearing, begin in the teens or early twenties. The cutaneous stigmata found in NF1 are much less prominent. Central nervous system tumours are common in NF2 and include meningiomas, gliomas and schwannomas. Juvenile posterior subcapsular lenticular opacities are also found. Linkage analysis has established that the inherited gene for NF2 is on the long arm of chromosome 22.

Tuberous sclerosis

This condition is inherited as an autosomal dominant trait but many cases are due to a new mutation. The typical clinical features include epilepsy, mental retardation and adenoma sebaceum. The epilepsy is due to small firm nodules over the surface of the brain which

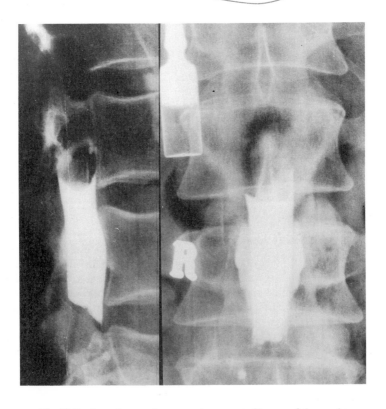

Fig. 12.2   A myelogram demonstrating a neurofibroma of the cauda equina. (Reproduced with permission from Walton 1985.)

may be quite numerous and these nodules may also be found in the white matter and in the periventricular regions. These nodules are aggregations of atypical glial cells; they frequently calcify and can then be easily identified on a CT brain scan. Even in the absence of calcification, an irregular ventricular outline can be reasonably diagnostic. Other cerebral malformations include neuronal heterotopias and microgyria. A small proportion of patients develop gliomas.

The condition usually presents in infancy with epilepsy and mental retardation. Some patients presenting with infantile spasms (p. 80) eventually turn out to have this condition. The skin manifestation, adenoma sebaceum, usually develops later as small discrete spots on the face, particularly around the mouth. These are not true adenomata but are small hamartomas. Other cutaneous manifestations include hypopigmented patches, which may be from a few millimetres to a few centimetres in diameter and may only become apparent when the skin is examined under Wood's light. Shagreen patches may also be found, usually in the lumbosacral region, and appear as a brownish elevated area of thickened skin. Café-au-lait spots and subungal fibromata also occur. Hamartomas (phakomata) may be found in the retina.

The diagnosis may not be apparent in an infant presenting with epilepsy and retardation since the cutaneous manifestations usually develop later and the EEG, although usually abnormal, has no characteristic features. However, a CT scan shows the widespread nodules, often best seen in the walls of the ventricles. In older children the presence of typical cutaneous manifestations makes the diagnosis obvious. In such cases the epileptic seizures are often intractable despite optimal anticonvulsant therapy. Many patients require institutional care and some die prematurely from gliomas.

Ataxia telangiectasia (the Louis-Bar syndrome)

This autosomal recessive condition presents in infancy with ataxia and mental retardation. The telangiectases may be found in the conjunctiva. Most of these patients have reduced or absent immunoglobulins, and in consequence are highly susceptible to infections from which many patients die in adolescence.

PARKINSON'S DISEASE

'An essay on the shaking palsy' was published by James Parkinson in 1817 and he described six patients with the syndrome which has been known ever since as Parkinson's disease or **paralysis agitans**. Three of these patients were only observed in the street and none were examined, so although James Parkinson recognised most of the

principal features of this condition, he mistook the bradykinesia for weakness and thought that the problem must lie in the high cervical spine. It was over 100 years before the involvement of the basal ganglia was recognised and only in the past two decades have the underlying biochemical abnormalities been elucidated.

Parkinson's disease is characterised by bradykinesia, rigidity, tremor and loss of postural reflexes. These features are the clinical mainfestations of degeneration of the dopaminergic pathways in the brain. All neuronal systems that depend on dopamine as a neurotransmitter are affected and although these are quite widely distributed throughout the brain, they are concencentrated in the basal ganglia and substantia nigra (Fig. 12.3). There is severe depletion of dopamine with an associated neuronal cell loss in the substantia nigra and, via the nigrostriatal pathways, a similar reduction in dopamine in the striatum, particularly the caudate nucleus and the putamen. The degenerative changes are associated with Lewy bodies; these intracellular, spherical, hyaline inclusion bodies are absolutely characteristic of Parkinson's disease but are not thought to be pathognomonic of it.

As with all degenerative conditions, the onset is insidious and by the time the patient seeks medical advice it is usually possible to establish a history of some months or even years. It most frequently presents in the fifties and sixties and affects both sexes. It may, however, occur at almost any age, though it is rather rare under the age of 30. Parkinson's disease usually presents in one of two ways, either with tremor or with bradykinesia and rigidity. As the condition slowly evolves, all the characteristic features of this disease become apparent.

The tremor of Parkinson's disease is characteristically seen at rest (static tremor) and nearly always starts in one arm and hand, but as it becomes more prominent so it may involve the feet, head and lips. It is virtually abolished by voluntary movement and for this reason, by itself, it has little effect on function, in striking contrast to the intention tremor of cerebellar disease which is absent at rest and becomes more prominent with co-ordinated movement. However, many patients with Parkinson's disease do have a fine action tremor which persists during movement but is not exacerbated by it. The tremor is typically rhythmical at about 6 per second, most frequently affecting the pronators and supinators of the forearm, and when this is combined with flexion and extension movements of the fingers, produces the well-recognised pill-rolling effect. As with all disturbances in motor function, the tremor is accentuated by stress and excitement.

The rigidity of Parkinson's disease is quite characteristic; it is present throughout the range of movement and in both directions of movement and is most easily appreciated in forearm pronation and supination. In the early stages it is often only found in one arm, but becomes more generalised with advancing disease.

Bradykinesia (slowness of movement) and difficulty in initiating movement (akinesia) are two of the striking features of Parkinson's disease and are not just due to the rigidity. The loss of facial expression, the monotonous low volume speech, the paucity of associated limb movements, often most obvious in walking, are all manifestations of this problem which are far more disabling than the tremor. The handwriting typically becomes much smaller (micrographia).

The loss of postural reflexes causes a considerable problem for patients with Parkinson's disease because of the tendency to fall which may occur as the patient intends to take a step forward, has difficulty in initiating this movement but nevertheless leans forward in anticipation, shifting the centre of gravity, and then falls over. The same thing occurs at the end of a run of festinant gait, a series of quick shuffling steps. James Parkinson described a particularly notable example of this in one of the patients whom he observed in the street.

As the disease slowly progresses, so all the typical features become apparent with an unblinking mask-like facies, a slight tendency to drool saliva because of difficulty in the control of saliva and not due to increased production, a low volume monotonous speech, some difficulty in swallowing, a stooping posture with lack of associated movements, a short shuffling gait with difficulty in initiating movement and the characteristic rest tremor.

In addition, many patients with Parkinson's disease develop some autonomic dysfunction with difficulty in controlling body temperature resulting in inappropriately profuse sweating, sometimes with orthostatic hypotension and sphincter disturbance. Despite their appearance, patients with Parkinson's disease do not have intellectual impairment in the early stages, but eventually a high proportion show evidence of cognitive perceptual and memory deficits and a small proportion develop a profound dementia, probably due to Alzheimer's disease. Recent work using monoclonal antibody staining for the protein ubiquitin, now known to be present in Lewy bodies, has shown, unexpectedly, that in demented

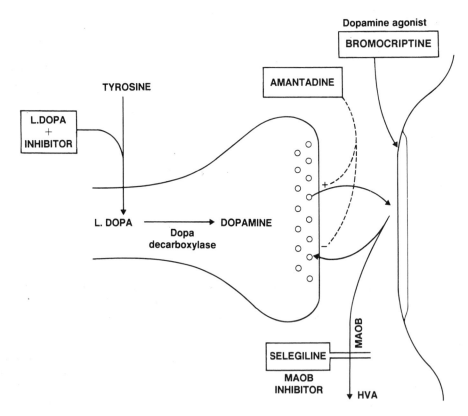

Fig. 12.3   Diagram of a dopaminergic nerve terminal to show the site of action of the principal drugs used in the treatment of Parkinson's disease (see text for details).

patients such Lewy bodies are found to be widespread throughout the cerebral cortex.

Differential diagnosis

The form of post-encephalitic parkinsonism which developed as a sequel to encephalitis lethargica in the 1920s has now virtually disappeared. In that condition the onset of the disease was generally earlier and progress more rapid than in the idiopathic variety. Limb contractures and dystonia often developed in advanced cases, along with emotional lability, dementia and psychiatric features such as paranoia and delusions. Oculogyric crises occurred only in this variety; these took the form of attacks of involuntary upward conjugate movement of the eyes with retraction of the upper lids and sometimes tilting backwards of the head (retrocollis). Clinical features superficially similar to those of parkinsonism can result from repeated head injury (the 'punch drunk syndrome' in professional boxers and steeplechase jockeys), in manganese poisoning, as a sequel to anoxia or in so-called atherosclerotic parkinsonism. The latter condition, seen usually in elderly hypertensive subjects with diffuse small vessel disease, gives some facial masking and stiffness of the limbs with a slow shuffling gait but without tremor. The plantar responses are usually extensor and signs of pseudo-bulbar palsy generally develop.

Treatment

Parkinson's disease requires continuous management from the time of diagnosis. There is no treatment available at the moment which alters the progress of the disease so that the management of the condition has to be seen against the background of a condition which is inevitably progressive. Unfortunately all the available drugs may be associated with considerable side-effects which limit their use. Since all treatment for this condition is symptomatic, there is no absolute necessity to start treatment as soon as the diagnosis is made, though usually by the time the patient seeks medical advice some treatment is needed. The drug treatment of Parkinson's disease falls into two groups, i.e. manipulation either of the dopaminergic system or of the cholinergic system. Some of the features of parkinsonism appear to be due to the imbalance between these two systems rather than just to depletion of dopamine.

Dopamine is synthesised in the nerve terminal from dopa by the action of dopa decarboxylase. Dopa in turn is formed from phenylalanine and tyrosine. Dopamine given orally would never reach the systemic circulation in significant concentrations, let alone the brain; it is possible to give dopa by mouth, although only levodopa crosses the blood-brain barrier; dextradopa is excluded, which is the reason for giving the levo isomer. About 90% of the drug when given orally is broken down outside the nervous system so that very large doses are required to achieve a useful concentration in the brain. For this reason, levodopa is given in combination with a dopa-decarboxylase inhibitor which itself does not cross the blood-brain barrier. This considerably reduces the breakdown of dopa outside the nervous system and therefore makes a much higher proportion of an orally administered dose available to the brain. Two dopa-decarboxylase inhibitors are available, benserazide which in combination with levodopa is marketed as Madopar®, and carbidopa which in combination with levodopa is marketed as Sinemet®.

Once dopamine has been released from the nerve terminal vesicles and has become attached to the receptor site, it is either taken up into the nerve terminal or cleared from the area by monoaminoxidase-B. The effect of the dopamine released can be enhanced by partially blocking its re-uptake which can be achieved with amantadine, an anti-viral agent which may also promote the release of dopamine. The alternative is to block the clearance of dopamine by inhibiting the monoamine-oxidase-B with selegiline. The final option in manipulation of the dopaminergic system is to treat the patient with a dopamine agonist which acts directly on the dopamine receptor; there are a number of such drugs available, but the only one widely used is bromocriptine.

The dopaminergic input to the striatum is normally in balance with the intrinsic striatal cholinergic system and many of the features of parkinsonism can be improved with anticholinergic drugs, of which the most widely used are benzhexol and orphenadrine.

Before the introduction of levodopa in the late 1960s, many patients with Parkinson's disease underwent stereotactic thalamotomy. This operation can be strikingly effective in controlling tremor but has little or no effect on bradykinesia and rigidity. It is now only rarely performed but retains a definite place for the younger patient with striking unilateral tremor but little or no bradykinesia and rigidity and no other contraindications such as hypertension. The use of surgery in these few patients may make it possible to delay the introduction of medication for some years.

There is some difference of opinion about the desirability of starting treatment with levodopa early or delaying it for as long as possible. After some years of levodopa therapy, patients develop side-effects, mostly dyskinetic movements and marked swings in performance known as the on-off phenomenon. This did not occur in parkinsonian patients before the introduction of levodopa and it is not known whether it is due to the drug itself or to the administration of the drug at a late stage in the disease. Until this question is satisfactorily answered, it seems prudent to delay starting treatment with levodopa for as long as possible in younger patients, but in older patients this is not necessary. In younger patients, particularly those with a tremor but little rigidity or bradykinesia, it is therefore reasonable to start treatment with an anticholinergic drug such as benzhexol or orphenadrine, though the side-effects of a dry mouth and blurred vision may limit the dose. These drugs should be used with caution in patients with glaucoma or prostatic symptoms. In younger patients with bradykinesia and rigidity but little or no tremor, anticholinergic drugs are less effective and treatment should be started with amantadine or selegiline in order to improve the intrinsic dopamine effect. Although a good initial response often occurs, it is seldom maintained. Starting treatment with levodopa should not therefore be unreasonably delayed.

Ideally, sufficient peripheral decarboxylase inhibitor should be given to block this enzyme's activity, and then sufficient levodopa to produce the clinical response. About 60–80 mg of inhibitor are required each day so that if small doses of levodopa are given, a preparation containing a 4:1 ratio of levodopa to inhibitor should be used (all the forms of Madopar® and Sinemet® Plus). If larger doses of levodopa are required, it may be more appropriate to use a 10:1 ratio (Sinemet 275). The therapeutic half-life of levodopa given orally is around three to four hours and this seems to shrink with time. This short half-life is the basis for many of the problems associated with the use of levodopa. If a large dose is given infrequently, the blood level rapidly rises to the point at which side-effects become evident and this is usually shown by the development of dyskinetic movements, which may be orofacial or may affect the limbs. These side-effects come on within 10–15 minutes of a dose and may continue for half an hour to an hour. As the blood level falls through the therapeutic range, the patient's symptoms may be under very satisfactory control with few side-effects, but after three to four hours the symptoms of Parkinson's disease start to reappear. This apparent fluctuation in response to levodopa is appropriately known as the 'peak-trough' effect. It is much less of a problem in the early stages of treatment but can become a major difficulty as the years go by. It can be minimised by giving multiple smaller doses throughout the day. The interval between doses need not necessarily be uniform since the response of most patients to oral levodopa does seem to vary throughout the day. After some years of treatment, most patients learn how to use this drug effectively and can be taught to observe the fluctuations in response.

As the disease progresses, the 'therapeutic window' seems to become narrower, peak-trough effects become more difficult to manage and the response to medication is less satisfactory. Most patients prefer to be slightly overdosed, with clinically evident dyskinesia, than to be underdosed, since when slightly overdosed they are much more mobile and therefore more functional, although the dyskinetic movements may be a source of embarrassment both to the patients and to their relatives. It should be noted that the few surviving patients with post-encephalitic parkinsonism are often peculiarly sensitive to levodopa and can sometimes tolerate very small doses only.

Every attempt should be made to optimise the dose of levodopa before adding any further medication. The addition of selegiline boosts the effects of each dose by about 20% and may allow longer intervals between doses. When selegiline is first added to the regime it is usually necessary to reduce the dose of levodopa to compensate for this effect. The addition of amantadine may also have a beneficial effect, although this response is often less evident after a year to 18 months.

Some authorities advocate the use of the dopamine agonist bromocriptine early in the course of treatment, but it is not known whether this avoids long-term problems with levodopa. Most clinicians use bromocriptine in the end-stage of the disease. A test dose of 1.25 mg should be given at night because a number of patients develop profound postural hypotension on bromocriptine. If this does not occur, the dose can be increased progressively and it is reasonable to establish the patient on 10 mg three times a day since it has a half-life of around eight hours. Levodopa can then be added to produce the optimum clinical response.

Physiotherapy and occupational therapy can be extremely valuable in improving the performance of patients with Parkinson's disease, though unfortunately the response is often short-lived unless the therapy is continued indefinitely.

SYRINGOMYELIA

Syringomyelia is a chronic and usually progressive disorder in which cavitation develops within the central grey matter of the spinal cord. This usually starts in the cervical cord and may extend over many segments. The clinical features are those of a central cord lesion with interruption of the reflex arc and impairment of pain and temperature appreciation due to involvement of the decussating fibres passing from the dorsal root entry zone to the spinothalamic tract on the other side of the spinal cord. As the cavitation becomes more extensive, so the anterior horn cells are involved and much later the lateral columns with involvement of the pyramidal tracts. The posterior columns are relatively preserved until the late stages of the disease.

In most patients this cavitation arises from a localised diverticulum of the central canal which then tracks up and down in the central grey matter, so that most transverse cord sections show a cavity alongside the central canal without an obvious connection, unless the section happens to pass through the diverticulum. These cavities contain CSF, and ependymal cells may be found in the walls, showing that they arise from the central canal. This appears to be a complication of a congenital anomaly at the craniocervical junction with prolapse of the cerebellar tonsils through the foramen magnum so that they come to lie posterolateral to the spinal cord. This is associated with obstruction to the foramina of Magendie and Lushka so that the respiratory and pulse pressure waves which displace CSF from the fourth ventricle through these foramina into the cisterna magna are instead transmitted down a patent central canal. A similar complication may follow arachnoiditis involving these foramina. Although this mechanism (communicating syringomyelia) accounts for the majority of patients with this condition, there are a number with syringomyelia who have no evidence of any anomaly at the craniocervical junction.

Syringomyelic cavities may also follow localised trauma to the spinal cord and were first recognised in the First World War following bullet and shrapnel injuries. In such cases they often extend upwards from the site of the cord lesion. They are more commonly seen now as a complication of extramedullary spinal cord tumours such as meningioma. How trauma and cord compression cause central cord cavitation is still obscure.

The initial symptoms are usually sensory; the patient becomes aware of an area of abnormal sensation, often around the shoulder girdle or in the arm. Sometimes the patient may notice that minor injuries to the hand, such as a burn when cooking, are not painful or that the temperature of bath water feels different on the two sides. If the cavitation starts in the upper cervical cord, the only physical sign may be impairment of pain and temperature (**dissociated anaesthesia**) over the back of the neck and across the shoulder. If it involves the middle cervical region a more extensive half-cape distribution of sensory impairment is found, associated with absent reflexes in the affected arm. Wasting of the small hand muscles may be found and occasionally patients present with a progressive loss of use of the hand. Extension of the syrinx into the medulla (**syringobulbia**) causes dissociated sensory loss in a 'balaclava helmet' distribution, with relative sparing of the snout area; this is due to involvement of the descending tract of the trigeminal nerve which extends down into the upper cervical region; the snout area relays largely to the main sensory nucleus in mid-pons. There may also be nystagmus, atrophy of one side of the tongue, and involvement of the sternomastoid and trapezius as well as weakness of palatal, pharyngeal and laryngeal muscles. There may also be a central Horner's syndrome.

As the disease progresses, so the area of dissociated sensory loss enlarges and wasting and weakness extend to involve most of the upper limb. Involvement of the lateral columns including the pyramidal tract causes a spastic paraparesis; initially there may be an extensor plantar response only, and as the disease progresses the more obvious signs of spasticity and pyramidal weakness develop. Involvement of Clarke's column may affect bladder function. Light touch and joint position sense are preserved until the very late stages of the disease.

Syringomyelia is the commonest cause of neurogenic arthropathy (**Charcot joint**) affecting the shoulder; the elbows and wrists may also be affected. The joint is very swollen with painless crepitus on movement and X-rays show gross disorganisation of the joint, loss of the head of the humerus and new bone formation (Fig. 12.4).

The clinical picture is usually sufficiently typical by the time the patient seeks medical advice so that diagnosis presents little difficulty. Plain X-rays of the craniocervical junction may show a congenital abnormality but are usually unhelpful. Magnetic resonance imaging is the investigation of choice, since this will show not only the tonsillar ectopia and the position of the fourth ventricle but will also show the size of the ventricles as a number of these patients have hydrocephalus; it may also show a cavity within the cord (Fig. 12.5). If this investigation is not available, a CT scan will show the size of the ventricles and thin axial slices through the foramen magnum may show descent of the tonsils alongside the upper cervical cord. A supine myelogram may also show the tonsillar ectopia as well as a swollen cord which is sometimes atrophic below the level of the syrinx. With large cavities and air as contrast medium, it may be possible to demonstrate a fluctuation in the size of the cord with tilting.

If an Arnold-Chiari malformation is demonstrated, and provided that there is no evidence of arachnoiditis, most patients will profit from a decompressive operation in which the foramen magnum is enlarged posteriorly and a laminectomy is carried out of C1 and C2. This procedure does not, however, improve the drainage of CSF from the fourth ventricle in the presence of arachnoiditis. In some cases it may be possible to drain large cavities with benefit.

The purpose of these procedures is to prevent further deterioration, though some patients do show some improvement especially when operated upon early in the course of the disease. It is therefore important to determine that the patient is actually deteriorating before proceeding to surgical intervention, which does carry an immediate perioperative risk. Not all patients with syringomyelia show progression of the disease and in some patients the condition remains static for many years.

SPINAL DYSRAPHISM AND SPINA BIFIDA

The neural tube evolves from a flat plate to a closed tube, separated from the skin by mesoderm, between the twentieth and thirtieth day of gestation. Failure of this fusion can cause a variety of defects and these may be associated with a number of other congenital abnormalities. The simplest form of spinal dysraphism is spina bifida occulta which is due to the failure of fusion of the spinal arches; this is quite a common abnormality in the lower lumbar and sacral regions and is not usually associated with any other malformation or neurological deficit. The failure of dorsal fusion may extend over several segments and may then be associated with cutaneous manifestations, sometimes only a hairy patch on the overlying skin and sometimes a blind sinus. There may be an associated intraspinal lipoma. Diastematomyelia may also occur; in this condition the spinal cord is split around a central bony spicule and the cord is often tethered distally. An even more extensive defect may be associated with a protrusion of the meninges through the defect presenting on the surface as a cyst and this cyst may contain spinal nerve roots and is known as a **meningocele**. If the spinal cord enters the cyst it is known as a **meningomyelocele**.

The greater the degree of abnormality, the greater the neurological deficit. Meningoceles are not necessarily associated with a neurological deficit although this is usually the case, while meningomyeloceles are always associated with significant neurological abnormalities, usually including loss of bowel and bladder sphincter control as well as weakness and sensory loss in the legs. Even in cases of occult spina bifida the presence of an intradural lipoma, of diastematomyelia or of a fibrous band tethering the cord with consequential stretching or compression of nerve roots can give neurological signs, such as deformity of one foot with localised weakness and sensory loss.

Most children with meningomyelocele also have hydrocephalus, either in association with an Arnold-Chiari malformation or aqueduct stenosis, so that closure of the defect in the lumbar region has to be accompanied by a shunting procedure to relieve the hydrocephalus.

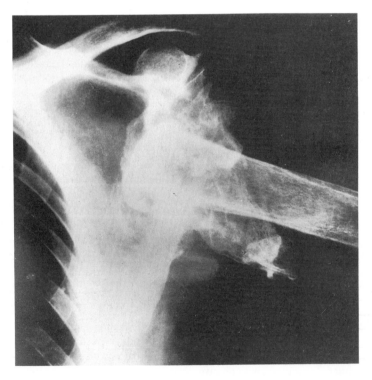

Fig. 12.4 Charcot's arthropathy involving the left shoulder joint in a patient with syringomyelia. (Reproduced with permission from Walton 1985.)

The diagnosis of spina bifida in its various forms can now be made early in pregnancy by ultrasound scanning and by amniocentesis for α-fetoprotein estimation in the amniotic fluid, thus allowing termination of a pregnancy of a severely affected fetus if that is the parents' wish. The criteria of selection of children for early surgery has aroused considerable controversy over the years; no general guidelines can be given and it is a matter which has to be discussed with the parents and considered carefully in each individual case. The more severely affected children will require many years of repeated operations for hydrocephalus and the associated problems of maintaining a shunt, procedures for bowel and bladder control as well as the treatment of limb deformities. However, techniques are improving all the time in all these areas and the less severely affected patients can now achieve a quality of life which is very much better than it was in the past.

Some patients with spinal dysraphism do not present until they are much older and then show progressive clinical deterioration. These patients should be investigated with magnetic resonance imaging or myelography. Abnormalities found in these patients include lipomata, diastematomyelia, tethered cords and dermoid cysts, all of which can be treated surgically with varying degrees of success.

BASILAR IMPRESSION OF THE SKULL

A congenital malformation of the occipital condyles of the skull can lead to the partial invagination of the first cervical vertebra into the foramen magnum. This results in an upward movement of the odontoid process of the axis with consequent compression of the lower cranial nerves, cerebellar tonsils, upper cervical nerve roots and the upper part of the spinal cord. In such individuals the neck is unusually short and there are typical radiological appearances. Thus the body of the atlas vertebra is tilted in relation to the skull and in lateral skull radiographs the tip of the odontoid process extends above a line drawn

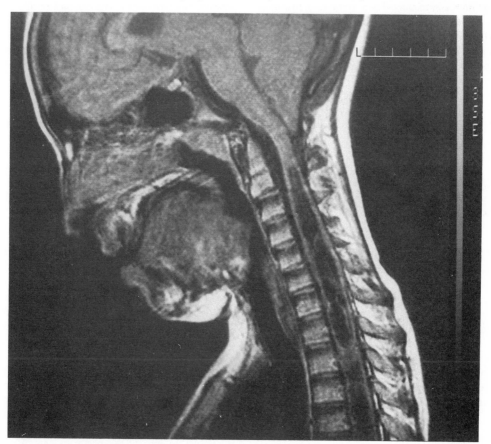

Fig. 12.5 Syringomyelia. Sagittal MRI, T1 weighted, to show a large cervical syrinx with tonsillar ectopia.

from the posterior margin of the hard palate to the posterior border of the foramen magnum (Chamberlain's line). The clinical features are variable in degree and severity, but include hydrocephalus (due to partial obstruction of CSF circulation through exit foramina of the fourth ventricle and basal cisterns), cerebellar ataxia in the limbs, and a spastic quadriparesis with posterior column involvement often giving severe loss of position and joint sense in both hands. Sometimes syringomyelia also develops. The clinical features of the condition can be mimicked by separation of the odontoid process from the axis vertebra, an occasional complication of rheumatoid arthritis. Once symptoms and signs have appeared they tend to progress, but the condition may be alleviated by surgical decompression, involving removal of the posterior border of the foramen magnum or excision of the odontoid peg. The syndrome is often called platybasia, as the skull base is flattened, but there are other causes of radiological platybasia (e.g. Paget's disease — see below). Basilar impression may be associated with congenital anomalies of the cervical spine (e.g. fusion of multiple cervical vertebrae — the Klippel-Feil syndrome), while such anomalies can in turn be associated with features suggesting a lesion in the neighbourhood of the foramen magnum, even when no significant degree of basilar impression is present. Mirror movements (a voluntary movement in one hand is copied involuntarily by the other) are common in cases of the latter type.

PAGET'S DISEASE AND OTHER SKELETAL ABNORMALITIES

The progressive thickening and distortion of bone which occurs in Paget's disease of the skull can produce neurological manifestations. Thus optic atrophy may result from compression of the optic nerves in their exit foramina and other cranial nerves can be similarly involved. Deafness due to eighth nerve involvement is particularly common. As a result of the platybasia caused by the disease, a clinical picture resembling basilar impression may develop. Other rare bony disorders which may give rise to overgrowth of skull and facial bones with consequent cranial nerve palsies include **leontiasis ossea** and **polyostotic fibrous dysplasia**. Paget's disease of the vertebral column is occasionally responsible for a progressive paraplegia due to spinal cord compression and a similar syndrome occurs infrequently in **achondroplasia**.

CRANIOSTENOSIS

This is an uncommon congenital abnormality due to premature fusion of the cranial bony sutures. It is characterised by an abnormal shape of the skull, optic atrophy, exophthalmos, and signs of increased intracranial pressure. Neurosurgical treatment (separation of the fused cranial bones) is often required early in life.

FACIAL HEMIATROPHY

This uncommon disorder of unknown aetiology (often called the Parry-Romberg syndrome) gives rise to a progressive atrophy of subcutaneous tissue, muscle, bone, and cartilage on one half of the face. Occasionally there is associated atrophy of the ipsilateral cerebral hemisphere.

VASCULAR MALFORMATIONS

Many developmental vascular anomalies of the nervous system have been described. The intracranial **arteriovenous angioma**, which is one of the commonest, will be considered in Chapter 17. **Arteriovenous malformations** (AVM) may also occur in the spinal canal. These either arise in the dura (dural AVM) or in the spinal cord itself (intramedullary AVM). These malformations may first be shown on magnetic resonance imaging or myelography and are often associated with markedly dilated veins over the surface of the spinal cord (see p. 280). The definitive investigation to define their full extent is angiography by selective catheterisation. The dural malformations are readily amenable to surgery or may be occluded at the time of the angiography by the injection of thrombotic material or selective embolisation. The treatment of intramedullary malformations is very much more difficult since the spinal cord derives its blood supply from the same vessels as the malformation and, therefore, any attempt to treat these lesions is usually associated with a substantial residual neurological deficit. Like intracranial arteriovenous malformations, spinal malformations present with subarachnoid haemorrhage or with neurological symptoms and signs which may be slowly progressive or episodic.

Another type of congenital malformation of small blood vessels in the brain stem (telangiectasia) can give rise to pontine or medullary haemorrhages and this may present as a rapidly evolving space-occupying lesion. Some of these patients improve markedly following surgical drainage of the haematoma.

One unusual but stereotyped cerebral vascular malformation is the **Sturge-Weber syndrome**. In this condition a subcortical angiomatosis of precapillaries, a lesion which eventually becomes calcified after a few years of life to give a characteristic radiological pattern outlining the gyri of the posterior part of one cerebral hemisphere, is associated with a port-wine naevus of the face on the same side. Often the eye on this side is also enlarged (buphthalmos or ox-eye). Usually these patients show a contralateral infantile hemiplegia and suffer from recurrent epileptiform convulsions. Some cases can be helped by removal of most of the affected cerebral hemisphere (hemispherectomy).

REFERENCES

Adams R D, Lyon G 1982 Neurology of hereditary metabolic diseases of children. McGraw-Hill, Washington

Adams R D, Victor M 1985 Principles of neurology, 3rd edn. McGraw-Hill, New York

Barnett H J M, Foster J B, Hudgson P 1973 Syringomyelia and other cord cavities. Major problems in neurology, Vol 1 (Walton J, series ed). Saunders, London

Calne D B 1970 Parkinsonism. Arnold, London

Fenichel G 1987 Neonatal neurology, 2nd edn. Churchill Livingstone, Edinburgh

Gamstorp I 1985 Paediatric neurology, 2nd edn. Butterworth, London

Gordon N, Schutt W 1976 Paediatric neurology for the clinician. Spastics International Medical Publications, Heinemann, London

Harding A E 1981 Friedreich's ataxia: a clinical and genetic study of 90 families with an analysis of early diagnostic criteria and intrafamilial clustering of clinical features. Brain 104: 589

Harding A E 1984 The hereditary ataxias and related disorders. Churchill Livingstone, Edinburgh

James C C M , Lassman L P 1972 Spinal dysraphism. Butterworth, London

Menkes J H 1985 Textbook of child neurology, 3rd edn. Lea & Febiger, Philadelphia

Riccardi V M , Mulvihill J J (eds) 1981 Neurofibromatosis: genetics, cell biology and chemistry. Advances in neurology, Vol 29. Raven Press, New York

Rosenberg R N 1986 Neurogenetics: principles and practice. Raven Press, New York

Walton J N 1985 Brain's diseases of the nervous system, 9th edn. Oxford University Press, Oxford

Yahr M D, Bergmann K J (eds) 1985 Parkinson's disease. Advances in neurology, Vol 45. Raven Press, New York

13. Trauma and the nervous system

The function of the various parts of the central and peripheral nervous system can be gravely disturbed by physical injury. Although penetrating wounds of the brain, spinal cord and peripheral nerves are often seen in war-time, they are relatively uncommon in civil practice. Nevertheless, closed head injuries (in which the skull is not penetrated), resulting from road, domestic and industrial accidents, are a major problem. Although the finer points of diagnosis and management in cases of severe craniocerebral injury are largely a matter for the neurosurgeon, every physician, accident surgeon and general practitioner requires a working knowledge of the nosology of the different types of head injury, of their clinical course and of their sequelae. To refer all patients with minor head injuries for neurosurgical advice would impose an impossible load upon these special units and it is essential that the physician or surgeon who may care for these patients initially should be able to recognise major complications. It may also be difficult to decide in an individual case whether neurological symptoms and signs have resulted from a head injury or whether the initial event had been a cerebral vascular accident, say, due to which the patient had fallen and injured the head. The clinical syndromes produced by injury to or compression of the spinal cord and peripheral nerves can also present difficult problems in diagnosis and management. This chapter will therefore deal first with head injuries, their effects, complications and sequelae, secondly with injury to the spinal cord, and thirdly with peripheral nerve lesions.

HEAD INJURIES

The immediate effects of head injury may be classified into three principal groups which are first, concussion, a temporary and largely reversible disorder of brain function which is not apparently associated with any striking pathological change in the brain; secondly, cerebral contusion or laceration, in which there is direct bruising or tearing of brain tissue; and thirdly, intracranial haemorrhage, either from tearing of the middle meningeal artery or its branches following skull fracture (extradural haemorrhage), subdural haematoma, which results from an injury to veins traversing the subdural space, and intracerebral haemorrhage or traumatic subarachnoid haemorrhage which often accompany cerebral contusion or laceration.

Concussion

There have been many attempts to explain the phenomenon of concussion; this produces the syndrome of impaired consciousness which follows a closed head injury. Probably it is due to a transitory disturbance of function in the brain stem reticular substance. Concussion can occur with or without skull fracture. Uncomplicated concussion most often results from blunt head injuries but even these may cause unexpected areas of focal brain haemorrhage or laceration, particularly in elderly patients suffering relatively minor blows to the head producing little or no impairment of consciousness. Depressed fractures of the skull (such as those produced by sharp, localised blows resulting, say, from a missile) may be associated with severe local brain injury but yet consciousness may not be lost. Extensive linear skull fractures are sometimes found in patients showing only the clinical features of concussion; on the other hand they too can be associated with contusion or laceration (see below) of the subjacent brain.

The patient who recovers from concussion is usually unable to recall the actual moment of injury and indeed his memory is often blank for several preceding seconds or much longer. The duration of this **retrograde amnesia** is not a satisfactory guide to the severity of the injury; much more reliable in this respect is the duration of the **post-traumatic amnesia** (i.e. the period for which memory is lost after the accident, corresponding to the duration of the concussion). Usually this period is much longer than that of observed unconsciousness. After a relatively severe injury the patient may be comatose with shallow, slow respiration, a feeble pulse, and widely dilated pupils; during recovery, after minutes or even several hours the pupils react, the pulse becomes stronger and the patient responsive. For some time, however, he is restless, confused and irritable, complains of headache and may vomit repeatedly. When coma is complete for more than a few hours it is likely that the injury has been more serious than simple concussion. Following a less severe injury the patient may merely be dazed for some minutes or hours and may undertake purposive activities of which he subsequently has no recollection; generalised headache and vomiting are common at this stage. Most patients recover from mild or moderate concussion within a few days or weeks, but headaches and other symptoms of the post-traumatic syndrome (see below) sometimes persist for weeks or months and occasionally for years.

Contusion and laceration

Cerebral contusion may take the form of localised bruising of the brain directly beneath the point of impact in a closed head injury. Alternatively, a contusion, or a laceration, which can be similarly produced, though it can, of course, result from a penetrating wound, may occur on the side of the brain opposite to the site of injury, due to a sudden thrust of the relatively mobile brain against the inner table of the skull (contrecoup injury). For example, injury to the frontal lobes or the anterior part of the temporal lobes can result from a blow to the back of the head. The term contusion has also been applied to a generalised cerebral disturbance more severe than concussion in which there are multiple small intracerebral haemorrhages as well as diffuse cerebral oedema, changes which result at least in part from a sudden violent movement of CSF along perivascular meningeal cuffs which penetrate the brain along the blood vessels. Mild and transient concussion on the one hand and this more severe form of pathological change (which may lead to irreversible demyelination in central cerebral white matter and other degenerative changes in the cortex) on the other, represent the two extremes of a continuum of severity. In the more severe cases the diffuse oedema which often develops immediately after the injury can be reduced by drugs, such as dexamethasone, by osmotic agents such as mannitol or by hypocapnia produced by hyperventilation.

The patient with a severe cerebral contusion is usually unconscious immediately, but becomes progressively more deeply comatose until he dies from respiratory and later cardiac arrest due to brain stem haemorrhage or infarction or medullary compression. Some patients remain unconscious and unresponsive but can neverthe-

less be kept alive for many weeks or months by careful nursing and sometimes by assisted respiration in what is often referred to as a persistent vegetative state. Usually in patients who show no significant recovery of awareness within a week from the time of injury there has been a degree of damage to the cerebral white matter or to the brain stem reticular substance which is incompatible with complete recovery; in rare instances, however, patients have recovered, though with considerable intellectual impairment, after months of unconsciousness. In less severely injured cases, there is often a period of several days during which the patient is comatose or semicomatose. There may be signs indicating damage to the brain stem (decerebrate posture and spasms, cranial nerve palsies) or to one or other cerebral hemisphere (focal convulsions, or hemiplegia), though these are often difficult to identify while the patient is unconscious. With returning awareness comes the stage of traumatic delirium, in which the patient may be noisy, unco-operative, confused and even violent. It is at this stage that symptoms or signs of focal brain damage often become apparent. Gradually, as improvement continues, the patient becomes more rational and orientated, though headache commonly persists, and symptoms of the post-traumatic syndrome appear. There may also be persisting aphasia, paralysis or cranial nerve palsies if the local injury has been sufficiently severe. If the cranial nerve injuries have been due to tearing of nerve trunks owing to skull fracture involving their exit foramina (as may occur particularly with the facial, auditory, abducent and optic nerves) the injury is often permanent. A sixth-nerve paralysis can occur, however, as a transient phenomenon following a relatively mild head injury, usually being a false localising sign due to cerebral oedema. The commonest cranial nerve palsy after head injury is loss of the sense of smell due to injury to the small perforating olfactory fibres as they pass through the cribriform plate. If these fibres are contused then recovery can occur after weeks or months, but if they are ruptured, then the loss of the sense of smell is permanent. Occasionally during the recovery phase, a Korsakoff syndrome (see p. 96), develops, but soon resolves. In other cases the initial injury has been so severe, and damage so widespread, that permanent intellectual impairment, or traumatic dementia, results. The so-called traumatic encephalopathy or **punch-drunk syndrome** of professional boxers, in which there is usually deterioration of memory and intellect, with tremor and slowness or poverty of movement resembling that of Parkinson's disease, is probably due to the cumulative effect of many episodes of cerebral contusion. In such cases a CT scan may demonstrate absence of the septum pellucidum. A similar syndrome has been described in steeplechase jockeys.

Intracranial haemorrhage

Multiple small intracerebral haemorrhages may be due to cerebral contusion, and sometimes more extensive and focal bleeding into brain tissue follows injury. It is also common to find bleeding into the subarachnoid space after a closed head injury, particularly if the skull has been fractured. It is, however, those haemorrhages into the extradural and subdural spaces, in which bleeding can continue for some time after injury, that are particularly important to recognise, as these require specific treatment.

An acute **extradural haematoma** can follow any head injury in which there has been a fracture of the skull vault involving one of the channels on the inner table in which lies the middle meningeal artery or one of its branches. The bleeding is arterial and the condition therefore develops rapidly. Typically in such a case there is a concussive head injury of moderate severity with recovery of consciousness within a few minutes or hours. For an hour or two the patient may then be reasonably alert, but subsequently he becomes increasingly drowsy and lapses into coma. In some such cases, signs of compression of one cerebral hemisphere (contralateral hemiparesis, homolateral fixed dilated pupil or third-nerve palsy, due to cerebral herniation and compression of the third nerve at the edge of the tentorium cerebelli) may develop. There are many cases in which no lucid interval occurs, and in which diagnosis must depend upon progressive deepening of unconsciousness following the injury. Early diagnosis is imperative as operation is usually curative; otherwise death soon results from brain stem compression and infarction.

An acute **subdural haematoma** (Fig. 13.1) is another complication of head injury, resulting from rupture of veins which traverse the subdural space. When this condition develops acutely, as it may after severe trauma at any age, the clinical picture differs little from that of extradural haemorrhage, but the prognosis, even after evacuation, is poor. However, since the bleeding is venous, the onset and development of the condition is much more often slow and insidious. Such cases of subacute or chronic subdural haematoma commonly present baffling diagnostic problems, but their recognition is equally important as the condition may readily be treated neurosurgically; if unrecognised and the bleeding continues it is eventually fatal, but some subdural haematomas do not progress, while some small haematomas may cause no persisting disability and do not necessarily require evacuation. Chronic subdural bleeding generally occurs in elderly patients in whom the subdural veins are fragile; it can follow a trivial injury, such as jarring the head or a minor knock, and sometimes seems to occur

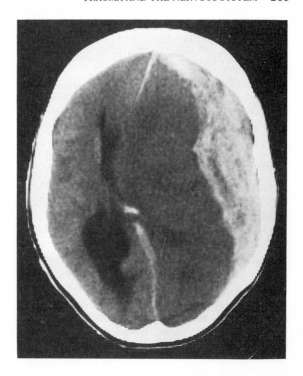

Fig. 13.1 An acute traumatic subdural haematoma, unenhanced axial CT scan. Note the blood adjacent to the falx cerebri.

spontaneously. 'Spontaneous' subdural bleeding is particularly common in patients receiving long-term anticoagulant therapy or in those with chronic liver disease. Typically the injury has no immediate ill-effects, but over the succeeding days or weeks the patient complains of vague headache, intermittent drowsiness and lapses of memory. There may be episodes of confusion, lack of attention to detail, failure of concentration, and long periods of apathy. Transient severe headache induced by change in posture, coughing or exertion is a notable feature in some cases, but by no means all. Drowsiness, headache and sometimes vomiting become progressively more severe, and the patient eventually lapses into stupor, intermittent mutism or even semicoma. Commonly the conscious level fluctuates, lucid intervals alternating with periods of confusion or stupor. Focal neurological signs, focal seizures, dilatation of the homolateral pupil and papilloedema can result, and eventually respiration and cardiac function are impaired. The CSF is often xanthochromic but contains no blood. Occasionally these patients present with seizures and the EEG may show unilateral suppression of alpha activity with unilateral slow activity. Rarely calcification occurs in a chronic haematoma. The CT scan is diagnostic. Evacuation of the clot usually results in a good recovery but may need to be repeated if the bleeding continues and the clot reforms. Occasionally in very chronic cases resection of the membrane lining the cavity, which by then is filled with serous yellow fluid rather than blood (a subdural hygroma), is needed to allow the compressed cerebral hemisphere to expand.

Management of the comatose patient

In the comatose patient, whether due to head injury, intracranial haemorrhage or some other cause, appropriate nursing care is essential if life is to be saved and undue disability avoided. The first essential is maintenance of an adequate airway. This is first achieved by turning the patient on to his side so that the tongue does not obstruct the oropharynx. Secretions and vomit, if present, should then be removed from the mouth, pharynx and upper respiratory passages, using suction if possible. If unconsciousness is at all prolonged it is wise to pass a nasal tube into the stomach and to aspirate the gastric contents so that the danger of inhalation of vomit can be avoided. If there is any difficulty in maintaining an airway, tracheal intubation is wise; if required for more than 5 days tracheotomy is necessary. Despite these precautions, comatose patients are particularly liable to develop pulmonary collapse and/or consolidation

Regular physiotherapy and the removal of secretions by suction through a tracheal catheter are therefore necessary. It is also usual to give prophylactic antibiotic therapy, usually at first with ampicillin, 250 mg every four hours, and the chest should be examined frequently. Care of the skin is equally as important as in paraplegic patients (see below), and if there is retention of urine, catheterisation will be required. The urine should also be examined frequently, beeause of the danger of urinary infection, and the urinary output must be measured to be sure that renal function is being maintained. If faecal incontinence is troublesome it is often preferable to give daily enemas. It is also important to maintain an adequate intake of fluid and of food if unconsciousness is likely to be prolonged. No particular steps are necessary in this connection as a rule if the patient is unconscious for 24 to 48 hours or less. Intravenous fluid may be necessary, monitored by the recording of central venous pressure to avoid the danger of pulmonary oedema. The serum electrolytes should be estimated daily and may subsequently indicate the need for intravenous therapy with correction of electrolyte imbalance. Later, if there is no vomiting, an adequate fluid and food intake can be achieved by intragastric tube feeding, which can be continued indefinitely until the patient is capable of taking adequate nourishment by mouth. Milk and various protein hydrolysate preparations are the basis of most meals given by tube, but care should be taken to see that vitamin supplements and adequate quantities of sodium and potassium are added. Intravenous feeding may also be required if unconsciousness is prolonged.

Complications and sequelae

Infection is an important complication of skull fracture, particularly if this is associated with scalp wounds. Cranial osteomyelitis may occur and can lead to extradural suppuration. Penetrating wounds carry the risk of infection of the meninges (meningitis) or of the brain tissue itself (suppurative encephalitis, cerebral abscess). Even when there is no wound of the scalp a skull fracture may involve the paranasal sinuses or middle ear. Organisms can then pass through a tear in the dura mater, causing meningitis; this complication should always be considered if there has been bleeding or leakage of CSF from the ears or nose and there may then be an indication for antibiotic therapy, followed later by surgical repair of the dural tear if the leak persists. Such a fistula should be suspected if clear watery fluid drips from the nose, particularly when leaning forwards; the fluid can be shown to contain glucose by appropriate tests, in contrast to rhinorrhoea in which the fluid does not contain glucose, and the fistula may then be localised by isotope ventriculography (see p. 35). In such cases air may enter the cranial cavity and even the cerebral substance, producing an encysted collection or **aerocele**. This can cause recurrent infection if a communication with the sinus or middle ear persists, Jacksonian epilepsy, or symptoms and signs of an intracranial space-occupying lesion.

The commonest cause of **post-traumatic epilepsy** is, however, a focal cerebral contusion or laceration which, having healed by the formation of a scar, may adhere to the inner surface of the dura. If the scar is large it can produce a cystic evagination of the lateral ventricle (traumatic porencephaly). About 5% of patients admitted to hospital with a head injury will develop epilepsy. The incidence of late epilepsy depends on four factors, a post-traumatic amnesia of greater than 24 hours, compound depressed fractures of the skull, focal neurological signs and the occurrence of fits in the first few weeks after the injury. If all these four factors apply, the incidence of late epilepsy is around 60% and this diminishes to around 3–5% if none apply. Although about 50% of patients who are going to develop epilepsy have their first fit within a year of the injury, in about a quarter it is delayed for four or five years. Patients at high risk should be treated with anticonvulsant drugs and may need to be given advice about their occupation or driving. Commonly post-traumatic fits are complex partial seizures and then the clinical features depend upon which area of the brain has been injured; in other cases in which, presumably, the epileptic discharge spreads rapidly throughout the brain, major convulsions occur.

The post-traumatic syndrome is a name applied to a constellation of disabling symptoms which may follow head injury. It is most common and persistent following cases of severe cerebral contusion and in these it may accompany post-traumatic dementia. Following simple concussion it is generally mild and of brief duration, but much depends upon the individual's premorbid personality. Whereas the condition clearly has an organic basis, emotional factors may be responsible for its exaggeration and perpetuation. Patients of good personality may recover quickly even after severe trauma, while those of less stable constitution are often considerably disabled for some time after a relatively trivial injury. The problem of financial compensation can greatly complicate prognosis and management. The characteristic features of the condition are first, headache, which is often persistent or paroxysmally severe; it is generally felt in the frontal and/or occipital regions, is most severe in the mornings, and is accentuated by coughing or by movement. Secondly, defects of memory and concentration and lack of interest are usual, as are periods of depression or anxiety and episodes of fear, panic or depersonalisation. Diminished tolerance of alcohol is common. Often, too, there is a complaint of giddiness or instability, which is not always true vertigo though the latter may occur particularly after sudden changes in the position of the head. Post-traumatic postural vertigo, a self-limiting disorder which may last for one or two years and which resembles benign positional vertigo, appears to be due to damage to the utricle and saccule of the internal ear. Syncopal attacks, accompanied by hysterical manifestations in some cases, are also frequent and are sometimes difficult to distinguish from post-traumatic epilepsy. These symptoms can persist for many weeks or months, and may even in occasional cases be permanent in some degree, but many patients recover completely in from six months to two years after the injury. The symptoms are nevertheless distressing and many subjects show considerable personality change from their premorbid state; appropriate management is often difficult, but reassurance and confident predictions of eventual recovery are all-important. When anxiety and depressive symptoms are prominent, treatment for a few months with anxiolytic and antidepressant remedies can be very helpful.

THE SPINAL CORD

The effects of a sudden penetrating injury to the spinal cord and those of cord compression are broadly similar, though certain clinical differences in effect stem from the fact that in the one case the lesion is sudden and in the other it is often more gradual.

Cord injuries

The spinal cord may be damaged by penetrating wounds resulting from missiles but more often it is injured through indirect violence. Thus severe flexion or hyperextension injuries of the neck can injure the cord, particularly when fracture-dislocation of the spine results. Even without fracture, however, the cord may be contused; this is particularly likely to occur in the cervical region when the anteroposterior diameter of the spinal canal is reduced by cervical spondylosis which may previously have been symptomless. Such sequelae can be particularly severe if the spinal canal is congenitally narrow. Falls from a height on to the feet or buttocks can also injure the spinal column and secondarily the cord. Sudden cord compression will also result from collapse and angulation of a vertebral body due, for example, to tuberculosis, a haemangioma or myeloma or a spinal metastasis.

The main pathological varieties of spinal cord injury are similar to those which affect the brain. Thus **spinal concussion** is generally a temporary but reversible disorder of function. In **spinal contusion** or bruising there are actual pathological changes including oedema and small focal haemorrhages, and the degree of eventual recovery is less complete as ascending and descending degeneration of spinal tracts takes place. **Laceration of the cord** implies an actual break in continuity which is irremediable, and symptoms resulting from such an injury show no improvement; furthermore, since penetrating wounds may cause laceration, there is the additional complication of possible infection, which can lead to meningitis or myelitis.

A spinal cord injury usually gives immediate flaccid paralysis and sensory loss in the limbs and trunk below the level of the lesion, with retention of urine and faeces. As spinal shock wears off, movement and sensation gradually return if the lesion is reversible, but if more severe, the patient remains paraplegic and the upper level of sensory impairment fails to recede. In such a case, reflex activity is eventually restored below the level of the lesion, the tendon reflexes become exaggerated, the plantar responses are extensor and automatic bladder and bowel activity are gradually established. Usually contractures of the hamstrings develop and there is a **paraplegia-in-flexion**, as tone is excessive in flexor muscles. Minimal cutaneous stimulation of the lower limbs often evokes painful flexor spasms which are a part of the primitive withdrawal reflex, and these are occasionally accompanied by the so-called mass reflex of autonomic activity with profuse sweating below the lesion and evacuation of the bladder and bowels. Paraplegia-in-flexion usually develops after a complete or almost complete cord transection, since the reticulospinal pathways which are responsible for an extensor hypertonus corresponding to that seen in the decerebrate posture, are interrupted. In partial lesions, however, in which the injury involves predominantly the pyramidal or corticospinal tracts, this extensor hypertonus predominates, to give **paraplegia-in-extension**, and the flexor withdrawal reflex, which depends upon short spinal reflex arcs, is partially suppressed. Many other clinical syndromes can result from incomplete spinal injuries. Of these, the Brown-Séquard syndrome, resulting from cord hemisection, is an example (see p. 172). The prognosis of spinal cord injuries must of course depend upon the severity of the injury; symptoms of spinal concussion generally resolve within at the most four weeks after the injury. Thereafter comparatively little further recovery of function is to be expected, but remarkable degrees of adaptation are sometimes possible.

Injuries of the **cauda equina** (the spinal roots below the termination of the spinal cord) are relatively uncommon. These usually produce total paralysis of the bladder, bowels and sexual function, with flaccid paralysis of the lower limbs; the actual distribution of muscular paralysis depends upon which roots are involved. Since regeneration of these roots can occur, the prognosis of cauda equina injuries is somewhat better than that of cord injury, provided the continuity of the neurolemmal sheaths of the injured roots is preserved.

Management of the paraplegic patient

The nursing and medical care of the patient who has paralysis of the lower limbs or of all four limbs can be considered under three principal headings. First proper care must be taken of the skin to prevent the development of pressure sores (bedsores); secondly, particular attention should be paid to the functioning of the bladder and bowels; and thirdly, contractures and deformities must be prevented as far as possible and physiotherapeutic measures must be utilised in order to make the best possible use of the voluntary activity, if any, which remains or returns in the weakened limbs. Pressure sores are due to prolonged pressure upon an area of skin which is at first reddened and then, as a result of ischaemia, it either becomes gangrenous or breaks down to form an ulcer. Loss of cutaneous sensibility and urinary or faecal incontinence leading to frequent wet or soiled beds are important contributory factors. The prevention of sores must depend first upon the posturing of the patient, with the assistance of special mattresses or foam-rubber cushions, secondly upon frequent turning, with a change of position every half-hour, and thirdly upon strict cleanliness of bed-linen with frequent washing and massaging of vulnerable skin areas. Various forms of skin protectives, such as barrier creams, may be helpful. Susceptible areas include the elbows, the skin over the scapulae, the sacrum and buttocks, the lateral aspect of the hips and the heels. Bedsores which extend down to bone or are associated with sinus formation may best be treated surgically with excision of necrotic tissue and closure of the defect with rotation flaps if necessary.

The patient with a total paraplegia, however caused, almost invariably develops retention of urine, though sometimes from the beginning there is retention with a dribbling overflow. Catheterisation is then essential. It is preferable to use a silastic catheter since this only needs to be changed every few months. Drainage should be continuous initially in order to avoid infection.

When infection develops, the urine should be cultured and appropriate therapy with urinary antiseptic drugs, or with antibiotics, is given depending upon the infecting organism and its sensitivity to these drugs as revealed by microbiological tests. Regular bladder washouts with dilute chlorhexidine solution are also useful. Every few days, the catheter should be removed, or intermittent catheterisation delayed, to see whether satisfactory evacuation of the bladder can be achieved either by voluntary effort, with the aid of manual compression above the pubis, or following the oral administration of 10–30 mg of bethanechol or an intramuscular injection of 0.25 mg of carbamylcholine (carbachol) or distigmine (Ubretid®, 0.5 mg). If a single injection has no effect, it can be repeated half an hour later, but if there is still no evacuation, the catheter should be reinserted and the procedure attempted again a few days later. Eventually, in most cases of spastic paraplegia, automatic bladder action becomes established, even if the paraplegia remains complete, within a few weeks or months and the bladder is then evacuated automatically every few hours, whenever the intravesical pressure reaches a certain level. In some cases, surgical resection of the bladder neck is needed to facilitate this process, as the internal urethral sphincter becomes greatly hypertrophied. Once automatic bladder action is established, the male patient can be helped by the use of disposable urinals made of plastic which prevent inadvertent wetting of his garments. Incontinence pads may be used in the female but are much less satisfactory. Following lesions of the cauda equina, or permanent flaccid paraplegia due to cord infarction, the bladder remains permanently atonic and in many cases evacuation is only achieved by means of abdominal contraction or manual compression. Intermittent self-catheterisation can be very useful in some patients, particularly if there is no loss of manual dexterity. Diversion procedures are now only very rarely performed. Permanent catheter drainage or suprapubic cystostomy are, however, rarely necessary.

Care of the bowels does not as a rule present as many problems as care of the bladder. Retention of faeces is usual in the initial stages and enemas are generally required every two or three days. Subsequently the patient usually regains some voluntary control over the act of defaecation, unless the cauda equina is damaged, when regular enemas may be needed indefinitely. Many paraplegic patients learn the technique of regular manual removal of faeces with a gloved hand, while others prefer a twice-weekly enema. Sexual function is also totally lost, as a rule, in the paraplegic patient. Under exceptional circumstances when the male partner of a marriage is paraplegic and a child is greatly desired, the intrathecal injection of a small dose of neostigmine may produce ejaculation and artificial insemination of the wife will then be possible. A female paraplegic patient may be able to have a child though delivery by Caesarian section will often be needed.

The posture of the patient is all-important in preventing muscular contractures and consequent skeletal deformity. Thus a cage is usually required to take the weight of the bedclothes which would otherwise cause foot drop. Splinting of the legs is also required in some cases in order to prevent hamstring contractures. When flexor spasms at the hips and knee develop, antispastic agents such as baclofen or dantrolene can be very helpful. Baclofen is a GABA agonist and probably works on the internuncial neurones in the spinal cord. Treatment should be started with 5 mg three times a day, increasing as appropriate to 60–80 mg a day. It should be used with caution in patients with epilepsy. Dantrolene is thought to work on the sarcoplasmic reticulum and to have little or no central nervous system effects. The starting dose is 25 mg three times a day and the dose may be increased to 400 mg a day according to response. Liver function should be monitored during the early months of treatment. Both these drugs are most effective in patients with pronounced spasticity and little in the way of weakness, sensory loss or cerebellar deficit. Some patients with profound weakness and spasticity may be worse off on these drugs since they need some spasticity to be able to stand or walk (the spastic crutch). The relief of spasticity in these patients and in those with cerebellar and sensory loss may result in an impairment of function. A single dose of baclofen given at night may relieve nocturnal spasms without impairing mobility during the day. Diazepam is an effective antispastic agent, but the accompanying sedation is often unacceptable. Intrathecal phenol injections may be very helpful in relieving severe spasticity, particularly in the legs, but this should be reserved for patients with little or no function so that any additional weakness that might result is not important. Intrathecal phenol is not to be used in patients with some useful preservation of bladder function.

Haematomyelia and central cord softening

Haematomyelia is a term which implies bleeding into the substance of the spinal cord. It can occur spontaneously in patients with bleeding disorders, or may result from small vascular malformations or telangiectases within the cord, while it rarely results from haemorrhage into a syringomyelic cavity. More often it is due to relatively minor injury to the spine. It almost always develops in the cervical region and may complicate cervical spondylosis, a condition in which there are multiple chronic central intervertebral disc protrusions. This causes narrowing of the cervical spinal canal, so that sudden hyperextension of the neck, as may occur following a sudden blow upon the forehead, produces sharp but transient compression of the spinal cord, which in turn can cause haematomyelia. The haemorrhage occurs as a rule in or around the central canal of the cord and can extend over several segments. In most such cases there is contusion and central softening of the cord without haemorrhage, but the clinical effects are similar.

As a rule, the patient with cervical haematomyelia or central cord softening experiences sudden weakness or total paralysis of all four limbs; this phase of spinal shock may pass off in a day or two, but spastic weakness of the lower limbs persists, sometimes affecting one leg more than the other if the bleeding is not entirely central and if one pyramidal tract is selectively compressed. As the bleeding or softening in the cervical cord extends into the anterior and posterior horns there is loss of the spinal reflexes innervated by the affected segments as well as atrophy and weakness of lower motor neurone type in the muscles innervated by the affected roots. Wasting of small hand muscles is particularly common. Furthermore, as in syringomyelia, decussating sensory fibres travelling to the spinothalamic tracts may be interrupted so that there is often some dissociated sensory loss in the upper limbs. If the lesion is extensive there will also be damage to the posterior columns of the cord giving impairment of position and joint sense and of vibration sense, particularly in the lower limbs. This clinical picture mimicking syringomyelia can also occur rarely in cervical myelopathy due to spondylosis without a clear history of trauma.

Prognostically, much depends upon the severity and extent of the injury; substantial recovery of function can occur in the three months after the injury but some lower motor neurone weakness and dissociated sensory loss in the upper limbs may persist, with residual spasticity in the legs. And if the cervical spinal canal remains narrowed as a result of spondylosis the spinal cord remains vulnerable and may be injured further by relatively minor trauma.

Spinal cord compression

Compression of the spinal cord can result from disease in the vertebral column or in the spinal canal itself. Apart from the injuries of the vertebral column which were described above, the commonest skeletal disorders to compress the cord are intervertebral disc protrusions, either acute or chronic, tuberculous spinal osteitis (Pott's disease), acute staphylococcal osteitis giving rise to extradural abscess, and primary or secondary neoplasms of the vertebral bodies. The commonest situation in which central disc prolapse compresses the cord is in the cervical region; a sudden soft protrusion of the nucleus pulposus may be responsible, but more often there are one or several chronic protrusions which have become calcified to produce bony hard ridges between the vertebrae (cervical spondylosis) and the clinical picture is one of slowly progressive spinal cord disease (**cervical spondylotic myelopathy**). In patients with Pott's disease, now rare in Western countries but once most common in children and young people, a paraplegia often develops abruptly; this often occurs, too, in older patients when a metastasis in a vertebral body causes a pathological fracture with sudden collapse and angulation. In spinal extradural abscess (see p. 220) there is usually acute spinal tenderness and the patient is usually febrile. This condition is a neurosurgical emergency; indeed it must be stressed that any syndrome of rapidly progressive weakness of the lower limbs requires immediate investigation in a specialised neurological or neurosurgical centre. Primary neoplasms of the vertebrae (osteoma, haemangioma, myeloma) and Paget's disease (osteitis deformans) usually give a more slowly progressive clinical picture. Conditions within the spinal theca which may compress the cord include arachnoiditis due to syphilis or to chronic trauma, extramedullary neoplasms such as meningioma or neurofibroma, and intramedullary lesions such as glioma and ependymoma (see Ch. 16), meningeal deposits of neoplastic tissue or of a reticulosis, and, exceptionally, congenital fibrous bands or developmental cysts (which are sometimes associated with spina bifida) or parasitic cysts.

The **clinical features** of spinal cord compression depend upon the level of the lesion and its rapidity of development. Not only must one consider the direct effects of pressure but also those which can result from a secondary alteration in blood supply. In general, how-ever, the symptoms and physical signs so produced can be classified into two principal groups which are first, those resulting from compression of nerve roots at the level of the lesion and secondly, those due to interference with the function of long ascending or descending tracts. The principal symptom of root compression is pain, which is generally aching in character, and radiates to the myotome, in contrast to numbness and paraesthesiae which are felt in the dermatome. If the motor roots are also involved there will be weakness, wasting, and sometimes fasciculation of the muscles which they supply. Interruption of the spinal reflex arc gives absence of the reflexes innervated by the segment being compressed. If the pressure develops asymmetrically, these phenomena can occur unilaterally at first. Compression of long tracts may give weakness and dragging of a leg and/or clumsiness of an arm and hand, again depending upon the situation of the lesion, and eventually a spastic paraplegia or quadriplegia will result. When the spinothalamic tract is involved, the patient often experiences unpleasant burning pain in a limb or on the trunk and some hypalgesia is generally found on examination with impairment of temperature appreciation. Similarly involvement of the posterior columns gives characteristic paraesthesiae below the level of the lesion, often with typical 'electric shocks' radiating downwards on movement of the neck, if the lesion is cervical; there is also impairment of position and joint sense, sometimes of light touch, and generally of vibration sense in the lower limbs. These so-called 'long-tract' symptoms and signs develop especially early when the lesion is intramedullary. As a rule, the pyramidal tract is most sensitive to pressure, possibly because of the comparative vulnerability of its blood supply, while the spinothalamic tracts are most resistant. Hence a slowly progressive lesion generally gives first signs of pyramidal tract dysfunction, next sensory phenomena of posterior column' type, and lastly those indicating a spinothalamic tract lesion.

Sphincter disturbances tend to develop late in compressive lesions, but may be the first manifestation of an intramedullary lesion. When a severe paraplegia has developed there is often excessive sweating below the level of the lesion. Disturbances of sphincter control appear early, however, in lesions compressing the cauda equina in which pain in the lower back is usual and there are also symptoms and signs of muscular weakness of 'lower motor neurone' type in the lower limbs. Cutaneous sensory loss is also apparent, its distribution varying depending upon which roots are involved; compression of lower sacral roots, for instance, often produces perianal and perineal anaesthesia. Some of the most difficult lesions to localise accurately on clinical grounds are those which compress both the lower spinal cord (the conus medullaris) and several roots of the cauda equina; in such cases, there are generally severe disorders of sphincter control, along with a combination of 'upper motor neurone' and 'lower motor neurone' signs in the lower limbs.

Accurate **clinical localisation** of the site of cord compression can be greatly helped by the presence of certain specific symptoms and physical signs. The distribution of root pain, or the situation of local spinal pain and tenderness may be valuable, while a 'sensory level' on the trunk, below which sensation is impaired, is also helpful. It must, however, be remembered that the actual site of the lesion may be several segments higher than that suggested by this sensory 'level'. Weakness of lower abdominal muscles, too, or selective absence of lower abdominal reflexes will localise the lesion to approximately the tenth dorsal segment of the cord. Reflex changes are also useful since an absent reflex marks the level of the lesion; thus absence of the biceps and radial jerks with exaggeration of the triceps jerk indicates a lesion of the fifth and sixth cervical segments, while absence of the knee jerks and retention or exaggeration of the ankle jerks indicates usually that the third or fourth lumbar segment is involved. In the lower limbs, too, the distribution of sensory impairment or muscular weakness may clearly indicate disease of specific motor or sensory roots. Thus perianal anaesthesia is diagnostic of lower sacral root involvement. In localising a lesion on the basis of these clinical features one must remember that the spinal cord is much shorter than the spinal column and ends at the lower border of the first lumbar vertebra. Thus the seventh cervical segment of the cord lies beneath the arch of the sixth cervical vertebra, the sixth dorsal segment beneath the fourth dorsal arch; under the tenth dorsal arch are the first and second lumbar segments, under the twelfth the fifth, while the sacral and coccygeal segments are opposite the body of the first lumbar vertebra.

Although these clinical features help to localise a spinal lesion, they are insufficient for the surgeon, should operative intervention be considered. Often when compression has occurred acutely, irreversible damage has taken place before the surgeon can operate. The results of removal of extramedullary tumours are, by contrast, usually good, if done sufficiently early. Although there are some causes of cord compression in which the results of surgical decompression are variable (e.g. cervical spondylosis), this is the only effective treatment in some patients (see p. 293). Examination of the CSF is of limited value in diagnosis since although the protein content of the fluid may be raised (see p. 31) and Queckenstedt's test may be positive, these findings are not invariable and the performance of a lumbar puncture may prejudice subsequent myelography. Radiography of the spine may indicate the cause of the compression, but the definitive investigation is myelography using water-soluble contrast medium with CT scanning at selected levels if appropriate. Future developments in magnetic resonance imaging may make these techniques obsolete.

Injuries to peripheral nerves and plexuses

A detailed description of the many clinical phenomena which can result from injury to or compression of peripheral nerves or plexuses is outside the scope of this volume, but the salient features of some of the lesions which most often occur in clinical practice will be described briefly. There are two principal types of lesion resulting from injury to nerve trunks. These are first, neurapraxia, a temporary and completely reversible block of nervous conduction which can last for days or even weeks without permanent pathological change; and secondly, neuronotmesis, in which there is interruption in continuity of nerve fibres with subsequent Wallerian degeneration, so that regeneration of nerve fibres is required before recovery can occur. In the early stages these two types of lesion may be indistinguishable, save by specialised methods of investigation (see pp. 35–38). Bearing this fact in mind it should be noted that a total lesion of a mixed motor and sensory peripheral nerve gives flaccid paralysis and eventual atrophy of the muscles which it supplies. There is also cutaneous sensory loss, though the area of anaesthesia and analgesia is often less than would be expected, as a result of 'overlap' from nerves supplying adjacent cutaneous areas particularly in root lesions; distal peripheral nerve lesions are more consistent in the distribution of the sensory loss they produce. Trophic changes (shiny skin, loss of sweating, indolent sores) may be seen in the extremities after complete peripheral nerve lesions. We shall now consider the clinical phenomena which result from lesions of some of the more important nerve plexuses and peripheral nerves. Direct trauma, pressure or irritation are usually responsible, and inflammatory lesions are comparatively uncommon. The condition often referred to in the past as an interstitial neuritis of individual peripheral nerves is generally due to pressure upon or ischaemia of the nerve trunk, although allergic or hypersensitivity neuropathies do occur.

The term mononeuritis or, more correctly, mononeuropathy is used to describe a single peripheral nerve lesion and this is most likely to be due to an entrapment of the nerve as it passes through muscle planes or down a fibro-osseous tunnel; the other common cause is external compression where the nerve lies between skin and bone. The term mononeuritis multiplex is used to describe more than one isolated peripheral nerve lesion and while this may be due to an entrapment or compression, it may indicate an underlying systemic disorder such as diabetes or one of the collagen or connective tissue diseases.

The **phrenic nerve** is derived from the third, fourth and fifth cervical anterior roots; compression or irritation of the nerve can cause an irritating, unproductive cough or hiccup, while a complete lesion gives paralysis of the diaphragm on the affected side. The nerve is usually paralysed as a result of lesions of the anterior horn cells of the cord or the anterior roots, as in poliomyelitis, the Guillain-Barré syndrome and spinal neoplasms, but may be injured in its peripheral course by penetrating wounds, malignant disease in the chest, or an aortic aneurysm.

The **brachial plexus** is formed from the anterior primary divisions of the fifth to eighth cervical and of the first thoracic nerves. Sometimes the plexus is prefixed, receiving contributions from the fourth cervical, or postfixed, with fibres from the second thoracic segment. The divisions split into anterior and posterior trunks which again unite to form three cords. The outer cord is formed from the anterior trunks of the fifth to seventh cervical nerves, the inner or lower cord from the anterior trunk of the eighth cervical and the entire contribution from the first thoracic while the posterior cord is formed from all the posterior trunks. The lateral head of the median nerve and the musculocutaneous nerve come from the outer cord, the medial head of the median nerve and the ulnar from the inner cord, and the circumflex and radial nerves from the posterior cord. The long thoracic nerve, which supplies the serratus anterior and is derived from the fifth to seventh cervical roots as well as the suprascapular nerve which innervates the spinati, and comes from the fifth and sixth segments, arise proximal to the brachial plexus.

The brachial plexus can be injured or compressed by penetrating wounds, by dislocation of the head of the humerus, by tumours in the root of the neck or by lesions causing compression at the thoracic outlet. Even more commonly it is damaged by traction injuries of the arm, perhaps in an infant during delivery, or in an adult on an operating table while anaesthetised. A common injury is one of the inner cord of the plexus due to hyperabduction of the arm at the shoulder; or alternatively downward compression of the point of the shoulder (as in motor cycle injuries) or a violent pull downward on the arm may tear the outer cord. Severe injuries may forcibly tear the spinal nerves or may even pull the anterior and posterior roots away from their attachment to the spinal cord. When this happens in the cervical region the symptoms and signs are similar to those of brachial plexus injury but the 'flare' response (see p. 179) indicates that the lesion in sensory fibres at least is proximal to the posterior root

ganglia. Myelography is useful when such an injury is suspected as it shows excessive filling of root 'sleeves' (meningoceles) at the appropriate level. It is important to recognise these cases in which no significant recovery is possible; in lesions of the plexus itself, even if severe, some recovery may result from nerve regeneration, even after extensive Wallerian degeneration, provided the damaged nerve trunks remain in continuity.

Injury to the outer cord gives paralysis of the biceps brachii and of the radial flexors of the wrist and fingers. An inner cord lesion, which may be due to shoulder dislocation, gives paralysis of all the small muscles of the hand with sensory loss along the ulnar border of the hand and forearm. The posterior cord is rarely injured. The two common varieties of *birth injury to the plexus* are first, Erb's paralysis, in which the contribution from the fifth cervical nerve is torn; and secondly, Klumpke's paralysis in which the first nerve is damaged. In Erb's paralysis there is paralysis of the deltoid, spinati, biceps and brachioradialis so that the arm hangs limply by the side, internally rotated with the forearm pronated. Klumpke's paralysis gives a 'claw' hand due to paralysis of small hand muscles with sensory loss down the inner side of the forearm. Whereas about 50% of cases of the Erb type recover, the prognosis of the Klumpke type is less good. Surgical treatment is of no value, but splinting of the arm to prevent overstretching of paralysed muscles can assist partial recovery.

A syndrome with clinical features of inner cord injury can result from compression or angulation of the cord as it crosses a *cervical rib* joining the transverse process of the seventh cervical vertebra to the first rib; a fibrous or cartilaginous band in the same situation may have a similar effect. Indeed, fibrous bands in this situation seem to present more often with neurological deficit whereas complete bony ribs present more frequently with vascular complications due to kinking and obstruction of the subclavian artery. Commonly there is aching pain down the inner arm and forearm; this is accentuated by carrying heavy weights in the hand, while weakness and wasting of all small hand muscles and sensory loss on the ulnar side of the hand and forearm develop slowly over months or years. Wasting sometimes begins in the lateral half of the thenar eminence giving difficulty in differentiation from a carpal tunnel syndrome (see below) in some cases. An ipsilateral Horner's syndrome due to pressure on the stellate ganglion occurs occasionally, but is more likely to indicate malignant infiltration of the plexus. This cervical rib syndrome, which is uncommon (many individuals have cervical ribs visible radiologically which do not give rise to symptoms) is one variety of the *thoracic outlet or costoclavicular outlet* syndrome. Similar compression of the inner cord of the brachial plexus and sometimes of the subclavian artery, leading rarely to aneurysm formation or to ischaemia or embolism of the hand, can be the result of narrowing of the space between a prominent first rib and the clavicle through which the neurovascular bundle to the upper limb must pass. Alternatively, distortion resulting from angulation of the cord as it crosses the scalenus anterior has been implicated. The syndrome has been attributed to drooping of the shoulders and may be aggravated by carrying heavy shopping bags. In some patients the symptoms can be relieved at least partially by appropriate physiotherapy and correction of posture. While it is true that the typical cervical rib syndrome as outlined above can occasionally result from other causes of compression in the costoclavicular outlet, it is evident that many symptoms previously attributed to this cause are due to other lesions, including cervical spondylosis and, in the case of acroparaesthesiae (see below), a common syndrome in middle-aged women, compression of the median nerve in the carpal tunnel. In diagnosing the thoracic outlet syndrome it is important to note that pain and paraesthesiae occur down the *inner* side of the arm and forearm, and that if motor weakness and muscle wasting are present these predominate in the small hand muscles. It is useful to roll the trunks of the brachial plexus beneath the examiner's fingers in the supraclavicular fossa, since this often reproduces the patient's pain and paraesthesiae on the affected side.

Isolated lesions of the **long thoracic nerve** are not uncommon and may result from an inflammatory lesion which is presumed to be autoimmune and which is akin to neuralgic amyotrophy (see p. 235). The result is 'winging' of the scapula due to paralysis of serratus anterior. When the patient pushes forward with the arm outstretched horizontally the scapula protrudes backwards like an 'angel's wing'.

When the **axillary** (**circumflex**) **nerve** is injured, as it may be by direct trauma, shoulder dislocation or by being involved in neuralgic amyotrophy (see p. 235), the deltoid muscle is paralysed and there is often a patch of sensory loss over the belly and insertion of the deltoid.

The **radial nerve** innervates the triceps, brachioradialis, the radial extensor of the wrist and the long extensors of the fingers. Hence a lesion of this nerve high up in the spiral groove in the humerus (crutch palsy) will cause paralysis of extension of the elbow together with wrist-drop and finger-drop. If the lesion is lower the triceps is often spared. Sensory loss is usually slight and is confined to a small area on the dorsum of the hand between the thumb and index finger, even though the nerve has a more extensive cutaneous innervation. The nerve is frequently damaged in its spiral groove when the humerus is fractured, or by pressure, as when the upper arm rests for a long period over the back of a chair (Saturday-night paralysis).

The **musculocutaneous nerve** is rarely injured alone but a lesion will result in paralysis of flexion of the elbow (biceps brachii and brachialis).

A lesion of the **median nerve** at the elbow gives paralysis of the radial flexors of the wrist and also of all the finger flexors except flexor digitorum profundus to the ring and little fingers. There is also weakness and wasting of the muscles of the outer half of the thenar eminence (abductor pollicis brevis and opponens pollicis). There is sensory loss over the radial part of the hand and on the palmar aspect of the thumb, index, middle, and half the ring finger. The distal part of the extensor aspect of these fingers may also be anaesthetic. Apart from direct trauma (as by a misplaced injection) the nerve can be compressed at the elbow as it passes through the pronator teres or in relation to the flexor digitorum sublimis; but these disorders are uncommon. A lesion at the wrist gives similar sensory loss, abductor pollicis brevis is weak and may be wasted, but the long flexors are normal. The **anterior interosseous nerve**, a branch of the median, may be constricted by a fibrous band between the two heads of pronator teres and this causes weakness of flexor pollicis longus and flexor digitorum profundus to the index and middle fingers. Many such lesions recover spontaneously, but the affected nerve should be explored surgically if recovery has not occurred within two or three months.

Lesions of the median nerve are often due to direct trauma, and causalgia is a particularly common sequel. *Compression of the median nerve in the carpal tunnel* is also a very common syndrome. It often results from excessive use of the fingers (as in housewives, women who knit a great deal and pianists) and is usually the result of a tenosynovitis of the flexor tendons, causing swelling of their sheaths and increased pressure beneath the carpal ligament. Local injuries of the wrist, rheumatoid arthritis, acromegaly and disorders which give rise to soft tissue swelling (pregnancy, myxoedema, nephrotic syndrome) can have a similar result. The condition is commonest in middle-aged women, but may occur in men. It is often bilateral but worse in the hand which is used more often (usually the right). The most typical symptoms are burning pain, aching or tingling and pins and needles in the fingers (acroparaesthesiae) which are worse in bed at night or in warm surroundings (due to vasodilatation and increased nerve compression). Symptoms often occur outside median nerve territory with paraesthesiae in all the fingers or aching pain and paraesthesiae in the forearm; however, physical signs are confined to median nerve distribution. Percussion of the median nerve at the wrist sometimes evokes tingling in the affected fingers while the application of a tourniquet to the arm at above arterial blood pressure gives ischaemic paraesthesiae in the fingers within one to three minutes (an abnormally short period). Often there is some sensory impairment over the tips of the thumb and radial three fingers, while the muscles of the lateral half of the thenar eminence may be weak or even wasted in advanced cases. Nerve conduction velocity studies demonstrate increased terminal latency due to conduction delay beneath the carpal ligament or a reduced amplitude of sensory nerve action potentials from the median-innervated fingers. The symptoms, which are disabling and can last for many years, may be relieved by rest or by the injection of hydrocortisone into the carpal tunnel; operative section of the carpal ligament will effect a permanent cure.

The **ulnar nerve** at the elbow lies behind the medial epicondyle of the humerus; a lesion at this level results in paralysis of the flexor carpi ulnaris, of flexor digitorum profundus to the ring and little fingers and of most of the small muscles of the hand save the lateral half of the thenar eminence and the two most lateral lumbricals. The hand is deviated radially, there is inability to flex the ring and little fingers completely and a 'claw-hand' results from paralysis of small hand muscles and from unopposed action of their antagonists. On testing there is inability to adduct the little finger, to adduct the thumb and to separate or oppose the fingers, while lumbrical weakness means that the terminal phalanges of the affected fingers cannot be fully extended. Sensory impairment is found over the palmar and dorsal aspects of the little finger and the ulnar half of the ring finger; it sometimes spreads up the palm as far as the wrist and rarely on to the medial aspect of the forearm. The nerve can be damaged at the elbow by penetrating injuries or fractures of the humerus or it may be subjected to repeated irritation in its groove behind the humerus in patients who have an unusually wide 'carrying angle' or arthritic osteophytes in this area; in some patients with shallow grooves, the nerve subluxes on full elbow flexion. In such cases, the nerve trunk becomes swollen, tender and fibrotic and surgical transposition, bringing it to lie in front of the epicondyle, is necessary. The nerve can also be temporarily compressed through leaning on the elbow for a long period, or by 'sleeping on the arm'. The ulnar nerve may also be compressed as it passes between the two heads of flexor carpi ulnaris (the cubital tunnel syndrome). In these patients the ulnar-innervated long finger flexors are usually spared and the treatment of choice is simple decompression. It is important to identify these patients since anterior transposition, which

carries a small risk of damage to the nerve, is unnecessary in such cases. In the region of the wrist the nerve may be injured particularly by penetrating injuries, and it is not uncommon for the median and ulnar nerves and several tendons to be severed, particularly when a hand is thrust through a glass door or window. The nerve may also be compressed in Guyon's canal by a ganglion and in these cases the palmar sensory branches are involved but the dorsal sensory branches may be spared. Atrophy and weakness of the interossei, lumbricals and adductor pollicis, with sparing of the hypothenar eminence and without sensory loss, can result from continuous or repetitive pressure on the medial side of the palm, a hazard of certain occupations, and is due to repeated trauma to the deep palmar branch of the nerve. A similar syndrome occasionally develops spontaneously without a history of trauma and may be found to be due to a ganglion compressing this branch. Nerve conduction velocity studies and measurements of terminal latency are often diagnostic.

Lesions of the intercostal nerves are unusual though they may be involved by neurofibromata. Occasionally patches of numbness occur, usually near the midline on the abdomen or close to the midline in the paraspinal region and this is due to an entrapment neuropathy of the perforating cutaneous branches as they pass through the fascial planes of the rectus abdominus and the paraspinal muscles respectively. A rare and intractable syndrome of intercostal neuralgia also occurs, sometimes without obvious cause, sometimes after thoracotomy.

The **lumbar plexus** is formed from the twelfth dorsal and first to fourth lumbar nerves, the **sacral plexus** from the fourth and fifth lumbar and first to third sacral nerves. Usually the two together are called the **lumbosacral plexus**. The principal nerves arising from the lumbar plexus are the femoral and obturator, while the greater part of the sacral plexus forms the sciatic nerve. Injuries of the lumbosacral plexus are relatively uncommon, but it can be damaged by undue pressure of the fetal head or by obstetric forceps during delivery (obstetric lumbosacral palsy); a syndrome which may result from this cause is unilateral paralysis of the anterior tibial and peroneal muscles due to a lesion of one lumbosacral cord. The commonest cause of involvement of the lumbosacral plexus is malignant infiltration.

A common clinical syndrome, known as **meralgia paraesthetica**, is due to compression of the lateral cutaneous nerve of the thigh as it passes beneath the lateral part of the inguinal ligament or as it traverses the fascia lata to reach its cutaneous distribution. It usually occurs in the obese, and in middle-age, but not invariably so, and can be unilateral or bilateral. The principal symptoms are an unpleasant burning ache, with superadded tingling or pins and needles, which are accentuated by standing for long periods, and involve much of the lateral aspect of the thigh. In this area there is often some hypalgesia and hypaesthesia. The condition, though benign, is often troublesome. Surgical decompression of the nerve may be necessary, but is not always completely effective in relieving symptoms. Repeated injections of local anaesthetic around the nerve at the inguinal ligament occasionally afford relief.

Lesions of the **obturator nerve** are uncommon but can follow hip dislocation or difficult labour. The adductor muscles of the thigh are paralysed, but as a rule there is no sensory loss. Rarely, the **genitofemoral or ilioinguinal nerves** may be injured directly, by a misplaced herniorrhaphy incision, during pelvic operations including appendicectomy, or by hip joint disease, giving pain in the groin and a flexed posture; local anaesthetic injection is the treatment of choice.

The principal effect of a lesion of the **femoral nerve**, which may result from penetrating wounds, from haematomas which sometimes appear to be spontaneous but are more common in patients with a bleeding diathesis, or from compression by pelvic neoplasms, is paralysis of the quadriceps with inability to extend the knee and loss of the knee jerk. There may also be some weakness of hip flexion owing to involvement of the iliacus and sensory impairment is usual over the medial and anterior aspects of the lower two-thirds of the thigh; if the saphenous nerve, a branch of the femoral, is also affected, the analgesia and anaesthesia also extend down the inner side of the leg and foot. In some cases of '*diabetic amyotrophy*' painful wasting of one quadriceps results from a localised ischaemic femoral neuropathy.

The **sciatic nerve** has two principal divisions which form the medial and lateral popliteal (tibial and common peroneal) nerves, respectively, and it divides at a variable point in the back of the thigh. It enters the buttock via the sciatic notch and then passes into the thigh midway between the greater trochanter of the femur and the ischial tuberosity. A complete lesion of the nerve gives paralysis of the hamstrings, resulting in inability to flex the knee, as well as paralysis of all muscles below the knee. The foot becomes flail, it cannot be dorsiflexed or plantar-flexed and the toes are immobile. The patient can walk but does so with a drop-foot and cannot stand on his toes. There is sensory loss over virtually the whole of the foot and also over the lateral and posterior aspect of the leg below the knee. The ankle jerk and the plantar response are absent. Damage to the sciatic nerve is generally due to gunshot wounds or other penetrating injuries of the buttock or thigh, though it may also be injured by pelvic or femoral fracture or a misplaced injection. Its constituent roots are often compressed by

lateral prolapse of an intervertebral disc, giving the syndrome of sciatica.

Lesions of the **lateral popliteal (common peroneal) nerve** are relatively common and usually result from repeated trauma to the nerve as it curls around the neck of the fibula; here it lies just beneath the skin and is particularly vulnerable. Compression by a tight garter or bandage, as a result of repeated crossing of the legs, or in workers who habitually sit with one leg folded beneath them (as in tailors or roofing workers) are common aetiological factors. A complete lesion gives paralysis of the dorsiflexors of the foot and toes and of the peroneal muscles, causing foot-drop with some degree of inversion. There is generally sensory impairment over the anterolateral aspect of the leg and foot, extending medially to the cleft between the fourth and fifth toes.

When the **medial popliteal (tibial) nerve** is injured, an uncommon event which is normally seen only after a penetrating wound, the muscles of the calf and of the sole of the foot are paralysed and the foot is partially dorsiflexed and everted. Sensory loss is usually noted on the sole of the foot and the plantar surface of the toes. Very rarely the **posterior tibial nerve** is compressed behind and below the medial malleolus giving sensory loss over almost the entire sole of the foot (the tarsal tunnel syndrome). Rarely, compression of **plantar** and **interdigital** nerves can give similar but less extensive pain and sensory loss (Morton's metatarsalgia).

In this chapter an outline has been given of the effects of trauma upon the central and peripheral nervous system. For more detailed information about the effects of injury to the skull, vertebral column and spinal cord, the reader is referred to textbooks of neurosurgery and orthopaedic surgery. In a case of peripheral nerve injury, a working knowledge of the anatomical relationships of the nerves and plexuses and of the innervation of the skeletal muscles and dermatomes is clearly needed for accurate diagnosis and localisation of the responsible lesion: some reference texts which may help in this connection are listed below.

REFERENCES

Cartlidge N E F, Shaw D A 1981 Head injury. Major problems in neurology, Vol 10 (Walton J, series ed). Saunders, London

Critchley E R 1988 Neurological emergencies. Major problems in neurology, Vol 17 (Walton J, series ed). Baillière Tindall, London

Donaldson J O 1989 Neurology of pregnancy, 2nd edn. Major problems in neurology, Vol 18 (Walton J, series ed). Baillière Tindall, London

Feiring E H 1974 Brock's Injuries of the brain and spinal cord and their coverings, 5th edn. Springer, New York

Guarantors of Brain 1986 Aids to the examination of the peripheral nervous system. Baillière Tindall, London

Guttman L 1976 Spinal cord injuries: comprehensive management and research, 2nd edn. Blackwell, London

Jennett B, Teasdale G 1981 Management of head injuries. F A Davis, Philadelphia

Kopell H P, Thompson W A L 1976 Peripheral entrapment neuropathies, 2nd edn. Williams & Wilkins, Baltimore

Rosenberg R N, Grossman R (eds) 1984 Neurosurgery. The clinical neurosciences, Vol 2. Churchill Livingstone, New York

Seddon H 1975 Surgical disorders of the peripheral nerves, 2nd edn. Churchill Livingstone, Edinburgh

Sunderland S 1978 Nerves and nerve injuries, 2nd edn. Churchill Livingstone, Edinburgh

14. Infection and allergy and the nervous system

The central nervous system, its meningeal coverings and its peripheral ramifications may be invaded by infective agents, of which bacteria, viruses, spirochaetes, fungal agents and parasites of various types are examples. Sometimes a bacterial infection of the nervous system, for instance, is but one part of a more widespread disease process; some viruses, on the other hand, the so-called neurotropic group, have a particular predilection for nervous tissue. In general infective agents produce an inflammatory response; inflammatory changes in the nervous system and particularly in and around its blood vessels can also be the result of an allergic or hypersensitivity response to an infective agent or foreign protein (e.g. serum) which is present elsewhere in the body but which has not invaded nervous tissue. Many nervous complications of general infections are probably due to pathological mechanisms of this nature, involving a number of cell-mediated or humoral immune mechanisms, while others are the direct result of circulating toxins which are produced by the infecting agent.

BACTERIAL INFECTIONS

Bacteria may enter the nervous system by direct spread from an infective focus in the cranial bones or vertebrae, as in patients with suppuration in the middle ear or paranasal sinuses, or osteomyelitis of a vertebra. This spread can be facilitated by injury producing a penetrating wound, or a fracture of the cranial vault with a tear of the adherent dura mater. Alternatively organisms can arrive via the blood stream, being derived from a remote focus of infection; commonly this spread is via the arterial system, when invasion of the nervous system is preceded by a phase of bacteraemia or pyaemia, but an alternative route is via the profuse anastomosis of vertebral veins through which infection may spread directly from the thorax or abdomen to the cranial cavity. The common bacterial infections of the nervous system so produced are meningitis, septic venous sinus thrombosis, intracranial abscess and spinal extradural abscess.

Meningitis

Although pachymeningitis (inflammation of the dura) can occur as a secondary effect of inflammation in the paranasal sinuses, middle ear or skull bones, the term meningitis is now generally used to identify inflammation of the leptomeninges (the arachnoid and pia mater). Viral meningitis is the commonest variety and in general it is less serious than the bacterial variety which embraces both the pyogenic and tuberculous forms. Pyogenic meningitis is invariably life-threatening and often difficult to recognise in its earliest stages, especially in children, and demands immediate treatment with appropriate antibiotics. The tuberculous variety is also eminently treatable if recognised early; it is now much less common in developed countries than it was 30 to 40 years ago but is still a serious problem in the third world. Meningitis due to fungal agents is uncommon, except in immunocompromised patients, and so too are the parasitic varieties, save in some tropical countries. Traumatic or aseptic meningitis can result from intracranial haemorrhage and some meningeal inflammatory changes occur in spirochaetal infections, in granulomatous processes such as sarcoidosis, and in patients with carcinomatosis.

Pyogenic meningitis

The commonest variety of pyogenic meningitis is **meningococcal meningitis** or cerebrospinal fever. The disease can occur in epidemic form and the organism enters the body via the nasopharynx, being spread by droplet infection. During epidemics many apparently unaffected individuals carry the organism. There is a preliminary phase of bacteraemia or even septicaemia before meningeal manifestations appear, and in a few cases acute meningococcal septicaemia is rapidly fatal due to adrenal haemorrhage (Friedrichsen–Waterhouse syndrome). More often the phase is asymptomatic but is followed by frontal and occipital headache of mounting severity with fever. Occasionally at this stage there are rose-red or purple spots on the skin of the trunk, but these are infrequent in sporadic cases. The classical features of the illness, including neck stiffness (see below), are not invariably present or easy to identify in young infants and children. On suspicion of the diagnosis it is important to consider giving parenteral benzylpenicillin before transfer to hospital. As headache worsens and becomes generalised, so drowsiness and confusion supervene and the patient may lapse into semicoma within 12 to 24 hours. Vomiting is frequent and often projectile in type.

On examination the patient tends to lie on one side with his eyes away from the light and the knees pulled towards the chin; he is irritable and resents interference, pulling back the bedclothes when an attempt is made to remove them. Generally the pulse rate is slow. Neck stiffness is almost invariable once meningeal inflammation is widespread and in severe and established cases there may even be neck retraction. Kernig's sign is usually positive (restriction of knee extension when the thigh is flexed). Paralysis of one or other sixth cranial nerve is sometimes seen and the patient who is sufficiently conscious then complains of diplopia. Usually, the deep tendon reflexes are depressed, but focal neurological signs are rare. Although the inflammatory process affects principally the leptomeninges (arachnoid and pia mater), so that suppuration is mainly confined to the subarachnoid space, there are secondary degenerative changes in the superficial areas of the cerebral cortex, brain stem and cranial nerves in some cases. Hence fits occasionally occur, particularly in childhood; in cases treated late or ineffectively, there may be residual diplopia or nerve deafness, and sometimes communicating hydrocephalus develops giving papilloedema and residual dementia, often with spastic paralysis of the limbs. Other rare complications include spread of infection to the brain or subdural space to give abscess formation.

The CSF is typically under increased pressure and is cloudy or frankly purulent. There are many pus cells present, the protein content of the fluid is increased but sugar is absent. Scanty meningococci may be found on a direct smear of the fluid stained by Gram's stain, and the organisms can be cultured, though they are difficult to grow. If no organisms are isolated in a case of pyogenic meningitis the infection is probably meningococcal.

Serious epidemics of meningococcal meningitis occurred in Britain at the end of the First World War and the beginning of the second. Another peak occurred in 1974 and yet another upsurge has occurred since 1984. There are many antigenically distinct groups of meningococci, the commonest in Britain being types B, C, A, Y and W135;

typing is possible using monoclonal antibodies. Two types of vaccine (one active against A and C, the other against A, C, Y and W) are at present available but none has yet been produced against type B. Chemoprophylaxis of contacts should be started as soon as possible after confirmation of the diagnosis; rifampicin is the drug of choice and should be given at least to members of the patient's family and other close contacts. Vaccination is only at present indicated in the case of infections other than with type B when epidemics occur in closed or semi-closed communities (e.g. schools and military camps).

The clinical picture of pyogenic meningitis due to other bacteria is similar. That due to the pneumococcus (*Streptococcus pneumoniae*) can also be due to a blood-borne infection, without clear evidence of an infective focus elsewhere, and the same is true of *Haemophilus influenzae* meningitis. In pneumococcal meningitis the organisms are seen in profusion in direct smears of CSF. About 90% of cases of meningococcal meningitis now survive with appropriate treatment, but the prognosis of pneumococcal meningitis is rather less favourable and there is a significant mortality rate; influenzal meningitis, which is particularly common in childhood, is less ominous, but can run a smoulderering course for some weeks even after the initial acute phase has been satisfactorily controlled. Meningitis due to the *streptococcus* or *staphylococcus* is usually due to a spread of infection from the middle ear or elsewhere, although there is a curiously localised variety of spinal staphylococcal meningitis in which the exact method of bacterial entry has not yet been determined. In neonates, a purulent meningitis is often found to be due to infection with *Listeria monocytogenes*. *E. coli* is another organism which occasionally causes meningitis, more often in neonates, less commonly in adults. Listerial meningitis is rare in adults, except in elderly individuals suffering from other debilitating diseases. *Enterobacteriaceae*, *Bacteroides*, *Klebsiella*, *B proteus*, and *Pseudomonas* are other organisms which are rarely the cause in sporadic cases.

Treatment General measures which are indicated in most cases include intensive nursing care and analgesics for the relief of headache; intravenous fluids are sometimes needed to correct dehydration or electrolyte imbalance, phenytoin to control or prevent seizures and intravenous mannitol (rather than steroids which may impair the host response to the organism) is occasionally needed to reduce intracranial pressure. The prognosis of meningococcal meningitis was transformed first by the introduction of the sulphonamides and later by the antibiotics. So many organisms are now sulphonamide-resistant that these drugs have been largely abandoned. The most satisfactory remedy for treatment of this condition is intramuscular benzylpenicillin G. Although very little penicillin normally penetrates the blood-brain barrier, substantial amounts can cross the inflamed arachnoid to enter the subarachnoid space, so that intrathecal therapy is unnecessary. The usual adult dose is 600 mg of benzylpenicillin given intramuscularly every two hours at first and later six-hourly; the total daily dose in children is 10–20 mg/kg, in the neonate 30 mg/kg. Treatment should be continued for at least seven days and sometimes longer, depending on the clinical response. Many now prefer to give treatment intravenously rather than intramuscularly, at least for the first few days (Table 14.1).

The treatment of **other varieties of pyogenic meningitis** is similar, provided bacteriological tests reveal that the organism is penicillin sensitive (Table 14.1). Until a bacteriological diagnosis has been made, intramuscular benzylpenicillin is probably still the most satisfactory initial treatment. Many authorities still favour the policy of giving 10 000 units (6 mg) of benzylpenicillin, well diluted in 10 ml of normal saline, by intrathecal injection as soon as turbid spinal fluid is found on lumbar puncture. Care must be taken not to exceed this dose in any single injection. The use of intrathecal treatment is steadily declining but many still hold the view that in pneumococcal, streptococcal, and staphylococcal meningitis, further intrathecal penicillin therapy is usually wise, at least for the first few days. Intrathecal injection should be repeated not more often than every 24 hours until a satisfactory reduction in the number of cells in the

Table 14.1 Antimicrobial chemotherapy of some of the common causes of acute bacterial meningitis. (Reproduced with permission from Juel-Jensen et al 1987.)

Organism	First choice	Second choice
Neisseria meningitidis *Streptococcus pneumoniae*	Benzylpenicillin i.v.: *adults* 4 mega units (2.4g) 4 hourly; *children* 50 000 units/kg (30 mg) 4 hourly In *s. pneumoniae*: If no response double dose	Chloramphenicol i.v.: *adult* 20–25 mg/kg 6 hourly, up to 4g/d; *children* 12.5 mg/kg 6–8 hourly. *Cave*: dangerous in neonates and infants
Haemophilus influenzae 'Gram-negative'	Chloramphenicol i.v. (dose, see above) Cefuroxime (or 3rd generation cephalosporin*) i.v.: *adult* 3 g, 8 hourly; *children* 200–240 mg/kg/d initially	Ampicillin i.v. 50 mg/kg 4 hourly Co-trimoxazole i.v.: *adults* 160 mg trimethoprim + 800 mg sulphamethoxazole 12 hourly; *children* 6 + 30 mg/kg/d. *Cave*: hypersensitivity to sulphonamide
Pseudomonas aeruginosa	Piperacillin i.v.: *adults* 4 g, 6–8 hourly; *children* 100–300 mg/kg/d or ceftazidime i.v.: *adults* 2 g, 8–12 hourly; *children* 30–100 mg/kg/d + tobramycin i.v.: *adults* 3–5 mg/kg/d; *children* 6–7.5 mg/kg/daily or netilmicin 4–6 mg/kg/daily in divided doses (8 hourly)	Ticarcillin or mezlocillin + gentamicin 5 mg/kg/d
Staphylococcus aureus	Flucloxacillin (or oxacillin or nafcillin USP): *adults* 3 g 6 hourly; *children* 300 mg/kg/d	Vancomycin i.v.[+]: *adults* 500 mg 6 hourly; *children* 40 mg/kg/d
Staphylococcus epidermidis	Vancomycin i.v.[+] + gentamicin 5 mg/kg/d + rifampicin: *adults* 1.2 g/d; *children* 20 mg/kg/d (penicillin-sensitive organism should be treated with benzylpenicillin i.v., dose as above)	
Listeria monocytogenes	Ampicillin i.v. (dose see above) (+ gentamicin i.v. for immunocompromised patients)	Chloramphenicol i.v. or co-trimoxazole i.v. (dose as above)
Streptococcus agalactiae (Group B)	Benzylpenicillin i.v.: *neonates* 150 000–250 000 units/kg/d (90–150 mg/kg/d)	

Note: In all cases, normal renal function is assumed. In renal failure dose must be reduced after the initial dose; as a rough guide:

$$\frac{\text{normal plasma creatinine}}{\text{patient's plasma creatinine}} \times \text{normal dose may be used}$$

*3rd generation cephalosporins such as cefotaxime or latamoxef.

[+]Intrathecal, intraventricular or intrashunt injection of vancomycin or gentamicin may be used (contact manufacturers for special preparation and dosage).

CSF is achieved and cultures become sterile. Often systemic penicillin must be continued for two or three weeks. If the organism identified is known to be insensitive or shown to be resistant to penicillin, then other antibiotics must be considered (see Table 14.1).

Erythromycin, for example, of which the dose is 250–500 mg, six-hourly, is best reserved for staphylococcal infections which resist penicillin, while chloramphenicol (250 mg, six-hourly) is also useful as a wide-range antibiotic, particularly in influenzal meningitis, but should only be used for relatively short periods as it is liable to produce blood dyscrasias. In influenzal meningitis it often combined with ampicillin. Gentamicin, 2–5 mg/kg daily in eight-hourly divided doses, given along with ampicillin or sodium carbenicillin, is probably the treatment of choice for bacterial meningitis due to *E. coli*, to *Pseudomonas aeruginosa* or to other Gram-negative organisms. Antibiotic therapy may have to be continued for many weeks in influenzal meningitis before the spinal fluid returns to normal. In listerial meningitis, chloramphenicol or ampicillin (150 mg/kg daily in divided doses) are the most effective.

Tuberculous meningitis

Tuberculous meningitis can arise as a complication of miliary tuberculosis when meningeal inflammation may smoulder for some weeks before becoming clinically apparent. It is therefore wise to examine the CSF in cases of miliary tubercle in order to determine whether subclinical meningitis is present. The disease can also develop in children with primary tuberculosis or in adults with pulmonary disease and is then usually due to an acute or subacute exudative reaction in the meninges following the rupture of a small cerebral or cerebellar tuberculoma into the subarachnoid space. Cerebral tuberculomas are usually small, although rarely one is of sufficient size to present as a space-occupying lesion; this is commoner in India than in Western countries.

The symptoms of tuberculous meningitis are similar in character but different in tempo from those of the pyogenic variety, although there are rare cases in which the onset is equally abrupt and progression just as rapid. In children and young adults previously vaccinated with BCG the illness is rare, but when it does occur it is often comparatively mild initially and is easily mistaken for benign lymphocytic meningitis. Another important diagnostic pitfall to recognise is that the sudden rupture of a small tuberculoma into the subarachnoid space in an individual already sensitised to the bacterial protein of the tubercle bacillus can give rise to an acute allergic meningeal reaction with a lymphocytic pleocytosis lasting for a few days and then resolving, only to be followed later by a more progressive meningitic picture as the organisms multiply in the subarachnoid space. Thus the illness can be biphasic with the initial phase again being suggestive of viral meningitis. More often, however, there is a period of several days or even weeks of fluctuating premonitory malaise, anorexia, vomiting, vague headache and disinterest, before sustained fever, persistent headache and signs of meningeal irritation become clearly evident. When present, retinal miliary tubercles, yellowish nodules about half the size of an optic disc, are diagnostic. It is important to recognise the disease early, since the longer it exists before treatment, the more probable are complications such as diplopia and communicating hydrocephalus or focal neurological signs (monoparesis or hemiparesis), which can result from cerebral infarction due to associated tuberculous arteritis. Adhesions in the spinal subarachnoid space may cause difficulty in treating the condition with intrathecal remedies, and spinal block sometimes develops; a rare variety almost confined to the spinal cord and causing a paraparesis is not uncommon in India. Similar adhesions around the brain stem can cause attacks of decerebrate rigidity, which generally imply a gloomy prognosis. The complications and sequelae of tuberculous meningitis are more severe than those of any other variety.

The cerebrospinal fluid, usually under increased pressure, is generally clear but a fine 'cobweb' clot often forms on standing. There is an increase in cells to about 100/mm^3 but their number can vary from 10 to about 1000. In the early stages some neutrophils are present but later most, if not all, are mononuclear. The protein content of the fluid is usually increased to about 1.0–4.0 g/l but much greater increases can result from subarachnoid block. The glucose content of the fluid is usually reduced to below 0.5 g/l. If tubercle bacilli are found in the fluid in centrifuged specimens stained by the Ziehl-Neelsen method, this clinches the diagnosis, but even with the most meticulous examination of specimens this is not invariably possible and culture with assessment of sensitivity to streptomycin and other drugs is invariably necessary. A rapid latex particle agglutination test which detects *M. tuberculosis* plasma membrane antigen is a quick and accurate aid to diagnosis.

Treatment The essential drugs in the treatment of tuberculous meningitis are streptomycin (1 g intramuscularly daily in adults, 200 mg–1 g in children), rifampicin (450–600 mg daily by mouth in adults and 10–20 mg/kg daily in children) and isoniazid (200–300 mg daily). Ethambutol (25 mg/kg body weight) is of little value in the treatment of meningitis. There is virtually unanimous agreement that intrathecal treatment is not now necessary but a few authorities still favour the administration of 0.1 g streptomycin intrathecally, daily for six or seven days and thereafter twice-weekly for three or four weeks in very severe cases in adults. In children, a proportionately lower intrathecal dose (25–50 mg) is given. Many authorities also give 20–30 mg of prednisone daily in addition, in an effort to prevent the development of adhesions in the subarachnoid space. In cases in which multiple subarachnoid adhesions and spinal block have developed despite treatment, it is sometimes necessary to give intrathecal streptomycin and 10–25 mg of hydrocortisone via cisternal puncture or even through burr holes in the lateral ventricles. Anticonvulsants may also be required, pyridoxine (10 mg daily) should be given to prevent isoniazid polyneuropathy and, if hydrocephalus develops, surgical treatment may be required. When the organism is resistant to the standard drugs mentioned above, ethionamide (10–15 mg/kg daily) and cycloserine (15 mg/kg daily) have been recommended but both are toxic and should be used only as a last resort.

Brucellosis

Meningoencephalitis is an uncommon but well-recognised complication of infection with *Brucella mellitensis, Brucella abortus* and *Brucella suris*. The clinical picture is usually that of a subacute or chronic meningitis but focal encephalitis giving a pseudotumoural clinical picture or epilepsy, aphasia, confusion or dementia may also occur. The CSF shows a mononuclear pleocytosis. Diagnosis rests upon serological tests and isolation of the organism from the fluid. These organisms are largely resistant to antibiotics but some strains are sensitive to tetracycline, gentamicin or kanamicin.

Sarcoidosis

The aetiology of Boeck's sarcoid remains unknown; while its pathological changes resemble those of tuberculosis save for the absence of caseation, it is probably unrelated to tuberculous infection. It is accompanied by a depression of cell-mediated immune mechanisms. While lymphadenopathy in the mediastinum or elsewhere, iridocyclitis and hepatic involvement are its more common manifestations, the nervous system is sometimes involved, resulting usually in a combination of chronic basal granulomatous meningitis on the one hand with multiple cranial nerve palsies, a pleocytosis and increased protein in the CSF, and sometimes a peripheral neuropathy or myopathy on the other. The granulomatous meningitic form can damage the optic nerves, the third, fourth and sixth nerves and less often the seventh and eighth; sometimes spinal cord involvement gives signs of a myelopathy. Focal granulomas occasionally develop within the brain or spinal cord, especially in the hypothalamus. However, some patients present simply with

features of raised intracranial pressure due to cerebral oedema or communicating hydrocephalus. In the later stages hypothalamic involvement, with obesity, diabetes insipidus, and impairment of recent memory are not uncommon. Temporary or sustained remission is often produced by large doses of steroids but maintenance treatment is often needed for several years.

Intracranial thrombophlebitis

Suppurative thrombophlebitis of intracranial venous sinuses most often affects the lateral, cavernous and superior longitudinal (sagittal) sinuses, due to centripetal spread of infection from the middle ear, skin of the face and frontal sinus, respectively. In all three conditions the patients have pyaemia and are acutely ill with high remittent fever. Lateral sinus thrombosis must be suspected in patients with otitis media who show this clinical picture without signs of meningitis or intracerebral spread of infection, while septic thrombosis of the cavernous sinus generally gives unilateral proptosis, chemosis of the conjunctiva and oculomotor paresis. In sagittal sinus thrombosis there may be oedema and tenderness of the scalp over the vertex and spastic weakness of one or both lower limbs; a subdural abscess not uncommonly results. Aseptic thrombosis of the lateral or sagittal sinuses may also complicate middle-ear disease but then causes the syndrome of 'otitic hydrocephalus' which can resemble that of 'benign intracranial hypertension' (see Ch. 12, p. 259).

Intracranial abscess

Localised suppuration within the cranial cavity can occur outside the dura mater, giving an *extradural abscess*. This condition is invariably the result of cranial osteomyelitis which in turn is usually due to infected scalp wounds, otitis media, or paranasal sinusitis. Generally there is a remittent fever and some tenderness over the overlying scalp, but symptoms and signs of increased intracranial pressure and CSF changes, if present at all, are minimal.

A **subdural abscess** or **empyema** is usually a sequel of frontal sinusitis but rarely results from middle-ear disease or septic thrombophlebitis; often the layer of pus extends over the whole of one cerebral hemisphere. Initially there is headache and tenderness over the affected frontal sinus or mastoid bone but subsequently the patient becomes drowsy or stuporose, his fever mounts and neck stiffness develops. Jacksonian seizures are frequent in the contralateral limbs and a hemiparesis or hemiplegia almost invariably develops. Usually there is a polymorphonuclear pleocytosis in the CSF with a marked rise in protein content. If not treated quickly by surgical evacuation this condition is soon fatal.

Abscess formation in the subarachnoid space is very rare and the commonest site for intracranial suppuration is within the brain substance itself, a **brain abscess**. In up to 30% of cases this is due to a direct spread of infection through adherent meninges from the bones of the middle ear, when the principal sites are the temporal lobe (upward spread) or one cerebellar hemisphere (lateral spread); about another 10% are due to frontal sinusitis, when the frontal lobe is usually involved. Of the remaining 60%, a few are due to penetrating injuries, but most are metastatic; in many of these the primary focus of infection is in the lung (bronchiectasis, empyema, lung abscess) but it may lie anywhere in the body. Brain abscesses are particularly liable to develop in patients with cyanotic congenital heart disease, even without bacterial endocarditis. The cocci are the organisms usually responsible. Pathologically there is an initial stage of focal necrosis and liquefaction, or suppurative encephalitis, but this is followed by proliferation of glial and fibrous elements, with eventual encapsulation of the abscess.

When a patient with otitis media or sinusitis notes the suppression of a previously profuse discharge and this is followed by headache, vomiting and confusion, it is reasonable to suppose that inflammation has spread intracranially. Often, however, the patient seems to recover from otitis, say, but remains unwell, with depression or irritability, vague intermittent headache and nausea, anorexia, weight loss and mild fever. Even in haematogenous cases, though the onset is occasionally acute, with focal seizures and neurological signs, there may be minimal headache and progressive personality change. If the signs and symptoms of infection have been masked by antibiotic therapy, the patient may be thought to be suffering from an intracranial tumour.

Usually, however, there is intermittent pyrexia, and symptoms and signs of increased intracranial pressure (headache, vomiting, papilloedema, bradycardia) develop steadily. Other manifestations depend upon the localisation of the abscess. There will be aphasia if a frontal or temporal lobe abscess involves the dominant hemisphere; a temporal lobe lesion often gives a quadrantic visual field defect and minimal weakness of the contralateral face and hand, while in frontal lobe abscess, intellectual impairment may be prominent and a contralateral hemiparesis is common. When the cerebellum is involved, headache is often suboccipital, nystagmus is seen and signs of cerebellar dysfunction (ataxia, dysmetria, etc.) are usually present in the ipsilateral arm and leg.

In the early stages, examination of the CSF can be helpful but this test is not without risk, and is certainly contraindicated if the intracranial pressure is clearly raised. Indeed on suspicion of such a lesion most authorities would now agree that the CT scan (Fig. 14.1) is the initial investigation of choice. If the CSF is examined, its pressure is usually increased and it contains up to 100 white cells/mm^3, of which many are lymphocytes, though some are usually polymorphonuclear; there is a moderate rise in protein, while the sugar content of the fluid is normal. The EEG may be helpful, revealing a striking focus of delta activity over the affected cerebral hemisphere, but the CT scan, with contrast enhancement, is usually diagnostic. Treatment, apart from systemic antibiotic therapy, is then neurosurgical. Systemic antibiotic therapy is now preferred and it is no longer felt necessary as a routine to instil antibiotic into the abscess cavity if drainage is satisfactory. Ampicillin and gentamicin are among the antibiotics most often employed, but much depends upon the nature and sensitivity of the organism responsible and metronidazole is commonly added in cases of otogenic abscess. Where possible the abscess is excised; in other instances it is drained. The mortality rate, despite treatment, was formerly about 30% but has now fallen to about 10% in many series; many survivors suffer from headaches, epilepsy (up to 50%) and residual limb weakness or ataxia according to the situation of the lesion.

Intraspinal suppuration

An **intramedullary spinal abscess** is a very rare condition of metastatic origin; it usually presents with initial paraesthesiae in the lower limbs followed by a flaccid paraplegia of rapid progression. Generally there is suppuration elsewhere in the body, but few cases are diagnosed in life, and the condition is difficult to distinguish from other forms of acute myelopathy and from rapidly-growing intramedullary neoplasms. It should be considered in patients presenting with signs of an acute spinal cord lesion, as improvement may follow surgical drainage.

Much more common and particularly important to diagnose is spinal **extradural abscess**. This can be due to tuberculous caries of the spine (Pott's disease), but a staphylococcal aetiology is now very much commoner. In about a third of all cases the condition is secondary to osteomyelitis of a vertebral body but in the remainder the infection, of metastatic origin, develops primarily within the extradural space. Suppuration and exuberant granulation tissue may extend over several segments of the spinal cord and eventually spread into the spinal muscles and soft tissues of the back. Compression of the cord and interference with its circulation are the most important complications.

The initial symptom is usually an ache in the affected area of the spine, followed by root pain and fever. Intense spinal tenderness follows, particularly in osteomyelitic cases, and paraesthesiae in the lower limbs followed by ascending paralysis subsequently develop. The diagnosis must be made early as paralysis, once present, may be irreversible while surgical exploration and drainage of the abscess, combined with appropriate antibiotic therapy, can be curative. Lumbar puncture (which usually demonstrates complete spinal block) and myelography have been considered essential for diagnosis and localisation, but should never be performed close to an area of spinal pain or tenderness in view of the risk of introducing organisms into the subarachnoid space. When clinical evidence has suggested that such a lesion is present in the lumbar region it has been thought wiser to introduce contrast medium cisternally. Even in osteomyelitic cases, spinal radiographs are often normal initially. As a result of the increasing availability of whole-body scanning and magnetic resonance imaging (MRI) it now seems likely that diagnosis of this condition by CT scanning and/or MRI will increasingly obviate the need for myelography.

Leprosy

Leprosy, an infectious disease due to *Mycobacterium leprae*, is endemic in some tropical countries, particularly Africa and India. It is characterised by a long incubation period, a prolonged remittent course and involvement of

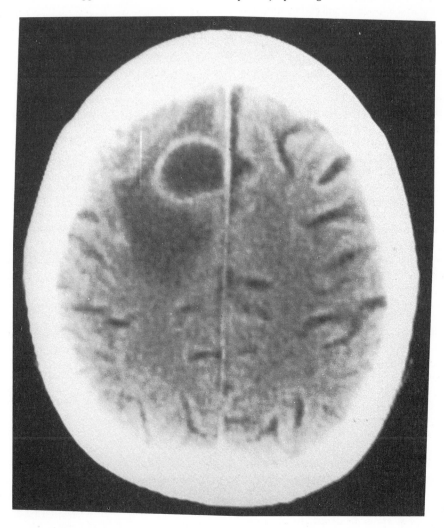

Fig. 14.1   Unenhanced axial CT scan showing a cerebral abscess in the medial part of the right frontal lobe with some surrounding oedema.

the skin, mucous membranes and peripheral nerves. The more acute and infectious or lepromatous form affects particularly the nasal mucosa and the skin; it is in the chronic tuberculoid form that the peripheral nerves are generally involved. In the beginning there are generally thickened, pigmented and anaesthetic areas of skin; later the areas of numbness extend, many peripheral nerves are thickened and tender and eventually there is destruction of the distal phalanges in the hands and feet with painless ulcers of the extremities.

This condition can be treated effectively with drugs of the sulphone group, of which the most effective is dapsone, given initially in a dosage of 25–50 mg twice weekly, increasing to a maximum of 400 mg twice weekly. It is now recommended that rifampicin should also be given for the first four weeks and clofazimine 100 mg three times daily for a year, while the dapsone is continued indefinitely.

VIRUS INFECTIONS OF THE NERVOUS SYSTEM

The so-called neurotropic viruses have in common the fact that they are visible only under the electron microscope, that they generally pass through filter candles and that they are intracellular parasites. They attack principally nerve cells and hence the main brunt of the pathological changes which they produce falls upon the grey matter of the central nervous system. However, it is now known that the distinction between neurotropic and non-neurotropic viruses according to whether or not the nervous system is the primary or secondary site of attack by the disease process is largely artificial. Most viruses which attack the nervous system do so after multiplying in other organs; involvement of the nervous system results from haematogenous spread or retrograde dissemination along nerve fibres after endocytosis at axonal terminals. Viruses are classified according to their nucleic acid content, size, sensitivity to lipid solvents, morphology and method of development in cells. The commoner viruses which may attack the nervous system are listed in Table 14.2, from which it will be seen that viruses certainly account for acute anterior poliomyelitis, various forms of encephalitis and encephalomyelitis, rabies, lymphocytic meningitis, herpes zoster and probably also for encephalitis lethargica. Others which are not normally neurotropic, such as those of mumps and glandular fever (infectious mononucleosis) may attack the nervous system, giving rise to an encephalitic or meningitic illness.

In recent years the concept of **'slow virus' infections** of the nervous system has aroused interest. Kuru, a progressive disorder characterised initially by cerebellar

Table 14.2 Viral infections of the nervous system (Reproduced with permission from Walton 1985 and modified from Johnson 1982.)

	Some representative viruses causing neurological disease in man and animals
RNA viruses	
Paramyxovirus	
Paramyxovirus	Parainfluenza virus
	Mumps virus
Morbillivirus	Measles virus
Rhabdovirus	
Lyssavirus	Rabies virus
Bunyavirus	California encephalitis virus
	Rift Valley fever virus
Reovirus	
Orbivirus	Colorado tick fever virus
Togavirus	
Alphavirus (formerly group A arboviruses)	Eastern encephalitis virus
	Western encephalitis virus
	Venezuelan equine encephalitis virus
Rubivirus	Rubella virus
Flavivirus (formerly group B arboviruses)	St Louis encephalitis virus
	Japanese encephalitis virus
	Murray Valley encephalitis virus
	Tick-borne encephalitis virus
	Louping-ill
	Yellow fever virus
	Dengue viruses
Picornavirus	
Enterovirus	Polioviruses
	Coxsackie viruses A and B
	Echoviruses
Cardiovirus	Encephalomyocarditis virus
Arenavirus	Lymphocytic choriomeningitis
DNA viruses	
Herpes viruses	Herpes simplex, types 1 and 2
	Varicella-zoster
	Cytomegalovirus
	Epstein-Barr virus (infectious mononucleosis)
Papova virus	Polyoma virus (progressive multifocal leucoencephalopathy)
Poxvirus	Vaccinia
	Variola
Retrovirus	AIDS
Unidentified presumed viral illnesses	Encephalitis lethargica
	Kuru
	Creutzfeldt-Jakob disease
	Scrapie

ataxia and confined to the natives of New Guinea, has been transmitted to the chimpanzee; the same is now true of subacute spongiform encephalopathy (Creutzfeldt-Jakob disease). Both conditions appear to be due to small transmissible but as yet unidentifed agents, presumed to be viruses, and show affinities with scrapie, a disorder of sheep, which has an incubation period, after inoculation, of at least nine months. In another rare disorder, progressive multifocal leucoencephalopathy (PML), which usually complicates Hodgkin's disease or other reticuloses, polyoma virus has now been identified in cerebral lesions. Cytomegalic inclusion body disease is another slow virus infection, while the acquired immune deficiency syndrome (AIDS — see below) is becoming an increasingly serious and ubiquitous infection which, though primarily systemic in its effects upon the immune system, produces major neurological complications. It has been suggested, without, as yet, good evidence, that some commoner conditions (e.g. multiple sclerosis) will eventually prove to be due to viral infection. Subacute sclerosing panencephalitis (SSPE) now appears to be due to the prolonged persistence of measles virus in the brain.

Acute anterior poliomyelitis

Three principal strains of poliomyelitis virus have been identified and are known as the Brunhilde, Lansing and Leon strains, of which the Lansing is probably the most virulent. Other closely-related enteroviral agents (e.g. the Coxsackie A7 virus) can occasionally produce a clinical picture like that of poliomyelitis. The virus attacks particularly the anterior horn cells of the spinal cord, around which collections of inflammatory cells are generally found in fatal cases, but the cells of motor brain stem nuclei and even those of the cerebral cortex may be invaded. It appears to enter the nervous system by travelling in a retrograde direction along peripheral and autonomic nerves. The usual portal of entry is the alimentary tract, although in some cases it may be the nasopharynx, particularly after recent tonsillectomy. In the latter cases there is a particular tendency for the bulbar nuclei to be involved.

As alimentary infection is derived from contaminated water or food, and flies are a common vector, epidemics tend to occur in summer and early autumn, though sporadic cases occur all the year round. The disease was once virtually confined to young children (hence the name 'infantile paralysis'), but in the 1940s and 1950s, particularly in countries like the USA, Britain and Scandinavia, where standards of hygiene had been improving, more older children and young adults were afflicted. This change was probably accounted for by the fact that fewer children were acquiring immunity as a result of subclinical infections in early life. The pattern has now changed even further as most children and young people have been effectively protected by inoculation and the incidence of the disease has declined sharply.

The incubation period is usually between seven and 14 days. During epidemics many individuals are infected and acquire immunity without developing symptoms (**subclinical cases**). A second group of patients experience a mild febrile illness without clinical evidence of nervous system involvement (abortive cases); in a third group there is a meningitic illness with headache, fever, neck stiffness and a CSF pleocytosis but no muscular paralysis (**non-paralytic cases**). The fourth group of patients in whom paralysis develops (paralytic cases) constitute a relatively small proportion of the whole. Excessive physical exertion or localised trauma to a limb (e.g. a prophylactic inoculation) during the pre-paralytic phase can promote paralysis of the affected member.

In non-paralytic cases or in the pre-paralytic phase of the paralytic form, headache, fever, neck stiffness and Kernig's sign are usual and there may be abdominal pain and widespread muscular pain and tenderness. Attempted spinal flexion is often painful. Sometimes after two or three days of fever there is apparent improvement for from 24 to 48 hours followed by a recrudescence of fever and the onset of paralysis, with muscle pain and tenderness. The distribution of muscular weakness is very variable. Typically it is asymmetrical, affecting perhaps one arm and the opposite leg, but any muscle group may be involved. Occasionally the weakness ascends, endangering life through respiratory paralysis. In a few cases the main brunt of the disease falls upon the brain stem (polioencephalitis), giving paralysis of facial, pharyngeal and/or laryngeal muscles. The combination of pharyngeal and respiratory paralysis which occurs in some such bulbar cases is particularly sinister because of the danger of inhalation of secretions or vomit, and tracheotomy and assisted respiration are then required. Once paralysis appears, it usually reaches its maximum distribution within 24 hours, but in a few cases it continues to progress for two or three days. Fortunately the extent of the weakness at the height of the illness does not always indicate the degree of permanent paralysis which will persist; some anterior horn cells are only temporarily affected, recovery occurring subsequently. This is the principal justification for using assisted ventilation in this disease. Nevertheless there is nearly always some residual paralysis, followed by muscular wasting and often fasciculation, contractures of paralysed muscles, bony deformity and failure of growth in the affected member. Rarely, progressive muscular weakness and atrophy develop many years later to give a clinical picture like that of progressive muscular atrophy (see p. 285).

It is difficult to assess accurately the mortality of the disease, in view of the many subclinical and abortive cases which occur. Furthermore, the mortality varied from epidemic to epidemic, having been as high as 25% of paralytic cases in some, but this was an exceptionally high figure and 10% was more usual. Respiratory paralysis and/or infection have generally been the cause of death, which is now much less common with modern management.

The CSF in the first two to three days of the illness generally shows an increase of polymorphonuclear leucocytes, but these are soon replaced by a lymphocytic pleocytosis, up to 200 or more cells per mm^3. A substantial rise in protein in the fluid persists much longer than the pleocytosis.

Diagnosis depends in the first instance upon serological and antibody tests and virus isolation. Monoclonal antibodies are now available which can not only distinguish infection with the various strains of the virus but can also identify natural infection as distinct from those rare cases which are due to oral vaccination.

Prevention of this disease is more satisfactory than any form of treatment. Passive immunisation with globulin gives temporary protection during an epidemic, but permanent immunity is only achieved either by acquiring a natural infection or by active immunisation. The Salk and British vaccines were partially effective, particularly in reducing the incidence of paralytic cases; these have now been supplanted by the Sabin type oral vaccine, utilising live but attenuated virus.

In treatment, complete and immediate rest is necessary in any suspected case since physical activity in the pre-paralytic phase increases the risk of severe paralysis. In patients without evidence of respiratory or bulbar paralysis (early evidence of impending respiratory insufficiency can often be identified by asking the patient to count aloud without taking a breath, when less than 15 is usually a warning sign) the important principles are to use analgesics and sedatives in the acute stage and active physiotherapy once this is over. When respiratory insufficiency is impending or established, intermittent positive pressure respiration, initially via an endotracheal tube, subsequently via a tracheostomy (with a cuffed tube when there is also bulbar paralysis) in an intensive care unit is needed. In the rare cases of bulbar paralysis without respiratory insufficiency, a tracheostomy will also be necessary to avoid the inhalation of secretions, and feeding via an oesophageal catheter or parenterally will be required until swallowing recovers.

Encephalitis lethargica

This disease is probably due to a virus, although no organism has ever been isolated. The principal site of pathological change is in the grey matter of the midbrain, particularly in the substantia nigra. The disease appeared in Europe in 1915 and occurred in epidemics up to the early 1920s, when its frequency began to wane. No epidemics have occurred since then, but some believe that sporadic cases still occur. Thirty years ago the illness was usually acute, beginning with headache, vomiting, convulsions and confusion; nowadays the condition probably presents, if indeed it occurs at all, in a more subacute or chronic form, with manifestations of post-encephalitic parkinsonism (see p. 193).

In the acute cases, there was characteristic lethargy and somnolence, sometimes amounting to stupor, during the day, but the patient was often awake, though confused and perhaps delirious, at night (reversal of sleep rhythm). Ocular palsies and pupillary changes were invariable, giving blurred vision and diplopia. Choreiform limb movements, tremor and tics involving facial and respiratory muscles were also seen. Sometimes parkinsonian features (mask-like face, festinant gait, tremor, oculogyric crises) were seen early, but more often did not appear until several years after the acute illness. Probably in these cases, even after many years, the causal organism persisted in the central nervous system. Indeed many patients with post-encephalitic parkinsonism gave no history of a previous recognisable encephalitic illness. Not only were neurological sequelae common in children particularly, after partial recovery from the acute disease, there were often severe behaviour disturbances, including cruelty, violence and moral and intellectual degeneracy. Some such individuals required permanent institutional treatment.

Only about 25% of patients afflicted by this disease in its acute form recovered completely. About one-third died within four weeks of the onset, but the remainder were usually disabled in the end by parkinsonism. The CSF was often normal, but there was sometimes a minimal pleocytosis and increase in protein.

Other forms of virus encephalitis and encephalomyelitis

Several specific varieties of encephalitis occurring in various parts of the world have been found to be due to viruses. In this group are the Japanese type B, St Louis, Russian spring-summer, Murray Valley, Venezuelan, Californian and Colorado varieties, in which infection is transmitted by the mosquito or by a tick. Equine encephalomyelitis, which occurs in the USA, is transmitted by the mosquito from a reservoir of virus in birds or in the wood-tick. Louping-ill, a virus disease of sheep, has also been known to cause an encephalitic illness in man in Great Britain. Although all these forms of encephalitis show differences from one another in clinical present-ation, course and mortality, each, except the Venezuelan, Californian and Colorado forms, gives an encephalitic illness characterised by headache, fever, a period of confusion, stupor or semicoma and/or rigidity or tremor of the limbs. In equine encephalomyelitis particularly there may be spastic paresis of the limbs, fits and permanent mental deterioration. Each of these con-ditions (and there are probably many more varieties as yet unrecognised) is likely, after an acute onset, to result in a relatively protracted illness, with fluctuating levels of consciousness; and the mortality can be as much as 60% in some epidemics. Though some patients recover com-pletely, a number show intellectual and physical residua which persist when the acute illness is over. In each type the CSF is abnormal; there is a lymphocytic pleocytosis in the Japanese B and St Louis types, and in louping-ill, but polymorphs predominate, often in large numbers, in the early stages of the equine variety. The Venezuelan form, which also occurs in the southern USA, is trans-mitted via the mosquito from a reservoir in horses, and like Colorado tick fever usually gives a mild and transient influenza-like illness with recovery in a few days. The Californian arthropod-borne bunyavirus infection is also mild as a rule but can cause an aseptic meningitis and very rarely a more severe encephalitis.

Similar, though usually relatively mild, encephalitic illnesses occur in Great Britain and continental Europe and only rarely is the causal virus identified except perhaps in the small proportion of cases of infectious mononucleosis in which an encephalitic illness develops, in mumps, in some Coxsackie or Echo virus infections and in herpes simplex encephalitis (see below). In Western Europe postinfective encephalitis (see p. 238) may be as common as the viral variety, although a mild and transient encephalitic illness sometimes occurs in influenza.

Herpes simplex encephalitis

While an encephalitic illness rarely complicates dissem-inated herpes simplex infection in infancy, in patients of all ages an explosive cerebral illness characterised by coma, hyperpyrexia and features (fits, hemiparesis) sug-gesting a lesion in one temporal lobe, may be due to infection with the virus but is not then associated with cutaneous manifestations. Subacute cases also occur, and indeed chronic limbic encephalitis is rarely due to this organism. The virus implicated is usually type I, the strain which causes oral and labial herpes, and not type II which is responsible for genital herpes. Often, because of the clinical picture in the commoner acute or hyperacute cases cerebral haemorrhage or abscess are suspected. However, CT or MRI scanning is usually diagnostic and the EEG often demonstrates a characteristic burst sup-pression pattern (see p. 34). The CSF is often normal but can show a mild pleocytosis and increase in protein. Herpes simplex virus may be cultured or identified on electron microscopy in biopsy specimens obtained from the necrotic temporal lobe; becasue of the focal features many such cases are explored neurosurgically. While operative decompression alone may save life and recovery may in the end be reasonably good, good results have been achieved in some cases with massive dosage of steroid drugs (e.g. dexamethasone 5 mg four times daily) but most authorities now favour antiviral chemotherapy with acyclovir. While such modern treatment has undoubtedly reduced the mortality rate, some survivors are left with severe defects of memory or even dementia.

Benign myalgic encephalomyelitis (the post-viral fatigue syndrome)

This name has been given to an encephalomyelitic illness which has occurred in outbreaks throughout the world. It has also been called 'epidemic neuromyasthenia' or, more often, the post-viral fatigue syndrome. No organism has been isolated consistently from such cases, even from the many which occurred in the Royal Free Hospital, London, in 1955. The illness usually begins with lassi-tude and malaise, headache, neck stiffness and general-ised muscular pain. Vertigo, vomiting and diplopia are common, as are bizarre disorders of concentration, behaviour and gait, with inordinate chronic fatigue, often suggesting hysteria. Indeed some have asserted that the condition is due to 'epidemic hysteria' as it has often occurred in closed communities (schools, convents, nurses' homes), especially in females. Paraesthesiae are frequent and there is variable limb paralysis and sensory loss with, however, preservation of deep reflexes. The EMG often shows a curiously intermittent pattern of voluntary muscular contraction. Rarely, there is an associated hepatitis. There is little or no fever and the CSF is always normal. The illness may run a prolonged relapsing course of months or years and during this period persistent fatigue is prominent. Recent studies utilising viral culture and monoclonal antibodies against VPI polypeptide have produced convincing evidence to suggest chronic enterovirus infection in many such patients (Yousef et al 1988). Depression is common and many patients improve with anti-depressive medication.

Subacute sclerosing panencephalitis

This subacute variety of encephalitis, which was previously called subacute inclusion body encephalitis (Dawson) and subacute sclerosing leucoencephalitis (van Bogaert), is clearly due to virus infection. Serological and other evidence has confirmed that it is usually a late effect of measles (or may rarely follow vaccination with attenuated measles vaccine) and that the measles virus has persisted in the brain and has undergone modification to make it behave like a 'slow virus'. The disease is commonest in infancy and childhood but can occur in adult life; nerve cell degeneration, gliosis and inflammatory changes occur in the cerebral cortex and many nerve cells and astrocytes contain inclusion bodies. The disease is characterised clinically by progressive dementia, spastic paralysis of the limbs and myoclonus, and generally runs a fatal course, usually within nine to 12 months. Retinal degeneration and pigmentation with visual failure occur in some cases. Rarely, partial remissions are seen and in exceptional cases incomplete recovery has occurred. The EEG is virtually diagnostic, revealing bizarre generalised repetitive slow-wave complexes separated by periods of comparative electrical silence (a so-called burst suppression pattern) and the CSF shows increased measles-specific immunoglobulin. No treatment is known to influence the course of this disease.

Rabies

Rabies in man follows a bite from an infected animal, usually a dog, rarely a cat, bat or fox, which excretes the virus in its saliva. The virus enters the nervous system along peripheral nerves and attacks nerve cells in which the characteristic acidophilic inclusions (Negri bodies) are eventually demonstrated. Rabies in animals is characterised first by a change in behaviour with perversion of appetite, excessive excitement, salivation and progressive paralysis with muscular spasms. The incubation period in man is from 28 to 60 days or even more; during this asymptomatic period, protective vaccination can prevent the development of the disease. The first symptoms are usually apprehension, depression and restless sleep. These are followed by pharyngeal spasm (hydrophobia) which soon extends to the muscles of respiration and then to those of the trunk and limbs, producing opisthotonos. Any attempt to drink brings on the spasms which are accompanied by profuse salivation and later succeeded by profound paralysis. Rarely, ascending paralysis

(the paralytic form) can be the presenting feature. Death may occur during the spasms or later, and is usually due to respiratory or cardiac failure. A serum fluorescent antibody test is diagnostic. The mortality rate is virtually 100% but very occasional patients treated with curarisation and assisted respiration have recovered.

Viral meningitis

Many virus infections can produce the clinical picture of an acute meningitis with a lymphocytic pleocytosis in the CSF and with little or no evidence to suggest involvement of the nervous parenchyma (i. e. meningoencephalitis). Apart from non-paralytic poliomyelitis mentioned above, the agents involved include those of acute lymphocytic choriomeningitis (see below), mumps, infectious mononucleosis, some viruses of the Coxsackie and Echo groups, louping-ill and the chlamydia of psittacosis among others. Most such cases run a benign course leading to complete recovery and these benign forms of lymphocytic meningitis account for about 50% of all cases of infectious meningitis seen in hospital in Britain.

Acute lymphocytic choriomeningitis

This benign disorder is due to an arenavirus which also afflicts mice, and the house mouse may be the source of the human disease which can occur sporadically or in small epidemics. The condition is commonest in childhood but also affects adults. The prodromal symptoms are those of fever and are rapidly succeeded by headache, drowsiness and neck stiffness. Severe disturbance of consciousness is uncommon and many patients are alert throughout; diplopia is an infrequent complication. The illness usually lasts for about a week but complete recovery is the rule. The CSF is usually under increased pressure and may contain 1000 or more cells per mm^3, of which most are mononuclear, though an occasional polymorph may be seen; the protein content of the fluid is raised and a 'cobweb clot' may form on standing. The sugar content of the fluid is generally normal; this helps in the differential diagnosis from tuberculous meningitis with which the condition is most often confused. It is impossible clinically to distinguish this condition from the other benign varieties of viral meningitis mentioned above. Specific CSF antibodies appear within a few days and immunofluorescent staining of cells in the fluid or the use of the ELISA test may be helpful; virus can be cultured from the fluid within a few days in most cases. Treatment, as in all cases of viral meningitis, is purely symptomatic; no antiviral agents currently available are known to be of value.

Neurological complications of some other viral infections

The commonest neurological complication of **mumps** is acute lymphocytic meningitis but encephalomyelitis, unilateral or bilateral nerve deafness, optic neuritis, facial palsy and severe generalised polyneuropathy have all been described. In infectious **mononucleosis**, meningitic, encephalitic, polyneuritic and myelitic forms have all been described, as well as ophthalmoplegia, facial palsy, optic neuritis, isolated peripheral nerve palsies and severe cerebellar ataxia; rarely the clinical picture can simulate the Guillain-Barré syndrome. Enterovirus 70 (EV70), closely related to the Coxsackie and Echo agents, usually causes **acute haemorrhagic conjunctivitis** but during epidemics in India has been found to give a radiculomyelopathy. **Cytomegalovirus infection** in infancy is well known to cause neonatal jaundice, hepatosplenomegaly, anaemia and thrombocytopenia but can also produce microcephaly, microgyria and/or other cerebral malformations as well as chorioretinitis, retinal calcification, cataract and optic atrophy. Less commonly the virus can cause meningitis or encephalitis in adults, especially in immunodeficient or immunocompromised subjects.

AIDS and the nervous system

Since 1979 much attention has centred upon the increasingly severe (and frequent) complications which have been reported as a result of the **acquired immune deficiency syndrome (AIDS)** which results from infection with a virus which was first described as human T-lymphotropic virus type III (HTLV-III) but which is now known as the human immunodeficiency virus (HIV). A related retrovirus (HTLV-I) is now known to be associated with tropical spastic paraparesis (Sever & Gibbs 1988). AIDS is the late result of HIV infection, occurring in some but not all individuals infected with the virus, and is due to severe T helper cell immunodeficiency. The commonest neurological complications are due to opportunistic infections (cerebral abscesses due to toxoplasmosis, progressive multifocal leucoencephalopathy, cryptococcal meningitis, candidal meningitis, cytomegalovirus encephalitis) or diffuse lymphomatous infiltration of the nervous system, but in adults a syndrome of progressive dementia is becoming increasingly common, as is an encephalopathy in infants born to HIV-positive mothers. Indeed, new neurological manifestations of this protean disease are being reported almost weekly and Table 14.3 lists most of those reported to date. Some, as will be seen, are focal, others non-focal or systemic affections of the nervous system. As yet no specific

Table 14.3 Nervous system complications of AIDS. (Reproduced with permission from Kennedy & Johnson 1987.)

Brain
Very common
  AIDS-dementia complex (? direct HIV brain infection)
Common
  Cerebral toxoplasmosis
  Cytomegalovirus (CMV) encephalitis
  Primary CNS lymphoma
Uncommon
  Progressive multifocal leucoencephalopathy
  Varicella-zoster virus (VZV) encephalitis and vasculitis
  Fungal abscess: *Candida* and *Cryptococcus* spp.
Rare
  Herpes simplex virus (HSV) encephalitis
  Tuberculosis (*M. tuberculosis*)

Leptomeninges
Common
  Aseptic meningitis (HIV)
  Cryptococcal meningitis
Uncommon
  Lymphomatous meningitis
  Tuberculous meningitis

Spinal cord
Common
  Vacuolar myelopathy (clinically part of the AIDS-dementia complex)
Uncommon
  Viral myelitis: VZV, HSV and CMV

Peripheral nerve and root
Common
  Distal, predominantly sensory polyneuropathy
Uncommon
  Segmental herpes zoster
  Mononeuritis multiplex
  Demyelinating motor polyneuropathies
  Polyradiculopathy (CMV, ? HIV)

vaccine is available and treatment with 3'-azide-2'-3' dideoxythymidine (AZT) has been shown to produce, at best, limited improvement in some cases and temporary arrest of the disease process in others.

Herpes zoster

In herpes zoster or shingles, the principal sites of pathological change are the posterior root ganglia and the sensory ganglia of the cranial nerves, but occasionally the grey matter of the spinal cord and brain stem is damaged. Intranuclear inclusions have been demonstrated in cases of this disease which is due to the varicella-zoster (VZ) virus which also causes varicella (chicken-pox). The condition can develop without apparent precipitating cause, and usually does so in elderly people, but it can occasionally be precipitated by spinal cord trauma, intervertebral disc prolapse, spinal tumour, subarachnoid haemorrhage, or radiotherapy to the nervous system. This course of events suggests some excitation by the precipitant concerned of a virus which was previously lying dormant in the nervous system.

The incubation period of the illness is about 14 days; the first symptom is usually continuous dull burning pain in the distribution of the affected nerve root or roots, and this mounts in severity. There is often cutaneous hyperpathia. Within three to four days an erythematous rash appears in the affected region and is followed by a vesicular eruption which dries within a few days leaving pigmented scars which may itch for a time. The pain and skin eruption are always unilateral. Persistent, severe pain may persist for weeks, months or even years after the initial illness, particularly in elderly people (post-herpetic neuralgia). Often the affected skin area becomes permanently anaesthetic and sometimes the anterior horn cells of the same segment of the spinal cord are also damaged, giving muscular weakness and wasting. Rarely there is evidence of damage to long tracts (pyramidal and spinothalamic), indicating a 'zoster myelitis'. Zoster of the ophthalmic division of the fifth cranial nerve is particularly unpleasant; the vesicles in the supraorbital region may spread to the cornea, leaving permanent scars. Oculomotor paresis can also occur. Herpes of the geniculate ganglion produces vesicles on the tympanic membrane or soft palate; often there is a watery or sanguineous discharge from the ear, homolateral deafness and facial paralysis and loss of taste on the anterior two-thirds of the tongue (the Ramsay Hunt syndrome). Sometimes there is also sensory loss on the affected side of the face. Rarely in severe herpes zoster there is some headache and neck stiffness indicating meningeal inflammation, and a herpes zoster encephalitis has been described but is uncommon.

The only antiviral agent which has been shown to produce rapid healing of skin lesions and relief of pain in a controlled trial is acyclovir. Steroids have been widely employed but are of no proven value. In post-herpetic neuralgia, carbamazepine in standard dosage is sometimes helpful but its results are unpredictable. Many patients who become depressed by the persistent pain are helped by antidepressant remedies and short courses of phenothiazines, while in some cases the repeated application of cooling sprays or electrical vibrators to the painful skin area or self-administered percutaneous electrical stimulation have produced lasting relief.

Behçet's syndrome

This is an uncommon syndrome of unknown aetiology, thought by many to be due to an as yet unidentifed virus but by others to be an autoimmune disorder, possibly precipitated by one or more viruses. It is characterised by ulceration of the mouth and genitalia, often with iritis, and runs a remittent course. Papilloedema, scleritis, arthropathy and pericarditis and multiple venous thromboses are other common manifestations. When the nervous system is involved the picture may be that of indolent meningitis or encephalomyelitis with variable headache, while parkinsonian features and cranial nerve palsies or fluctuating spastic weakness of the legs may occur, sometimes suggesting multiple sclerosis. The CSF usually demonstrates a lymphocytic pleocytosis (up to 100 or more cells/mm^3) and a rise in its protein content. When nervous manifestations arise the ultimate prognosis is poor and treatment of little avail, although steroids have been recommended.

SPIROCHAETAL INFECTIONS OF THE NERVOUS SYSTEM

The principal spirochaetal agents which may invade the nervous system are first, and most important, the *Treponema pallidum* of syphilis, secondly the leptospirae of Weil's disease and of canicola fever, and thirdly the *Borrelia burgdorferi* of Lyme disease.

Neurosyphilis

Invasion of the nervous system accounted in the past for many of the deaths due to syphilis. The three principal pathological changes resulting from nervous involvement by the spirochaete are meningeal, vascular and parenchymatous. Meningeal and vascular symptoms appear relatively early, often during or just after the secondary stage and within one to five years of the primary infection; these can generally be treated effectively. Manifestations of parenchymatous cerebral and spinal cord disease, which usually develop in the tertiary and quaternary stages of the illness, do not appear for some 10 to 20 years, or exceptionally even later; treatment of these is less effective, though improvement can nevertheless be expected in many cases. The secondary manifestations of syphilis are more acute and florid, and tertiary manifestations (gummata, skeletal involvement) more common, in populations and communities in which syphilis is a relatively recent acquisition. When the disease has been present in a community for hundreds of years the quaternary or parenchymatous neurosyphilitic manifestations are more frequent. Tertiary syphilis is now very rare in Great Britain, but quaternary neurosyphilis still occurs. However, because of early and effective identification and treatment of primary infections, the overall incidence of neurosyphilis has declined in most developed countries.

Asymptomatic neurosyphilis is not uncommon. These are cases in which there are no symptoms or signs of nervous disease but nevertheless there are changes in the CSF (pleocytosis, raised protein, positive VDRL or equivalent reaction) indicating disease activity. In addition to the VDRL test, the treponema immobilisation test and even more sensitive fluorescent treponemal antibody absorption (FTA-ABS) tests are now used in most laboratories, and the IgM and IgG immunoglobulin fractions in the fluid are usually increased. The positive serological reactions reveal that the nervous system has been invaded, while the cell count usually parallels the degree of activity. Marked CSF abnormality usually heralds the eventual development of clinical neurosyphilis. If the fluid is normal in every respect it can reasonably be assumed that the nervous system is not affected by active disease.

An acute **meningitic illness** (luetic meningitis) can occur in the secondary stage of the illness, within two years of the primary infection. It causes fever, headache and neck stiffness, sometimes with confusion or semicoma and even papilloedema. There are usually many hundreds of lymphocytes per mm³ in the CSF and the serological reactions are strongly positive. The clinical picture resembles that of lymphocytic or early tuberculous meningitis; it usually responds well to anti-syphilitic treatment.

The term **meningovascular syphilis** is applied to a group of clinical manifestations of luetic infection which generally appear between two and five years after the primary infection. They result from subacute or chronic inflammatory changes in the leptomeninges (arachnoiditis) on the one hand or from a syphilitic endarteritis of cerebral and/or spinal cord arteries on the other. The symptoms may be those of subacute meningitis with intermittent headache, low fever and neck stiffness, but more often basal arachnoiditis causes strangulation of one or more cranial nerves to give clinical signs of a cranial nerve palsy. The third and sixth nerves are particularly vulnerable; and even today when the disease is rare this diagnosis must be considered in all patients presenting with isolated palsies of one or both of these nerves. Sometimes affection of the eighth nerve gives unilateral or bilateral deafness, while optic chiasmal arachnoiditis can give progressive bilateral, but often asymmetrical, visual failure. Manifestations of communicating hydrocephalus are also sometimes seen and convulsions are not uncommon. The arterial changes, if involving cerebral, brain stem or cerebellar arteries, can cause infarction, particularly if a vessel is suddenly occluded, and the clinical effects are indistinguishable from any episode of cerebral 'thrombosis' (see pp. 271–276). Hemiplegia, monoplegia, aphasia and vertigo may

all occur. The arteries of the spinal cord may also be involved; one presentation is with an acute transverse cord lesion or so-called luetic transverse myelitis. Sometimes the arterial changes are more insidious and the pyramidal tracts, supplied by the peripheral branches of the anterior spinal artery, suffer increasing ischaemia so that a gradually progressive spastic paraplegia develops (Erb's syphilitic spastic paraplegia). Arachnoidal and vascular lesions may be combined in the cervical region; strangulation of nerve roots caused by the arachnoiditis gives weakness and wasting of upper limb muscles, while in the lower limbs there is a spastic paraplegia, due to ischaemia of long tracts. This condition, which can resemble motor neurone disease (see p. 284) has been called luetic amyotrophic lateral sclerosis, or, because of macroscopic changes in the cervical meninges, pachymeningitis cervicalis hypertrophica. The CSF in meningovascular syphilis is always abnormal, showing a lymphocytic pleocytosis, an increase in protein, positive serological reactions and marked changes in the immunoglobulins (see p. 31).

Tabes dorsalis

Tabes dorsalis (locomotor ataxia) is one of the parenchymatous forms of neurosyphilis, in which the spirochaetes have invaded nervous tissue, though they cannot always be demonstrated at autopsy. The principal pathological change is degeneration at the entry zone of the posterior spinal roots, with secondary involvement of ascending fibres in the posterior columns of the cord. Typically, patients experience 'lightning pains' which are probably due to posterior root gliosis. These are often described as 'like red hot needles sticking into the legs'. Generally, too, there is severe sensory ataxia, and the unsteadiness is therefore worse in the dark. Paraesthesiae, particularly in the lower limbs, and subjective numbness are also common. Sometimes transient episodes or 'crises' occur; their aetiology is not fully understood. In laryngeal crises there is spasm of the vocal cords with stridor and difficulty in breathing; in gastric crises acute upper abdominal pain and vomiting occur, lasting perhaps for several days, while renal (like renal colic) and rectal (rectal pain and tenesmus) crises have also been described. Urinary symptoms (delayed or difficult micturition) are not infrequent and the normal sensation indicating a need to micturate may eventually be lost, while impotence is also frequent.

On physical examination, tabetic patients show a typical ataxic, high-stepping gait, and Romberg's sign is positive. The Argyll Robertson pupil is almost invariable. The pupils are small, irregular and unequal, they fail to react to light but do so on accommodation convergence;

there is atrophy of the iris and loss of the ciliospinal reflex (dilatation of the homolateral pupil on pinching the skin of the neck). Bilateral optic atrophy, with pallor of the discs and concentric constriction of visual fields, is seen in about 10% of patients. Ptosis is usual, contributing to the characteristic long, drooping, 'tabetic facies'. There is often loss of superficial pain sensibility (i.e. to pinprick) over the bridge of the nose, the centre of the sternum, the perineum, and variably over the lower limbs. Deep pressure over the Achilles' tendons is often painless. Generally the deep tendon reflexes, and certainly those in the lower limbs, are depressed or absent and there is severe impairment of position and joint sense and of vibration sense in the legs. Loss of pain sensation can lead to a degenerative arthropathy (Charcot's joint) in the feet, ankles or knees.

In early cases of tabes the serological reactions are usually positive in the blood and CSF and the latter generally shows a pleocytosis. In 20% of late or so-called 'burnt-out' cases, the tests are negative and the CSF may be normal. These investigations are nevertheless important in distinguishing between tabes dorsalis and various peripheral neuropathies; in so-called diabetic pseudo-tabes there may actually be pupillary changes as well as peripheral nerve involvement. Tabes dorsalis is the least satisfactory syphilitic condition to treat, as there is often little or no improvement. Nevertheless, treatment should certainly be given (see below).

General paresis

General paresis (general paralysis of the insane or GPI) is a form of progressive dementia, in which there are extensive inflammatory and degenerative changes throughout the cerebral cortex, and the *treponema pallidum* is usually found in the brain at autopsy. In the beginning the symptoms can consist of little more than impaired memory and concentration, and undue fatigue. Subsequently, however, judgement and personality deteriorate with increasing neglect of responsibility and personal hygiene. Often the patients are confused and apathetic with a poor memory for recent events, combined with a singular lack of insight and concern. A grandiose variety is uncommon, but such patients are often euphoric, hypomanic and have delusions of great personal power or ability. They may confabulate wildly, describing in detail personal experiences which have no foundation in fact. The latter manifestations probably occur particularly in individuals of previously extroverted personality. In due course all patients become grossly demented and bed-ridden. There are a few in whom the disease presents more acutely with headache, sudden confusion, convulsions and focal neurological signs (aphasia, hemiparesis, etc.) but this variety of the illness is uncommon. Physical examination reveals evidence of a clear-cut dementia; Argyll Robertson pupils are usual but not invariable. There are commonly tremors of the lips,. tongue and out-stretched hands, the tendon reflexes are, generally exaggerated, and often the plantar responses are extensor. Occasionally the lower limb reflexes are absent and there are other features reminiscent of tabes dorsalis, when the condition is usually called **taboparesis.** **Juvenile paresis** is general paresis due to congenital syphilis, and developing usually in adolescence. The clinical manifestations are similar to those in the disease of late onset, except that the pupils, though unresponsive to light, are often dilated; the prognosis is poor even with vigorous treatment. General paresis must be distinguished from other causes of dementia arising in the presenium (see p. 99). This is most readily achieved by means of CSF examination. The fluid is always abnormal in untreated cases; the serological reactions are positive, there is a lymphocytic pleocytosis and the protein content is raised. The condition, if untreated, is fatal within a few years, but most cases improve with treatment and 50% or more may recover completely.

Penicillin is the sheet-anchor of treatment for neurosyphilis, and is in the view of most neurologists the only drug required. An average course of treatment is 600 mg of benzylpenicillin (penicillin G) or procaine penicillin given intramuscularly each day for 21 days. In patients allergic to penicillin, erythromycin 500 mg four times daily for 15 days, is probably the alternative drug of choice, but three courses of treatment should be given at monthly intervals. Alternatively cephaloridine 2 g daily for 21 days may be used. Often the course of treatment must be repeated at three-monthly intervals, on two or possibly three occasions, until the CSF cell count and protein content revert to normal and the serological reactions become negative. It is not nowadays considered necessary to begin treatment with small doses of penicillin as Herxheimer reactions (exacerbation of symptoms at the commencement of treatment) are extremely rare. If such a reaction does occur it may be terminated rapidly by the use of prednisone or dexamethasone. Penicillin is almost invariably curative in meningovascular syphilis, but in general paresis and tabes dorsalis recovery is often incomplete. Carbamazepine, phenytoin and steroids have all been tried in an attempt to relieve the lightning pains of tabes dorsalis but none of these is universally effective.

Leptospirosis

In leptospirosis icterohaemorrhagica (Weil's disease) the organism, derived usually from rat's urine, attacks principally the liver (giving hepatitis and jaundice) and the kidneys (giving nephritis) but occasionally there are also symptoms and signs of a lymphocytic meningitis. A meningitic illness, clinically indistinguishable from other varieties of lymphocytic meningitis may, however, be the predominant or sole manifestation of canicola fever, which is due to *Leptospira canicola*, an organism which is generally carried by dogs. Hence this diagnosis should be considered in all cases of lymphocytic meningitis, particularly if the patient has been in contact with a sick dog. Although these leptospira are moderately sensitive to penicillin and this antibiotic should certainly be given to such cases in appropriate dosage, it does not appear to have much influence upon the clinical course of the illness in most cases and treatment therefore depends upon general principles of dietary and nursing care.

Lyme disease

Lyme disease was originally described in 1975 as a form of juvenile arthritis which followed the skin lesions of erythema chronica migrans resulting from bites by ticks of the *Ixodes* species. Soon it became apparent that neurological manifestations were common and include facial palsy, lymphocytic meningitis, painful polyradiculoneuritis, mononeuritis multiplex, brachial neuritis, a Guillain-Barré-like syndrome, chronic fatigue and a relapsing encephalomyelitis resembling multiple sclerosis. The condition has been shown to be due to infection with the spirochaete *Borrelia burgdorferi* and usually responds to treatment with antibiotics; while the organism is sensitive to penicillin, either tetracycline 250 mg four times daily for 10 days or ceftriaxone 2 g daily appear to be the treatment of choice (Pachner & Steere 1985, Halperin et al 1987, Parke 1987).

FUNGAL INFECTIONS

Fungal disorders of the central nervous system are rare. **Actinomycosis** has been known to cause a subacute purulent meningitis of invariably fatal termination in certain cases, and in others vertebral involvement has resulted in extradural abscess formation with spinal cord compression. **Cryptococcosis (Torulosis)**, due to *Cryptococcus neoformans (Torula histolytica)*, a yeast-like organism, is the commonest fungal infection of the nervous system but is also uncommon. It gives the clinical picture of a subacute or chronic and fluctuating meningitic illness which sometimes lasts for many months with increasingly severe headaches, confusion and neck stiffness. There is usually papilloedema and sometimes cranial nerve palsies occur. The condition often develops in patients with reticulosis or other debilitating illnesses, but can arise *ab initio* in the apparently healthy. This diagnosis should always be considered when the clinical picture suggests tuberculous meningitis, intracranial sarcoidosis, or carcinomatosis of the meninges. Although in the past the condition was generally fatal, effective treatment, in the form of amphotericin B or 5-fluorocytosine, is now available. Miconazole may be even more effective. The organism may be recognised in direct smears of the CSF or it can be grown on Sabouraud's medium or identified by a specific antibody reaction.

Primary amoebic encephalomyelitis, acquired by bathing in water infested with amoebae, has been reported to cause either a mild meningitic illness or a fatal meningoencephalitis in childhood. Amphotericin B and/or the other agents which are effective in cryptococcosis appear to be effective in treatment.

PARASITIC DISORDERS OF THE NERVOUS SYSTEM

Malaria

Cerebral symptoms are not uncommon in malignant tertian malaria (due to *Plasmodium falciparum*), particularly in children. The manifestations are probably due to blockage of cerebral capillaries by parasitised red cells. Commonly the onset is abrupt with high fever (up to 40°C), severe headache, neck stiffness and sometimes focal neurological signs (hemiplegia, aphasia). In some cases there is papilloedema, and clinical differential diagnosis from cerebral tumour or abscess may be difficult. The prognosis of cerebral malaria is grave, the mortality being as great as 50%. The appropriate emergency treatment is intravenous quinine.

Toxoplasmosis

This condition, due to the protozoon *Toxoplasma gondii*, is usually congenital, being transmitted from the mother in utero. Often the infection in adults is asymptomatic, though some experience an acute or subacute illness with fever, headache and a skin rash when first affected. The encephalomyelitis which is the commonest manifestation of this disease in infancy usually causes fits, hydrocephalus, intracerebral calcification and chorioretinitis. In some babies the disease runs an acute and fatal course, in others it becomes arrested leaving permanent mental handicap with a recurrent tendency to convulse, but some few children survive with minimal disabilities. The diagnosis may be confirmed serologically; pyrimethamine or spiramycin appear to be of benefit in treatment.

Trypanosomiasis

This disease occurs in African (*Trypanosomiasis gambiense* and *rhodesiense*) and South American (*Trypanosomiasis cruzi*) forms. The African form, sleeping sickness, is transmitted by the tsetse fly. After a long incubation period, there is a febrile illness followed by meningitic symptoms, irritability, indifference, somnolence and eventually after some months by coma and death. The South American form (Chagas disease) is a more acute illness, commoner in children and less grave in outlook, but often followed by mental defect and residua like those of cerebral palsy; it may also cause myositis.

Trichiniasis

This disease is contracted usually through eating inadequately-cooked pork containing the larvae of the *Trichinella spiralis*. The larvae are released in the intestinal tract, mature and produce further larvae which penetrate the intestinal wall and enter the blood stream. The common clinical features at this stage are fever, puffiness of the eyelids, and severe generalised muscular pain and often weakness, indicating invasion of the muscles. Respiratory difficulty due to diaphragmatic involvement is common. Sometimes fits or paraplegia result from blockage of cerebral or spinal blood vessels. Though the disease is occasionally fatal the illness usually resolves within a few days or weeks and the larvae become encysted. During the acute stage there is usually a striking eosinophilia and the parasites can be identified in muscle biopsy sections.

Cysticercosis

This disorder is contracted by eating food which has been contaminated with tapeworm ova, usually those of *Taenia solium*. The ova are converted into the larval form of the parasite which then penetrates the intestinal wall and enters the circulation to reach the brain, muscles and subcutaneous tissues. The larva becomes encysted to form a cysticercus which may then calcify and often has a characteristic oval shape which can be recognised on radiographs. Rarely, a hypertrophic myopathy results. Cysticercosis of the brain often causes epilepsy but a racemose form has also been described in the cerebral ventricles (particularly the fourth) which can result in either repeated attacks of lymphocytic meningitis or in intermittent or progressive hydrocephalus suggesting the presence of a posterior fossa tumour.

Bilharzia

Involvement of the nervous system in bilharzia or schistosomiasis, which results, especially in the Orient and Middle East, from bathing in infested water, is relatively uncommon. When it occurs, *S. japonicum* shows a predilection for the cerebral hemispheres causing headache, papilloedema and focal neurological signs. *S. haematobium* and *S. mansoni* attack the spinal cord, usually causing an incomplete transverse myelopathy. Praziquantel is the treatment of choice.

NEUROLOGICAL COMPLICATIONS OF SPECIFIC INFECTIONS

Disorders due to specific exotoxins

The principal infecting organisms which produce exotoxins with an affinity for nervous tissue are diphtheria, tetanus and botulism.

Diphtheritic polyneuropathy

The exotoxin of the diphtheria bacillus gives a polyneuropathy which generally begins in the musculature nearest to the point where the infecting organism is located. Since this is usually the tonsillar fossa, larynx or nasal mucosa, the muscles most often paralysed initially are those of the pharynx, larynx and soft palate, with resulting dysphagia, dysarthria or dysphonia, or nasal speech. Sometimes the external ocular muscles are affected. When the organism has contaminated a limb wound, then the weakness may begin in the muscles of that limb. Whatever the site of infection, the weakness may remain localised, but in other instances it spreads to involve the muscles of all four limbs and those of the trunk. The physical signs of generalised muscular weakness with absent deep tendon reflexes and variable sensory impairment are typical of any polyneuropathy, save for the almost constant involvement of bulbar muscles. Frequently the initial manifestations of diphtheritic polyneuropathy are observed within seven to 10 days of the onset of the infection, and weakness can be profound and generalised in two to four weeks. Recovery soon begins to occur spontaneously and is often complete, though variable muscular weakness and depression of tendon reflexes sometimes persist. Fortunately as a consequence of prophylactic inoculation, diphtheria is now a rare disease.

Tetanus

This condition is due to the exotoxin of the tetanus bacillus, which, being an anaerobic organism, flourishes only in deep penetrating wounds. The exotoxin enters the central nervous system by travelling along the sheaths of the peripheral nerves from the site of the injury. If the amount of toxin produced is large there is also rapid dissemination via the blood stream. This toxin blocks inhibitory neurones thus disturbing the normal regulation of the reflex arc so that intense muscular spasms are produced by minimal sensory stimulation. The incubation period of the illness varies from three or four days to as long as several weeks after the injury. The longer the incubation period, the better the prognosis, as the development of symptoms within a few days after the injury usually implies a massive infection. Usually the first symptom is one of trismus or inability to open the jaw; this is followed by stiffness of the neck, dysphagia, spasm of the facial muscles (risus sardonicus) and eventually by rigidity of the abdominal muscles and of all the limbs. Noise or minimal sensory stimulation of any kind may then provoke intense and generalised muscular spasms, with arching of the back (opisthotonos). Between spasms the muscles remain rigid and the tendon reflexes are brisk. Hyperpyrexia often develops; death can result from heart failure, asphyxia or exhaustion. If the patient survives the first critical days the spasms gradually lessen in frequency and severity and recovery eventually occurs, though some stiffness may persist for several weeks. The disease can occur in a less severe or localised form when bacteria are present in fewer numbers, or when the patient has previously received prophylactic inoculations. In such cases the rigidity and spasms may remain localised to the limb or part of the body in which the original injury occurred and can persist for several weeks or months. In cephalic tetanus, following a facial wound, in addition to spasm of facial and jaw muscles, facial paralysis and ophthalmoplegia often develop on the side of the face nearest to the injury. A neonatal form also occurs when tetanus spores infect the umbilical cord.

The affected patient must be nursed in isolation, if possible in an intensive care ward. Some authorities still recommend an intravenous injection of 10 000 units of tetanus antitoxin but most prefer to give 250 IU of human tetanus immune globulin intrathecally. Muscle spasms are eliminated by tubocurarine chloride given in doses of 15 mg repeated as necessary up to a daily total of 150–650 mg, while artificial respiration is maintained with intermittent positive pressure equipment through a tracheostomy tube. Naso-oesophageal or intravenous feeding will be required, antibiotics are usually necessary to avoid secondary infection, and hyperthermia and/or hypotension which are not uncommon complications require appropriate treatment. The overall mortality rate has now fallen to less than 30%; some degree of muscular weakness may persist for many months in some cases but in those who survive, complete recovery is the rule in the majority.

Botulism

This condition follows ingestion of the exotoxin of *Clostridium botulinum* and in the older child or adult is always acquired from infected foodstuffs, particularly tinned food. Infantile botulism which occurs rarely world-wide but which is commonest in California, has been shown to be due, in infants between one and six months of age, to colonisation of the gut by spores derived from dust or soil; these spores subsequently multiply and produce botulinum toxin. The toxin has a direct effect upon the neuromuscular junction, inhibiting acetylcholine release. Symptoms usually develop within 24 to 48 hours after eating the tainted food. The first symptoms are usually vomiting and diarrhoea, followed by blurring of vision (due to pupillary dilatation), diplopia, ptosis, dysphagia, dysarthria and weakness of jaw muscles. Death is due to respiratory paralysis or bronchopneumonia. The infantile condition usually presents with poor sucking, difficulty in swallowing, a weak cry and weak head movements with variable limb and respiratory muscle involvement. Between 20 and 60% of adult cases are fatal but the prognosis in infantile cases is often surprisingly good and gradual recovery within a few weeks is usual. The toxin can be destroyed by cooking tinned food for a few minutes and prophylaxis is much more satisfactory than treatment.

Even though antitoxin is of greater prophylactic than therapeutic value, 50 000 units of a polyvalent serum is nevertheless recommended in adults, along with penicillin to destroy surviving organisms in the gastrointestinal tract. In severe cases artificial respiration and nasal feeding may be needed. Sustained improvement may follow the administration of guanidine hydrochloride 20–50 mg/kg body weight in divided doses daily for several days, but side-effects of this treatment can be troublesome and 4-aminopyridine given by single or repeated intravenous injection in a dose of 0.35–0.5 mg/kg body weight is generally preferred.

Saxitoxin poisoning

Eating mussels or other shellfish contaminated by dinoflagellates of the genus *Gonyaulax* ('the red tide') can cause saxitoxin poisoning, producing paraesthesiae, muscular weakness, ataxia, headache and vomiting within 1–12 hours after ingestion. Fatalities are very rare, most patients recovering in 24–72 hours.

Other neurological complications of specific infections

In certain cases of **typhus fever** and other disorders due to rickettsial infection, nervous symptoms are prominent.

Headache, sleeplessness and delirium may indicate an encephalitic element of the general infection but in addition, focal neurological signs (hemiplegia, aphasia, dysarthria, facial paralysis) occasionally develop and are most probably due to occlusion of cerebral vessels by so-called typhus nodules (foci of perivascular inflammation). In **typhoid fever**, delirium and confusion are common, but meningitis or cerebral abscess can rarely result from direct invasion of the nervous system by the typhoid bacillus. Rarely, too, the bacillus of **dysentery** or even the *Entamoeba histolytica* of amoebic dysentery are responsible for intracranial abscess formation. A form of encephalopathy can also complicate whooping cough; in such cases multiple cerebral petechial haemorrhages may be demonstrated and are possibly due to violent bouts of coughing. The clinical manifestations include convulsions, which may be repetitive and fatal, and focal neurological signs such as aphasia and hemiplegia. A similar syndrome, of unknown aetiology, but occasionally following non-specific or banal infections, has been called **acute toxic encephalopathy** and may be related more closely to post-infectious encephalitis (see p. 237). It occurs chiefly in young children, sometimes in small epidemics and is characterised by delirium or coma, convulsions, variable paresis of the limbs, and signs of meningeal irritation. The condition may be fatal but when recovery does occur it is often complete. A specific sub-variety is called **acute toxic encephalopathy with fatty degeneration of the viscera (Reye's disease)** and causes similar clinical manifestations in childhood along with hypoglycaemia and evidence of hepatic dysfunction; it is probably of viral origin. There is evidence of diffuse mitochondrial damage in brain, liver and kidney in such cases along with an inability to metabolise salicylate; many affected children were found to have been treated with aspirin, which should not be given to young children. Yet another variant may be associated with opsoclonus (jerky spontaneous ocular movements) and myoclonus and is called **subacute myoclonic encephalopathy**. The CSF is usually normal in such cases.

While a depressive syndrome of considerable severity is a common sequel of **influenza**, cases of post-influenzal encephalomyelitis have been described; most are probably due to viral invasion of the brain, but others may be allergic in origin and related to the forms of encephalomyelitis which may complicate childhood exanthemata (see p. 238). Subacute influenzal myositis has also been described. The principal neurological complication of **acute rheumatism** is **rheumatic chorea**, which was mentioned in Chapter 9 (p. 157). Probably this condition is a form of rheumatic encephalitis, although the pathological changes in the brain in such cases are non-specific and the condition is not usually a complication of acute rheumatism but rather an alternative manifestation of

rheumatic disease. It can affect the face and all four limbs or may be hemiplegic in distribution. Severe cases also show mental confusion, restlessness and emotional lability. The involuntary movements of characteristic type sometimes persist for some months or years and may recur, especially in pregnancy (chorea gravidarum), but as a rule recovery is complete. In the acute stage, bed rest, preferably in a quiet room, is needed and relief of restlessness as well as some improvement in the involuntary movements may be achieved with drugs such as chlorpromazine, haloperidol or diazepam in appropriate dosage. One further neurological symptom which deserves mention is the **meningism** or occipital headache and neck stiffness which occasionally complicates infective illnesses and particularly pneumonia in childhood. Under such circumstances, lumbar puncture may be necessary to exclude meningitis, but the CSF is normal and the neck stiffness is difficult to explain.

ALLERGIC, HYPERSENSITIVITY AND AUTOIMMUNE DISORDERS

Many disorders of the central and peripheral nervous systems which were once thought to be due to unidentified infective agents are now known to result from an allergic or hypersensitivity response occurring within the nervous substance but affecting particularly the blood vessels and connective tissue elements. The pathological changes in such cases can be regarded as inflammatory in the broadest sense and often occur as the secondary effect of an infective agent which has not invaded the nervous system itself but has precipitated a cell-mediated or humoral immune response. In other instances the neurological manifestations are but one element of a clinical syndrome resulting from a generalised disorder of blood vessels and connective tissue. The neurological sequelae of prophylactic inoculation and the nervous complications of the common childhood exanthemata constitute an important group of disorders falling into this category; in most instances the neurological syndrome so produced is one of encephalomyelitis. This condition is generally considered along with the other so-called demyelinating diseases and will be described in Chapter 15. The principal conditions which warrant consideration here are serum neuropathy, 'shoulder girdle neuritis', postinfective polyneuritis or polyradiculoneuropathy and the neurological complications of the 'collagen', 'collagen-vascular' or 'connective tissue' diseases.

Serum neuropathy

Serum neuropathy or neuritis is a condition which can follow the injection of foreign serum (e.g. antitetanic serum, antidiphtheritic serum). It is usually but one manifestation of the syndrome of serum sickness which may follow some days or weeks after such an injection, and in which fever, nausea and joint pains are usually the most prominent clinical features. The neuropathy generally affects cervical nerve roots and gives weakness and wasting of a group of muscles around the shoulder girdle, sometimes with localised sensory loss. Though some cases recover, in others, particularly when a single peripheral nerve seems to be involved (e.g. the nerve to serratus anterior), the weakness is permanent. The condition now generally called **neuralgic amyotrophy**, but often entitled in the past **shoulder-girdle neuritis**, is similar and must be distinguished from the clinical syndrome once designated by the outmoded term **brachial neuritis**; most cases so diagnosed 20–30 years ago were the result of prolapse of a cervical intervertebral disc (see p. 289). Neuralgic amyotrophy is a disorder of sudden onset which can follow an acute non-specific infection (e.g. influenza) or may complicate any febrile illness (e.g. pneumonia); occasionally it develops during pregnancy, after relatively minimal trauma or without apparent precipitating cause. The first symptom is a severe burning pain which generally develops over the shoulder and spreads down the arm to a variable extent. It can persist for several days making sleep impossible except with the aid of powerful analgesics and sedatives. Within a few days the patient becomes aware of muscular weakness and certain muscles (deltoid is a typical example) are found to be completely paralysed. The weakness may be limited to a single muscle (e.g. serratus anterior) but is sometimes much more extensive. When the latter is the case, muscular involvement is patchy, some being profoundly weak, others comparatively spared both clinically and electromyographically. Areas of sensory loss are often found, but are much less striking than the motor deficit. Gradually the pain improves and some return of muscular function occurs during the succeeding weeks or months; in most cases recovery is eventually complete, but some permanent weakness occasionally persists. No treatment, apart from analgesics, and later, remedial exercises and splinting where necessary, appears to be of any value.

Postinfective polyneuritis (the Guillain-Barré syndrome)

Postinfective polyneuritis or polyradiculoneuropathy is the term now used to describe the condition once entitled infectious polyneuritis. It is more often called the Guillain-Barré syndrome and is one of the commonest causes of the clinical syndrome of ascending paralysis (Landry's paralysis). The principal pathological change in such cases is an autoimmune inflammatory response within multiple spinal roots, so that the disorder is a radiculopathy (polyradiculitis) as well as a peripheral neuropathy. Thus, lymphocytic infiltration is often found in peripheral nerves as well as in the roots. There is evidence to suggest that the nerves are attacked by lymphocytes which have become specifically sensitised to peripheral nerve protein, but that humoral factors (circulating immune complexes) also play a major role in pathogenesis. The neuropathy is demyelinating in type although in long-lasting cases some secondary axonal degeneration occurs.

The condition can follow a preceding infective illness or may develop without apparent antecedent infection. Sometimes the first symptom is one of weakness in the feet and legs, which within a few hours or days spreads up the lower limbs and trunk giving an ascending flaccid paralysis. In acute cases the motor weakness ascends rapidly to involve the upper limbs, muscles of respiration and bulbar musculature; assisted respiration and tracheotomy may be necessary. Hence rapidly increasing and ascending paralysis is a clear indication for admission to a unit where intensive care facilities are immediately available. More often weakness begins in the proximal muscles of the limbs. In some cases there are accompanying paraesthesiae and sensory loss with an ascending sensory 'level' on the trunk but usually motor symptoms and signs predominate. There are subacute cases in which the paralysis increases slowly over the course of several weeks or even months, in which despite a complaint of paraesthesiae, sensory loss cannot be demonstrated, and in which the march of the disease process apparently becomes arrested when the weakness and sensory loss has reached the mid-dorsal or lower cervical level. In occasional cases weakness begins in the muscles innervated by the cranial nerves (cranial polyneuritis), again without significant sensory impairment. The so-called Miller Fisher syndrome of ophthalmoplegia, ataxia and areflexia is generally believed to be a variant of this condition although in some cases there are symptoms and signs of involvement of the brain stem parenchyma justifying its identification as a separate syndrome.

Eventually in most cases there is usually spontaneous remission and the motor and sensory changes regress, until complete recovery occurs within the course of a few months, but in the more acute cases the condition constitutes a severe danger to life. Typically all the tendon reflexes in the affected limbs are lost and the paralysed limbs remain flaccid throughout; the plantar responses, when obtainable, are flexor. Though sensory loss is often minimal or absent, when present it usually affects all modalities of sensation; sphincter control is sometimes impaired, though not usually so early or as completely as in transverse myelitis (see p. 238) which may present a similar clinical picture but in which the plantar responses are extensor. In the occasional cases of cranial polyneuritis it may be difficult to distinguish the disorder from bulbar poliomyelitis and from neoplasms or granulomas of the basal meninges. In postinfective polyneuritis, after the first few days of the illness the CSF typically shows a substantial increase in protein content (0.1 = 1.0 g/l) but there is generally no pleocytosis (*dissociation albuminocytologique*). Slowing of nerve conduction is found early in the course of the illness. Although many patients with this disease recover completely, residual weakness and sensory impairment of some degree persist in some. For many years steroid drugs were widely used in treatment but several well-designed controlled trials have shown them to be of no value, unlike their proven beneficial effect in subacute or chronic relapsing autoimmune polyneuropathy (p. 295) of demyelinating type. However there is now increasing evidence to suggest that plasmapheresis can be very helpful in acute cases; when respiratory insufficiency threatens, assisted respiration in an intensive care unit is necessary. Once improvement begins, a vigorous programme of rehabilitation should be planned.

Neurological complications of the 'collagen' or 'connective tissue' diseases

Many of the 'neurological' complications of the 'collagen' diseases, using neurological in its broadest sense to imply those disorders which fall into the province of the neurologist, affect the voluntary muscles. The principal conditions of this type, namely polymyositis and dermatomyositis, occurring alone or in combination with other conditions such as rheumatoid arthritis or systemic sclerosis are considered in Chapter 18. Polyneuropathy also occurs occasionally in association with rheumatoid arthritis. Chorea, as a form of rheumatic disease, has already been mentioned and cranial arteritis as well as other autoimmune arteritides are discussed in Chapter 17. The major disorders of the connective tissue group which remain are **systemic lupus erythematosus and polyarteritis nodosa** and so-called **mixed connective tissue disease**. Each of these disorders can give symptoms and signs of nervous disease by producing pathological changes in small blood vessels in the central or peripheral nervous system. Thus in systemic lupus erythematosus, focal lesions in the brain or brain stem may cause epilepsy, chorea, limb paresis, vertigo or cranial nerve palsies, while paraplegia due to spinal disease has been described. In occasional cases, too a symmetrical polyneuropathy develops. Polyneuropathy (see Ch. 18) is even more common in polyarteritis nodosa, but can be asymmetrical

or may give a clinical picture suggesting multiple peripheral nerve lesions (mononeuritis multiplex). More rarely, there are symptoms and signs indicating multiple lesions of the brain, brain stem or spinal cord. Whether systemic lupus or polyarteritis is the cause, there will usually be associated clinical features in such cases (including fever, multiple arthropathy, albuminuria, increased serum immunoglobulins, raised ESR) to indicate the nature of the underlying disease, but these features are sometimes unobtrusive and 'collagen' disease should always be considered in patients with obscure neurological syndromes which run a subacute or remittent clinical course.

REFERENCES

Adams R D, Petersdorf R G 1980 Pyogenic infections of the central nervous system. In: Isselbacher K J et al (eds) Harrison's principles of internal medicine, 9th edn McGraw-Hill, New York, Ch 368

Behan P O, Currie S 1978 Clinical neuroimmunology. Major problems in neurology, Vol 8 (Walton J, series ed). Saunders, London

Halperin J J, Little B W, Coyle P K, Dattwyler R J 1987 Lyme disease: cause of a treatable peripheral neuropathy. Neurology 37: 1700

Johnson R T 1982 Viral infections of the nervous system. Raven Press, New York

Juel-Jensen B E , Phuapradit P, Warrell D A 1987 Bacterial meningitis. In: Weatherall D J , Ledingham J G G, Warrell D A (eds) Oxford textbook of medicine, 2nd edn, Oxford University Press, Oxford, Section 21, p 21.129

Kennedy P G E, Johnson R T (eds) 1987 Infections of the nervous system. Butterworth, London

Menkes J H 1985 Textbook of child neurology, 3rd edn. Lea & Febiger, Philadelphia

Pachner A R, Steere A C 1985 The triad of neurologic manifestations of Lyme disease: meningitis, cranial neuritis, and radiculoneuritis. Neurology 35: 47

Parke A 1987 From new to old England: the progress of Lyme disease. British Medical Journal 294: 525

Pennybacker J B 1951 Abscess of the brain. In: Feiling A (ed) Modern trends in neurology, 1st series. Butterworth, London, Ch 10

Russell W R 1956 Poliomyelitis, 2nd edn. Arnold, London

Sever J L, Gibbs C J (eds) 1988 Retroviruses in the nervous system. Annals of Neurology 23: suppl

Spillane J O (ed) 1973 Tropical neurology. Oxford University Press, London

Walton J N 1985 Brain's Diseases of the nervous system, 9th edn. Oxford University Press, Oxford

Wood M J, Anderson M 1988 Neurological infections. Major problems in neurology, Vol 16 (Walton J, series ed). Saunders, London

Yousef G E, Bell E J, Mann G F, Murugesan V, Smith D G, McCartney R A, Mowbray J F 1988 Chronic enterovirus infection in patients with postviral fatigue syndrome. Lancet i: 146

15. Demyelinating diseases

The demyelinating diseases are a group of disorders of the nervous system characterised pathologically by a destructive process affecting the myelin sheaths of nerve fibres within the brain and spinal cord. Although grey matter can be secondarily involved, these are primarily white matter diseases. The principal conditions which fall into this group are acute disseminated encephalomyelitis, acute haemorrhagic leucoencephalitis, neuromyelitis optica, multiple sclerosis and diffuse cerebral sclerosis. Central pontine myelinolysis, in which massive demyelination occurs in central areas of the pons, is now known to be a metabolic disorder (see Ch. 19). Whereas it now seems likely that autoimmune mechanisms within the nervous system account for most cases of acute encephalomyelitis, and similar factors can play a part in multiple sclerosis, much information about the aetiology and pathogenesis of these disorders is still lacking, so that an aetiological classification of the separate disease entities within the group is still impossible. Clinical differentiation can also be difficult; although the natural history of a chronic relapsing case of multiple sclerosis is quite different from that of encephalomyelitis following measles, in other instances there may be no means of distinguishing between an acute episode of multiple sclerosis on the one hand and an encephalomyelitic illness on the other. Pathologically, too, there are similarities between the changes in the nervous system in each of these diseases. Between the acute perivascular inflammatory and demyelinating lesions which occur in encephalomyelitis, and the massive confluent areas of demyelination of diffuse cerebral sclerosis, there exists a spectrum of pathological change which can occur in varying permutations and combinations in each of these conditions. Sometimes the axis cylinders within areas of demyelination are destroyed early, in others they survive for some time, but the overall pattern of pathological reaction is broadly similar; this does not imply identity of aetiology, as the nervous system has only a limited repertoire of pathological responses and myelin destruction may result from many noxious agents. Thus no clear-cut definition of the demyelinating diseases is at present possible, and some of the clinical syndromes customarily identified (of which neuromyelitis optica is a good example) may be artificially defined. Certainly several conditions traditionally classified as forms of cerebral diffuse sclerosis (such as metachromatic leucodystrophy due to aryl sulphatase deficiency and X-linked recessive adrenoleucodystrophy, once equated with Schilder's disease, are now known to be due to specific inborn metabolic abnormalities and are more properly referred to as dysmyelinating disorders.

ACUTE DISSEMINATED ENCEPHALOMYELITIS

Acute disseminated encephalomyelitis is an acute inflammatory disorder of the brain and/or spinal cord of variable clinical course and severity, in which the principal pathological changes are perivascular cellular infiltration and perivenous demyelination in the white matter of the brain or spinal cord. Pathologically the condition differs from the various viral forms of encephalitis (see p. 224) which are essentially polioclastic (i.e. involving grey rather than white matter). The syndrome can follow smallpox vaccination, inoculation against rabies or other protective inoculations, or a non-specific 'influenzal' infective illness; alternatively it may develop during one of the childhood exanthemata, while on occasion such an illness occurs without there being any clinical evidence of preceding or concurrent infection. Probably this is an autoimmune response of the nervous system to many antigenic agents, many of them viral; the disorder closely resembles experimental allergic encephalomyelitis which can be produced in animals by injecting brain emulsion or purified encephalitogenic factor with Freund's adjuvant. Indeed it is now generally accepted that the condition is due to a hypersensitivity response of the nervous system to viral multiplication or the products of viral injury and there is evidence that both lymphocyte-mediated and humoral mechanisms are important in pathogenesis. Recent work suggests that the distinction between this condition and the viral encephalitides is less absolute than was once thought as in some such cases active virus can be isolated from brain tissue.

The clinical picture of the illness is variable; sometimes it is primarily encephalitic with headache, drowsiness, confusion and possibly convulsions, but in other cases the disease process appears to be confined to the spinal cord and a syndrome of transverse or ascending myelitis results. Indeed, now that neurosyphilis is comparatively rare, post-infective encephalomyelitis and multiple sclerosis are the most common causes of the syndrome of **transverse myelitis**. Less often the clinical features indicate that the disease process is involving brain-stem structures or cerebellar connections, to give ataxia, nystagmus, vertigo and cranial nerve palsies. In such a case, differential diagnosis from an acute episode of multiple sclerosis is difficult if not impossible, and may depend wholly upon follow-up studies. In yet other cases there may be involvement of motor and sensory roots as well as the spinal cord and the condition resembles the closely-related acute postinfective polyneuritis (the Guillain-Barré syndrome). Often the question as to whether or not the spinal cord is involved depends upon the plantar responses. It will now be convenient to consider the clinical features of the different varieties of encephalomyelitis.

Post-vaccinal encephalomyelitis was most common after primary smallpox vaccination in children of school age, and was known in epidemics to affect as many as 1 in 2500 vaccinated individuals. Now that smallpox has been eradicated and vaccination has therefore been abandoned the illness has disappeared. Many affected patients had a relatively mild encephalitic illness which began with headache, neck stiffness, drowsiness, fever and vomiting and lasted for only a few days. In others convulsions occurred and there was stupor and later deepening coma. The condition had to be distinguished from post-vaccinal encephalopathy which, particularly in infants and young children, caused transient drowsiness and convulsions, often lasting for no more than 24 to 48 hours. Often symptoms and signs of spinal cord involvement were seen; hemiplegia was comparatively rare but often there was ascending flaccid weakness of the limbs with loss of tendon reflexes and paralysis of the bladder and bowels. Indeed, in occasional cases, a myelitic picture of this nature occurred without headache, neck stiffness or clouding of consciousness. The disease was fatal in up to 30% of cases, although the prognosis was probably influenced favourably by steroid therapy. In the remaining cases eventual recovery was often complete, although neurological signs, intellectual deterioration and personality change could persist for some years and were rarely permanent. A similar illness is seen less often after prophylactic inoculation against pertussis and more rarely still after diphtheria or tetanus vaccine. All of the features described (encephalitis, myelitis and polyradiculitic syndromes) can also occur in the encephalomyelitis which followed antirabic inoculation in between 1 in 1000 and 1 in 4000 individuals treated with vaccines prepared in animal brain or spinal cord. The incidence of this complication has been reduced progressively since vaccines grown in duck embryos or in tissue culture in human diploid cell cultures have been used.

A common variety of **post-exanthematous encephalomyelitis** is that which complicates *measles*, though this condition has declined greatly in incidence with the falling incidence of measles world-wide following the widespread use of prophylactic inoculation. A similar disorder may also occur following *chicken-pox* (varicella) or *German measles* (rubella), and very rarely in *scarlet fever* (scarlatina). The neurological complications of mumps and glandular fever are probably due to direct invasion of the nervous system by the causal virus, causing lymphocytic meningitis and occasionally encephalitis (p. 224) while those of whooping cough (pertussis encephalopathy) are more probably due to repeated episodes of cerebral anoxia developing during bouts of coughing. The encephalomyelitis of measles usually develops some two to four days after the rash appears but can even antedate it; it has been known rarely to develop in contacts who do not develop a rash. The usual pattern of the illness is one of encephalitis which, if mild, gives headache, neck stiffness, drowsiness and confusion for a few days, but if severe there are convulsions and deepening coma. Less commonly an acute hemiplegia develops, or a cerebellar ataxia of acute onset, while some few cases develop a transverse myelitis or polyradiculitis. About 10% of cases end fatally; many recover completely but a few remain disabled by hemiplegia, paraplegia, fits or dementia. In chicken-pox the clinical picture is broadly similar but most cases of encephalitis complicating this illness are mild and recover completely, while cerebellar ataxia occurs in an unusually large proportion. An explosive encephalomyelitic illness can occasionally complicate rubella, but more often in this disease the encephalitic or myelitic illness, if it occurs, is mild and transient.

The form of **postinfective encephalomyelitis** which can follow non-specific infective illnesses or which may occur without clinical evidence of preceding infection, is even more protean in its manifestations. Sometimes the picture is that of severe disseminated encephalomyelitis with deepening coma, convulsions and flaccid paraplegia, or the illness may be mild with headache, drowsiness, fever and transient limb or bulbar pareses.

Alternatively, a transverse myelitis may be the presenting feature, while in many cases the disease process affects the brain stem, giving nystagmus, impairment of conjugate ocular movement, dysphagia, facial weakness and variable long-tract signs. As mentioned above, the clinical features may be indistinguishable from those produced by an initial episode of multiple sclerosis. There may also be difficulty in diagnosis from viral encephalitis. While herpes simplex encephalitis (see p. 225) usually gives a hyperacute clinical picture suggesting a focal lesion in one temporal lobe, some patients show a non-specific acute encephalitic picture and the diagnosis may depend upon fluorescent antibody studies. Other specific varieties of viral encephalitis (e.g. the St Louis type) occur in endemic areas. The view that many cases previously regarded as examples of postinfective encephalomyelitis may result from viral infection is gaining ground. In early childhood the condition which has been called 'acute cerebellar ataxia of infancy' is probably a variant of encephalomyelitis and can also occur in a subacute form.

The changes in the cerebrospinal fluid in all varieties of encephalomyelitis are similar, though by no means diagnostic. There is a variable pleocytosis, usually lymphocytic, but in acute cases polymorphonuclear leucocytes are present for a few days; the protein and immunoglobulin content of the fluid is invariably raised.

In comatose patients, tube-feeding, parenteral fluids and even tracheostomy with or without assisted respiration may be needed, with nursing in an intensive care unit and surface cooling if hyperpyrexia occurs. Prednisone with or without azathioprine or other immunosuppressive agents should be given in appropriate dosage, although in acute childhood encephalopathies, high-dose dexamethasone may be preferred to control cerebral oedema. Antibiotics are generally needed to control secondary infections and anticonvulsants may also be needed to control seizures, often in the short-term, less often indefinitely if attacks recur. When there is evidence of residual brain or spinal cord damage, a planned programme of rehabilitation may be required.

ACUTE HAEMORRHAGIC LEUCOENCEPHALITIS

This condition, also called acute necrotising haemorrhagic leucoencephalopathy, is a fulminating form of acute encephalomyelitis. A closely related condition is brain purpura which can be fatal within a few hours and is probably due to an acute hypersensitivity reaction affecting cerebral blood vessels. In haemorrhagic leucoencephalitis the pathological changes are those of widespread vascular necrosis with perivascular haemorrhage in the cerebral white matter and with large areas of demyelination which may be confluent. The onset of the illness is often apoplectiform, with headache, convulsions and coma which deepens rapidly. The physical signs are often unilateral in the first instance so that an onset with hemiplegia is not infrequent. Death often occurs within 24 to 48 hours; comparatively few cases are recognised during life, but CT or MRI scanning can be very helpful as the clinical features may mimic those of massive cerebral infarction or cerebral abscess. If the CSF is examined it usually shows a neutrophil pleocytosis and a moderate rise in protein. The clinical picture is similar to that of herpes simplex encephalitis, although pathologically the two conditions are quite different. Recent evidence suggests that the herpetic condition is the commoner of the two and that haemorrhagic leucoencephalitis is now very rare. Possibly in some cases of myelitis of exceptionally acute onset, the pathological process in the spinal cord is similar.

NEUROMYELITIS OPTICA

Neuromyelitis optica (Devic's disease) is not a separate disease entity, as the clinical features typical of this syndrome can occur as one episode in the course of multiple sclerosis. Rarely, too, cases of postinfective encephalomyelitis present in this way and the neurological manifestations of systemic lupus erythematosus can, even more rarely, produce a similar picture. The symptoms of the condition, which is relatively common in Japan, are, however, sufficiently distinctive for it to be accepted as a distinctive syndrome even though its pathogenesis and nosological status remain uncertain. The condition may develop at any age and in either sex. Typically it begins with pain in the eyes and visual loss which may be unilateral at first but usually involves the other eye within hours or days. Blindness may rapidly become complete with subsequent slow regression but in other cases some useful vision is retained throughout. Usually the optic discs are swollen and the visual fields show bilateral central scotomas, though one eye is often more severely affected than the other. Soon afterwards the typical picture of a transverse myelitis appears with flaccid paralysis of the limbs, loss of sphincter control, absence of tendon reflexes, extensor plantar responses, and an ascending sensory 'level' below which all forms of sensation are impaired. Sometimes the spinal cord symptoms precede the visual loss, and possibly some cases of bilateral retrobulbar neuritis without other neurological signs are abortive examples of this syndrome. The CSF shows simply a non-specific rise in protein and mononuclear cells with raised IgG. The disorder is fatal within a few weeks in some cases, others make a slow but complete recovery; one may then assume in retrospect that the pathological process was probably one of acute encephalomyelitis. However, some patients have residual visual loss and optic atrophy with paraparesis, and many of these eventually turn out to be suffering from multiple sclerosis. Probably all cases of this syndrome should be treated initially with high-dose prednisone.

MULTIPLE SCLEROSIS

Multiple or disseminated sclerosis is a disease of obscure aetiology characterised clinically by symptoms which indicate the presence of multiple lesions in the white matter of the brain and spinal cord (Fig. 15.1). In most cases the disease process extends episodically, with remissions of variable duration separating the relapses, but in other individuals it presents as an intermittently progressive disease with spastic paraparesis and/or signs of cerebellar or brain-stem disease. Although there are many relatively mild cases in which relapses occur at intervals of several years and even then are comparatively transient and only slightly incapacitating, it is equally true that in some others the disease is inexorably progressive, producing almost total disability and rarely death within two to three years of the onset. Eventually most patients are disabled by progressive paraplegia and/or ataxia. Pathologically there are multiple plaques of demyelination and gliosis of varying age throughout the nervous system (Fig. 15.1); these mainly involve the white matter of the brain and cord and are often perivenous or periventricular in distribution, but the grey matter is sometimes involved as well. There seems to be little doubt that during remissions of the disease some remyelination can occur within the plaques, though

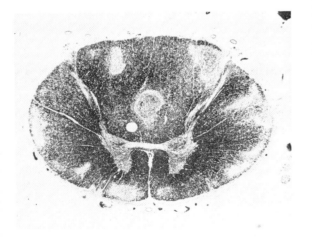

Fig. 15.1 Multiple sclerosis: spinal cord, T9.
(Reproduced from Walton 1985 with permission)

some of the clinical improvement may result from the resolution of oedema around areas of acute or subacute demyelination or from the restoration of conduction in axons suffering reversible damage.

The **aetiology** of the disease remains obscure. It is commonest in temperate climates, being rare in the tropics, and although it is principally a disease of the white races it does appear sometimes in Negroes living in Europe or North America. It occurs equally in the two sexes and usually begins between the ages of 20 and 40, although it occasionally develops in the first and second decades or in the fifth and sixth. Its prevalence in temperate zones is between 50 and 150 per 100 000 population. It certainly occurs more often in several members of a family than could be accounted for by chance, usually in sibs, but parent–child transmission has been reported. There is a 25–50% concordance for clinical MS in monozygotic twins and a much lower concordance in the dizygotic. Conjugal cases occur very rarely. Probably there is an inherited susceptibility to the agent or agents which account for the demyelinating process. There is some evidence that this susceptibility may be related to the presence of certain histocompatibility antigens. The determinants HLA-A3 and HLA-B7 are significantly more common in MS patients than in controls; the increased frequency of these may be related to a high incidence of the mixed-leucocyte culture determinants DW2 and DR2. These relationships do not, however, seem to account for the geographical distribution of the disease. The rarity of conjugal cases is against an infective theory of aetiology, and there is no convincing evidence to indicate that the disease is due to infection by a virus or spirochaete. However, recent work has suggested that the condition probably represents a hypersensitivity response on the part of the nervous system to the presence of one or more common viral agents, occurring in a genetically susceptible individual. There seems to be some evidence that the environmental agent (possibly viral) may be acquired in childhood as migrants appear to retain the risk of developing the disease associated with their mother country. Antibody studies have suggested that the measles virus may sometimes be the environmental agent but several other viruses have also been suggested as precipitants. Other theories implicating excessive dietary animal fat, heavy-metal poisoning, vasospasm or venous thrombosis also have adherents but have not won general acceptance. Current opinion favours the view that hypersensitivity plays a major role. Although evidence in favour of this hypothesis is much less convincing in this disease than in acute encephalomyelitis, it receives modest support from the fact that the total γ-globulin and oligoclonal IgG are generally increased in the CSF. It is also apparent that relapses can repeatedly follow infective illnesses in some individuals, and they have also been described after prophylatic inoculation. The fact that onset or relapse may also follow trauma and/or emotional stress is much less easy to explain.

The **clinical manifestations** of the disease can be very variable, depending upon the situation and intensity of the pathological changes. A single discrete initial lesion can produce many different symptoms and signs depending upon its site, but if multiple lesions occur simultaneously in eloquent areas of the nervous system a much more specific clinical picture will result. This variation in spatial distribution of the areas of demyelination is responsible for the remarkable clinical pleomorphism of the disease. Symptoms due to a single localised lesion almost always remit within a few days or weeks as do those attributable to multiple lesions which have developed acutely. In such cases, numerous relapses may occur after intervals of months or years, each followed by a partial remission, but each leaving in its wake further evidence of permanent neurological deficit upon which each succeeding manifestation is superimposed. In the end the clinical picture is often indistinguishable from that observed in cases which from the beginning are recognised as harbouring multiple and widespread lesions, all progressing inexorably at much the same rate. The relapsing type with multiple acute or subacute episodes is commoner in young patients, whereas in cases with an onset in middle life the course of the disease is more often slowly progressive and the brunt of the disease process usually falls upon the spinal cord. Although it is possible that in a few cases the disease becomes arrested, and that in fewer still a remission may be complete and permanent, most cases eventually follow a final common path of increasing ataxia and/or spasticity, immobility, respiratory or urinary infection and death.

Although it is a truism that almost any symptom of neurological disease can at some time be observed in cases of multiple sclerosis, there are certain symptom-complexes which occur particularly often, usually as the presenting features of the disease.

One of the most frequent initial symptoms is *visual failure*, which is generally unilateral but occasionally bilateral, and is the result of *retrobulbar neuritis*. There is often pain in the eye with progressive blurring or dimming of vision over a period of several hours or days. Often vision is totally lost but spontaneous improvement generally occurs and recovery may be complete within a few weeks or months, although a central scotoma sometimes remains. In the acute stage the optic disc is usually swollen, but subsequently waxy pallor of the temporal half of the disc or optic atrophy is seen. An alternative presenting symptom, which can also antedate other neurological manifestations by several years, is *diplopia*, lasting for several hours or days. Occasionally this is due to involvement of the nucleus of one of the oculomotor nerves, but more often it is of central or internuclear type, occurring without an objective ocular palsy. A sign almost pathognomonic of this disease is one form of internuclear ophthalmoplegia, sometimes called Harris's sign, or ataxic nystagmus, in which, on lateral gaze, there is gross nystagmus in the abducting eye and failure of medial movement of the adducting eye.

An alternative mode of onset is with *transient weakness or loss of control of the limbs*. The weakness can take the form of a monoparesis or hemiparesis, but paraparesis is more common. There is weakness and clumsiness of the affected limb or limbs with difficulty in walking. Frequently, the weakness is asymmetrical so that even in the presence of clear-cut signs of pyramidal tract dysfunction in both legs the patient may complain that one leg only 'drags' and often insists that the other is normal. In mild or early cases the weakness may only become apparent after walking or standing for long periods. Physical examination during the episode reveals either spasticity with increased reflexes and extensor plantar responses, or cerebellar ataxia. These initial manifestations may resolve over a few days or weeks to be succeeded by other manifestations in the subsequent months or years.

Sensory symptoms are also common as primary manifestations. Paraesthesiae in a limb lasting for a few days can easily be overlooked; often these spread in a typical manner, indicating centrifugal spread of a plaque of demyelination in the posterior columns of the cord. In such a case the tingling and numbness may spread up one leg and down the other or from an arm to the trunk and then to the face and leg on the same side of the body. Often there are 'tight-band' sensations or feelings of swelling in the affected member (see p. 169). The so-called 'useless hand' syndrome is often due to such a lesion which so impairs proprioceptive sensation in one hand that the patient is virtually unable to use it even though motor power remains intact. On examination there is impairment of position and joint sense, of vibration sense and two-point discrimination in the affected limb or limbs, while if the legs are involved, Romberg's sign will be positive. Lhermitte's sign is often present too. Less frequently the patient observes, particularly on entering a hot bath, that pain and temperature sensation is diminished in one leg, and examination reveals the clinical features of a partial Brown-Séquard syndrome, indicating the presence of a plaque of demyelination in one lateral column of the spinal cord. Sensory symptoms almost invariably remit over the course of a few weeks or months.

Symptoms indicating primary *involvement of brainstem structures* are also common. One mode of presentation is with an acute episode of vertigo and vomiting due to involvement of vestibular centres; evidence of sensory or motor long-tract lesions is occasionally seen in such cases. More often as the vertigo abates the patient also complains of diplopia, and ataxic nystagmus is often found. Alternatively, there is sometimes an ataxia of relatively acute onset with signs of cerebellar disease affecting the co-ordination of all four limbs; this is generally associated with severe nystagmus on lateral gaze and with dysarthria (Charcot's triad). A similar constellation of signs may also develop at a later stage in established cases. Combined lesions involving cranial-nerve nuclei and long tracts are also seen, sometimes in bewildering variety. Unilateral facial paralysis occurs rarely and may be difficult or impossible to distinguish from Bell's palsy unless there are other signs. Facial myokymia (a slow rippling movement of the muscles of one side of the face) is a rare manifestation. Some patients develop a unilateral facial anaesthesia, presumed to be due to a plaque at the point where the sensory root of the trigeminal nerve enters the brain stem. This generally resolves within about three months but can be followed months later by tic douloureux on the same side of the face and later still by evidence of spinal cord disease. Tic douloureux (see p. 57) can also develop in patients who have suffered from the disease for some years.

As already mentioned, many patients demonstrate a *slowly progressive weakness and clumsiness of the limbs.* When this occurs in younger patients there is usually clinical evidence of widespread lesions. Thus it is common to find in such individuals temporal pallor of the optic discs (even without a previous history of retrobulbar neuritis), nystagmus, cerebellar ataxia, and spastic weakness of the limbs with absent vibration sense at the ankles. In the common intermittently progressive form of multiple sclerosis which begins in middle life the main brunt of the disease falls upon the pyramidal tracts in the spinal cord, and the signs are those of a spastic paraparesis with impaired or absent perception of vibration in the lower limbs, but without any evidence of cranial nerve involvement.

A transient increase in the severity of both symptoms and signs may occur due to vasodilatation as after a hot bath or physical exertion (Uhthoff's symptom). This can be especially striking in patients with scotomas in the visual field in whom exertion or heat may cause a marked increase in visual symptoms followed by a return to the previous state after rest or cooling.

Acute episodes of multiple sclerosis can involve almost any area of the central nervous system. Thus the onset may be explosive with headache, vomiting, vertigo and facial pain and with a succession of symptoms indicating severe involvement of the brain stem, optic nerves or spinal cord. Indeed an episode indistinguishable from other forms of transverse myelitis may occur. Rarely a cerebral illness with mental changes, convulsions, aphasia, hemiplegia or hemianopia develops at the onset. Under such circumstances, differentiation from acute encephalomyelitis can be difficult or impossible. Even in subacute or chronic cases, plaques of cerebral demyelination occasionally cause recurrent focal or major fits.

Tonic seizures (brief and often painful episodes in which the limbs on one side adopt a posture reminiscent of tetany and which are often precipitated by movement or sensory stimulation) occasionally occur; as with focal or generalised epilepsy, these attacks respond to anticonvulsant medication.

Mental symptoms are not infrequent. Often features of emotional elaboration of symptoms suggesting hysteria are present at the outset and may mask the organic nature of the illness. Euphoria is the prevailing mood of many patients, but some are depressed; in the late stages a progressive dementia sometimes develops.

Sphincter involvement is common; urgency or precipitancy of micturition is a constant feature in most established cases, but as the paraplegia advances, urinary retention with overflow is common and even faecal incontinence occasionally develops.

The **prognosis** of the disease is variable. Many patients live for as long as 30 to 50 years from the onset, while a few die within one to three years. The prognosis is much more favourable in patients who are not significantly disabled within five years of the onset or in those presenting with sensory symptoms or with relapses followed by complete remission. An onset with cerebellar ataxia or the development of cerebellar signs at any stage imply a more serious outlook. However, the disease runs a very indolent or benign course in almost 20% of patients. A few who suffer episodes of retrobulbar neuritis or other attacks strongly suggestive of multiple sclerosis even remain symptom-free indefinitely. The average duration of the disease is from 20 to 30 years; the final state of the bedridden incontinent patient, racked by painful flexor spasms of the lower limbs and shaken by febrile episodes of intercurrent infection, can be one of the most distressing in medicine.

The **cerebrospinal fluid** may be normal, particularly in chronic or advanced cases. During an acute episode there is occasionally a moderate mononuclear pleocytosis of up to 50 cells/mm^3 and the protein content of the fluid is often raised to between 0.5 and 0.9 g/l. Over 50% show an increase in the total γ-globulin content of the fluid, but between 70 and 90% have an increased percentage (in relation to the total protein) of oligoclonal IgG, especially in acute cases or during relapses. Radioimmunoassay generally reveals an increased concentration of the P1 fragment of myelin basic protein in the fluid.

Electrophysiological techniques are now known to be of considerable diagnostic value. Delay in the conduction to pattern-evoked visual potentials (visual-evoked responses or VERs) from the eye to the cerebral cortex may give evidence of subclinical optic nerve demyelination, even in the absence of a history of retrobulbar neuritis. Measurement of auditory evoked potentials and of both cerebral and spinal somatosensory potentials have proved of lesser value but are helpful in detecting unsuspected conduction delay indicative of demyelination in some cases. VER recording has been shown to detect clinically silent lesions in the optic nerves or more particularly in the visual pathways in about 70% of patients in whom clinical evidence has suggested that the disease process is confined to the spinal cord, while the recording of somatosensory potentials can also reveal evidence of unsuspected lesions in about 50%. The **CT scan** shows in many cases areas of reduced density, presumed to be plaques of demyelination, in the cerebral white matter. There is now good evidence to show that magnetic resonance imaging (MRI) is an even more sensitive and accurate method of identifying and localising plaques (Fig. 15.2).

The **diagnosis** in a typical case in which there has been a remittent course and the clinical features indicate the presence of lesions widely disseminated throughout the central nervous system, is not difficult. It is indeed a useful axiom that this disease should not be diagnosed when all the symptoms and signs can be accounted for by a single lesion. Whereas this rule must often be ignored in the presence of one of the typical symptom-complexes described above, it is a useful guide. Acute episodes may mimic epidemic vertigo, meningovascular syphilis and

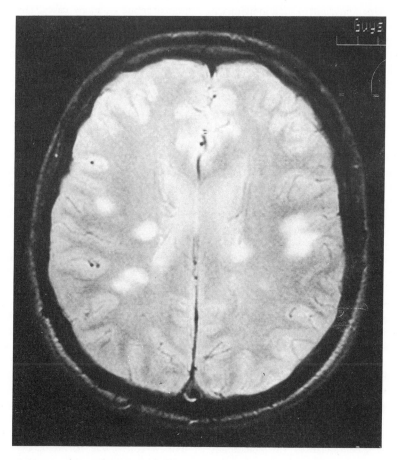

Fig. 15.2 Axial MRI to show multiple white matter lesions typical of multiple sclerosis, T2 weighted.

even encephalitis; the first of these can only be recognised by the course of the illness and then not with certainty, but the other two conditions will generally be identified by CT or MRI scanning or CSF examination. Distinction from acute encephalomyelitis can be particularly difficult but the latter is usually a monophasic self-limiting disease. In the more chronic cases, diagnosis from the familial ataxias is made by virtue of the consistent pattern of inheritance and stereotyped clinical pattern of the latter group of diseases, while motor neurone disease is identified by the presence of muscular wasting and fasciculation, features which are very rare indeed in multiple sclerosis, in which the lower motor neurones are hardly ever involved. Subacute combined degeneration can occasionally be mimicked and when 'posterior column' and 'pyramidal' symptoms and signs predominate, examination of the blood and estimation of the serum B_{12} are obligatory. In patients who present with a progressive spastic paraplegia it is sometimes impossible to exclude spinal tumour and cervical spondylosis with certainty except by myelography, and in such individuals the diagnosis of multiple sclerosis may have to be made by exclusion, although a raised oligoclonal in the CSF will give valuable confirmatory evidence.

Management of the disease requires exceptional tact and judgement. Because of its public image as a progressive and incurable disorder it may be wise in initial attacks, when there is a strong probability of total and prolonged remission, to use such terms as 'neuritis' in discussion with the patient, but when the disease enters upon a progressive course or if the patient asks 'Is it MS?' it is unjustifiable to withhold the diagnosis. But even then it is wise to stress the very benign course of the illness in many cases and to explain that whereas the disease is not at present curable , many forms of treatment are available to modify its course or to alleviate its effects. Every effort should be made to help the patient to continue in his or her normal occupation for as long as possible. As the condition advances, continuing encouragement combined with vigorous physiotherapy, including active and passive movements and re-educational walking exercises, may long postpone recourse to a wheelchair and/or the bedridden state. Calipers, walking aids and other appliances may all be invaluable and the advice of an occupational therapist upon appropriate aids, modifications, where necessary, to the patient's home, types of wheelchair for indoor and outdoor use and other aids to daily living for both patient and spouse or other family members can be invaluable.

Many forms of treatment can be considered for various specific manifestations or complications; the attachment of weights to the arms, isoniazid or, in the last resort, stereotaxic thalamotomy have been used with benefit for the control of intention tremor. However, stereotaxic surgery does have the considerable disadvantage that because the disease has already produced multiple lesions in the nervous system, the addition of yet another, surgically induced, may relieve the tremor while accentuating any deficits of speech or intellect which may be present. Spasticity may be partially relieved by drugs such as diazepam, dantrolene or baclofen, while in more severe cases, intrathecal phenol or hypertonic saline can be valuable in controlling flexor spasms. Some workers have claimed benefit from electrical stimulation of the spinal posterior columns through percutaneous or implanted extradural electrodes but others regard this method, which is still experimental, as being of dubious value. Propantheline and related remedies have been widely used in controlling urgency of micturition; however, it is now considered sensible, when urinary problems are troublesome, to carry out video cystometrograms to determine the nature of the problem. Oxybutinin (1–3 tablets daily) seems likely to be even more helpful than propantheline in many cases. However, some patients ultimately require catheter drainage, while others are now being helped by implanted artificial sphincters. Carbamazepine or other anticonvulsants are usually effective when tonic fits occur. In the later stages the skin, bladder and bowels require attention as in paraplegia from any cause and antibiotics are regularly needed to control urinary or other infections.

Assessment of the effects of specific treatment in a disease like MS which is often subject to remissions and relapses is exceptionally difficult but a number of helpful disability rating scales have been introduced and found helpful by Schumacher, Kurtzke and others. Innumerable controlled and uncontrolled trials have been carried out with a variety of remedies including azathioprine, cyclophosphamide, plasma exchange, interferon and total lymphoid radiation, and none has been shown to be universally effective. Nevertheless there is general agreement that high-dose steroid therapy (prednisone is now preferred to ACTH and is usually given for a few weeks, and certainly for not more than three months) is beneficial in acute relapses. Many authorities now prefer enteric-coated prednisolone (60 mg daily, then 45 mg, 30 mg, 20 mg, 10 mg each for five days over a total period of 25 days). Others prefer to admit patients with severe relapses to hospital for five days of intravenous methylprednisolone 500 mg daily. A few patients seem to be steroid-dependent, improving while on treatment and relapsing when it is withdrawn, but it must be stressed that in the great majority of patients, the hazards of long-term treatment far outweigh any possible advantages. Azathioprine and other immunosuppressive agents have also been claimed to be of benefit in short-term trials but recent major controlled trials have failed to demonstrate benefit from long-term treatment. A gluten-free diet, and the use of linoleic acid supplements, as well as hyperbaric oxygen are other measures which have been recommended but which are now generally agreed to be of little or no value.

DIFFUSE CEREBRAL SCLEROSIS AND THE LEUCODYSTROPHIES

Diffuse cerebral sclerosis was first described by Schilder in 1912 under the title of **encephalitis periaxalis diffusa.** Pathologically it was thought to be characterised by a progressive massive demyelination of the cerebral white matter, usually beginning posteriorly and spreading more or less symmetrically throughout the two hemispheres but sparing the arcuate fibres of the occipital lobes. Macroscopically the affected white matter became greyish, rubbery and translucent, and microscopically there was accumulation of sudanophilic lipid derived from the degenerating myelin. Clinically the condition was described as beginning usually in childhood with progressive visual failure, focal or generalised fits, aphasia, mental deterioration and variable degrees of paresis of the limbs, leading eventually to total blindness, dementia and spastic quadriplegia. Rarely the onset was sudden with headache, stupor and convulsions. The condition was progressive, uninfluenced by treatment and usually ended fatally in the first decade within one to three years of the onset. The CSF commonly showed an increase in its protein content, the EEG diffuse slow activity.

The nosological status of Schilder's disease has become confused over the years because the condition has not been properly distinguished either clinically or pathologically from a number of other progressive white matter diseases, often occurring in infancy and childhood, which have in the past been classified as diffuse cerebral sclerosis but which are now known to be disorders of the metabolism of myelin or to be the result of storage of abnormal chemical substances in the cerebral and spinal white matter and sometimes even in peripheral nerves. These are now classified as the **leucodystrophies.** Most of these conditions are genetically determined whereas Schilder's disease occurs sporadically and is not believed to be due to a specific gene. Another important development has been the discovery that many male patients previously diagnosed as examples of Schilder's disease also show adrenal atrophy pathologically and some also have the clinical features of Addison's disease. This condition, now known to be due to an X-linked gene, is known as **adrenoleucodystrophy** (Addison-Schilder's disease or sudanophilic leucodystrophy with adrenal atrophy and bronzing of the skin (the latter is a common feature). It has also become evident that many other cases of what was once called Schilder's disease are due to acute cerebral multiple sclerosis. Indeed some authorities are now suggesting that Schilder's disease, in which the lesions are indistinguishable histologically from those of multiple sclerosis, may simply be an acute variant of the latter disease occurring exceptionally in childhood; yet another variant, in which concentric areas of demyelination are found in the white matter of the cerebral hemispheres, is sometimes called Baló's concentric sclerosis. Nevertheless, histological similarity cannot be taken to imply a common aetiology as the cerebral changes in adrenoleucodystrophy, now known to be an inherited metabolic disorder, are also indistinguishable. Thus the nosological status of Schilder's disease remains uncertain; however, this diagnosis is still appropriate in children or young adults presenting with a rapidly progressive course suggesting progressive degeneration of the posterior parts of one or both cerebral hemispheres in whom CT or MRI scanning and subsequent pathological examination reveals one or more sharply outlined areas of massive confluent demyelination, especially when arcuate fibres are spared.

Of the other leucodystrophies, there is another form of sudanophilic leucodystrophy of infantile onset and X-linked recessive inheritance which usually presents with disorganised ocular movements and cerebellar ataxia; in this condition, **Pelizaeus-Merzbacher disease**, the pathological changes are again similar to those of Schilder's disease but the adrenals are spared. In autosomal recessive **metachromatic leucodystrophy** (p. 186) due to arylsulphatase deficiency, there is diffuse demyelination with the accumulation of metachromatically staining granules in the white matter of the brain and peripheral nerves. In childhood, dysarthria, spasticity, athetoid movements and dementia begin at about the age of two years and there are signs of polyneuropathy with slowing of peripheral nerve conduction. Death occurs within six months to three or four years after the onset. The CSF protein is usually raised and peripheral nerve biopsy may give diagnostic findings. An adult-onset form occurs giving rise to progressive dementia, spasticity and subclinical polyneuropathy. The features of **globoid cell leucodystrophy** (Krabbe's disease) are not very different except that the onset is usually in the first six months of life with irritability, convulsions, spasticity, optic atrophy and progressive dementia, death occurring as a rule within a few months. There is a substantial rise in the CSF protein and marked slowing of nerve conduction. Large globoid cells containing cerebroside are found in areas of degenerating white matter in the brain, spinal cord and peripheral nerves. The condition is due to an autosomal recessive gene causing a deficiency of galactocerebroside B-galactosidase.

REFERENCES

Adams R D, Victor M 1985 Principles of neurology, 3rd edn. McGraw-Hill, New York

Behan P O, Currie S 1978 Clinical neuroimmunology. Major problems in neurology, Vol 8 (Walton J, series ed.). Saunders, London

Fishman R A 1980 Cerebrospinal fluid in diseases of the nervous system. Saunders, Philadelphia

Hallpike J F, Adams C W M, Tourtellotte W W 1983 Multiple sclerosis. Chapman & Hall, London

Matthews W B, Acheson E D, Batchelor J R, Weller R O 1985 McAlpine's Multiple sclerosis. Churchill Livingstone, Edinburgh

Menkes J H 1985 Textbook of child neurology, 3rd edn. Lea & Febiger, Philadelphia

Millar J H D 1971 Multiple sclerosis: a disease acquired in childhood. Thomas, Springfield, Ill.

Walton J N 1985 Brain's Diseases of the nervous system, 9th edn. Oxford University Press, Oxford

16. Neoplasms and the nervous system

About 1% of all deaths are due to intracranial tumours. These occur in great variety; most are locally malignant and constitute about 15% of all malignant tumours occurring in man. Of these, most arise primarily within the cranial cavity and, being invasive, cannot be completely removed surgically, but many are metastatic from a malignant neoplasm growing elsewhere in the body which has given secondary deposits within the brain or meninges or in the bones of the skull. There are, however, a number of benign neoplasms which may grow within the skull and it is particularly important that these should be recognised as they can generally be removed in whole or in part at operation, with excellent results. The proportion of intraspinal tumours which compress the spinal cord and are benign is very much higher, and diagnosis of these removable growths is even more imperative. The symptomatology of intracranial neoplasia is very variable, as it depends not only upon the character of the neoplasm but also upon its situation and rate of growth, There are limitless permutations and combinations of these three factors which may influence the clinical picture. However, intracranial tumours usually produce a number of general symptoms, upon which the specific features produced by different varieties of tumour arising in individual situations are superimposed. Before considering these general symptoms and some of the more common and important tumour syndromes, it is first necessary to formulate a working classification of tumours of the nervous system in order to provide an understanding of the basic pathological features of intracranial and intraspinal new growths and to give an approximate outline of their relative incidence.

CLASSIFICATION OF NEOPLASMS IN THE NERVOUS SYSTEM

In the absence of any convincing evidence about the aetiology of intracranial or intraspinal tumours, they are at present classified according to their cells of origin. Of the **primary neoplasms**, those arising from the nerve cells and fibres themselves or from their cells of embryonic origin (neuroblastomas and neurocytomas) are rare. Commonest are the gliomas, of which the most malignant is the glioblastoma multiforme, the least invasive the astrocytoma. According to the popular Kernohan classification all gliomas are called astrocytomas and are graded I to IV according to the characteristics of the predominant cells in the tumour; grade I is the least, and grade IV the most anaplastic and malignant. Accurate grading can be difficult, as in a single tumour it may be possible to find certain cells characteristic of glioblastoma and others which are those of a typical slowly-growing astrocytoma, so that a tumour cannot be more benign than is indicated by the small amount of tissue that is removed by needle biopsy, but can well be more malignant. The rapidly-growing medulloblastoma, a common malignant tumour of the posterior fossa in infancy and childhood, which tends to metastasise, usually in the subarachnoid space, but sometimes to long bones, is probably best classified with the gliomas, although its predominant cell is very different from the astrocyte and its precursors. Other tumours of the nervous supporting tissues are first, the relatively slow-growing and benign oligodendroglioma, which has a particular tendency to calcify, and the ependymoma, which arises from the ependymal cells lining the cerebral ventricles or the central canal of the spinal cord.

Of the primary neoplasms which arise in the meninges, the benign meningioma is the most common, but occasionally a fibrosarcoma, a reticulum cell sarcoma, or a melanoma may arise in this situation. In considering growths which arise from organs which are attached to or lie in close relationship to the brain, but are not strictly a part of it, there are the adenomas of the pituitary gland (the hypophysis), pinealomas, papillomas of the choroid plexus and glomus tumours which arise from the glomus jugulare. Neoplasms of developmental origin ('rest cell' tumours) include: the craniopharyngioma which arises from remnants of Rathke's pouch; haemangioblastomas which are usually found in the cerebellum; arteriovenous angiomas or hamartomas (which are more properly regarded as vascular malformations rather than tumours); chordomas, which arise from remnants of the primitive notochord and occur around the pituitary fossa and clivus or in the sacral region; lipomas in the corpus callosum or spinal canal; epidermoid (cholesteatoma) and dermoid cysts, some of which are teratomas; and an uncommon tumour called a colloid cyst which is generally found in the third ventricle and arises from vestiges of the primitive paraphysis. Primary neoplasms of the cranial or vertebral bones which secondarily involve the brain or spinal cord are relatively uncommon. These include osteomas, osteogenic sarcomas, osteoclastomas, and haemangiomas of vertebral bodies. Lastly, in considering primary tumours, one must remember those which grow from or in relation to nerve trunks, as these may form upon cranial nerves or spinal nerve roots to give symptoms and signs indicating the presence of an intracranial or intraspinal tumour. By far the commonest is the neuroma, neurilemmoma, neurinoma or neurofibroma (as it is variously called), which grows from Schwann cells or perineural fibroblasts; usually a neoplasm of this type takes the form of an encapsulated swelling upon a nerve, but occasionally it infiltrates between nerve fibres, with which it becomes inextricably intermingled to give a plexiform neuroma. This latter type of growth is seen particularly on peripheral nerves. Neurofibromas sometimes grow in relation to nerve plexuses or single peripheral nerves outside the central nervous system, when they give a clinical picture indicating a peripheral nerve or plexus lesion (see Ch. 13) and there is usually a palpable swelling over the nerve trunk. Fibrosarcomas also occur occasionally on or in peripheral nerves.

Tumours arising outside the cranial cavity may affect the brain or other intracranial structures in a number of ways. The most common are secondary carcinomas arising as blood-borne metastases from tumours elsewhere in the body, of which lung, breast, kidney, ovary and skin (malignant melanoma) are the most common. Intracranial deposits may occur in diseases of the lympho-reticular system which include Hodgkin's disease, the non-Hodgkin lymphomas (the majority of which are monoclonal B cell neoplasms) and lymphatic leukaemias. The meninges are the most frequently involved, deposits within the brain parenchyma are rare. However, primary intracerebral lymphomas have been described. Intracranial structures may also be involved by direct invasion from tumours lying outside the cranial cavity; the most common is a nasopharyngeal carcinoma invading the base of the skull but tumours may also arise in the paranasal sinuses. Involvement of the skull vault or base of the skull by secondary deposits (lung, prostate, breast and thyroid) and by myelomatosis, may cause headache

and cranial nerve palsies as their initial manifestations. Finally, systemic neoplasms may affect the nervous system without there being any evidence of metastases; these are known as the non-metastatic paraneoplastic syndromes (see p. 265).

It is important to remember that certain conditions which are not strictly neoplastic can give a clinical picture suggesting the presence of a space-occupying lesion within the skull or spinal column. That this is true of cerebral abscess has already been mentioned (see p. 219) but in such individuals there is usually clinical evidence of infection. In others, however, an intracranial or intraspinal mass of inflammatory origin develops in an indolent manner without such clear clinical evidence. This is true of certain granulomas (gumma, tuberculoma, sarcoidosis) and parasitic cysts (e.g. cysticercosis). Arachnoidal cysts of developmental origin are rare in the cranial cavity, more common in the spinal canal.

There is much evidence to suggest that the relative incidence of intracranial tumours has changed considerably over the years. Thus the once common granulomas (gumma, tuberculoma) are now rare in Western Europe and in the USA (though not in parts of Asia) and the incidence of metastatic tumours is increasing. The most common intracranial tumours are gliomas, metastases and meningiomas in that order. In adult life, most gliomas are supratentorial, and over half are glioblastomas; more males than females are affected. In childhood, most gliomas occur in the posterior fossa and are generally either medulloblastomas, cerebellar astrocytomas or pontine gliomas. Gliomas developing in adult life are most common in middle-age; but in women with increasing age there is an increasing probability that a supratentorial neoplasm will be a meningioma. In the spinal canal, gliomas are comparatively rare and neurofibromas, which occur at any spinal level and equally in the two sexes, are much more common. Spinal meningiomas usually occur in the dorsal region, and nearly always in women. An outline of this classification with approximate figures of incidence are given in Table 16.1.

INTRACRANIAL TUMOURS

The pathophysiology of increased intracranial pressure

We must first consider the means by which intracranial tumours alter brain function and so give rise to symptoms and signs. The brain and its membranes are contained within the rigid bony skull; hence an evolving tumour must displace normal intracranial contents. If the tumour grows very slowly, some compensation for its presence can occur, partly by displacement of CSF and reduction in the venous spaces and partly by accommodation of the brain itself. Eventually this compensation fails and the intracranial pressure rises, often in association with the development of cerebral oedema. This decompensation may be quite rapid so that a tumour present for many years may present ictally; about 5% of tumours have a stroke-like presentation. More rapidly developing tumours and other space-occupying lesions are much less well tolerated as exemplified by a patient with a small haematoma who may present with a dense neurological deficit, possibly in coma. As would be expected from the principles elucidated in Chapter 4 (pp. 53–54), headache is an almost invariable accompaniment. In extreme cases the pressure is raised to such a degree that there is increased resistance to the entry of blood into cerebral

arteries, so that the cerebral blood flow is reduced. This increased arterial resistance leads in turn to a reflex raising of arterial blood pressure in an attempt to overcome it, so that temporary hypertension develops, the so-called Cushing effect. Rarely blood flow may be reduced sufficiently for infarction to occur. The local cerebral oedema which is almost invariable in the immediate vicinity of an intracranial tumour contributes to the increasing intracranial tension. Not only is the pressure of the CSF increased in the spinal theca but in all extracranial extensions of the subarachnoid space. Thus the pressure in the meningeal sheaths around the optic nerves also rises; this in turn leads to diminished venous return from the retinae, with engorgement of

Table 16.1 Classification of intracranial and intraspinal tumours

	Approximate incidence in cranium
I. *Primary tumours*	
1. Neuroblastomas and neurocytomas	Rare
2. Gliomas and other supporting cell tumours	
a. Glioblastoma	
b. Astrocytoma	
c. Medulloblastoma	40%
d. Oligodendroglioma	
e. Ependymoma	
3. Meningeal tumours	
a. Meningioma	15%
b. Fibrosarcoma and reticulum cell sarcoma	
c. Melanoma	Rare
4. Tumours of secretory or glandular tissues	
a. Pituitary adenomas	
b. Pinealoma	8%
c. Papilloma of choroid plexus	
d. Glomus tumours	
5. Tumours of developmental origin	
a. Craniopharyngioma	
b. Haemangioblastoma	
c. Arteriovenous angioma	10%
d. Chordoma	
e. Epidermoid and dermoid cysts	
f. Colloid cyst of third ventricle	
6. Primary tumours of cranial vertebral bones	
a. Osteoma	
b. Osteogenic sarcoma	Rare
c. Haemangioma of vertebral body	
7. Tumours of nerves and nerve roots	
a. Neurinoma (neurofibroma) and plexiform neuroma	10%
II. *Secondary tumours*	
1. Intracranial and intraspinal metastases	
a. Carcinoma (lung, breast, kidney, thyroid, ovary, colon)	
b. Sarcoma	15%
c. Melanoma	
2. Tumours involving cranial bones, vertebral bodies and meninges	
a. Carcinoma of nasopharynx and paranasal sinuses.	
b. Metastatic carcinoma of bone (lung, prostate, breast, thyroid)	
c. Multiple myelomatosis and solitary myelomas	
III. *Granuloma* (gumma, tuberculoma, sarcoid, parasitic invasion)	2%

retinal veins, swelling of the optic nerve heads or discs (papilloedema) and in severe cases, retinal haemorrhages and exudates around their edges. Another effect of increased intracranial pressure is compression of the respiratory and cardiac centres in the brain stem so that both respiration and the heart rate become slower; a full, slow pulse is characteristic. In severe cases with progressive deterioration, brain-stem centres (the reticular substance) can be so compressed as to cause coma. In these later stages, respiration becomes irregular or of Cheyne-Stokes type and eventually ceases altogether, while a terminal tachycardia, rather than bradycardia, is common.

The severity of the symptoms of increased intracranial pressure depends not only upon the size and rapidity of growth of the tumour but also upon its situation. Thus a slowly-growing meningioma in one or other frontal region will produce few pressure symptoms, at least initially, when manifestations of focal cerebral dysfunction predominate. Growths in the posterior fossa, however, which interfere with the free circulation of CSF at an early stage, either through aqueductal pressure, or through blockage of foramina in the fourth ventricle, give symptoms of raised pressure very early.

Additional complications may arise as a result of herniation of brain tissue under the free edge of the falx cerebri, through the tentorial notch, or the foramen magnum. The falx is the longitudinal and vertical fold of dura mater which separates the medial surfaces of the two cerebral hemispheres, while the tentorium is the horizontal fold whose curved free edge encircles the upper brain stem, and which separates cerebrum from cerebellum. A mass in either cerebral hemisphere can cause a gradual extrusion of a part of the hemisphere across the free edge of one of these folds. Downward displacement of the medial aspect of the temporal lobe through the tentorial notch is particularly important. As the third (oculomotor) cranial nerve crosses this notch, it is often compressed, and the first sign of herniation may be a fixed dilated pupil, ptosis or later a complete third-nerve palsy on the side of the lesion. Subsequently there is compression of the upper brain stem with stupor or coma and occasionally ipsilateral pyramidal signs develop due to compression of the contralateral crus cerebri against the opposite free tentorial edge (Kernohan's sign). If tentorial herniation is allowed to increase or to persist unchecked then tearing of small perforating arteries and veins can cause haemorrhages in the midbrain (median raphe haemorrhages); when such lesions occur, damage is generally irreversible. Reduction of the pressure below the tentorium, say by lumbar puncture, will increase the herniation, giving a rapidly fatal termination to the illness owing to brain-stem compression.

The risks of lumbar puncture are equally great when there is a tumour in the posterior fossa, but then it is herniation of the cerebellar tonsils through the foramen magnum (a pressure cone), with compression of the medulla oblongata, which is responsible. Patients with posterior fossa tumours and incipient coning may present with occipital headache and a stiff neck; these features may be misinterpreted as suggesting meningitis for which a lumbar puncture would be the appropriate investigation, but if this procedure were performed in such a case it could result in coning and death.

General symptoms

Since all cerebral tumours, whatever their character and situation, can be expected to increase the intracranial pressure, the characteristic symptoms and signs so produced appear eventually in almost every case. They are headache, vomiting and papilloedema.

The **headache** is of little localising value, although it is sometimes unilateral and then generally affects the side of the head upon which the tumour is situated. More often it is frontal or occipital or both. It may be more severe posteriorly in patients harbouring posterior fossa tumours, but this is not invariable. It is often intermittent and usually 'throbbing' or 'bursting' in character. It is generally most severe on waking and tends to improve as the day wears on; typically it is made worse by coughing, stooping or straining at stool. But these features are not invariable and in some cases the pain is vague and indefinite.

The **vomiting** experienced by patients with intracranial neoplasms often has no specific characteristics though it tends to be worse in the mornings, like the headache, and is sometimes precipitate and projectile, occurring without preceding nausea.

Papilloedema, though a characteristic physical sign, does not as a rule produce symptoms in the early stages. Typically the retinal veins are distended, the optic disc is pinker than normal, the physiological cup is obliterated, and the edges of the disc (including its temporal edge) are blurred. There is, of course, some blurring of the nasal edge of the disc in many normal persons. As papilloedema increases, haemorrhages may be seen in 'flare' formation around the disc and the patient will often complain of some visual obscuration, or of seeing haloes around lights. These are ominous symptoms, as is transient blindness occurring in one or other eye, say on stooping, since although gross papilloedema can exist without apparent impairment of visual acuity, visual failure, when it comes, is often rapid, complete and irreversible, due to occlusion of the central retinal artery.

The increased intracranial pressure and/or hydrocephalus produced by a tumour in any site can cause mental symptoms and false localising signs. **Mental symptoms** may take the form of progressive apathy leading in the end to stupor and coma, but earlier there is often evidence of mild dementia with impairment of memory, intellect and social adaptation. Later there may be incontinence of urine and faeces. Confusion and disorientation in time and place are common and occasionally there is a fully-developed Korsakoff syndrome (see p. 96). The commonest **false localising signs** are a unilateral or bilateral sixth-nerve palsy (due to pressure upon the nerve trunks in their long intracranial course), a partial third-nerve paralysis (due to tentorial herniation) or an extensor plantar response on one or both sides due to brain-stem compression.

It will next be appropriate to describe the various **modes of clinical presentation** of intracranial tumours. As in most nervous diseases the physical signs are generally of most assistance in localising the lesion, whereas one is dependent upon the clinical history in attempting to identify the nature of the growth. As a rule the onset is relatively rapid when the tumour is a glioblastoma, a medulloblastoma or a metastasis, but when it is an astrocytoma, an oligodendroglioma, a meningioma, an acoustic neuroma or pituitary adenoma, the symptoms usually develop insidiously. In many cases, and particularly when the tumour is a supratentorial glioma or meningioma, the clinical picture is one of progressive focal symptoms and signs indicating cerebral compression or destruction, combined with features of increased intracranial pressure. In other instances, particularly when the tumour is slow-growing, the focal symptoms progress insidiously but there are no clinical features indicative of raised pressure when the patient attends for examination. Another common history is one of focal or generalised epileptiform seizures which may precede other symptoms of a space-occupying lesion by months or years, so that even in the absence of any physical signs, late-onset epilepsy requires investigation to exclude an underlying structural abnormality, particularly if the attacks have focal features.

Another common group of cases is that in which there are symptoms and signs clearly indicating raised pressure, but there is no clinical evidence whatever to indicate the situation of the neoplasm. While this may be the case in a patient harbouring a glioblastoma, even in one cerebral hemisphere, it is particularly common in children with medulloblastomas and in adults with tumours in the posterior fossa or in the upper brain stem or third or fourth ventricle in whom the raised intracranial pressure is due to obstruction to the circulation of CSF causing hydrocephalus rather than to the size of the tumour itself. A final but important group of cases is that in which the

symptoms of indefinite headache, intermittent giddiness, vague memory loss and lack of concentration are ill-defined but nevertheless progressive. These are the most difficult cases of all, as the clinical picture is easily confused with that of emotional illness. Under these circumstances it is often difficult to decide how far investigations should be pursued in an attempt to demonstrate or exclude an intracranial neoplasm. Cases of this type are unfortunately common and it is in just such an individual that diagnostic errors are particularly easy. Hence before discussing specific tumour syndromes it will be appropriate to consider a number of cardinal points of value in the management of patients in whom the diagnosis of intracranial tumour is suspected.

Management of the tumour suspect

When the patient's history suggests that an intracranial tumour may account for his symptoms, a careful physical examination is of course imperative. If papilloedema is observed as well as a hemiparesis in a patient with a few weeks' history of increasing headache and drowsiness, it is not difficult to conclude that a glioblastoma in one cerebral hemisphere is the most probable diagnosis, while, alternatively, unilateral ataxia will point to one lateral cerebellar lobe as the most likely site. Focal (partial) epilepsy, too, suggesting the presence of a lesion near to the motor or sensory cortex, is of great localising value. It is when the physical signs are minimal or indefinite that difficulties arise. In such a case the importance of palpation, percussion and auscultation of the skull should not be overlooked. A localised area of bony tenderness or hyperostosis is sometimes present in the skull overlying a meningioma, while in young children with tumours in the posterior fossa, there may be separation of the cranial sutures and a typical 'cracked-pot' note on percussion, as in hydrocephalus from any cause. Similarly, a cranial bruit or enlarged arteries in the scalp or, more commonly, arterial or venous bruits in the neck may suggest the presence of an intracranial arteriovenous angioma.

If clinical examination is uninformative, the next investigations indicated are radiography of the skull and chest. The plain films of the skull may reveal a shift of the pineal gland from the midline, enlargement of the sella turcica (due to a pituitary tumour), flattening of the sella and erosion of the clinoid processes (due to raised intracranial pressure), intracranial calcification, or erosion of the internal auditory meatus on one side (in a patient with an acoustic neuroma). In the chest film a shadow indicating the presence of a silent bronchogenic neoplasm will suggest that the intracranial lesion is probably a metastasis. A CT scan is the most useful investigation and, if readily available, obviates the need for plain skull films in most cases as it will not only localise the neoplasm but will often suggest a pathological diagnosis, whether it be in a cerebral hemisphere, a ventricle or the posterior fossa. The EEG is an unreliable guide to the location of intracranial tumours and may be misleading. Gamma-encephalography may be helpful in patients with a known primary tumour elsewhere and with suspected cerebral metastases, but it should not be used as a screening test for primary intracranial tumours since these lesions are often not visualised by this technique. Lumbar puncture is contraindicated in patients with suspected cerebral tumours since it does not provide any very useful information and may well cause additional problems. A CT brain scan may give all the information that is required to make a decision about surgery (Figs. 16.1 and 16.2), but angiography may be required for accurate information about the blood supply of the neoplasm, particularly with tumours around the pituitary fossa which may involve the carotid artery or its major branches, in very vascular tumours including meningiomas and especially in arteriovenous malforma-

tions. If these facilities are not available, the patient should be transferred to a neurological or neurosurgical unit where the appropriate investigations can be carried out.

Although it is difficult to generalize, surgical exploration should be considered in all cases in which a tumour appears to be at all accessible, and particularly if there is any possibility, however remote, that it may be benign. If the preliminary investigations are strongly indicative of a malignant infiltrative astrocytoma, a simple needle biopsy through a burr-hole may be sufficient to establish the diagnosis. Small deep lesions are now accessible to this technique with the use of stereotactic apparatus. When doubt exists, particularly in superficial lesions, a formal biopsy carried out under direct vision via a trephine hole or craniotomy may be necessary. But if the presence of a glioma is confirmed and unless the pressure is greatly raised, indicating that decompression is necessary as a life-saving procedure, exploration and partial removal for internal decompression may be better avoided as some patients deteriorate rapidly after this procedure. Temporary but prolonged improvement may be

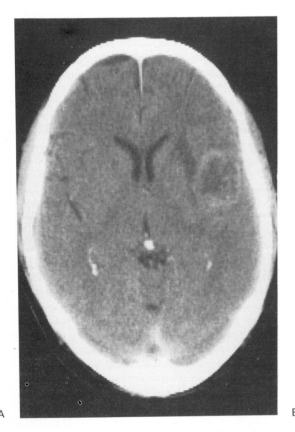
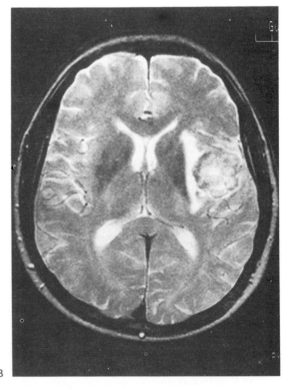

A   B

Fig. 16.1   Malignant left hemisphere glioma. **A** Contrast enhanced CT scan. **B** Axial T2 weighted NRI scan.

achieved with high doses of steroids (e.g. dexamethasone 4 mg four times daily at first with subsequent lower maintenance doses) which reduce cerebral oedema.

Radiotherapy, even with newer improved techniques, is not invariably indicated in cases of cerebral hemisphere glioma since the duration and quality of survival of the patient may be little improved thereby. However, in some patients with slowly-growing gliomas a course of radiation treatment is undoubtedly worthwhile but it has little value in patients with highly malignant and rapidly growing tumours. Circumstances vary so much from one patient to another that each deserves individual consideration in this respect. In most patients with cerebral metastases this treatment certainly deserves consideration. Cases have been described in which a primary bronchial carcinoma and a single cerebral metastasis have been removed successfully, but this is exceptional as most metastases are multiple. Often, however, it is a single large metastasis which produces the patient's symptoms and even if a primary growth is demonstrated in the lung or elsewhere, the intracranial growth usually takes precedence with respect to treatment. Partial or complete removal may be fully justified in such cases followed by radiotherapy if histological examination demonstrates that the neoplasm is likely to be radiosensi-

tive, as improvement may follow for several months or occasionally even longer. Even when metastases are multiple and inoperable (particularly when the primary tumour is in the lung or breast) remarkable and sustained improvement, at least for a time, can often be achieved by the use of steroids. Cytotoxic drugs given systemically have also been shown to have a markedly beneficial though temporary effect in some patients with gliomas and metastases and particularly in children with medulloblastomas. The aim must always be not just to prolong life but to relieve suffering and improve the quality of life.

Tumour syndromes

Having considered the general symptomatology and the management of cases of suspected intracranial tumour, it will now be appropriate to describe briefly a number of the syndromes which may result from specific tumours in different parts of the cranial cavity.

Glioma

Between the rapidly-growing glioblastoma on the one hand, and the insidiously invasive astrocytoma on the other, many types of gliomatous tumour are seen, each with its own pathological characteristics and rate of growth. As the clinical history of the illness produced by such a lesion depends upon its rate of development, it is impossible to describe fully all the possible variations in clinical presentation and course which can be observed in such cases. Typically, however, the patient with a glioblastoma gives a history of increasingly severe headache, drowsiness, nausea and vomiting, with or without focal or generalised epileptic attacks and often with recent disorders of memory, of speech or of movement of the limbs; usually in such a case the duration of the illness is measured in weeks. By contrast, in the patient with a slowly-growing astrocytoma, it is common to obtain a history of occasional major seizures and of vague headache or failure of concentration, beginning some years previously and not causing undue alarm until some new symptom (dysphasia, monoparesis, vomiting) makes its appearance. Much depends, of course, upon the situation of the tumour. Those in the **frontal lobe** often produce progressive dementia without other localising features until the motor cortex or speech area is irritated or invaded, when focal (partial) epilepsy, or hemiparesis or dysphasia will result. Rarely there are episodes of turning of the head or eyes away from the side of the lesion (adversive attacks). Occasionally a contralateral grasp reflex can be elicited. Lesions in the anterior part of the **temporal lobe** may produce initially any of the features of temporal lobe epilepsy (attacks of fear, *déjà vu*, unreality,

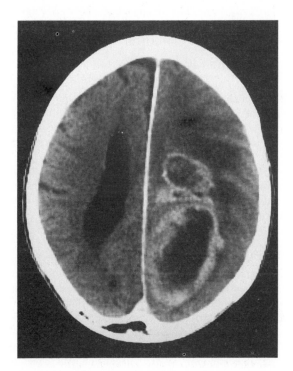

Fig. 16.2 Malignant left hemisphere glioma with central necrosis. Contrast enhanced CT scan.

hallucinations of smell or taste, and lip-smacking or chewing) while the proximity of the face and arm areas of the motor cortex means that focal seizures affecting the contralateral face and hand or else weakness of the hand and arm often occur. Should the lesion extend more posteriorly, there may be an upper quadrantic visual field defect, or Wernicke's aphasia if the dominant hemisphere is involved. Lesions of the **parietal lobe** generally result in impairment of the appreciation of the finer and discriminative aspects of sensibility in the opposite limbs, while disorders of the body image (see p. 67) may occur in non-dominant, and apraxia and agnosia in dominant hemisphere lesions. Formed auditory or visual hallucinations can be experienced if a tumour is present in the auditory or visual association areas of the cortex, but when, as rarely happens, it involves the **occipital lobe**, visual hallucinations are generally crude (e.g. unformed flashes of light) and a contralateral homonymous hemianopia, either partial or complete, is invariable. Involvement of the **thalamus and basal ganglia** usually leads to contralateral patchy impairment of all forms of sensation, somnolence and a dense hemiplegia due to damage to the internal capsule, while tumours of the **corpus callosum** are characterised particularly by progressive apathy, disorders of memory and ultimately dementia, followed usually by generalised convulsions and later still by unilateral and then bilateral pyramidal signs.

When a glioma develops in the **midbrain** (Fig. 16.3), symptoms and signs of increased intracranial pressure develop early owing to hydrocephalus due to aqueductal compression, but in addition there is generally impairment of conjugate ocular deviation upwards or laterally or both, with bilateral ptosis and/or ophthalmoplegia and variable long-tract signs. Gliomas of the **pons or medulla** tend to be particularly slow-growing and are commonest in children; diplopia is usually the first symptom and is followed by other cranial nerve palsies, often combined at first with contralateral sensory or pyramidal signs ('crossed paralysis') but subsequently the 'long-tract' signs are bilateral. Perhaps remarkably, it is well-recognised that temporary remission of symptoms and signs, often for weeks but rarely for months, sometimes occurs in such cases. Gliomas rarely develop in an **optic nerve or the chiasm**, again usually in children, or in adults with neurofibromatosis, and cause progressive unilateral visual failure with optic atrophy and a visual field defect which tends to be unusual in outline. Astrocytomas of one **cerebellar hemisphere** are particularly common in childhood but do occur in adult life. In such cases the intracranial pressure is increased early, but there is usually evidence of cerebellar ataxia in the limbs on the side of the tumour with nystagmus on lateral gaze to the

same side. When the growth involves central cerebellar structures (the vermis and roof nuclei) the patient's gait is very unsteady (disequilibrium or truncal ataxia) but there may be no nystagmus and no clear evidence of ataxia in the limbs when these are tested individually.

Occasionally multiple areas of gliomatous infiltration can develop, apparently simultaneously, throughout the brain and brain stem (**gliomatosis cerebri**). In such a case the clinical picture, indicating the presence of multiple lesions, may suggest a diagnosis of multiple metastases. Microgliomatosis cerebri is a name sometimes given to the rare diffuse **reticulum cell sarcoma** of the brain which presents similarly.

Medulloblastoma

This common tumour of infancy and early childhood grows almost invariably in midline cerebellar structures and has the property of seeding throughout the meningeal space so that tumour cells may be discovered in the CSF. Metastases outside the nervous system (e.g in bone) sometimes develop, particularly after operative treatment. The characteristic clinical picture is one of progressive ataxia, with frequent falls, followed by drowsiness and vomiting in a young child. Papilloedema is almost invariable and the cranial sutures are separated at an early stage. The treatment of choice is surgical removal of as much of the tumour as possible followed by radiotherapy and chemotherapy.

Oligodendroglioma

These uncommon tumours, which usually grow in one cerebral hemisphere, and particularly in the temporal lobe, are remarkably benign, and most patients experience intermittent focal or generalized seizures for several years before additional symptoms appear. They often calcify and a punctate area of calcification seen on a skull radiograph can be virtually diagnostic. Some such lesions can be completely removed, depending upon their location.

Ependymoma

This rare intracranial tumour is most often found in the fourth ventricle; it rapidly produces symptoms and signs of raised intracranial pressure and other signs are rare although there may be evidence of cerebellar dysfunction or of compression of long tracts in the brain stem. Positional vertigo, occipital headache and morning vomiting are common in the early stages, and may indeed be the only symptoms, while nystagmus with variable neck stiffness or vertigo provoked by attempted neck flexion

A

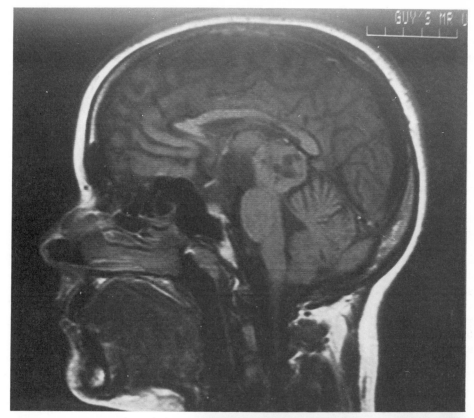

B

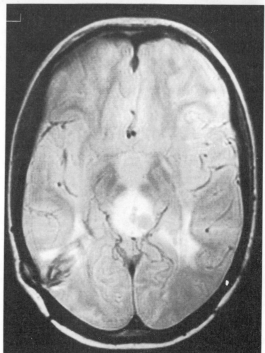

Fig. 16.3 Midbrain glioma. **A** Sagittal MRI, T1 weighted. **B** Axial MRI, T2 weighted.

are often the only physical signs. Some such tumours, particularly if pedunculated, can readily be removed surgically.

Meningioma

A meningioma compressing one cerebral hemisphere (Fig. 16.4) may produce a clinical picture indistinguishable from that resulting from an astrocytoma arising in a similar situation, although focal epilepsy seems to be particularly common with these benign neoplasms. There are, however, several specific syndromes which have been recognised as being due to meningiomas arising in particular situations. The **olfactory groove meningioma** which lies beneath one frontal lobe typically gives unilateral anosmia and dementia, often with inappropriate jocularity (*Witzelsucht*) due to frontal-lobe compression. As it extends posteriorly it can compress the ipsilateral optic nerve to give unilateral optic atrophy, and when this is combined with contralateral papilloedema, this combination of signs is known as the Foster Kennedy syndrome. A **parasagittal meningioma**, growing between the two cerebral hemispheres, typically compresses the foot and leg areas of the motor or sensory cortex in one or both cerebral hemispheres, giving focal

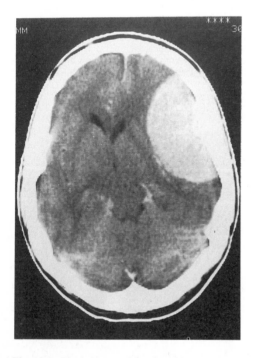

Fig. 16.4 Meningioma arising from the pterion, contrast enhanced CT scan. Note the hyperostosis and displacement of ventricles.

seizures in one or rarely both legs and/or a spastic paraplegia. Urinary incontinence sometimes occurs. A meningioma in the **cerebellopontine angle** can cause a clinical picture indistinguishable from that resulting from an acoustic neuroma (see below), while a similar tumour growing above the sella turcica (**parasellar meningioma**) typically produces progressive unilateral and later bilateral visual failure with a visual field defect indicating chiasmal compression. The meningiomas which arise from the **sphenoidal ridge**, on the lesser wing of the sphenoid, protrude into the orbit to produce unilateral proptosis, optic atrophy (due to compression of the optic nerve), ptosis and diplopia (due to involvement of the oculomotor nerve). Rarely a growth arising from the basal meninges may gradually involve multiple cranial nerves as they approach the exit foramina by which they leave the skull (**meningioma en plaque**). Many meningiomas can be removed totally, others only partially, but all deserve to be considered for surgery. Meningiomas occasionally recur after apparently total surgical removal and rarely show sarcomatous malignant change.

Pituitary adenomas

There are two principal varieties of pituitary adenoma (Figs. 16.5 and 16.6) which produce similar neurological signs but have different endocrinological effects. An adenoma of the acidophil cells gives rise to gigantism if it develops before puberty and to acromegaly afterwards, while most chromophobe adenomas eventually produce signs of hypopituitarism. About three-quarters of all patients with pituitary tumours have elevated blood prolactin levels, including about half those patients presenting with acromegaly. However, most of the latter patients do not show galactorrhoea and amenorrhoea. Some patients with these clinical features, however, have a microadenoma secreting prolactin and these do not cause neurological signs or symptoms. Basophil adenomas are uncommon and do not usually grow sufficiently large to give symptoms or signs of an intracranial space-occupying lesion. They produce the endocrine features of Cushing's syndrome which is, however, more often produced by over-activity of the adrenal cortex. Many of these patients are first seen by endocrinologists, but acidophil and chromophobe adenomas may present to neurologists or ophthalmologists with headache and visual field defects; sometimes acromegaly is unrecognised until these features develop. Both tumour types are generally large enough to cause expansion of the sella turcica and also tend to extrude above the sella to compress the medial aspect of both optic nerves and the chiasm. A bitemporal hemianopia is the typical field defect but many variations are seen. Occasionally a

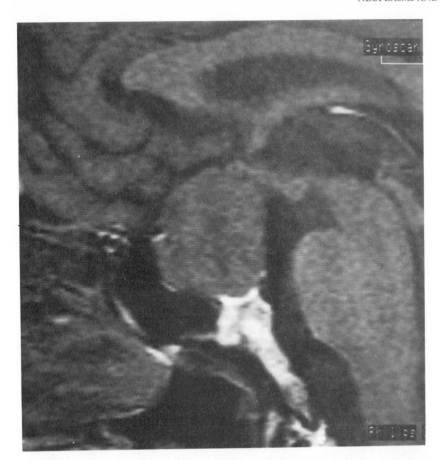

Fig. 16.5 Large pituitary adenoma with suprasellar extension, sagittal MRI, T1 weighted.

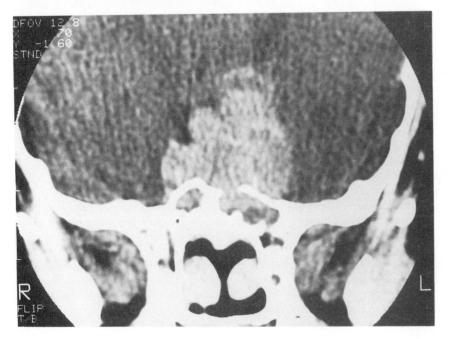

Fig. 16.6 Large pituitary adenoma with suprasellar extension and invasion of the sphenoid sinus on the left through a defect in the floor. Coronal CT scan.

chromophobe adenoma expands rapidly due to infarction when it outstrips its own blood supply; it may then compress one third nerve and the optic nerve to give sudden severe headache, unilateral blindness, a third-nerve palsy and sometimes subarachnoid haemorrhage (the syndrome of 'pituitary apoplexy').

Investigation includes plain skull films with coned views of the pituitary fossa and these usually show expansion of the fossa, often with the appearance of a double floor on lateral views. The visual fields should be accurately charted so that the effects of treatment can be quantitatively assessed. CT scanning or magnetic resonance imaging (Figs. 16.5 and 16.6), particularly in the coronal plane, will show the size of the tumour and any suprasellar extension or erosion of the tumour into the sphenoid sinus. Most of these patients are hypothyroid and will require thyroid replacement. Small tumours, even those with modest suprasellar extension, can be removed by a transnasal approach. The larger tumours with major suprasellar extension or with lateral extension out of the fossa are probably best approached through a frontal craniotomy and removed under direct vision. Post-operative radiotherapy reduces the risk of recurrence and should be given to all patients with larger tumours, particularly if the surgical removal has not been complete. In addition to thyroid replacement, some patients require continuous treatment with cortisone post-operatively and a few patients also need testosterone.

Pinealoma, papilloma and glomus tumour

Tumours in the region of the pineal gland are rather uncommon and usually occur in children or young adults. Although commonly referred to as **pinealomas**, they are of several different types. The most common is a germinoma, which is histologically similar to the seminoma of the testicle or dysgerminoma of the ovary. It may be locally invasive and sometimes these tumours present in the hypothalamus with diabetes insipidus. Tumours arising from other cell types in the pineal gland are rare. The next most common tumour in this region is an astrocytoma, but teratomas, ependymomas and meningiomas may also occur. These patients present with symptoms of raised intracranial pressure due to hydrocephalus caused by compression of the aqueduct. Pressure on the corpora quadrigemina and upper midbrain causes a defect of upward conjugate gaze and failure of convergence (Parinaud's syndrome). Larger tumours may give rise to cerebellar signs. Precocious puberty may occur in a small percentage of children with large lesions, particularly boys.

Papillomas of the choroid plexus may arise in the lateral or third ventricles but are more common in the fourth ventricle; they usually present with the features of raised intracranial pressure due to hydrocephalus without other specific features, but occasionally they cause intraventricular and subarachnoid bleeding. The characteristic manifestations of the rare **chromaffinoma of the glomus jugulare** are multiple lower cranial nerve palsies (deafness, facial palsy, dysphagia, hemiatrophy of the tongue), combined sometimes with a vascular polyp in the inner ear or a palpable mass anterior to the mastoid bone.

Craniopharyngioma

This relatively common tumour, arising from developmental remnants of Rathke's pouch, may be solid, but more often produces a cholesterol-containing cyst which is suprasellar in situation. It compresses the optic chiasm to give unilateral or bilateral optic atrophy and progressive visual-field defects, and also extends upwards into the hypothalamus. In childhood it can give delayed physical and sexual development (pituitary infantilism), or diabetes insipidus; in some cases symptoms do not develop until early adult or even middle life, when diminished libido, mental dullness and signs of hypopituitarism develop. The sella turcica is generally enlarged but shallow, unlike the typical ballooning produced by a pituitary adenoma, and there is calcification in the tumour, visible radiologically in up to 50% of cases. Few such tumours can be removed completely but often partial excision or drainage of a cyst produces substantial benefit, sometimes for several years.

Haemangioblastoma

This tumour occurs almost invariably in one cerebellar hemisphere in children or young adults and gives symptoms indistinguishable from a cerebellar astrocytoma. It may be familial and is often associated with angiomatosis of the retina or abdominal organs (Lindau-von Hippel disease). Polycythaemia is often present.

Arteriovenous angioma

The characteristic clinical features produced by these vascular malformations which will be further considered in Chapter 17, are epilepsy, subarachnoid haemorrhage, focal neurological signs, depending upon their situation, and a cranial bruit. Small vascular malformations (hamartomas) may remain silent for many years before producing epileptic attacks as their only clinical manifestation.

Chordoma

This soft jelly-like tumour, arising from remnants of the primitive notochord, usually grows either between the basisphenoid and the anterior aspect of the brain stem, or in the sacral canal. When it develops intracranially there are typically multiple cranial-nerve palsies associated often with extensive erosion of the base of the skull; in the sacrum it produces signs of involvement of multiple roots of the lower cauda equina.

Epidermoid or dermoid cysts

These rare pearly tumours or cholesteatomas are most commonly found in the posterior fossa, and are usually indistinguishable clinically from other posterior fossa tumours. Diagnosis is generally made at operation.

Colloid cyst of the third ventricle

This uncommon tumour arises within the third ventricle from vestigial remnants of the primitive paraphysis. Usually it produces clinical features indicating merely a progressive increase in the intracranial pressure, but the presence of such a lesion may be suspected when the patient experiences intermittent hydrocephalus· with attacks provoked by change in posture; in such cases it seems that the pedunculated cyst may act as a ball-valve, giving intermittent blockage of one or both foramina of Monro. These cysts are easily identifiable on the CT scan which shows a spherical highly dense lesion in the third ventricle on the unenhanced scan. Most can readily be removed surgically.

Neurofibroma (neurinoma)

This relatively common intracranial neoplasm is sometimes single, sometimes multiple; in the latter case the patient is usually suffering from neurofibromatosis, and other stigmata of the disease will generally be apparent (see p. 189). Whereas in the cranial cavity these neoplasms can grow upon the fifth or seventh nerves, the commonest site by far is the eighth or acoustic nerve (the acoustic neuroma). This tumour is commonest in middle-aged and elderly patients (except in individuals with neurofibromatosis). Unilateral nerve deafness is almost invariable and may be associated with some indefinite giddiness, but true paroxysmal vertigo is uncommon. Next in frequency as signs are nystagmus and unilateral facial sensory loss (an absent corneal reflex is sometimes the initial sign); later as a rule comes homolateral facial paresis or twitching due to compression of the facial nerve. Minimal cerebellar ataxia on the side of the lesion is often observed and there may be pyramidal signs which are usually contralateral but occasionally ipsilateral. The protein content of the CSF is often greatly raised and radiographs commonly demonstrate erosion of the internal auditory meatus. Neuro-otological studies (audiometry and caloric tests — see p. 47) are valuable aids to early diagnosis in such cases though the tumours are readily identifiable on CT or MRI scanning (Fig. 16.7), particularly if a small volume of contrast is given intrathecally and the patient is positioned so that the contrast material pools in the internal auditory meatus. Hearing may sometimes be preserved in patients with small tumours if a combined otological and neurosurgical approach is made.

'Pseudotumour cerebri' (Benign Intracranial Hypertension)

Benign intracranial hypertension is a clinical syndrome rather than a diagnosis and the term is best reserved for those patients in whom extensive investigation fails to reveal an underlying cause. The condition usually presents in overweight young women complaining of headache who are found to have bilateral papilloedema. The CT scan shows no evidence of a mass lesion, the ventricles are either normal in size or small and slit-like and there is relative obliteration of cortical sulci. Lumbar puncture shows normal CSF under increased pressure and the removal of CSF is effective both in relieving the headache and in reducing the papilloedema. Although in some patients it is a benign condition which is self-limiting, in many patients it is not at all benign because of the threat to vision produced by the papilloedema and the fact that the tendency to raised pressure persists. The acute stage can usually be managed by repeated lumbar punctures and a diuretic such as frusemide, which not only reduces the extracellular fluid volume within the brain but also reduces the production of CSF. It may be helpful to chart the area of the blind spot quantitatively to monitor progress. When the severity of the papilloedema is sufficient to be a threat to vision (see p. 109) and if these patients fail to respond to the initial treatment it is very rarely necessary to undertake surgical decompression. Steroids should be avoided because although they are very effective in the early stages, some patients become steroid-dependent and cannot withdraw the drugs without suffering a recurrence of the problem; these patients are particularly prone to develop the long-term complications of steroid therapy. A lumboperitoneal shunt is the appropriate treatment in patients who require continued CSF drainage.

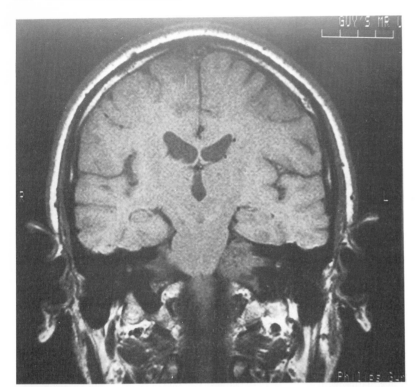

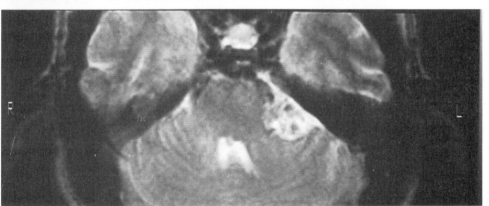

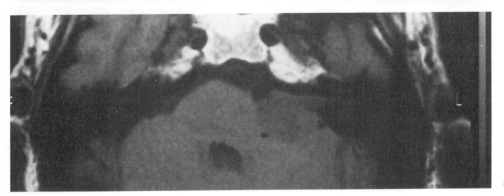

Fig. 16.7 Left acoustic neuroma.
A Coronal MRI, T1 weighted.
B Axial MRI, T2 weighted.
C Axial MRI, T1 weighted.

Conditions which may initially mimic benign intracranial hypertension include mass lesions without focal deficit, particularly if associated with obstructive hydrocephalus. This may also occur in basal meningitis due to sarcoid, fungal infections, tuberculosis or carcinomatous meningitis. The very high CSF protein that occurs in some patients with tumours such as spinal ependymomas may obstruct CSF drainage at the arachnoid villi and cause raised intracranial pressure. All these conditions are excluded by CT scanning and CSF analysis. It is important to exclude venous sinus thrombosis, which may occur during pregnancy or in the postpartum period or as a complication of taking the oral contraceptive pill. It may also develop in patients who become severely dehydrated or in the venous sinuses adjacent to infected air sinuses, for example lateral sinus thrombosis complicating mastoiditis. Cortical venous thrombosis may be associated with venous infarction, haemorrhage and epilepsy, but thrombosis in the major venous sinuses without such complications can produce a clinical picture indistinguishable from that of benign intracranial hypertension. The appropriate investigation to diagnose sinus thrombosis is venous phase digital subtraction angiography. Other rare causes of conditions mimicking benign intracranial hypertension have been described including steroid withdrawal, particularly in children, and intoxication with vitamin A and/or with tetracycline.

Intracranial metastases

Intracranial deposits secondary to extracranial malignant disease are generally carcinomatous, and the most common sites of primary growths which spread to the cranial cavity are the lung, breast, kidney, ovary and colon, although occasionally the primary tumour may be in some other organ. Sarcomas too may metastasise to the brain, as may malignant melanomas. The meninges or rarely the brain substance itself may be involved in the lymphoreticuloses (lymphoma and lymphatic leukaemia); this is becoming increasingly common in patients whose systemic disease is effectively treated by chemotherapeutic agents which do not cross the blood-brain barrier. The clinical picture produced by one or more intracranial metastases can be very variable, but does not appear to be dependent in any sense upon the nature or situation of the primary growth. Subarachnoid haemorrhage is a rare complication of intracranial metastases except that it frequently occurs in cases of malignant melanoma when the metastatic deposits are very numerous and very vascular; cytological study may then demonstrate melanin-containing cells in the CSF. In many cases the manifestations of intracranial disease precede those attributable to the primary tumour and the symptoms and physical signs usually resemble closely those produced by a glioblastoma in one or other cerebral hemisphere, or by a rapidly-growing tumour in the posterior fossa. Thus while the syndrome of morning headache and vomiting with postural vertigo and nystagmus, if occurring in a young person, may suggest an ependymoma of the fourth ventricle (see p. 254), in the middle-aged or elderly patient this clinical picture is more likely to be due to a metastasis (often from a bronchial carcinoma) in this situation.

The discovery of an opacity in a chest radiograph may be the first indication that the tumour is metastatic. Although cerebral metastases are frequently multiple (Fig. 16.8) it is comparatively uncommon, though not unknown, for the symptoms of physical signs to indicate the presence of more than one lesion. On occasion the clinical picture is even more indefinite, with vague headache, forgetfulness, lack of concentration, depression and intermittent confusion. Rarely, too, there are widespread carcinomatous deposits in the leptomeninges and the clinical picture is then one of headache, severe neck stiffness, confusion and sometimes paresis of one or more cranial nerves (*carcinomatosis of the meninges*). In such a case there is generally a moderate pleocytosis and rise in protein in the CSF, the sugar content of the fluid is

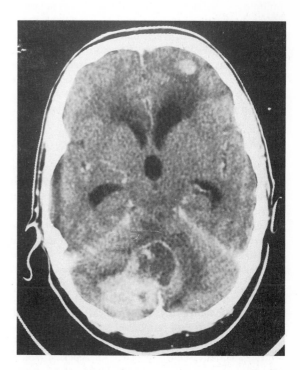

Fig. 16.8 Multiple cerebral metastases, large partially cystic lesion in the posterior fossa and a small left frontal lesion. Contrast enhanced CT scan.

greatly diminished and malignant cells can be recognised by cytological techniques.

Carcinomatous deposits in the bones of the skull may produce headaches and tenderness of the scalp, but only rarely do neurological signs result from involvement of the underlying brain. It is not uncommon, however, for a *nasopharyngeal carcinoma* to erode the base of the skull and to destroy multiple cranial nerves in succession, at first unilaterally and later bilaterally. Hence in any case in which there is progressive paralysis of the third, fourth, fifth, sixth or seventh nerves and later perhaps of those arising from the lower part of the brain stem, this diagnosis should be strongly suspected. A tumour mass may be felt in the nasopharynx but often nasopharyngeal biopsy is necessary in order to confirm the diagnosis. A somewhat similar picture, in which deafness and involvement of multiple lower cranial nerves on one side develop gradually over a period of months or years, may be the result of invasion of the cranial cavity by a *glomus tumour* arising from the glomus jugulare. A carcinoma in the maxillary sinus can also involve multiple cranial nerves, while a malignant neoplasm in the ethmoid sinus more often gives an asymmetrical proptosis with lateral displacement of the eye. Proptosis is also occasionally seen as a result of a *myeloma* of the orbit, although in general, multiple myelomatosis involving the skull does not cause neurological symptoms and signs. As mentioned above, deposits of *lymphoma, lymphosarcoma* and of *leukaemic cells* may involve the cerebral substance giving clinical manifestations similar to those of single cerebral tumours or multiple metastases, but more often develop in the meninges, compressing the brain or spinal cord or giving a clinical picture like that of meningeal carcinomatosis.

Intracranial granulomas and parasitic cysts

A *gumma* is now a rare lesion, although this diagnosis should be suspected when a patient with proven syphilis develops clinical features suggesting the presence of an intracranial space-occupying lesion. *Tuberculomas* are also uncommon, except in parts of Asia, and while the rupture of such a lesion into the subarachnoid space can cause tuberculous meningitis, they are rarely of sufficient size to give symptoms of focal brain disease. Cysticerci within the brain are an occasional cause of epilepsy, and in Britain were once seen particularly in those who had served in the Forces in India; typical calcified 'oval' lesions were sometimes recognised radiologically. Occasionally cysticerci of racemose type form in the cerebral ventricles and are then responsible for repeated attacks suggesting lymphocytic meningitis, followed by a progressive or intermittent hydrocephalus of the type which occurs in any patient with an intraventricular tumour.

Endarteritis with single or multiple infarction of the brain can be the result of meningovascular syphilis, connective tissue disease (Ch. 14) or other forms of arteritis (Ch. 17). *Sarcoidosis* is another well-recognised cause of granulomatous meningitis which often presents with either hydrocephalus or multiple cranial nerve palsies and occasionally sarcoid granulomas develop in the brain parenchyma. The commonest site is in the hypothalamus but they rarely occur elsewhere and may be multiple.

SPINAL TUMOURS

The tumours which arise within or encroach upon the spinal cord can be divided into three groups. These are: first, those which arise in the bones of the spinal column or in the extradural space (extradural tumours); secondly, those which lie within the dura mater but outside the spinal cord (intradural-extramedullary); and thirdly, those which grow within the substance of the spinal cord itself (intramedullary). In a general hospital, about 40% of all spinal space-occupying lesions are extradural, and of these the majority are **metastases**, although deposits of a reticulosis, extradural granuloma (due, for example, to sarcoidosis or tuberculous spinal caries), chordoma (in the sacral region) or a haemangioma or myeloma of a vertebral body can produce similar effects. Intradural-extramedullary tumours constitute about 50% of all spinal growths and intramedullary neoplasms about 5%. The common intradural-extramedullary tumours are first, the **neurofibroma** (Fig. 16.9), and secondly the **meningioma**. A neurofibroma may occur at any level of the spine and in either sex. It grows from a spinal root or nerve to give a mass which lies partly inside and partly outside the spinal canal, eroding the intervertebral foramen and adjacent vertebral pedicles (a 'dumb-bell' tumour). Meningiomas are nearly always found in the dorsal region and usually in women. The commonest intramedullary tumours are the **glioma** (Fig. 16.10) and the **ependymoma**. Arteriovenous angiomas may arise in the dura or in the cord itself (p. 258). The differentiation is important because dural angiomas may be embolised or removed surgically whereas intramedullary malformations are usually inoperable. Intramedullary metastases are very rare.

Although the clinical presentation of a spinal tumour will clearly depend upon its character and situation, the initial symptoms are usually those of compression of one or more spinal roots, of the spinal cord, or more often of both. If the tumour is intramedullary there is progressive destruction or distortion of long tracts resulting in motor and sensory change in the limbs and trunk below the level of the lesion, depending upon which pathways are principally involved; impairment of sphincter control usually appears comparatively early and may be the presenting symptom. Extradural growths are particularly liable to give pain of a persistent aching character in the back at the level where the tumour is situated; sometimes, if spinal roots are compressed, the pain radiates along the dermatomes innervated by the roots concerned. These symptoms are often present for some time before symptoms and signs of spinal cord compression appear, but this is not invariable and if a carcinomatous deposit causes collapse of a vertebral body, a sudden paraplegia may result. Pain in root distribution is also a character-

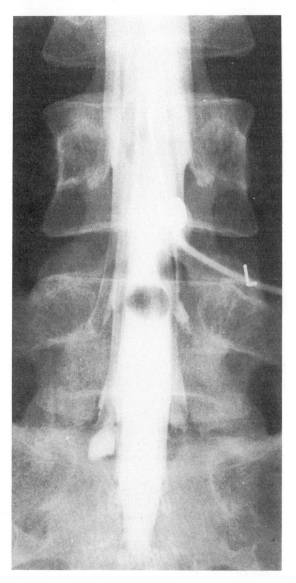

Fig. 16.9 Lumbar myelogram showing a neurofibroma.

istic symptom of an intradural-extramedullary tumour, particularly the neurofibroma, but is not invariable, and the clinical picture may be predominantly that of progressive spinal cord compression, as described in pp. 208–209. If the tumour is situated in the cervical region there will often be muscular wasting, weakness and sensory loss in one or both arms, indicating a lesion of one or more spinal roots or nerves, in addition to the evidence of spinal cord disease, but if it is dorsal in situation these signs are unobtrusive and it may be impossible clinically to determine whether the lesion is intramedullary. A Brown-Séquard syndrome can be an early result of an extramedullary tumour, but a clinical picture suggesting syringomyelia of unusually rapid progression generally implies that the lesion is intramedullary, and very probably an ependymoma. When the neoplasm lies below the termination of the spinal cord, the characteristic clinical features of involvement of one or more roots of the cauda equina are seen and there is often some pain over the lumbosacral region. Urinary retention and impotence usually develop and if the lower sacral roots are involved there is generally perianal or 'saddle' anaesthesia. A tumour at the eleventh and twelfth thoracic or first lumbar level can compress not only the roots of the cauda equina but also the conus medullaris to give a combination of upper and lower motor neurone signs. The commonest tumours involving the cauda equina are a neurofibroma, an ependymoma of the filum terminale, or a chordoma which may produce massive erosion of the sacrum, clearly visible radiologically. Rarely a solitary sacral myeloma produces similar effects.

The accurate diagnosis of spinal tumours is of the greatest importance, as so many are benign and can be successfully removed; if irreversible damage due to restriction of blood supply to the cord or by compression has not occurred, most patients recover completely. On suspicion that a tumour may be present, the first obligatory investigation is radiography of the spine, which may reveal excessive separation of the pedicles or bony erosion. If there are good clinical reasons for suspecting a spinal neoplasm, it is preferable for a patient to be transferred to a neurosurgical unit for the definitive investigation which is myelography or magnetic resonance imaging. A lumbar puncture should not be undertaken as this sometimes makes it difficult to obtain a satisfactory myelogram; it does not provide sufficiently useful information to justify the procedure and in some patients causes a marked deterioration in function of the spinal cord, probably due to a change in the pressure gradient across a spinal block. If this occurs as a result of myelography done in a neurosurgical unit, surgical decompression can be undertaken without delay. It is

A

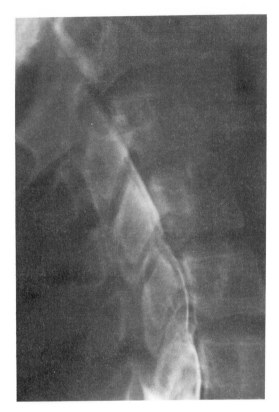

B

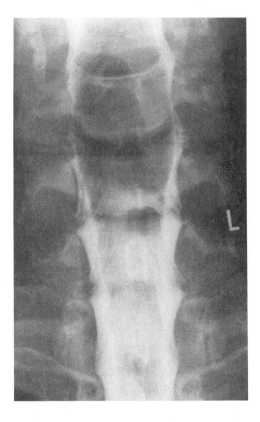

C

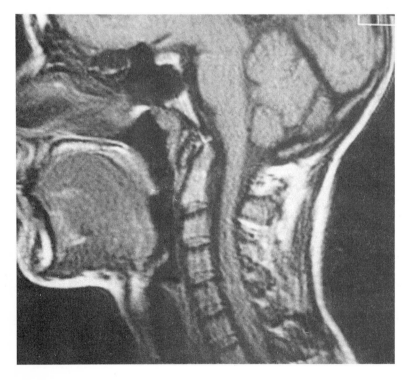

Fig. 16.10 **A** and **B**
Lateral and
anterior-posterior iohexal
cervical myelograms
showing an
intramedullary glioma
between C4 and C6 in a
patient with
neurofibromatosis.
C Lateral magnetic
resonance scan of the
cervical region showing
the same lesion.

often useful to carry out a few CT scan cuts through a lesion seen on myelography; much more information is obtained if there is already contrast in the theca than from scans done without contrast. Unfortunately the diagnosis of an intramedullary neoplasm cannot always be substantiated by myelography, even though in many such cases the spinal cord is seen to be expanded. It is, however, the extramedullary lesions which are particularly important to recognise, as these are so eminently treatable, and in this myelography rarely fails.

NEUROLOGICAL COMPLICATIONS OF MALIGNANT DISEASE

A number of specific neurological manifestions may develop in patients with malignant disease which are not due either to direct involvement of the nervous system or to the development of metastases within the brain or spinal cord. The symptoms of nervous disease can indeed antedate those attributable to the primary growth. The precise aetiology of these disorders is obscure, but they are most likely to be due to an immunological process related to proteins produced by the tumour. Support for this comes from the finding of Purkinje cell antibodies in patients with cerebellar degeneration. It must be stressed that clinical evidence of the neurological complication may appear months or rarely even years before the manifestations of the neoplasm responsible become apparent. The primary neoplasm is usually a bronchogenic carcinoma, less often one of ovary or breast. Carcinomas elsewhere rarely cause paraneoplastic syndromes but neurological complications of this type have now been described in occasional cases of malignant disease in many different sites and also in some patients with reticulosis.

The most common paraneoplastic syndrome is a peripheral sensorimotor neuropathy which may be acute and in that case is largely demyelinating or else it may be much more chronic and insidious in which case the pathological process is a mixture of axonal degeneration and demyelination. The clinical features are those of a peripheral neuropathy with early loss of reflexes, glove and stocking distribution of sensory loss with distal weakness in the arms and legs (p. 293). The distribution between motor and sensory involvement is very variable and almost pure sensory peripheral neuropathies sometimes occur. Carcinomatous neuromyopathy presents with proximal limb girdle weakness, suggesting a primary myopathy, but the underlying abnormality is usually a neurogenic lesion. An encephalomyelitis may also occur, almost always due to carcinoma of the lung; again the clinical manifestations are very variable. In **limbic encephalitis** the lesions are concentrated in the limbic system, the amygdala and hippocampus, resulting in severe memory difficulties. Brain-stem encephalitis principally involves the medulla affecting the lower cranial nerves, causing a bulbar palsy, and this is usually associated with eye movement disorders, particularly nystagmus, as well as long tract signs including extensor plantar responses. A pure cerebellar degeneration is another well-recognised syndrome, though it is rather rare and it is sometimes difficult to know how hard to search for an underlying neoplasm in patients presenting with such a clinical picture. If the Purkinje cell antibody test in peripheral blood proves to be a reliable marker, it may be possible to use this test to determine which patients should be thoroughly investigated for the presence of an underlying neoplasm.

Other paraneoplastic syndromes include the myasthenic-myopathic syndrome (the Lambert-Eaton syndrome, p. 300) as well as dermatomyositis and polymyositis (p. 306).

Unfortunately in almost all these syndromes, removal of the primary neoplasm may not result in much improvement in the neurological deficit. However in the Lambert-Eaton syndrome and in dermatomyositis, temporary improvement may follow steroid treatment and immunosuppression even while the malignant process is progressing.

REFERENCES

Adams J H, Corsellis J A N, Duchen L W 1984 Greenfield's neuropathology, 4th edn. Arnold, London

Adams R D, Victor M 1985 Principles of neurology, 3rd edn. McGraw-Hill, New York

Hankinson J, Banna M 1976 Pituitary and parapituitary tumours. Major problems in neurology, Vol 6 (Walton J, series ed.). Saunders, London

Henson R A, Urich H 1982 Cancer and the nervous system. Blackwell, Oxford

Hughes J T 1978 Pathology of the spinal cord, 2nd edn. Lloyd-Luke, London

Moseley I 1988 Magnetic resonance imaging in diseases of the nervous system. Blackwell, Oxford

Northfield D W C 1973 Surgery of the central nervous system. Blackwell, Oxford

Rosenberg R N, Grossman R 1984a Neurosurgery. The clinical neurosciences, Vol 2. Churchill Livingstone, Edinburgh

Rosenberg R N, Heinz R 1984b Neuroradiology. The clinical neurosciences, Vol 4. Churchill Livingstone, Edinburgh

Rosenberg R N, Schochet S S 1984 Neuropathology. The clinical neurosciences. Churchill Livingstone, Edinburgh

Russell D S, Rubinstein L J 1977 Pathology of tumours of the nervous system, 4th edn. Arnold, London

Thompson R A, Green J R (eds) 1976 Neoplasia in the central nervous system. Advances in neurology, Vol 15. Raven Press, New York

Walton J N 1985 Brain's diseases of the nervous system, 9th edn. Oxford University Press, Oxford

17. Vascular disorders of the nervous system

Disease in the cranial and/or spinal blood vessels can have profound effects upon the functioning of the nervous system. Indeed the clinical syndromes or 'strokes' produced by disorders of the cerebral circulation are the commonest neurological disorders. In 1952, 170 000 people in the USA died of cerebral vascular accidents, and many more were left crippled in body or in mind by a stroke or series of strokes which were not sufficiently severe to end their lives. While many patients so afflicted are elderly, these disorders are nowadays seen with increasing frequency in patients under the age of 60 and even in young adults. Although cerebral vascular disease usually produces symptoms and signs indicating a disorder of brain function, 'stroke syndromes' are not specific diseases, but rather they produce stereotyped combinations of clinical features which can be caused by many different diseases of the cerebral arteries and veins and which only secondarily affect the behaviour of the nervous system. Most are complications of hypertension and atherosclerosis, while other cardiovascular factors, including disease of the heart and great vessels, and variations in the systemic blood pressure, may play a part in their genesis. Hence one must always bear in mind the possibility, in any patient manifesting a cerebral vascular syndrome, that the primary abnormality may lie in the heart or kidneys. In this chapter, the common vascular disorders of the brain are first considered and then the much less common vascular syndromes of the spinal cord are described.

CEREBRAL VASCULAR DISEASE

The commoner cerebral vascular accidents fall into two principal categories, namely spontaneous intracranial haemorrhage on the one hand and cerebral infarction or ischaemia on the other. The word spontaneous is taken to exclude intracranial haemorrhage resulting from an obvious traumatic cause, which is usually evident in cases of extradural haemorrhage and in subdural haematoma (see pp. 203–204), though the latter condition masquerades in many guises and is a common pitfall for the unwary. About 80% of cerebral vascular accidents are the result of infarction or ischaemia (50% 'thrombotic', 30% 'embolic') while primary cerebral haemorrhage accounts for approximately 10% and subarachnoid haemorrhage for about 6–8% of all cases.

Spontaneous intracranial haemorrhage

The two principal varieties of intracranial haemorrhage are first, primary intracerebral haemorrhage, which is usually of hypertensive origin and secondly, subarachnoid haemorrhage, which generally results from the rupture of an intracranial aneurysm or angioma. The term 'subarachnoid haemorrhage' is often a misnomer, as in at least 50% of cases the haemorrhage involves brain tissue and is not purely subarachnoid in situation; furthermore, in many cases of primary cerebral haemorrhage the bleeding extends into the cerebral ventricles or subarachnoid space; this can cause considerable diagnostic difficulty in some cases.

Primary intracerebral haemorrhage

This condition is responsible for the classical stroke or apoplexy. It usually arises as a result of rupture of small perforating arteries, either in the putamen and internal capsule (the territory of the lenticulostriate artery), in one cerebellar hemisphere, or in the pons. Hypertension is the most important cause and the condition often begins during exertion or emotional stress when the blood pressure is at its height. Little is known of the pathological changes in the blood vessels which finally account for the arterial rupture, though micro-aneurysms on small arteries are often present within the brain in hypertensive patients; it seems that rupture of such a micro-aneurysm frequently initiates the haemorrhage. Much rarer causes include exposure to severe cold, drug abuse, delayed apoplexy after relatively minor head injury and bleeding due to ischaemic infarction or following carotid endarterectomy as well as arteritis and amyloid angiopathy, bleeding diseases and vascular malformations or undetected primary or secondary neoplasms. It appears that such haemorrhage occurring, as it may, in the non-hypertensive individual, is due to either (a) an acute and severe rise in blood pressure; (b) an acute rise in cerebral blood flow after relief of focal arterial obstruction ('reperfusion'); or (c) reperfusion of ischaemic or injured tissues (Caplan 1988). The condition is commonest in the elderly (60–80 year age group) but can occur in severely hypertensive individuals at any age. There is a rapid outpouring of arterial blood and, after ploughing up the brain tissue surrounding the site of origin of the haemorrhage, this often enters the ventricular system; if the bleeding is massive, death may occur within a few hours. More often the patient, without prodromal symptoms, complains of a sudden ill-defined sensation that something is wrong within the head. Within a few moments the face becomes twisted, weakness of one arm and leg and headache develop and consciousness is soon lost. The period of evolution of the stroke is rarely as brief as that seen in cases of cerebral embolism and onset is usually less abrupt than in subarchnoid haemorrhage; the full clinical picture can take up to half to one hour to develop. By this time the patient is usually deeply comatose, with stertorous respiration, neck stiffness, a slow, bounding pulse, deviation of the head and eyes away from the side of the lesion, and a dense, flaccid hemiplegia. Vomiting and incontinence of urine and faeces are usual. Occasionally 'decerebrate attacks', or generalised or focal convulsions occur at the onset. When the cerebellum is the site of the haemorrhage, the clinical picture may be indistinguishable from that produced by a severe cerebral haemorrhage, but if the bleeding is less quick to develop or is not too extensive, the early clinical features are vertigo, repeated vomiting and ataxia, often of truncal or central type; sometimes, however, unilateral ataxia confirms localisation to one cerebellar hemisphere. When the primary site of bleeding is the pons, the patient is usually comatose from the beginning, but in addition there is often inequality of the pupils, of which one may be pinpoint in size, with hyperpyrexia and a quadriplegia rather than hemiplegia.

About 80% of patients die, some within the first 24 hours, the remainder during the next few days. A fluctuant clinical course, and clinical features indicative of recurrent bleeding, are not usually seen; deterioration is generally remorseless in severe cases. Of the patients who survive, about half remain helpless neurological cripples, but there are some in whom the haemorrhage is relatively small, loss of consciousness brief, and residual disability comparatively slight. These cases are, however, difficult to recognise clinically and to distinguish from those with cerebral infarction.

Unfortunately, cerebral haemorrhage presents a gloomy picture therapeutically. Save in exceptional cases little, apart from nursing and other supportive care, can be done, though steroids may be used to reduce cerebral oedema. In selected cases surgical evacuation of the intracerebral clot, after localisation by CT scan and/or angiography or ventriculography, can occasionally be of benefit, but this procedure is only justifiable in less severe cases and in younger conscious patients. It is especially helpful in patients with cerebellar haemorrhage who survive the first few days. Lumbar puncture is of no therapeutic value and carries considerable risks of tentorial or cerebellar herniation. The administration of powerful hypotensive agents after the haemorrhage has occurred is not indicated, as lowering the blood pressure, in the presence of widespread vascular spasm (which is an almost invariable concomitant of intracranial haemorrhage) may give rise to the further complication of infarction. Clearly, prevention of cerebral haemorrhage (through the effective treatment of hypertension), rather than treatment, must be the aim.

Subarachnoid haemorrhage

This is the second major category of spontaneous intracranial bleeding and therapeutically it is much more hopeful. In about 85% of cases the condition results from rupture of an intracranial aneurysm on a major artery of the circle of Willis, while in about 10% an arteriovenous angioma is present. The remaining 5% of cases include patients with intracranial neoplasms, cerebral venous sinus thrombosis, blood diseases, and other conditions of which the subarachnoid bleeding is symptomatic. So-called berry aneurysms, the commonest cause, are probably due to the coexistence of a congenital defect in the media of a cerebral artery with an early atheromatous lesion in the intima which breaches the internal elastic lamina. Mycotic aneurysms are now rare and syphilitic arterial dilatations virtually non-existent. Aneurysms are particularly common at arterial bifurcations and are multiple in about 16% of cases. Their commonest sites are upon the internal carotid artery, below or near its bifurcation, the region of the anterior communicating, and the middle cerebral artery, but they can arise upon any intracranial artery.

The patient, who may be a young adult or even a child, but who is usually between 40 and 60 years of age, is suddenly struck down by an intense and catastrophic headache. Consciousness may be lost at the outset, and convulsions are common, but often the senses are retained, though the patient is drowsy and confused and complains bitterly of headache. The headache, which is usually frontal or occipital in situation at first, then mounts in severity and becomes generalised, severe neck stiffness and other symptoms and signs of meningeal irritation become apparent and vomiting is usual. Papilloedema is sometimes seen immediately or within a few days or weeks, but a more typical, if uncommon, sign observed on ophthalmoscopy is a brick-red subhyaloid haemorrhage, spreading outwards from the edge of one or both optic discs. In many cases there s evidence of damage to cranial nerves or to the brain itself. Unilateral or both optic discs. In many cases there is evidence of damage to cranial nerves or to the brain itself. Unilateral Depending upon the situation and severity of any intracerebral extension of the haemorrhage, aphasia, a monoparesis, hemiparesis or hemiplegia may be found. Similar signs are sometimes the result of coexistent cerebral infarction which is a common complication of subarachnoid haemorrhage and which usually results from arterial spasm, less often from tearing or compression of sulcal arteries by the force of the effused blood in the subarachnoid space. Rarely, bleeding breaches the arachnoid and produces a subdural haematoma. When the patient is comatose with a dense hemiplegia, clinical diagnosis from primary intracerebral haemorrhage with rupture into the subarachnoid space can be difficult or impossible and will depend usually upon the patient's age and upon the presence or absence of evidence of severe hypertension and atherosclerosis. However, in the initial stages of the illness, transient arterial hypertension is common, resulting probably from hypothalamic compression, and temporary albuminuria and glycosuria can also result from this cause.

Although in many cases the diagnosis is self-evident, a lumbar puncture is usually necessary for confirmation, and also in order to distinguish the condition from disorders such as meningitis or cerebral abscess, with which it may occasionally be confused, particularly if the onset is less abrupt than usual. However, the procedure is not without risk because of the danger of tentorial or cerebellar herniation, especially if there is an intracerebral extension of the haemorrhage or oedematous swelling, say, of one cerebral hemisphere secondary to infarction. Hence it is generally wise, especially in patients with focal neurological signs, to begin with a CT scan which will usually demonstrate blood in the subarachnoid space and/or cerebral substance (Fig. 17.1) before deciding whether lumbar puncture is needed to confirm the diagnosis. When it is done, the CSF is found to be deeply and uniformly bloodstained, unlike the early tingeing with blood, disappearing as the fluid flows, which can result from damage to vertebral veins caused

by the exploring needle. Furthermore on centrifuging, the supernatant fluid is found to have a faint orange tinge (due to oxyhaemoglobin) within four to six hours of the onset, and becomes deeply yellow or xanthochromic (due to bilirubin) within 30 to 48 hours.

With conservative treatment, including bed rest, sedation and relief of headache by appropriate drugs, along with prophylactic antibiotics given to avoid respiratory and urinary infection, between 40 and 50% of patients die within eight weeks of the ictus. Of these, some two-thirds die from the effects of the first bleed, often within 24 hours, but the remaining one-third succumb to a second, more catastrophic haemorrhage, which is particularly liable to occur within the second week after the first attack. Unconscious patients clearly require catheterisation and maintenance of an adequate airway, but if spontaneous respiration ceases, assisted ventilation is rarely if ever justified. Induced hypothermia is now known to be dangerous, hypotension even more so, because of the risk of increasing cerebral ischaemia. Antifibrinolytic drugs such as epsilon aminocaproic acid and tranexamic acid have had a considerable vogue but their use appears to be declining and there is no convincing evidence that they influence outcome. About 10% of those patients who are still alive eight weeks after the onset will die of recurrent bleeding before six months have elapsed and another 10% in the subsequent months or years. Of the long-term survivors, only one-third are symptom-free, while another third have severe and disabling sequelae, including hemiparesis, headache, epilepsy and psychoneurosis, and the remainder have less severe residual symptoms. The usual methods of physical and psychological rehabilitation appropriate in the management of stroke patients suffering residual disability should be employed. Some neurosurgeons give prophylactic anticonvulsant therapy for one or two years to all patients, more especially to those with evidence of intracerebral haemorrhage or infarction, but most neurologists prefer to await events and only give these remedies following the first epileptic seizure.

It is now clear that the prognosis of the condition can be radically improved in many cases by the judicious application of surgical methods of treatment. Nothing can at present be done to save those patients who die within the first two or three days, as surgical procedures carried out on the unconscious patient at this time carry almost a 100% mortality. And there are also some patients who for reasons of age and general condition are unsuitable candidates for surgery. But most who survive beyond the first few days should be considered as potential surgical candidates. First, however, the surgeon must know the situation and nature of the lesion responsible for the haemorrhage. He must also know whether there are complications such as cerebral infarction or intracerebral or subdural haemorrhage. Unfortunately clinical examination is of little help; for although it is reasonable to conclude in a hemiplegic patient that the bleeding point will probably be on the opposite side, it is usually impossible to localise a bleeding aneurysm or angioma, or to distinguish between the clinical effects of intracerebral haemorrhage and of cerebral infarction in such cases. Thus everything depends upon the results of the CT scan and cerebral angiography, which should be performed as soon as possible after the first bleed, subject to the caveats that the CT or MRl scan sometimes gives all the diagnostic information which the surgeon needs, or alternatively that in the comatose patient early angiography in the presence of generalised severe arterial spasm can be so risky that a few days of delay may be justified. Both carotid and both vertebral arteries should be visualised because of the possibility that multiple aneurysms may be present and also in an attempt to study the collateral circulation. If arteriography gives negative results, as it does in 10–20% of cases, this may mean that the causal aneurysm has clotted. There is some evidence that in cases with negative arteriograms the prognosis is somewhat better than the average. If, however, an aneurysm or angioma, or some other causal lesion is demonstrated, the surgeon can decide whether the lesion is surgically accessible and will then choose his time to operate depending upon the size and situation of the lesion and the age and condition of the patient. The most appropriate time is often at about seven days after the haemorrhage, when there is a chance of preventing those fatal recurrent haemorrhages which are particularly common in the second week and the arterial spasm which greatly increases the risks of surgical treatment because of the danger of infarction, has usually passed

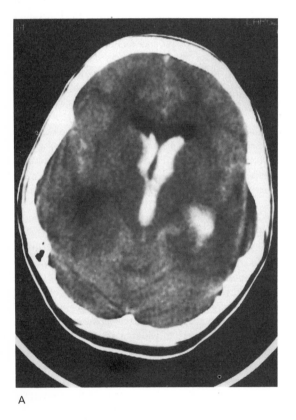

A

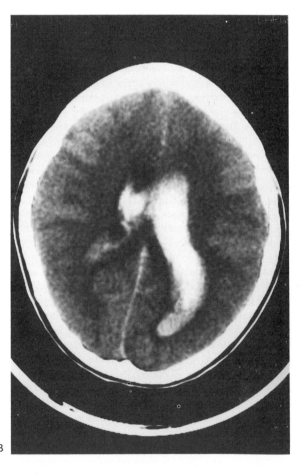

B

Fig. 17.1 A and **B**   Unenhanced axial CT scan of a patient who presented with the typical features of subarachnoid haemorrhage and who was found to have an intracerebral haematoma with extension into the ventricles and subarachnoid space.

off. The CT scan or angiogram may also demonstrate complications of aneurysmal rupture such as intracerebral or subdural haematoma which require surgical treatment in their own right. The use of hypothermia as an aid to anaesthesia has been a valuable aid in such cases as it reduces cerebral metabolism. With further improvements in surgical and anaesthetic techniques it is reasonable to predict further reduction in the mortality and morbidity of this condition.

Cerebral ischaemia and infarction

Cerebral ischaemia, or impairment of the blood supply to the brain, can be produced by:

1. a sudden fall in blood pressure and consequentially in cerebral blood flow (ischaemic anoxia — see p. 315), however caused;
2. occlusion or stenosis of one of the arteries supplying blood to the brain, whether caused by atherosclerosis, endarteritis or some other cause; and
3. obstruction of such an artery by a substance carried to it from elsewhere by the circulation — cerebral embolism.

In strict pathological terms, ischaemia is generally used to indicate a process which is temporary and wholly reversible, infarction to identify one in which ischaemia leads to death of brain tissue.

Infarction of the brain can be caused by the sudden embolic occlusion of a cerebral artery, by the gradual thrombosis of an artery, or by a combination of arterial narrowing with other factors which cause the blood supply of a part of the brain to be reduced below a critical level. Atherosclerosis, hypertension, heart disease (including cardiac dysrhythmia), single or multiple episodes of profound hypotension, and less often increased coagulability of the blood (as in pregnancy or in patients taking oral contraceptive drugs which contain oestrogen), haemoconcentration (due to dehydration) and an increase in circulating red cells (as in polycythaemia vera) are some of the principal aetiological factors.

Cerebral embolism

In cerebral embolism the onset is usually abrupt and if the artery blocked is a major one, loss of consciousness or even sudden death may occur. In less severe cases, consciousness is retained but the patient develops a hemiplegia or other evidence of a rapidly developing focal cerebral lesion. Headache is not usually a feature. When a minor artery is blocked there may simply be transient confusion, speech disturbance or monoparesis, a 'little stroke', which clears up rapidly owing to establishment of the collateral circulation. Indeed in many cases of cerebral embolism, even those with a complete hemiplegia, there is rapid improvement, leading sometimes to complete recovery within a few days or weeks, though some patients do remain seriously disabled. For every embolus there must be a source, generally in the heart or great vessels. Cerebral embolism in subacute bacterial endocarditis and in mitral stenosis is a well-recognised complication, but the frequency of its occurrence following mural thrombosis in the chambers of the heart after cardiac infarction, as well as embolism from thrombi forming on atheromatous plaques in the aorta and carotid arteries, were less well appreciated until comparatively recently. Less common causes include the prolapsing mitral valve (which may give vegetations on the valve leaflets which can cause cerebral embolism in young adults) and atrial myxoma (a rare condition largely limited to females). Recent evidence indicates that attacks of recurrent cerebral ischaemia (see below) are usually due to repeated micro-embolism either of platelet thrombi or of cholesterol derived from breakdown of an atheromatous plaque. The presence of a bruit over one of the major vessels in the neck may indicate a localised stenosis due to a plaque or mural thrombus from which such emboli can arise. Hence in any patient with a sudden onset of a hemiplegia or of less striking focal signs, a careful search should be made for a source of emboli, and particularly for evidence of cardiac disease. This is very important, as cerebral embolic episodes are for obvious reasons likely to be multiple and it is now evident that the danger of a major stroke can sometimes be averted by cardiac or arterial surgery or by treatment with aspirin or anticoagulant drugs.

Cerebral thrombosis

The remaining conditions which cause cerebral infarction have for long been grouped together under the broad general heading of 'cerebral thrombosis'. This title is often a misnomer, as there are many cases in which no actual arterial occlusion can be demonstrated. The condition is commonest in patients over 60 years of age but is nowadays occurring with increasing frequency in patients who are aged between 40 and 60 or even younger. Characteristically, the patient retires to bed perfectly well and wakes up next morning to find that one arm and leg are paralysed and perhaps that he cannot speak; or he may not discover the weakness until he attempts to stand and the leg gives way. Often there is no headache and no serious impairment of consciousness, though mild or moderate confusion is common. Rarely, headache is severe and has been attributed to compensatory vasodilatation in anastomotic vessels, or to cerebral oedema causing an increase in the intracranial pressure.

Much depends upon the size of the infarct and its situation. If it is large, the patient may be comatose, owing to swelling of the affected hemisphere, while if the brain stem is affected, rather than the cerebral hemisphere, vertigo, vomiting and diplopia are often prominent features. A mild attack of confusion, and transient weakness or numbness of one arm may be the only evidence of a small infarct. The differential diagnosis between a large infarct and a small intracerebral haemorrhage is difficult clinically but has become much easier with the advent of the CT scan, especially with contrast enhancement. Before scanning became generally available, examination of the CSF was thought to help as the fluid usually contains frank blood or a good many red cells in a cerebral haemorrhage. But even in cerebral infarction, red cells may be present and a slight to moderate rise in white cells and in the protein content of the fluid is not uncommon. Because of the potential risk of cerebral or cerebellar herniation, lumbar puncture is now generally thought to be contraindicated when full scanning facilities are available. Even angiography is now less widely used for diagnostic purposes, though the use of digital and magnification techniques has greatly improved the visualisation of small arterial occlusions in such cases. But angiographic visualisation of arterial stenosis and/or occlusion is still regarded as essential if surgical treatment is contemplated.

The size and anatomical delimitation of the infarct and hence the neurological signs depend upon many factors. In some typical cases angiography or autopsy reveal a large thrombus in, say, the internal carotid, vertebral or basilar artery or in one of their distal branches, giving an infarct in the expected distribution. In many others, however, no arterial thrombosis is demonstrated, although arterial narrowing produced by atheroma is widespread, affecting some arteries more than others, and the infarct may lie in the territory supplied by the narrowest of these vessels. In some such cases a fall in blood pressure may have been the final precipitating factor which produced infarction without arterial occlusion, due to a selective fall in blood flow through a particularly narrow vessel. Sometimes a cardiac infarct can present with cerebral symptoms in this way, or else the reduction in blood pressure which occurs during sleep or results from treatment with hypotensive drugs may be sufficient to tip the scales. Hypotension resulting from severe haemorrhage (as from the gastrointestinal tract) or from a prolonged or unusually severe episode of cardiac dysrhythmia may have a similar effect. On the other hand, paradoxically, similar infarcts may develop in hypertensive patients when the blood pressure is increased. Another important determining factor is the efficiency of the collateral circulation through the circle of Willis and through arterial anastomoses in the meninges. Furthermore, the importance of narrowing of, or thrombosis in, the main trunks of the carotid, vertebral and basilar arteries has been increasingly recognised, as these processes may cause reduced blood flow, embolism, or a spread of thrombosis to their distal branches. Atheroma is one important aetiological factor, but both transient hypotension and hypertension clearly play a part. Hence one must guard against the over-enthusiastic use of hypotensive drugs in patients who are atherosclerotic as well as hypertensive. However, since severe hypertension precipitates spasm of small arteries and arterioles which in turn contribute to infarction, in such cases a moderate reduction in the blood pressure should be achieved. Indeed there is now substantial evidence to indicate that the effective treatment of hypertension is reducing the incidence and severity of both cerebral haemorrhage and infarction.

There is also evidence to indicate that in hypertensive patients with 'small vessel disease' rather than the 'large vessel disease' due to atheroma which usually causes large areas of infarction, small cystic spaces which are tiny infarcts ('lacunes') may occur in either the internal capsule or brain stem. Such tiny lesions have been shown to be associated with certain clinical syndromes (**lacunar strokes**) including:

1. 'unilateral ataxia and signs of pyramidal tract dysfunction on the same side, involving the leg more than the arm',
2. a 'pure motor hemiplegia' (without sensory dysfunction),
3. a 'pure sensory stroke' and
4. the so-called 'dysarthria-clumsy hand syndrome' (dysarthria with cerebellar ataxia in one arm).

These syndromes have been shown respectively to be due to:

1. a lacune in the contralateral internal capsule,
2. a lacune either in the opposite side of the pons or in the opposite internal capsule,
3. a pontine lacune, and
4. a lacune in the contralateral posterolateral thalamic nucleus.

These lesions are so small that they may not be demonstrable by CT scanning, even with enhancement, but they may be more readily visualised in MRI scans.

Transient ischaemic attacks

While transient hypotension or a reduced cerebral blood flow resulting, say, from episodes of cardiac dysrhythmia, certainly account for some transient ischaemic attacks, whether these involve the cerebral hemispheres or the brain stem, most seem to be due to recurrent micro-embolism. The emboli consist either of platelets or of cholesterol and arise from mural thrombi or from atheromatous plaques in the large vessels in most cases. The consistency of the clinical pattern of the attacks is probably accounted for by laminar flow in the cerebral arteries which determines that a particle becoming free in the lumen at the same point usually reaches the same peripheral branch of the vessel. These attacks are particularly common in patients with carotid or vertebrobasilar insufficiency and were previously attributed erroneously to hypertensive encephalopathy or to vascular spasm. Patients with stenosis or even occlusion of one internal carotid artery often experience at frequent intervals over several days, weeks or months, recurrent brief attacks of weakness or paraesthesiae in the contralateral limbs, and particularly in the hand and arm. Often there are episodes of transient blindness in the homolateral eye ('amaurosis fugax') owing to involvement of the ophthalmic artery, a branch of the internal carotid. Micro-emboli can sometimes be seen in the retinal arteries in such cases. Pulsation in the affected internal carotid artery may be reduced on palpation in the tonsillar fossa, and the arterial pressure in the retinal arteries on the same side is also often reduced on ophthalmodynamometry. A systolic bruit over one common or internal carotid artery is a valuable sign, often indicating carotid stenosis. Patients suffering from basilar insufficiency experience similar transient attacks involving many brain-stem structures, now on one side of the body and now on the other, and including such features as vertigo, diplopia, transient hemianopia or bilateral blindness due to posterior cerebral artery insufficiency, paraesthesiae and weakness of one limb, of one arm and leg, or of all four limbs. Circumoral paraesthesiae, also involving the tongue, sometimes occur, as they do in basilar migraine or hypocalcaemia secondary to hyperventilation. Another uncommon manifestation is transient total blindness of cortical type due to a plaque at the termination of the basilar artery causing ischaemia in the distribution of both posterior cerebral arteries. It is important to recognise the significance of these symptoms early, since total occlusion of the artery can produce a complete hemiplegia (in carotid occlusion) or quadriplegia and death (in basilar occlusion). Doppler ultrasonography can be very helpful in demonstrating reduced blood flow through a stenosed artery, but in order to demonstrate stenosis or occlusion of the major arteries in the neck, and to slow collateral circulation, four-vessel arteriography carried out by aortic arch catheterisation is usually needed (Fig. 17.2). The intracranial arteries must also be visualised since management may have to be modified if there are intracranial as well as extracranial stenoses or occlusions. One syndrome which has been defined by this method is the so-called 'subclavian steal syndrome'. If the subclavian artery is occluded at its origin, then blood may travel in a retrograde manner down the ipsilateral vertebral artery in order to supply the arm. In such cases the radial pulse and arterial blood pressure are usually reduced in the affected arm, there is often a bruit in the root of the neck, and exercising the arm may give rise to manifestations of vertebro-basilar insufficiency due to brain stem ischaemia.

The natural history of recurrent cerebral ischaemia is variable. Some such patients do go on to suffer major episodes of infarction but in others the attacks cease spontaneously, despite complete occlusion of the affected major vessel, due to the increased efficiency of collateral arterial channels. Thus the external carotid artery can sometimes supply intracranial structures by means of retrograde flow through the ophthalmic when the internal carotid is totally occluded. When the subclavian artery is occluded at its origin or when an arterial stenosis in the neck is demonstrated, surgical thrombo-endarterectomy may abolish the ischaemic attacks and restore normal blood flow; but a totally occluded internal carotid artery can only rarely be disobliterated surgically. When a stenosis or occlusion is demonstrated in a situation which is not surgically accessible (e.g. in the carotid siphon) then there may be an indication for giving aspirin or anticoagulant drugs, particularly if the emboli responsible for the ischaemic attacks seem likely to consist of platelets and not cholesterol.

The syndromes of the cerebral arteries

Many eponymous clinical syndromes have been attributed to the occlusion of individual cerebral arteries. Of these, some occur consistently, and in a stereotyped manner, while others are rare. The fact that many cases of unquestionable cerebral infarction do not fulfil the diagnostic criteria of these classical syndromes demonstrates the variability in distribution of some of the cerebral arteries and of the anastomotic channels which exist in the meninges. In general, however, perforating arteries are true end-arteries and occlusion of these vessels can often be recognised clinically. A diagrammatic representation of the cortical distribution of blood from the major cerebral arteries is given in Figure 17.3.

Internal carotid artery thrombosis   The syndrome of transient ischaemic attacks resulting from stenosis of this vessel has already been described. When complete occlusion occurs, however, there is often a complete contralateral hemiplegia, with aphasia if the dominant

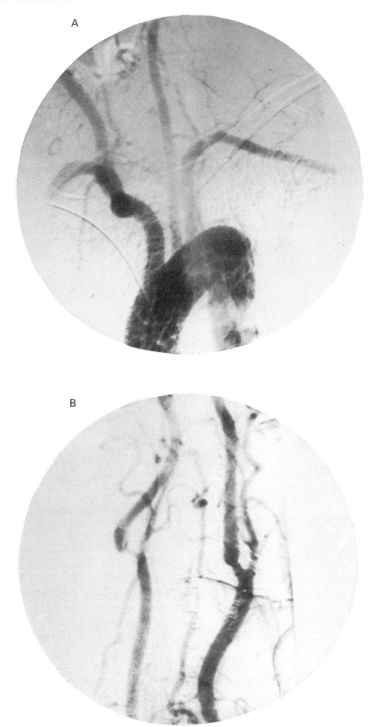

Fig. 17.2   Digital subtraction angiogram following intravenous injections of contrast medium. **A** The aortic arch and its major branches. **B** The major vessels of the neck angled to show the carotid bifurcations; there is bilateral internal carotid artery stenosis, more marked on the left side.

hemisphere is involved. Alternatively, if the collateral circulation is satisfactory, the clinical features may resemble those of middle cerebral artery occlusion, while on occasion, symptoms are transient, and disability trivial. Occlusion of this artery has replaced meningovascular syphilis as the commonest cause of hemiplegia in adults in the third and fourth decades. It may complicate pregnancy or oral contraceptive medication and can follow trauma to the neck. Rarely kinking of the vessel in the neck or fibromuscular hypoplasia of its wall appear to be contributing factors. A carotid arteritis with occlusion, sometimes due to a spread of inflammation from cervical lymph nodes, may account for some cases of acute infantile hemiplegia. Occlusion of a perforating branch of the *posterior communicating artery*, itself a branch of the internal carotid, causes infarction of the subthalamic nucleus (corpus Luysii), giving contralateral hemiballismus. Occlusion of the *anterior choroidal* branch of the internal carotid is often asymptomatic but can give contralateral hemianopia, hemiplegia and hemihypalgesia.

The middle cerebral artery   Occlusion of the main trunk of the middle cerebral artery (Fig. 17.4) gives a contralateral hemiplegia and sensory loss of cortical type. When the obstruction lies more distally, weakness involves mainly the face, arm and hand. Broca's aphasia is common, Wernicke's less so, but the latter does occur at times, and a hemianopia is occasionally seen due to infarction of the optic radiation in the temporal lobe.

The anterior cerebral artery   When the main trunk of this artery is occluded, this results in a contralateral hemiplegia with crural dominance (i.e. greater weakness of the leg than of the arm). Cortical sensory loss and aphasia are often present. When Heubner's artery, a penetrating branch which supplies the anterior limb of the internal capsule, is occluded, there is paralysis of the contralateral face and upper limb and often some sensory loss of spinothalamic type in the contralateral limbs.

The posterior cerebral artery   The principal effect of thrombosis of this artery is a contralateral homonymous hemianopia. When perforating branches to the thalamus are involved, a contralateral thalamic syndrome may develop, while lesions of the dominant visual association area occasionally cause visual agnosia.

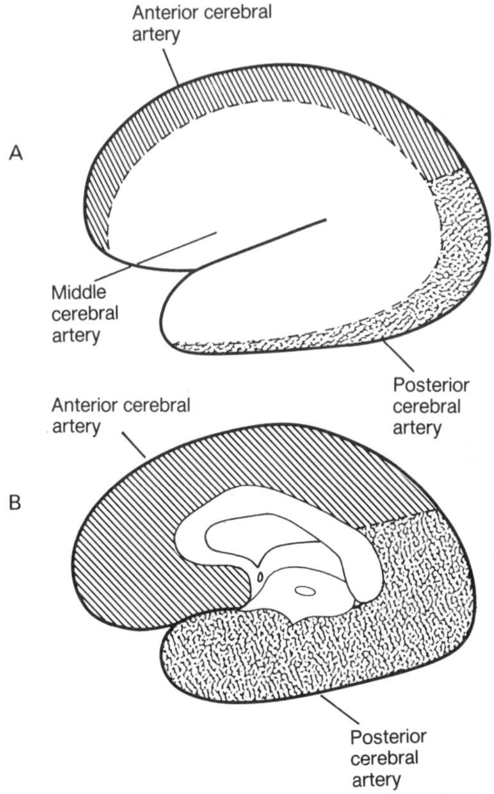

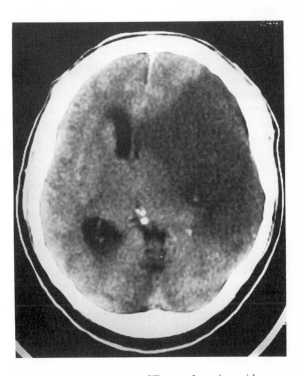

Fig. 17.3 A diagrammatic representation of the distribution of blood flow from the three major cerebral arteries to the cerebral hemispheres.

Fig. 17.4 Unenhanced axial CT scan of a patient with a large left middle cerebral artery infarct associated with swelling of the hemisphere and displacement of the lateral ventricle.

The basilar artery   Transient ischaemic attacks attributable to vertebro-basilar insufficiency were described above. Total occlusion of the basilar artery is generally soon fatal, with loss of consciousness, a decerebrate state, or quadriplegia, but a myriad of clinical syndromes can occur as a result of occlusion of its individual perforating branches. Thus Weber's syndrome consists of a unilateral third cranial nerve palsy and a contralateral hemiplegia. The Benedikt syndrome is a third-nerve palsy with ipsilateral cerebellar ataxia. A paralysis of the sixth and seventh cranial nerves on one side with a contralateral hemiplegia constitutes the Millard-Gubler syndrome, while the Foville syndrome consists of a sixth-nerve palsy, paralysis of conjugate ocular deviation to the side of the lesion, and again as a rule, a contralateral hemiparesis. Occlusion of the internal auditory artery may give sudden unilateral deafness and severe vertigo. Apart from these classical syndromes, many other clinical phenomena may be attributable to basilar artery insufficiency, including such features as cranial nerve palsies in various combinations, ipsilateral cerebellar signs, and contralateral hemiplegia or hemianalgesia.

The superior cerebellar artery   The characteristic features of superior cerebellar artery occlusion are first, ipsilateral cerebellar ataxia, often with choreiform movements; and secondly, contralateral hemianalgesia with preservation of finer sensory modalities.

The posterior inferior cerebellar artery   Occlusion of this branch of the vertebral artery gives a typical clinical picture which is one of the commonest brain-stem vascular syndromes (Wallenberg's syndrome). In fact it more often results from a thrombus in the vertebral artery itself and not in its posterior inferior cerebellar branch. The onset is usually abrupt with vertigo and vomiting, and sometimes with pain in one side of the face. There is often dysphagia at the onset and the palate is paralysed on the side of the lesion, while there are also 'cerebellar' signs in the limbs on this side. An ipsilateral Horner's syndrome is often present, and there may be dissociated anaesthesia to pain and temperature on the same side of the face and over the opposite half of the body below the neck. This sensory loss is, however, variable and a complete contralateral hemianalgesia is more common.

Although many other syndromes of the cerebral arteries have been described, these are the commonest. It is particularly important to recognise the nature of transient ischaemic attacks as these can often be treated effectively.

Prognosis

Cerebral infarction is fatal in up to 20% of cases. When the infarct is small or the causal ischaemia relatively transient, complete recovery can take place within a few days and this occurs in about 20% of patients. In the remaining 60% some degree of disability persists. For instance, up to 20% later develop focal or generalised seizures as a sequel of the illness. Indeed it seems likely that some cases of 'epilepsy of late onset' are due to pre-existing, symptomless or unrecognised, cerebral infarction. Even after a complete hemiplegia has developed, remarkable degrees of recovery may be seen and most patients are eventually able to walk after some weeks or months, although in cases of middle cerebral or carotid occlusion there is often little recovery of function in the affected hand. Aphasia, too, can recover to a surprising extent, either spontaneously or with appropriate speech training which may have to be continued in selected cases for many months. Recovery from brain-stem vascular syndromes is also virtually complete in some cases. The prognosis is particularly favourable in 'posterior inferior cerebellar artery thrombosis' in which after a few months the only residual signs may be a Horner's syndrome on one side and a contralateral hemianalgesia; occasionally persistent dysphagia is troublesome. Recurrent infarction occurs after a greater or lesser period in about half the survivors, but the remainder remain free from such episodes, often for several years.

Treatment

When a patient is comatose or semicomatose as a result of an ischaemic stroke, the normal measures necessary in managing the unconscious patient are required. There is no evidence that high-dose steroids, glycerol, low molecular weight dextran, barbiturates, antispasmodic, vasodilator or other vasoactive drugs are of any value. Most authorities now agree that anticoagulant therapy is of no value in the established stroke and of little benefit even in evolving infarction. However, long-term anticoagulant therapy has been shown to reduce the incidence of subsequent embolic strokes in patients with cardiac conditions (such as auricular fibrillation and mitral stenosis) which have caused one or more such episodes. Undoubtedly, too, anticoagulants can reduce or even abolish transient ischaemic attacks; the favoured treatment in such cases is now aspirin, 150 mg daily, and there is some evidence that the latter remedy may also be of prophylactic benefit in individuals thought to be at risk from stroke who have not suffered any such episodes. In relation to prophylaxis, the control of hypertension is fundamental and hypercholesterolaemia should be treated by dietary or other means.

Surgical methods of treatment remain controversial. Many neurologists and neurosurgeons continue to advise carotid endarterectomy in patients with transient ischaemic attacks associated with internal carotid artery stenosis in the neck but no adequately controlled trials of this treatment have yet been concluded and the procedure carries a significant morbidity. Surgical disobliteration of the occluded segment of the subclavian artery in patients with the 'subclavian steal' syndrome is, however, generally curative. However, a recent multicentre randomised controlled trial of extracranial-intracranial anastomosis (involving anastomosis of one superficial temporal artery with the trunk of the ipsilateral middle cerebral via a temporal trephine hole) failed to demonstrate any benefit in patients with intracranial arterial stenosis or occlusion in the relevant arterial territory.

Finally, the invaluable role of physiotherapy, occupational therapy and other methods of rehabilitation must be stressed. Exercise, re-education, the provision, where appropriate, of walking aids, toe-raising springs or calipers, and other appliances, adaptation to the home and domestic environment, speech therapy in the aphasic, anticonvulsant drugs in the management of post-hemiplegic epilepsy, antibiotics for the management of complications, attention to diet and vitamin intake in the confused elderly subject, and instruction of relatives and home-helps; all these and many more are invaluable. Treatment in a specialised unit and well-organised out-patient physiotherapy and occupational therapy department after discharge from hospital improves the outcome. Special attention should be paid to shoulder pain and immobility in the hemiplegic patient. The risk of deep venous thrombosis in the legs and of consequent pulmonary embolism should also be recognised. The treatment of aphasia and apraxia or agnosia may require special skills, but even in these cases, as in those who are paralysed, untrained volunteer helpers can play a valuable role. With appropriate and intensive treatment, many patients with strokes, of whatever age, can resume a useful life in society despite residual disability. Many problems may require to be resolved relating to employment, driving of motor vehicles, hostel or hospital residential care, and the like, but can only be determined in the light of the patient's progress and the doctor's experience of similar cases.

Moya-Moya disease

This rare condition, originally described in Japan, but subsequently recognised in Western countries, is one in which there is spontaneous occlusion of the major vessels of the circle of Willis so that the cerebral hemispheres are supplied with blood through a network of small vessels resembling the rete mirabile of lower mammals. The cause is unknown; the clinical manifestations include variable focal neurological deficits, convulsions and subarachnoid haemorrhage. The condition is seen especially in children and young adults, and is commoner in females.

Hypertensive encephalopathy

This term identifies a disorder of acute onset in which severe arterial hypertension is associated with headache, nausea, vomiting, confusion, convulsions and stupor or coma. Usually the condition occurs only in patients with malignant hypertension or in the terminal stages of chronic nephritis; papilloedema and advanced retinopathy are invariably present. Focal neurological symptoms and signs are not a part of this syndrome as a rule but imply the presence of complicating factors such as 'thrombosis', embolism, or haemorrhage.

Cerebral atherosclerosis

This term is used to describe the progressive degenerative disorder which results from widespread atheroma of the cerebral vasculature with consequent intermittently-progressive ischaemia of the brain. It ultimately gives an irreversible dementia (multi-infarct dementia) but the progress of the disorder is invariably step-like, and it is unwise to accept this diagnosis as a cause of dementia arising in the presenium or in the elderly unless there have been transient episodes of confusion, paraesthesiae, aphasia or paresis, to indicate that one or more 'little strokes' have occurred. In the late stages dementia is severe, the patient is doubly incontinent, but often has a voracious appetite, and may have few signs of neurological abnormality save for brisk tendon reflexes and extensor plantar responses.

A clinical picture which develops in some such cases is that of **pseudo-bulbar palsy**. This syndrome is characterised by over-emotionalism, often with pathological laughing and crying and gross lability of the affect, along with spasticity of the muscles of speech and swallowing, due to bilateral pyramidal tract lesions in the upper midbrain or cerebral hemispheres. Some dysarthria and dysphagia and pathological over-emotionalism are often seen too in the syndrome of so-called **atherosclerotic parkinsonism** in which hypertensive and atherosclerotic patients show little if any facial masking, but commonly demonstrate a shuffling gait, similar to that of paralysis agitans, and progressive rigidity of the limbs; usually, however, they also show evidence of dementia, the deep tendon reflexes are greatly exaggerated, and the plantar responses extensor. Pathologically and clinically pseudo-bulbar palsy and atherosclerotic parkinsonism are closely related.

Cerebral venous sinus thrombosis

The effects of suppurative thrombosis of intracranial venous sinuses have already been described (see p. 219). Aseptic thrombosis of the cavernous sinus is rare but this pathological process can occur, apparently spontaneously, in the lateral or sagittal sinuses, causing a syndrome closely resembling that of benign intracranial hypertension, or pseudotumour cerebri. The characteristic features are headache and papilloedema in a patient whose consciousness is often unimpaired, who may have no localising neurological signs, and is often found to have normal cerebral ventricles on CT scan or ventriculography. The condition can complicate otitis media or malignant disease, it may develop during pregnancy or after head injury, and sometimes occurs spontaneously, particularly in young and rather obese women. Cortical thrombophlebitis in childhood or in pregnancy is often different in its presentation and may give focal fits and neurological signs (e.g. hemiplegia) which can resolve unusually rapidly. However, when thrombosis of the sagittal sinus is extensive, the patient may be semicomatose and has fits and focal neurological signs (hemiparesis or paraplegia) due to venous infarction of the superior aspect of the cerebral cortex; subarachnoid haemorrhage sometimes occurs as a result. Headache is usual in the conscious patient and papilloedema usually develops due to the associated increase in intracranial pressure consequent upon impaired CSF absorption, and alternating attacks of Jacksonian epilepsy, occurring sometimes on one side, sometimes on the other, are thought to be characteristic. Anticonvulsant drugs are required in most cases because of the frequency of fits. The role of anticoagulant therapy is controversial since venous infarction is so often associated with intracerebral or subarachnoid haemorrhage, but if the CT scan shows no evidence of bleeding, some authorities recommend a short course of heparin if the diagnosis is made early, in the hope of preventing propagation of the clot (Donaldson 1989). In general terms the principle favoured is to give anticoagulants when all available evidence suggests that thrombosis is confined to the sinus, but not when there is evidence of cortical venous infarction. In acute and severe cases there is a significant mortality, but if the patient survives the first one to two weeks, recovery is often remarkably complete.

Temporal, giant-cell or cranial arteritis

This condition, which is commonest in patients over 60 years of age, is related to the other diseases of the 'collagen' or connective tissue group. Characteristically the patient suffers general malaise with vague aches and pains in the limbs and joints, fever and loss of appetite. There is also temporal headache and tenderness of the neck and scalp. The temporal and occipital arteries are nodular, tender and sometimes thrombosed. Sometimes there is little clinical evidence of disease in the temporal arteries and the presenting features are those of polymyalgia rheumatica (see p. 307). Polyneuropathy is also an uncommon but well-recognised manifestation. The most important complication is occlusion of the central retinal artery; this condition is the commonest cause of sudden unilateral blindness in the elderly. If the disease is not treated the second eye can be involved afterwards. Rarely, the carotid, cerebral and coronary arteries are affected to give cerebral or cardiac infarction. The erythrocyte sedimentation rate is invariably raised and the condition responds rapidly to steroid therapy.

Other 'collagen' or 'connective tissue' diseases

Occasionally polyarteritis nodosa and systemic lupus erythematosus produce neurological symptoms due to involvement of the small arteries of the brain or spinal cord (see p. 236). There is also a rare form of diffuse granulomatous angiitis of the cerebral vessels of unknown cause which affects young people and usually progresses to a fatal termination in about two years. Thrombotic microangiopathy (thrombotic thrombocytopenic purpura) is another rare condition in which fever, haemolytic anaemia, convulsions, confusion and variable pareses of the limbs may occur due to blockage of capillaries in the brain and elsewhere by platelet thrombi. The condition runs a fulminant course, there is thrombocytopenia and a high erythrocyte sedimentation rate, and treatment with steroid drugs is usually ineffective.

Buerger's disease

Thromboangiitis obliterans has been thought to involve the cerebral vasculature to give a clinical picture which is dominated by fits, progressive dementia and variable palsies of the limbs but most cases so diagnosed have proved to be suffering from atherosclerosis.

Pulseless disease (Takayasu's disease)

This is a condition, first described in Japan, in which non-specific arteritis of the aortic arch occurs in young people and results in slow progressive occlusion of medium-sized arteries. No limb pulses may be palpable. As the carotid and vertebral arteries are involved, symptoms and signs of progressive or repeated cerebral infarction commonly appear in such cases. True pulseless disease is rare in Great Britain and the USA, but a similar syndrome may occur in middle-aged or elderly patients due to atherosclerosis.

A

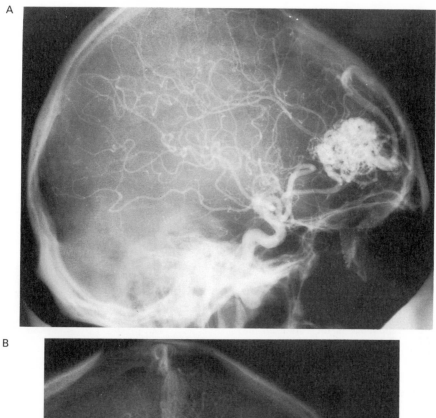

B

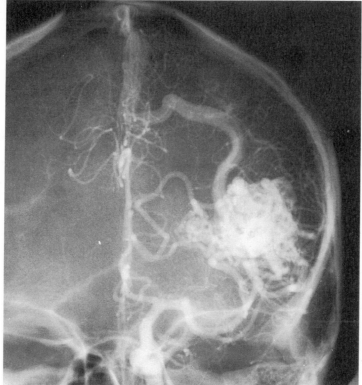

Fig. 17.5 A and **B**   Angiogram demonstrating a left frontal arteriovenous
malformation. Note the large draining vein into the superior sagittal sinus and the arterial
supply from dilated branches of the anterior and middle cerebral arteries.

Unruptured saccular aneurysms

Unruptured aneurysms of the cerebral vessels often give no symptoms, but they can simulate basally-situated space-occupying lesions if they become large enough to compress cranial-nerve trunks or other important structures. A supraclinoid aneurysm of the internal carotid artery is a common cause of an isolated third-nerve palsy, while a suprasellar aneurysm can be responsible for chiasmal compression and hence for appropriate visual-field defects. An aneurysm within the cavernous sinus may give paralysis of the third, fourth and sixth cranial nerves on the affected side, along with sensory loss in the distribution of the first and second divisions of the ipsilateral fifth nerve. If an aneurysm in this situation ruptures, pulsating exophthalmos develops and a loud bruit can be heard over the affected eye. A similar carotico-cavernous fistula rarely follows head injury in the absence of an aneurysm.

Arteriovenous angioma

Small angiomas in the substance of the cerebrum may produce no symptoms until they bleed, resulting in subarachnoid haemorrhage. Others are associated with headaches closely resembling migraine, often strictly limited to the side of the head upon which the angioma lies, while yet others give rise to focal fits and neurological signs (aphasia, hemiparesis) as they expand in size. Large angiomas (Fig. 17.5) are occasionally big enough to starve the surrounding brain of blood, resulting in dementia. A cranial bruit is often heard on the scalp overlying the intracranial lesion or over the appropriate internal carotid artery in the neck. Similar angiomas of the brain stem and posterior fossa are comparatively rare, but can be responsible for repeated episodes of brain-stem dysfunction occurring over a period of several years, resembling in some respects attacks of vertebro-basilar insufficiency and in others, repeated brain-stem episodes of multiple sclerosis. Angiomas of the spinal cord are mentioned below.

Sturge-Weber syndrome

This is a congenital malformation of precapillaries in the cerebral cortex, involving as a rule one parietal and occipital lobe and giving a characteristic radiological pattern of subcortical calcification outlining the cerebral gyri (see p. 198).

VASCULAR DISORDERS OF THE SPINAL CORD

By comparison with cerebral vascular disease, disorders of the spinal vasculature are relatively uncommon.

Spinal subarachnoid haemorrhage

This rare variety of subarachnoid haemorrhage causes sudden and severe pain in the back. This spreads into the arms and legs, depending upon which spinal roots are principally affected through being in close proximity to the bleeding point. Headache and neck stiffness often develop subsequently if the haemorrhage is sufficiently extensive and extends to the cranial subarachnoid space. There may be neurological signs of variable extent in the limbs, depending upon the aetiology of the bleeding and the amount of damage to the spinal cord and/or nerve roots which has taken place. The commonest cause is an arteriovenous angioma of the spinal cord (Fig. 17.6) but it can also be symptomatic of a cauda equina tumour, such as an ependymoma of the filum terminale or even a neurofibroma (see p. 263).

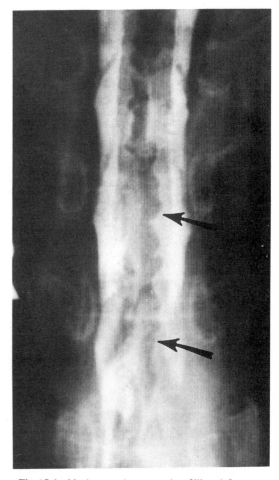

Fig. 17.6 Myelogram demonstrating filling defects due to tortuous blood vessels on the surface of the spinal cord in a patient with an arteriovenous angioma of the cord.

Intramedullary spinal haemorrhage is an extremely rare event; this spontaneous variety of haematomyelia gives a clinical picture resembling that of the traumatic condition (see p. 207). It is usually the result of bleeding from small vascular anomalies (angiomas, telangiectases) within the cord.

Anterior spinal artery thrombosis

The anterior spinal artery, formed by the fusion of branches from each vertebral artery at the level of the foramen magnum, descends in the anterior median fissure of the spinal cord and supplies, by means of its perforating branches, the greater part of the spinal cord apart from the posterior columns. The latter area receives its blood supply from two posterior spinal arteries which are also branches of the vertebral arteries and descend on the posterolateral aspect of the cord but which are smaller and less constant. Throughout the dorsal region the anterior spinal artery receives contributions from radicu-

lar arteries which are derived from the intercostals and in the lumbar region lumbar arteries also contribute. Indeed the most important artery supplying the cord below the D10 segment is the great anterior medullary artery of Adamkiewicz which arises from the lumbar aorta. Thrombosis of the anterior spinal artery gives massive infarction of the spinal cord with a complete flaccid paraplegia, retention of urine and sensory loss to pain and temperature below the level of the lesion. Only some light touch and position and joint sense may be retained. The condition is generally due to atherosclerosis and hence occurs in the elderly. When it develops in the upper cervical region there is a complete quadriplegia with respiratory paralysis, and death follows rapidly. More often the upper level of the paralysis and sensory loss is at about the D10 dermatome and in such a case occlusion of the artery of Adamkiewicz may be responsible. The latter syndrome is an important immediate complication of a dissecting aneurysm of the aorta which occludes the mouths of its branches. The paraplegia is

A
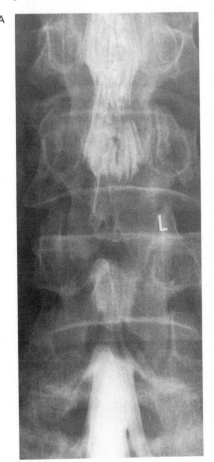

B
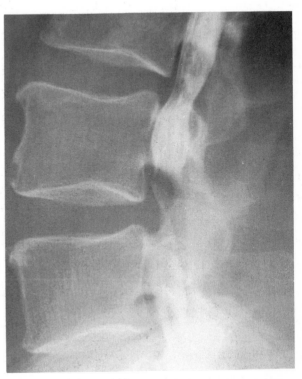

Fig. 17.7 Iohexal myelogram demonstrating lumbar canal stenosis. **A** anteroposterior; **B** lateral view.

irreversible and many patients so afflicted soon die from urinary or respiratory infection.

It has, however, become increasingly clear that a syndrome of incomplete infarction due to embolism or occlusion of radicals of the anterior spinal artery is not as uncommon as was once believed, and in such a case there is paresis rather than paralysis and partial recovery often occurs. Indeed a syndrome of combined but asymmetrical lower and upper motor neurone weakness confined to the lower limbs with variable sensory loss, in which myelography gives normal findings, is often due to an **ischaemic myelopathy**. Other patients prove to have episodes of transient spinal cord dysfunction comparable to transient cerebral ischaemic attacks, often following exertion ('intermittent claudication of the spinal cord'). Intermittent ischaemia or 'claudication' of the cauda equina is even more common. Such patients usually complain of pain or paraesthesiae in one or both legs occurring on exertion and relieved by rest but have normal peripheral pulses. Examination after exercise may demonstrate motor weakness, loss of reflexes and/or sensory loss which disappear with rest. Radiography and myelography in such cases usually demonstrate either a bony stenosis of the lumbar canal (Fig. 17.7) or a central disc protrusion, and the condition can be cured by surgical laminectomy and decompression.

Spinal venous thrombosis

A form of subacute necrotising myelopathy, giving a slowly ascending paraplegia, has been attributed to widespread thrombosis of vertebral veins, but is rare. It is particularly liable to occur in patients with chronic cor pulmonale, and myelography may demonstrate dilated veins on the surface of the cord. Some authors believe that this syndrome is due to a venous angioma rather than to venous thrombosis.

REFERENCES

Adams R D, Victor M 1985 Principles of neurology, 3rd edn. McGraw-Hill, New York
Barnett H J M, Stein B M, Mohr J P, Yatsu F M 1986 Stroke: pathophysiology, diagnosis and management. Churchill Livingstone, Edinburgh
Caplan L 1988 Intracerebral hemorrhage revisited. Neurology 38: 624
Donaldson J 0 1989 Neurology of pregnancy, 2nd edn. Major problems in neurology, Vol 18 (Walton J, series ed). Saunders, London
Hughes J T 1978 Pathology of the spinal cord, 2nd edn. Lloyd-Luke, London
Hutchinson E C, Acheson J 1975 Strokes: natural history, pathology and surgical treatment. Major problems in neurology, Vol 4 (Walton J, series ed). Saunders, London
Marshall J 1976 The management of cerebrovascular disease, 3rd edn. Churchill, London
Moseley, I 1988 Magnetic resonance imaging in diseases of the nervous system. Blackwell, Oxford
Rosenberg R N, Grossman R G, Schochet S S, Heinz E R, Willis W D Jr 1984 The clinical neurosciences. Churchill Livingstone, New York
Toole J F 1984 Cerebrovascular disorders, 3rd edn. McGraw-Hill, New York
Walton J N 1956 Subarachnoid haemorrhage. Livingstone, Edinburgh

18. Disorders of the lower motor neurone and voluntary muscles

The so-called neuromuscular disorders embrace a large and important group of diseases and symptom-complexes. They are characterised by weakness and/or wasting of the voluntary muscles, due to disordered function of the lower motor neurones or of the muscles themselves. Many of these conditions are chronic, progressive, and relatively uninfluenced by treatment, but others, which are superficially similar, can be treated effectively. Hence differential diagnosis between these disease entities is very important, and apart from the clinical criteria which are of value and which will be outlined below, certain special investigations, including techniques of electrodiagnosis and muscle biopsy (see pp. 36 and 27) have an important place. The first step in diagnosis must be to identify the site of the pathological change; the lesion may lie in the motor nuclei of the cranial nerves, in the anterior horn cells of the spinal cord, in the spinal roots or nerves; in the peripheral nerves or plexuses, in the neuromuscular junction, or in the skeletal muscles themselves. The co-existence of abnormalities of sensation can be of considerable assistance in precise identification. Next it is necessary to determine if possible the nature and aetiology of the pathological process. Unfortunately there are still many such diseases whose aetiology and pathogenesis remain obscure. Several of those of known cause have been considered in previous chapters. Thus muscular weakness and/or atrophy is a striking feature of many cases of acute anterior poliomyelitis, of postinfective polyradiculitis, and of 'collagen' disease affecting the peripheral nerves (see pp. 223, 235 and 294). Involvement of the anterior horn cells of the spinal cord, with resulting muscular atrophy, is often found, for example, in syringomyelia, and amyotrophy due to lesions in the cord or peripheral nerves occurs in some of the hereditary ataxias (see p. 188). Furthermore, intra- and extra-medullary spinal neoplasms (see p. 262) or traumatic disorders of the spinal cord, roots, plexuses or peripheral nerves (see pp. 209–213) may have a similar effect. This chapter will consider those common conditions not previously mentioned.

THE MOTOR NEURONE DISEASES AND SPINAL MUSCULAR ATROPHIES

Four principal conditions can provisionally be classified in this group. The first is a progressive genetically-determined disorder of the anterior horn cells, occurring either in infancy, childhood or adolescence, or in adult life. The second is adult motor neurone (or motor system) disease, the third the neuronal sub-variety of peroneal muscular atrophy and the fourth is scapuloperoneal muscular atrophy.

Progressive spinal muscular atrophy (SMA)

The most severe form of this condition (**Werdnig-Hoffman disease**, also known as acute infantile spinal muscular atrophy or SMA type I), which typically begins in the first six months of life, but can also be present at birth, affects babies of either sex. It is inherited as an autosomal recessive trait, so that it often affects more than one member of a sibship. Indeed the number of affected children in any one family often seems to exceed the expected one in four incidence. Usually the parents observe that the child is not moving his limbs normally, that he is unable to hold up his head or to sit, that he is generally limp and 'floppy' and when picked up he tends to slip through the hands. Gradually muscular weakness and generalised hypotonia increase, affecting first the muscles around the shoulder girdle and pelvis and later those of the chest wall, so that there is a characteristic indrawing of the lower ribs at the diaphragmatic attachment on inspiration. The infant, who is at first sight healthy and well-nourished, is seen to lie in a typical posture with the arms abducted on either side of the head, and with the legs abducted and externally rotated at the hips. Later there is weakness of the muscles of deglutition, and fasciculation in the tongue is seen. Most affected children die from respiratory infection before the end of the first or second year of life. Unfortunately there is no specific treatment.

In some other patients and families also demonstrating autosomal recessive inheritance, the condition presents with muscular weakness and hypotonia resembling that seen in Werdnig-Hoffmann disease in the second six months of life or in the second year. The paralysis is less severe than in the acute variety and often the disease process appears to arrest leaving the child severely crippled by muscular weakness, contractures and secondary skeletal deformity. These children, who may never be able to walk or even sit unsupported, often survive into the second or third decade; in them orthopaedic measures and appliances designed to reduce contractures and deformity are particularly important and must be started early. Some authorities regard this as a separate sub-variety of SMA (SMA type II) and classify it separately from juvenile SMA (SMA type III), while others suggest that this condition represents only the most severe end of a spectrum of varying severity in the subacute or chronic variety of SMA which may begin in childhood or adolescence. The latter view is based upon the observation of severe late infantile and benign juvenile cases within the same sibship. In the juvenile cases weakness may first appear in the proximal limb muscles later in the first decade or even in the second or third, when the picture is easily mistaken for that of muscular dystrophy (these are cases of 'pseudo-myopathic' spinal muscular atrophy, the so-called **Kugelberg-Welander syndrome**). In such cases the weakness involves proximal muscles of the lower and upper limbs giving postural changes, a waddling gait, and other features like those of muscular dystrophy. However, some muscles (e.g. deltoid) which are often spared in the early stages of a dystrophic process are commonly involved early and fasciculation may be seen in the tongue or elsewhere. Many such cases have undoubtedly been regarded in the past as examples of muscular dystrophy and the true diagnosis has only become apparent when modern methods of investigation (e.g. electromyography and muscle biopsy) have been employed. The distinction is not academic, as benign spinal muscular atrophy of childhood, adolescence, and early adult life can arrest temporarily, rarely permanently, or seems to run a more benign course than does muscular dystrophy, and the patients can sometimes be improved by vigorous physiotherapy. It is now evident that many patients thought to have developed limb-girdle muscular dystrophy in later adult life are in fact suffering from a similar autosomal recessive benign spinal muscular atrophy. In such cases diagnosis from motor neurone

disease (see below) rests upon the family history, the absence of signs of upper motor neurone dysfunction, the relative symmetry of the muscular weakness and wasting and its onset usually in proximal rather than distal limb muscles.

Motor neurone disease (MND)

This is a disease of adult life which usually begins after the age of 40, though it appears occasionally in younger individuals. In Britain, the USA and most Western countries it is usually sporadic, occurring equally in the two sexes. Its prevalence has been variably reported to be between 2.5 and 7 per 100 000 of the population. However, a rare form of the disease which is inherited by an autosomal dominant mechanism has been described, but in such families the condition is often clinically atypical and it may run an unusually benign course. In the Chamorro people on the island of Guam and in other parts of the Western Pacific, a severe form of the disease is very common and is often associated with features of parkinsonism and dementia (the parkinsonism-dementia complex) in affected individuals. This condition is not clearly inherited by a simple Mendelian mechanism though a genetic predisposition is still postulated. There is general agreement that an environmental factor is important but its exact nature is still a matter of dispute. A toxic substance present in the cycad nut is the most popular candidate.

The pathogenesis of the sporadic condition is obscure; cases of progressive muscular atrophy with muscular wasting progressing in a previously wasted limb or limbs have been described as developing many years after an attack of paralytic poliomyelitis and occasionally after encephalitis lethargica, while trauma has been implicated as a precipitating factor in isolated instances, but the significance of these observations remains doubtful. A 'slow virus' infection has been postulated but all attempts to isolate a virus from such cases have been unsuccessful so that the progressive degenerative changes which occur in the motor nuclei of the cranial nerves, in the anterior horn cells of the spinal cord, and in the pyramidal tracts remain unexplained. Even though minor pathological changes have been discovered in sensory pathways in certain cases, it is a diagnostic axiom that clinically-recognisable sensory disturbances are absent. Although they merge with one another, three distinctive clinical syndromes, namely progressive bulbar palsy, amyotrophic lateral sclerosis (ALS) and progressive muscular atrophy, have been described as typifying the variable clinical presentation of the disease. Some confusion has resulted from the fact that in the United Kingdom ALS is used to identify one clinical sub-variety of the disease, MND to embrace all three different types of clinical presentation, while in the USA, ALS is used as the generic term identifying the entire spectrum. In progressive bulbar palsy the motor cranial nerve nuclei are predominantly affected, in amyotrophic lateral sclerosis the pyramidal tracts, and in progressive muscular atrophy the anterior horn cells of the cord, but in almost all cases there is eventually evidence of lesions in all three sites.

Progressive bulbar palsy

The first symptom of this condition is often dysphagia, and dysarthria soon follows, though difficulty in speaking may come first. Indeed isolated dysarthria of gradual onset in the absence of other symptoms and signs should always suggest the diagnosis when appearing in middle or late life. Food, particularly solid particles, sticks in the back of the throat, choking is frequent and later there is often regurgitation of fluid down the nose owing to palatal paralysis; the voice, as well as being slurred, acquires a nasal quality. On examination there is paresis of palatal, pharyngeal and tongue muscles; atrophy and profuse fasciculation of the tongue are evident (Fig. 18.1), and the jaw jerk is exaggerated. Fasciculation is also observed as a rule in shoulder girdle muscles and there are usually signs of pyramidal tract dysfunction in the limbs. Often features of pseudo-bulbar palsy (see p. 277) due to bilateral pyramidal tract involvement accompany those of true bulbar palsy due to lower motor neurone lesions. The disease is progressive, leading to complete bulbar paralysis with the serious nursing problems which this entails, along with weakness and spasticity of the limbs. Tracheostomy and tube-feeding may ultimately be necessary. Most patients die from respiratory infection within one or two years.

Amyotrophic lateral sclerosis

The usual presenting symptom in this disorder is difficulty in walking due to stiffness of the legs, or else dragging of one leg with subsequent involvement of the other. Physical examination reveals a spastic quadriparesis with strikingly increased tendon reflexes in all four limbs and extensor plantar responses. There is no abnormality of sensation and the abdominal reflexes are often retained until late in the course. In the early stages there are few indications of lower motor neurone dysfunction but there is generally some fasciculation in the shoulder girdle and thigh muscles and subsequently muscular atrophy appears. However, the clinical picture is sometimes one of bilateral pyramidal tract disease for

some years before signs of lower motor neurone lesions develop. Symptoms and signs of bulbar paralysis appear late; in these cases it is spasticity and weakness due to the upper motor neurone lesions which are the principal cause of disability. Nevertheless weakness of the bulbar muscles ultimately causes death in most cases, often in two to five years from the onset.

Progressive muscular atrophy

In this, the most benign presentation of motor neurone disease, the first symptom is usually weakness of muscles in one hand or forearm; less commonly leg muscles are first affected, when a progressive foot drop is the usual manifestation. The weakness progresses insidiously; at first the only symptom may be clumsiness of fine movements of the fingers (inability to fasten buttons, to sew or to write) but subsequently the grip is affected or wrist drop develops, and the weakness spreads up the

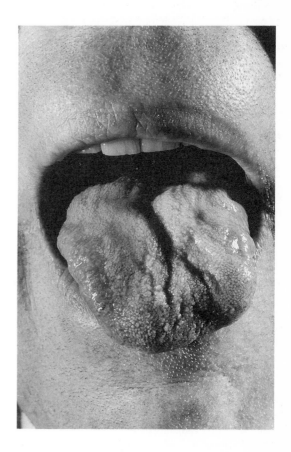

Fig. 18.1 Atrophy of the tongue in motor neurone disease. (Reproduced with permission from Spillane & Spillane 1982.)

arm. In the early stages, fasciculation is often scanty, but later it becomes prominent. There may be considerable difficulty in distinguishing the early manifestations of this disease from those due to cervical root, peripheral nerve or plexus lesions, but subsequently it becomes clear that the distribution of muscular weakness and wasting (Fig. 18.2) is more extensive than could be accounted for by involvement of a single peripheral nerve or of one or two motor roots. Eventually there is extensive involvement of the muscles of the limbs and trunk, but the signs are usually asymmetrical at first. Because of extensive muscular atrophy, the tendon reflexes subserved by the affected muscles are commonly lost, and evidence of pyramidal tract involvement is often lacking for some time, but in the end the plantar responses usually become extensor and bulbar palsy eventually develops in most cases. The absence of sensory loss generally serves to distinguish this condition from peripheral neuropathy, but when fasciculation is scanty, diagnosis from a predominantly motor polyneuropathy can be difficult if not impossible. Electromyography typically shows evidence of denervation, often with 'giant' motor units due to re-innervation of previously denervated muscle fibres by sprouts from surviving neurones. Muscle action potentials produced by peripheral nerve stimulation are often reduced in amplitude due to loss of functioning motor units, but motor and sensory conduction velocities are usually normal until late in the course of the disease. The natural history of this condition is variable; the average duration of the illness before it ends fatally, again as a rule from respiratory infection, is between 18 months and five years, but in some proven cases in which weakness and wasting has been confined to the extremities for many years the total duration has been as long as 10 or 20 years or even longer.

Treatment

Although research into this condition is moving apace, no form of drug treatment has yet been shown to be consistently successful in modifying its course. Pyridostigmine benefits swallowing temporarily in some cases, as may cricopharyngeal sphincterotomy, and diazepam or baclofen are sometimes helpful in reducing spasticity. Regular moderate exercise is useful in the early stages in maintaining morale, though intensive physiotherapy in such a progressive disease is commonly frustrating for both patient and therapist. Calipers, toe-springs, 'lively' splints and other appliances are useful at different stages in many cases and most patients eventually require wheelchairs. Some develop diaphragmatic weakness with consequential respiratory insufficiency and are greatly helped by portable respiratory support devices or even

continuous assisted ventilation, though this is only justified, as a rule, in order to prolong useful life, to reduce disability and to improve the quality of life when mobility is reasonably preserved. As swallowing difficulty increases, tracheostomy with a cuffed tube and tube-feeding (or even in the end gastrostomy) may be needed to avoid inhalation of secretions and to maintain nutrition. Antibiotics are commonly needed to treat intercurrent infection but most patients ultimately die from combined respiratory failure and infection. This is one of the most tragic diseases which any doctor is called upon to manage and in the end, when home nursing no longer proves feasible, this is one of the commonest disorders, other than terminal cancer, requiring hospice care.

Peroneal muscular atrophy (Charcot-Marie-Tooth disease)

This clinical syndrome was described in Chapter 12. The condition, which embraces the so-called Roussy-Levy syndrome, is now more often called hereditary motor and sensory neuropathy (HMSN), type I being the hypertrophic demyelinating form which is the commonest and usually the most benign with total restriction of weakness to distal limb muscles. The axonal variety (type II) is much less common and it, like the neuronal (distal spinal muscular atrophy) type, ultimately spreads to involve proximal muscles. The first symptoms are usually those of unilateral or bilateral foot drop. Subsequently the calf muscles are involved so that there is severe weakness of dorsiflexion, plantar-flexion, inversion and eversion of the feet and there is a striking atrophy of all muscles below the knee. The picture of an 'inverted champagne bottle' limb, with bilateral pes cavus, in which the thin legs contrast strikingly with the normal thighs, is characteristic. In most cases the intrinsic muscles of the hands are also affected to give a bilateral 'claw hand', but the muscular involvement does not often spread to involve the upper arms. Except in the neuronal type there is often loss of vibration sense in the lower limbs, but impairment of cutaneous sensibility is uncommon.

Scapuloperoneal muscular atrophy

This rare disorder, of dominant inheritance, is usually due to anterior horn cell disease. However, an X-linked myopathic variety, scapuloperoneal muscular dystrophy (the Emery-Dreifuss type) also occurs. In the legs the changes resemble those of peroneal muscular atrophy, while in the upper limbs there is winging of the scapulae. Both the neuronal and myopathic varieties are much more benign than progressive muscular atrophy, with which they are often confused.

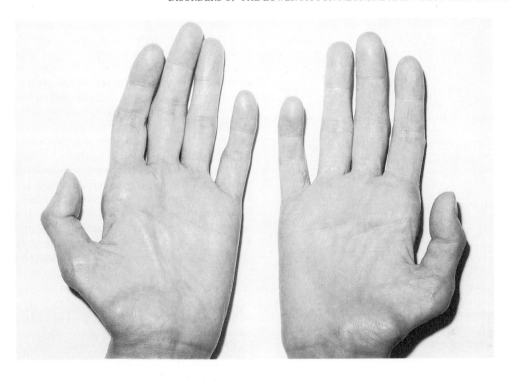

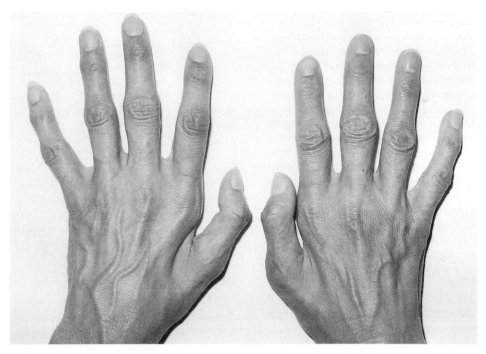

Fig. 18.2   Severe bilateral wasting of all the small hand muscles in a case of progressive muscular atrophy.

LESIONS OF MOTOR CRANIAL NERVES, OF SPINAL ROOTS AND OF PERIPHERAL NERVES

Many disorders which could be considered under this heading have already been described. Thus dysfunction of the nerves to the extrinsic ocular muscles was discussed in Chapter 8 (pp. 115–117). Infective and allergic conditions involving spinal roots were described in Chapter 14 (pp. 234–236), while trauma to roots, plexuses and peripheral nerves was considered in Chapter 13 (pp. 209–213). There remain to be considered some abnormalities of the facial nerve which were not considered in detail in Chapter 9, the clinical effects of intervertebral disc prolapse, of cervical spondylosis, and the differential diagnosis of disorders causing pain in the arm or wasting of the small hand muscles.

Facial paralysis

A lower motor neurone lesion of the facial nerve can be distinguished from an upper motor neurone type of facial palsy by the fact that in the former all the facial muscles on one side are equally affected, while in the latter the weakness involves principally the muscles of the lower face, and movement of those around the eye is comparatively unimpaired. A complete unilateral facial palsy can be due to a nuclear lesion, as in poliomyelitis, multiple sclerosis, pontine infarction or tumour, or rarely, motor neurone disease. It can also result from lesions of the nerve trunk in its intracranial course, when it is involved in cranial polyneuropathy, constricted by granulomatous inflammation in the subarachnoid space (meningitis, sarcoidosis, meningovascular syphilis), compressed by a tumour (e.g. acoustic neuroma) or aneurysm or infiltrated by a reticulosis or carcinomatosis of the meninges. The commonest conditions giving facial palsy due to damage to the nerve in its course through the temporal bone are otitis media and herpes zoster of the geniculate ganglion (the Ramsay Hunt syndrome). In its extracranial course the nerve may be damaged by disease of the parotid glands; bilateral facial palsy is a rare presenting feature of acute leukaemia or sarcoidosis.

The commonest variety of unilateral facial palsy is, however, **Bell's palsy** which can occur at any age and in either sex and is of unknown aetiology, although a swelling of the nerve in the narrow bony canal above the stylomastoid foramen has been postulated as its cause. It may follow exposure to cold or a draught but often arises without apparent precipitating cause. Viral and auto-immune causes have been proposed but remain unconfirmed. Often the patient awakens to find that he is unable to close the eye on the affected side, that the

furrows on this side of the forehead are lost, and that the mouth is drawn over to the sound side (Fig. 18.3). Occasionally there is hyperacusis in the ipsilateral ear due to involvement of the nerve to the stapedius. In some cases the paralysis is incomplete; when this is so, if there is no progression over the course of the first two or three days, complete recovery generally occurs within one to two weeks. More often the paralysis remains complete for two or three weeks and then begins to recover; and recovery then is complete as a rule within two or three months. In a comparatively small number of cases there is actual division of certain nerve fibres (neuronotmesis) and regeneration is necessary. In such a case recovery may take several months and even then is generally incomplete, as some of the regenerating nerve fibres go astray. Commonly in such a case a degree of permanent facial contracture develops, a factor which improves the appearance of the face while at rest, though paralysis is

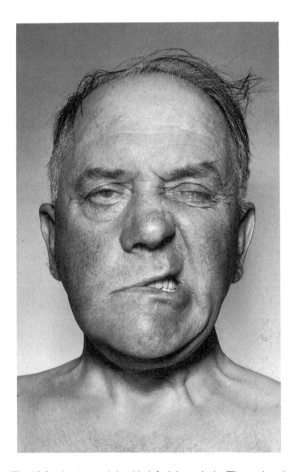

Fig. 18.3 An acute right-sided facial paralysis. The patient is trying to close his eyes and show his teeth. (Reproduced with permission from Spillane & Spillane 1982.)

still evident on movement (e.g. smiling). Occasionally, too, clonic facial spasm (see below) is a sequel. Another rare complication is involuntary lacrimation during eating (the syndrome of 'crocodile tears') due to the fact that regenerating autonomic fibres intended for the salivary glands reach the lacrimal glands instead. During the acute stage, it may be necessary to protect the cornea of the eye which cannot be closed. The cosmetic appearance can be improved by elevating the tissues of the affected side of the face with strips of transparent adhesive tape (e.g. Sellotape®). Treatment with steroid drugs or ACTH has been advocated but is only of value if given immediately after the onset, and surgical decompression of the facial canal is usually performed too late to help, as it is only done when it is evident that spontaneous recovery is not taking place. Unfortunately, electromyography gives relatively little information of prognostic value until about three weeks after the onset. However, if electrical conduction in the facial nerve can be demonstrated one week after the onset of paralysis this is a good prognostic sign. Electrical stimulation of the paralysed muscles has often been used but is of dubious value and may increase contracture. In long-standing facial paralysis, cosmetic plastic surgery has a limited but definite place. Some patients suffer repeated attacks of Bell's palsy, now on one side of the face and now on the other, but this is relatively uncommon. Recurrent familial facial palsy associated with congenital fissuring of the tongue is called Melkersson's syndrome.

Hemifacial spasm

This condition, also called clonic facial spasm, is commonest in middle-aged or elderly women. It gives intermittent fine twitching in one orbicularis oculi which later spreads to involve the remaining facial muscles on the same side. The spasms can eventually be quite powerful, and rapidly though irregularly repetitive. In the early stages it may resemble a tic and is certainly accentuated by emotional stress, but tics are usually bilateral so that the strictly unilateral movements of hemifacial spasm are diagnostic. The condition differs from the slow rippling movements of facial myokymia which may be a rare manifestation of multiple sclerosis. The EMG is often helpful in demonstrating 'grouped' motor unit discharges (each consisting of two or three motor unit action potentials) which repeat rhythmically. Eventually in some cases and after many years progressive facial paralysis may develop on the affected side and the movements cease. The condition is embarrassing and inconvenient and little influenced by drugs although diazepam has been thought to damp down the movements. The condition was formerly thought to be due to a benign irritative lesion of unknown aetiology involving the trunk of the nerve in its long canal and, in consequence, surgical decompression of the nerve was widely advocated and practised. Others recommended alcohol or phenol injection of the nerve trunk or operative partial division of the nerve, but these methods reduced the movements at the expense of causing a partial facial paralysis. Recent work has shown that by far the commonest cause is intracranial kinking or compression of the trunk of the nerve by an aberrant intracranial artery; operative decompression in the posterior fossa has proved curative in many cases.

Prolapsed intervertebral disc

The intervertebral disc consists of an outer fibrocartilaginous ring, the annulus fibrosus, and a central semifluid portion, the nucleus pulposus. As a result of a degenerative process of unknown aetiology, the annulus fibrosus may be breached, allowing the nucleus pulposus to herniate through the gap so formed. If this gap lies posteriorly in the annulus, as is usual, the prolapsed disc may encroach either upon the spinal canal (a central protrusion) or upon an intervertebral foramen (a lateral protrusion). An acute lateral prolapse of a cervical disc will usually compress a spinal root or nerve, giving the clinical syndrome of brachial neuralgia, while a similar lateral protrusion of a lumbar disc is the commonest cause of sciatica. An acute central protrusion in the cervical region causes sudden compression of the cervical cord, with symptoms and signs of partial, or even complete, paraplegia or quadriplegia depending upon the size of the protrusion and the level of the lesion, while in the lumbar region a similar acute prolapse may give a cauda equina syndrome of acute onset. Dorsal disc protrusions are comparatively rare, but when they do occur (Fig. 18.4), the spinal canal is so narrow in this situation that there is generally evidence of spinal cord compression.

The clinical syndromes resulting from disc prolapse can occur in either sex, but are more common in men; they are most often observed in middle and late life, as increasing age contributes to disc degeneration, but may occur in early adult life. Trauma plays an important role, as symptoms may develop first after sudden exertion (a twisting movement, hyperextension of the neck, straining to lift a heavy object). Almost certainly such traumatic incidents do no more than to precipitate prolapse of a degenerating disc which would eventually have ruptured spontaneously.

The first symptom is generally pain in the neck or back, with tenderness over the spinous processes of the affected vertebrae and with pain and tenderness in the spinal muscles (owing to protective spasm). This is why the first symptoms of an acute intervertebral disc prolapse are commonly attributed to 'stiff neck', 'fibrositis' or 'lumbago'. Movements of the affected area of the spine may be intensely painful. When the protrusion is central, weakness and paraesthesiae in the lower limbs and retention of urine are often seen immediately. If the lesion is cervical there will be signs of a symmetrical paraparesis, while if it is lumbar, there are usually lower motor neurone and sensory signs in the lower limbs indicating involvement of multiple roots of the cauda equina. In a laterally-situated prolapse in the cervical region, pain of an intense burning character spreads over the shoulder and down the arm, along the dermatome innervated by the affected root. In the lumbar region the pain travels down the back of the thigh and leg and often into the foot, although occasionally in a case of high lumbar disc protrusion it radiates down the front of the thigh. Typically the pain is made worse by movement, and by coughing or by straining, which temporarily increase the pressure in the spinal canal. Often, too, it is worse when the patient is warm in bed at night. Peripheral nerves (e.g. the sciatic) which receive contributions from the affected root, are tender and painful when stretched. When the lesion is cervical, lateral flexion of the head towards the side of the prolapse is painful (Spurling's sign) while in sciatica, straight-leg

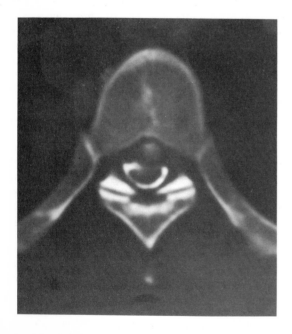

Fig. 18.4 Calcified prolapsed cervical disc. Iohexal in the subarachnoid space outlines the spinal cord which is indented by the disc anteriorly.

raising on the affected side is restricted and painful (Laségue's sign).

Compression of a motor root by the prolapsed disc often produces in due course muscular weakness, fasciculation, atrophy and reflex changes, depending upon which root is involved; affection of the sensory root gives subjective numbness and paraesthesiae and objective sensory loss in the appropriate dermatome. In the cervical region, the commonest levels of disc prolapse are at C5-6, in which case the fifth cervical root is involved, and at C6-7, giving compression of the C6 root. In either case, the deltoid, biceps and brachioradialis muscles may be weak or atrophic and the biceps and radial jerks are commonly depressed. In the lumbar region the sites of election are L4-5 (L5 root) and L5-S1 (S1 root). In either event a partial foot drop may result, but when the disc protrudes at the higher level the pain usually radiates down into the dorsum of the foot and the reflexes are intact, while compression of the S1 root gives pain along the outer border and sole of the foot and an absent ankle jerk. In a case of acute disc prolapse, spinal radiographs are often normal, but sometimes the affected disc space is narrowed. A moderate rise in the CSF protein (up to 1.0 g/l, or more if there is a complete block) is not uncommon.

Commonly with rest and analgesics alone the symptoms of an acute disc prolapse resolve within a few days or weeks, but exertion may cause a recurrence of symptoms, often after months or years. When bed rest fails, immobilisation in plaster or in a plastic cervical collar or lumbar support may· be needed; alternatively, either intermittent or continuous spinal traction may be tried. Manipulation has many advocates, and is occasionally very successful, though in the cervical region particularly, it carries some risk of damage to the spinal cord. Myelography (which is less successful in demonstrating lateral rather than central protrusions) followed by surgical decompression of the spinal cord, affected root(s) or spinal nerve(s) and removal of the prolapsed fragment of nucleus pulposus, are usually indicated if there is evidence of severe muscular weakness, extensive sensory loss or impairment of sphincter control, or in cases of prolapsed lumbar disc in which all other measures have failed to relieve pain.

Cervical spondylosis

This term is utilised to describe the chronic changes which occur in the cervical spine as a result of long-standing multiple or single intervertebral disc lesions, and which can cause a variety of symptoms and physical signs due to compression of cervical nerve roots and of the spinal cord (cervical myelopathy). This name should not be given to the syndrome of acute cervical disc prolapse, either central or lateral. When part of an intervertebral disc has been prolapsed for some time the protruding portion becomes at first fibrotic but later is calcified and bony-hard. A firm bar of tissue is thus created along the posterior aspect of the disc (and often on its anterior aspect as well); this is usually associated with overgrowth of the margins of the contiguous vertebrae to give bony spurs or osteophytes (so-called lipping) (Fig. 18.5). Commonly these bars and lips also encroach upon the intervertebral foramina, and this encroachment is shown in oblique radiographs of the spine. These changes are usually observed at several levels. The resulting changes in spinal radiographs are often referred to as indicating 'osteoarthritis'. Such appearances are found in many manual workers and in fewer sedentary workers after middle-age; some have no neurological symptoms and signs. Hence, it follows that these radiological changes are often found coincidentally in patients with other neurological diseases, including

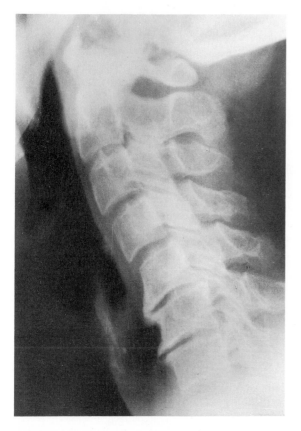

Fig. 18.5 Lateral radiograph of cervical spine demonstrating cervical spondylosis with severe narrowing of the C5–6 and C6–7 disc spaces and anterior and posterior 'lipping'.

multiple sclerosis, syringomyelia, motor neurone disease, and even spinal tumour; therefore it is unwise to assume that spondylosis necessarily accounts for the patient's symptoms even though this may ultimately prove to be the case.

The syndrome of **cervical myelopathy** resulting from spondylosis is a disorder of middle- and late-life and is much commoner in men than in women. There may have been symptoms in the past (episodes of stiff neck, or 'neuritis' in the arms) to indicate previous acute incidents of disc prolapse, while even in the chronic stage the patient sometimes complains of intermittent pain or stiffness in the neck, or of pain down one or both arms. Variable degrees of wasting and weakness of upper limb muscles, sometimes with fasciculation, may be observed on one or both sides, but these changes are not invariable and often unobtrusive; most symptoms are referable to the lower limbs. The muscles usually involved in the arms are the spinati, deltoid, biceps and triceps, as the roots which are most often compressed are those of the C5, 6 and 7 segments; involvement of intrinsic hand muscles is very rare but can result from ischaemia of anterior horn cells due to cord compression above the D1 segment. A common and valuable sign is inversion of the biceps or radial reflexes. The biceps jerk is said to be inverted if tapping the biceps tendon produces contraction of the triceps; while the radial jerk is inverted if a tap on the brachioradialis tendon produces no contraction of this muscle, but finger flexion. These signs, if present, imply that there is a lesion of the C5 or C6 segment of the cord, breaking the reflex arc for reflexes which utilise these cord segments, but at the same time compressing the pyramidal tract to give exaggeration of those reflexes whose pathways pass through lower segments. The usual symptoms and signs in the lower limbs are those of progressive spastic paraparesis, which is often, but not always, asymmetrical at first.

This syndrome is probably the commonest cause of a spastic paraparesis developing in late middle-life. Usually the patient describes a gradual onset with dragging and stiffness of one leg or with some aching pain in the limb after walking any distance. Paraesthesiae are relatively uncommon, but very occasionally 'electric shocks' in the trunk and legs on flexion of the neck (Lhermitte's sign) are experienced; this symptom is, however, much more common in multiple sclerosis. On examination there are signs of a spastic paraparesis with exaggerated tendon reflexes and extensor plantar responses. Absence of vibration sense in the lower limbs is common, due to posterior column involvement, but sensory loss of spinothalamic type is seen less often. In other words, the syndrome can mimic cervical cord compression due to a tumour or a focal cord lesion resulting from any cause.

The symptoms are usually slowly progressive, but less rapidly than in a case of cord tumour, while the absence of remissions is helpful in distinguishing the condition from multiple sclerosis. Prolonged clinical arrest is, however, seen in some patients. Diagnosis in the end depends upon myelography, which reveals in such cases one or, more often, several indentations of the column of contrast medium opposite the affected disc spaces. The cord is often compressed between the disc protrusion anteriorly and an infolded ligamentum subflavum posteriorly (Fig. 18.6). An ever-present danger in cases of this type is complete quadriplegia due to cervical cord contusion, which, as a result of narrowing of the cervical canal, may follow a relatively mild hyperextension injury of the neck. In the average case, although disability slowly increases, the patient is not totally disabled and

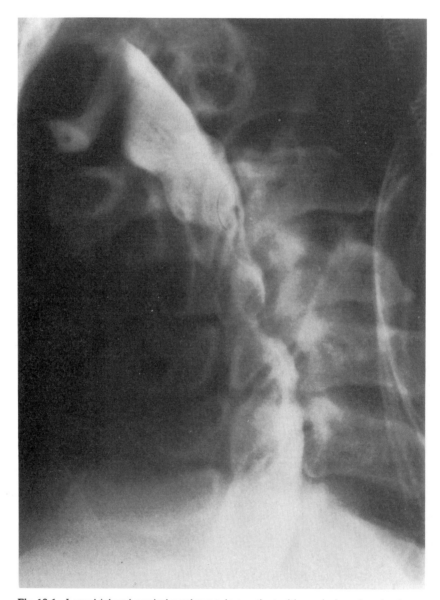

Fig. 18.6 Lateral iohexal cervical myelogram in a patient with cervical myelopathy due to spondylosis showing anterior indentation of the theca by osteophytes and chronic disc protrusions at C3–4, C4–5 and C5–6 with maximum cord compression at C4–5. Note the posterior indentations produced at the same levels by the ligamentum subflavum with further consequential narrowing of the spinal canal (the neck is extended).

often the symptoms of cord compression seem after a time to become no worse. Although often used, a cervical collar is of little value except in relieving pain.

The purpose of surgical intervention for cervical spondylosis is to prevent further deterioration and patients should be warned that they may be no better after an operation; indeed any improvement may be considered a bonus though this does, of course, often occur. It is therefore necessary to ensure that the patient is deteriorating before considering an operation since many of these patients may remain stable for many years. If the patient is deteriorating rapidly, then operative intervention should not be delayed. If the compression is at one or two levels, then the preferred procedure is an anterior approach with removal of the disc and fusion of the vertebrae (the Cloward operation). Instability of the cervical spine with subluxation is also treated by interbody fusion. A posterior decompression by laminectomy may be more appropriate for patients with a narrow canal over several segments and hypertrophy of the ligamentum subflavum.

The causes of pain in the arm

It is convenient at this point to mention briefly some important causes of the syndrome of brachial neuralgia or pain in the arm. The anatomical situation of the cause of the pain must first be considered; the conditions mentioned have all been discussed previously. Among the spinal disorders which may cause pain of root distribution in the upper limb are poliomyelitis, syringomyelia, multiple sclerosis and intramedullary tumour (intramedullary lesions); shoulder girdle neuritis (neuralgic amyotrophy), arachnoiditis and extramedullary tumours (extramedullary lesions); acute cervical disc prolapse, cervical spondylosis, and neoplasia in a vertebral body (lesions of the spinal column). Outside the spinal column, the commonest causes are cervical rib (pain down the inner side of the arm), or the ill-defined but closely related costoclavicular outlet syndrome due to kinking of the inner cord of the brachial plexus by a fibrous band, tumours (i.e. neurofibroma or metastases in the root of the neck) of the brachial plexus or peripheral nerves, and, at the wrist, compression of the median nerve in the carpal tunnel. A bronchogenic carcinoma at the apex of the lung (Pancoast's superior pulmonary sulcus tumour) is a not infrequent cause of pain in the arm associated with an ipsilateral Horner's syndrome due to involvement of the stellate ganglion. Pericapsulitis of the shoulder joint, giving an immobile painful joint or one with only slight restriction of movement but with a tender capsule, is often associated with pain at the insertion of the deltoid and occasionally with painful brawny swelling of the hand (the shoulder-hand syndrome or reflex dystrophy of the upper extremity); the latter, if long-standing, may lead to atrophy and decalcification of bones (Sudeck's atrophy). Often, too, patients referred to neurological clinics with pain in the forearm, spreading down the dorsum into the fingers, prove to be suffering from a 'tennis-elbow' syndrome with local tenderness over the common extensor origin at the lateral epicondyle of the humerus or at the neck of the radius.

The causes of wasting of small hand muscles

The conditions which cause wasting of the small muscles of the hands can be similarly classified. The commonest spinal cord lesions to have this effect are haematomyelia, poliomyelitis, motor neurone disease, syringomyelia and spinal muscular atrophy. A similar effect may result from an extramedullary tumour at the D1 level, or from arachnoiditis, but is very rare in cervical spondylosis or acute disc lesions as the D1 root is not commonly compressed. Wasting of all the small hand muscles can be the result of any lesion of the inner cord of the brachial plexus; common lesions at this site include birth injury (Klumpke's paralysis), a hyperabduction injury during anaesthesia, compression by the head of the humerus following shoulder dislocation, tumours of the brachial plexus, and compression by a cervical rib or by a fibrous band in the thoracic outlet. All the small hand muscles become atrophic as a rule in cases of motor polyneuropathy as in peroneal muscular atrophy (hereditary motor and sensory neuropathy), but when there is an ulnar nerve lesion, those of the lateral half of the thenar eminence are spared, while the latter muscles are selectively involved when there is a lesion of the median nerve (as in the carpal tunnel). Hence atrophy of all the small hand muscles usually indicates disease of the D1 segment of the cord, of the D1 root, of the inner cord of the brachial plexus, or a diffuse disorder of peripheral nerves or anterior horn cells; atrophy of the lateral half of the thenar eminence generally indicates a median nerve lesion, while sparing of those muscles but atrophy of the others, giving a 'claw hand,' indicates an ulnar nerve lesion. The presence or absence of sensory signs, and their distribution, are of additional value in differential diagnosis. Wasting and weakness of these muscles is rare in myopathies but may occur late in limb-girdle muscular dystrophy; it is, however, an early sign of the rare distal form and, sometimes, of inclusion body myositis.

Peripheral neuropathy (polyneuropathy)

This condition, often in the past entitled peripheral neuritis or polyneuritis, is more properly called peripheral neuropathy or polyneuropathy, as inflammatory changes are rarely discovered in the affected nerves except in postinfective cases. Pathologically there are two principal varieties. In one the process is one of axonal degeneration; surviving nerve fibres conduct at a normal rate but the muscle action potential evoked by stimulation of a motor nerve, or the sensory nerve action potential evoked on stimulating a sensory nerve, is reduced in amplitude. In the second type the neuropathy is demyelinating and conduction velocity is slowed. Any process of recurrent demyelination and remyelination may result eventually in Schwann cell proliferation and nerve hypertrophy. In severe axonal neuropathy there is often secondary demyelination, while primary demyelination ultimately causes axonal damage as a rule, so that in many cases there is evidence of both types of process.

Nevertheless, nerve conduction studies, and sometimes sural nerve biopsy, may help to determine the nature of the predominant pathological process, thus giving a clue to aetiology. The neuropathies constitute a group of clinical syndromes of multiple aetiology in which there are features indicating simultaneous involvement of many peripheral nerves. The clinical picture of sensorimotor neuropathy is therefore one of weakness of lower motor neurone type with eventual atrophy, in the peripheral limb muscles; there is usually symmetrical sensory impairment in 'glove and stocking' distribution, and the tendon reflexes are absent. In contradistinction to 'glove and stocking' sensory loss of hysterical origin, that due to polyneuropathy does not usually show a sharp margin between the area of sensory impairment and that of normal sensation, but the change is gradual. Furthermore, a 'flare' response (p. 179) following a scratch is absent in polyneuropathy if sensory fibres are severely involved, but is present in hysteria. Sometimes motor fibres are predominantly affected (motor neuropathy) and sometimes sensory (sensory neuropathy). Often the affected skeletal muscles, particularly those of the calves, are tender. While distal weakness in the upper and lower limbs is the rule, paradoxically postinfective polyneuropathy (the Guillain-Barré syndrome — see p. 235) often affects proximal upper and lower limb muscles first and the neuropathy is predominantly motor, so that in subacute cases the clinical picture may superficially resemble that of a myopathy such as polymyositis. Many variations in the clinical picture occur from case to case and depend in part upon the aetiology of the illness. It is therefore essential initially to classify and define the known causes of this syndrome according to present knowledge. A provisional classification, which is not intended to embrace all types but simply some of the more important, is given below.

Classification

1. *Infective*: leprosy, infectious mononucleosis.
2. *Postinfective*:
   a. due to specific exotoxins — e.g. diphtheria;
   b. postinfective (probably allergic) — the Guillain-Barré syndrome, serum neuropathy;
   c. complicating specific infections — typhoid fever, dysentery, etc.
3. *Metabolic*:
   a. nutritional — vitamin B_1, B_6 or B_{12} deficiency, alcoholism, pregnancy, etc.;
   b. heavy-metal poisoning — arsenic, mercury, gold, copper, thallium, etc.;
   c. other poisons — triorthocresylphosphate, isoniazid, acrylamide, vincristine, thalidomide, nitrofurantoin, chloroquine, clioquinol, disulfiram, *n*-hexane, phenytoin, organic poisons;
   d. diabetes mellitus;
   e. hyperinsulinism;
   f. myxoedema;
   g. acromegaly;
   h. uraemia.
4. *Vascular*: polyarteritis nodosa; systemic lupus erythematosus; other 'collagen' or 'connective-tissue' diseases; leukaemia and dysproteinaemias.
5. *Genetically-determined*: peroneal muscular atrophy (HMSN types I and II); Dejerine-Sottas disease (HMSN type III); hereditary sensory neuropathy; heredopathia atactica polyneuritiformis (Refsum's); neuropathy in metachromatic leucodystrophy and Krabbe's disease; neuropathy in primary amyloidosis; acute porphyria.
6. *Unknown aetiology*: carcinomatous neuropathy; critical illness neuropathy; chronic progressive polyneuropathy.

Most of the infective and postinfective varieties of polyneuropathy have already been described (see pp. 235–236). They are mainly demyelinating in type. In **leprosy** the clinical picture is one of progressive involvement of individual peripheral nerves with thickening of the nerve trunks and patchy cutaneous anaesthesia. Isolated palsies of single peripheral nerves (the facial or, say, the median or ulnar) or a symmetrical sensorimotor neuropathy are occasional complications of infectious mononucleosis. The polyneuropathy due to **diphtheria** exotoxin usually begins within 10 days of the acute infection and first involves muscles near to the infected area, so that dysphagia and palatal palsy are often the first manifestations; in more severe cases, a symmetrical polyneuropathy of all four limbs develops in about four to six weeks. The **Guillain-Barré syndrome** is the commonest cause of acute ascending paralysis, but more often gives a subacute, predominantly motor, symmetrical neuropathy first involving proximal limb muscles and associated with a raised CSF protein. Indeed, a rise in the protein content of the fluid is a feature common to many varieties of polyneuropathy, especially when demyelinating, but the values recorded in the postinfective cases are generally the highest of all. A polyneuropathy of nonspecific type can also complicate many specific infective disorders. In most of these the neuropathy should probably be regarded as postinfective and autoimmune in character. A form of subacute or chronic demyelinating neuropathy, immunologically related to the Guillain-Barré syndrome, which is steroid-responsive but commonly relapses and eventually gives rise to marked hypertrophy of peripheral nerves, has been called **recurrent** or **relapsing polyneuropathy**. It has been known to relapse during pregnancy.

In the metabolic group of cases, the predominantly axonal polyneuropathy resulting from a **deficiency of vitamin B$_1$** (thiamine) is well recognised. Sensory symptoms generally predominate, and the condition begins with paraesthesiae in the hands and feet; these are followed by pain and tenderness of calf muscles and by bilateral foot drop, weakness of the grip and later wrist drop. There is peripheral blunting of all forms of sensation and often excessive sensitivity of the skin of the feet. This syndrome can be the result of a primary dietary deficiency of vitamin B$_1$; in such a case there may also be tachycardia, enlargement of the heart and peripheral oedema, giving the fully-developed syndrome of beriberi. In less severe cases the polyneuropathy develops alone. The condition sometimes begins during pregnancy, following hyperemesis gravidarum, or may result from the anorexia which occasionally accompanies depression or chronic anxiety or is the predominant symptom of anorexia nervosa. Polyneuropathy due to vitamin B group deficiency is not uncommon even in developed countries in elderly people living alone on inadequate diets. The neuropathies of **pellagra** and of pyridoxine deficiency are similar; the sensory neuropathy of **vitamin B$_{12}$ deficiency** (see Ch. 19) is usually relatively minor in relation to the evidence of spinal cord dysfunction. The polyneuropathy which frequently complicates **chronic alcoholism** is due to thiamine deficiency and not to the alcohol itself; it only develops as a rule when the consumption of alcohol has increased to such an extent that it interferes with the intake of food. Pain and cutaneous hyperaesthesia are particularly severe in alcoholic neuropathy. Wernicke's encephalopathy (see p. 311) and the Korsakoff syndrome (see p. 96) may also be present. The polyneuropathies resulting from

heavy-metal poisoning are similar. Thiamine, as coenzyme A, is important in pyruvate metabolism; heavy metals, by competing with thiamine for certain essential SH groups, interfere with this activity and hence produce polyneuropathy through conditioned thiamine deficiency. Lead poisoning in adults (see p. 320) commonly gives a neuropathy which begins with localised weakness of one muscle group (e.g. wrist drop) but polyeuropathy due to other heavy metals such as arsenic is more often generalised. A variety of polyneuropathy due to mercury poisoning (from the use of teething powders) which disappeared once these powders were abandoned, was called pink disease (acrodynia). This condition produced in infants profound irritability, hypotonia of the limbs, weight loss and a reddened, scaly condition of the hands and feet. Thallium, which has been used in homicidal attempts, typically produces severe sensorimotor polyneuropathy, mental changes (confusion and sometimes dementia) and severe loss of hair (depilation).

Triorthocresylphosphate, a cholinesterase poison, which was an occasional contaminant of illicit alcoholic liquors in America in the 1930s, produced many cases of severe axonal polyneuropathy, in which paralysis and sensory impairment were often permanent (Jamaica ginger paralysis). It caused a more recent 'epidemic' of polyneuropathy in Morocco, due to the use of lubricating oil for cooking purposes. A similar syndrome may follow the use of **apiol**, taken to procure abortion. In recent years, many drugs have been found to cause polyneuropathy; **isoniazid** is one example. Usually in such cases the neuropathy recovers in a few weeks or months after the offending drug has been withdrawn. Isoniazid produces its effect through conditioned pyridoxine deficiency and sensitivity to the drug in this respect is geneticallydetermined, as some people excrete it quickly, others slowly. The exact mechanism by which other drugs and certain **industrial organic poisons** such as acrylamide produce polyneuropathy is unknown. The neuropathy following **sulphonamide therapy** is probably due to hypersensitivity and is in many cases related to that which may complicate polyarteritis nodosa or systemic lupus erythematosus (see below). **Thalidomide**, now withdrawn from the market, gave a peculiarly painful distal sensory neuropathy, while **vincristine** (used for the treatment of malignant disease) and **chloroquine** give a mixed sensorimotor neuropathy with axonal degeneration, as does **nitrofurantoin**, particularly if given to patients with a high blood urea. **Clioquinol**, often used to treat traveller's diarrhoea, was also shown after prolonged usage to produce a severe polyneuropathy with optic nerve damage, especially in Japan, and a similar syndrome believed to be due to dietary cyanide in cassava root is the cause of the **tropical ataxic neuropathy** seen in Nigeria and other parts of Africa. Sensorimotor axonal neuropathy can also be caused by **disulfiram** (Antabuse®, used in the management of alcoholism), **n-hexane** which is used in the leather industry and in certain plastic glues ('glue-sniffers' neuropathy) and even rarely after the prolonged ingestion of phenytoin given as an anticonvulsant. **Organochlorine insecticides** are another uncommon cause. Among the many other drugs which have been implicated are misonidazole, ethambutol, perhexilene, amiodarone and sodium cyanate.

Peripheral neuropathy is a common and important complication of **diabetes mellitus**. Two principal clinical varieties exist. One, which is particularly common in the elderly, produces pain and cramp in the calves, symptoms which are particularly troublesome at night. The ankle and/or knee jerks are absent and there is some impairment of the appreciation of vibration at the ankles. The second form, which usually occurs in younger patients, is a more severe and generalised form of mixed axonal and demyelinating polyneuropathy, affecting power and sensation in all four limbs. It has been suggested that the first type is due to atherosclerosis of the vasa nervorum, the second to some as yet unidentified metabolic disorder associated with diabetes. Whether this is so remains to be proved; however, most cases of both clinical types improve when the diabetic condition is controlled. In the syndrome of **diabetic amyotrophy** wasting and weakness develop most often in one or both quadriceps muscles and rarely in other muscle groups; there may also be pain in the affected muscles. It is usually due to a localised ischaemic femoral neuropathy and also tends to improve when the diabetes is controlled. A rare diabetic autonomic neuropathy with diarrhoea, impotence and dysuria has also been described. Another rare variety of polyneuropathy, which is, however, predominantly motor in type and may therefore mimic motor neurone disease, is an occasional complication of **hyperinsulinism** due to an adenoma of the islets of Langerhans. Bilateral compression of the median nerves in the carpal tunnel is a common complication of **myxoedema** and **acromegaly** but in both these conditions and in thyrotropic hormone deficiency and pituitary gigantism, sensorimotor polyneuropathy has also been described as a rare complication.

Amyloid neuropathy occurs in three distinctive inherited varieties, usually in genetic isolates in various parts of the world. The Portuguese variety produces progressive weakness and sensory loss in the limbs, and is often associated with autonomic dysfunction and trophic ulceration of the feet. The Rukavina and van Allan varieties are very rare; the former usually presents with a bilateral carpal tunnel syndrome due to thickening of the median nerves, the latter with sensorimotor neuropathy, nephropathy and peptic ulcer. Occasionally a neuropathy with deposits resembling amyloid in the peripheral nerves may complicate **multiple myelomatosis**. An association between peripheral neuropathy and episodes of abdominal pain and mental confusion, during which port-wine coloured urine is passed, favours a diagnosis of **acute porphyria**, which will be considered further in Chapter 19 (p. 323). Now that patients with chronic renal disease survive longer than they once did, a specific sensorimotor axonal neuropathy due to **uraemia** is increasingly common; the condition is improved by effective dialysis but may relapse as the blood urea rises.

The varieties of peripheral neuropathy which complicate cases of 'collagen' disease depend in part upon pathological changes in the vasa nervorum; they are predominantly demyelinating in type. Asymmetrical involvement of multiple peripheral nerves (mononeuritis multiplex) is a common feature of **polyarteritis nodosa**, while a symmetrical polyneuropathy develops in some cases of **rheumatoid arthritis** and **systemic lupus erythematosus** (see p. 236). Steroid therapy may then not only control the primary illness but also the neuropathic syndrome. Polyneuropathy is also an occasional complication of leukaemia, reticulosis and of the dysglobulinaemias.

As previously mentioned (see p. 189) a progressive peripheral neuropathy can be inherited. This is the case in the **peroneal muscular atrophy syndrome** and the closely related **Dejerine-Sottas disease** (see p. 189). Polyneuropathy associated with nerve deafness and cerebellar ataxia occurs in **Refsum's disease** in which an abnormal lipid (phytanic acid) accumulates in the peripheral nerves (see p. 188). Similar abnormal collections of lipid may impair peripheral nerve function in metachromatic leucodystrophy and in Krabbe's disease (see p. 186). Polyneuropathy is also one feature of a-α-lipoproteinaemia (Tangier disease) and of a-β-lipoproteinaemia (the Bassen-Kornzweig syndrome). In **hereditary sensory neuropathy** a progressive degeneration of posterior root ganglia gives progressive peripheral sensory loss, often accompanied by perforating ulcers of the feet and necrosis of phalanges (often called acrodystrophic neuropathy or Morvan's syndrome).

Finally there are certain varieties of peripheral neuropathy of unknown aetiology. A progressive polyneuropathy of demyelinating type is a common complication of **bronchogenic carcinoma** and less commonly of malignant disease in other sites. Sometimes the symptoms and signs of the peripheral nerve disorder precede those of the primary neoplasm by months or even years. Although some of the earliest cases described were examples of pure sensory neuropathy, in most cases the affection is predominantly motor, though variable peripheral sensory loss is often found. Numerous clinical variations occur, but a common story is one of vague pain in the legs on exertion, followed by gradual diminution and eventually loss of the lower limb reflexes and then by foot drop and sensory changes. Myopathic changes are sometimes present in addition, thus giving a neuromyopathy. A negative chest X-ray is never sufficient to exclude the diagnosis of bronchogenic carcinoma, and the primary neoplasm may appear in subsequent radiographs. In rare cases, the neuropathy remits after successful removal of the primary growth, but the nature of the relationship between the malignant disease and the neuropathy remains unexplained. Another polyneuropathic syndrome, so far unexplained and described only recently as developing in patients under prolonged treatment in intensive care units, has been called 'critical care' or 'critical illness' neuropathy. The final category included in our provisional classification is chronic progressive polyneuropathy. Many cases exist in which a progressive polyneuropathy develops without obvious cause. The number of cases so classified is steadily diminishing and there is evidence to suggest that some of these, and particularly cases of recurrent demyelinating polyneuropathy (see p. 236) are steroid-responsive. Certainly when there is slowing of nerve conduction indicating demyelination, when the CSF protein content is raised and when no cause for the neuropathy is evident, steroids deserve a trial. Probably, however, many causes of polyneuropathy are yet to be identified. Now that new drugs are continually being introduced into medicine and new toxins (e.g. insecticides) are to be found in man's environment the possibility of a toxic or metabolic cause should always be considered in cases for which no valid explanation can be found.

Treatment

Where the cause is known, treatment consists, whenever possible, in removing any toxin or poison from the patient's body or environment or alternatively in treating the primary disease to which the neuropathy is secondary. Thus in leprous neuritis the appropriate drug treatment of leprosy is indicated, while if the neuropathy is drug-induced, the causal drug should be discontinued and another substituted. And in patients with diabetes mellitus, for example, proper control of the diabetes is essential. In treating heavy-metal poisoning, chelating agents such as sodium EDTA may be required, and when there is evidence of addiction to alcohol or other drugs, the appropriate treatment of addiction is required and nutritional deficiency, whether general or of specific vitamins, should be managed as described in Chapter 19.

The treatment of the Guillain-Barré syndrome is described on pp. 235–236. In relapsing or recurrent demyelinating polyneuropathy or in that complicating connective tissue disease, prednisone or prednisolone in standard dosage (60 mg daily in an adult with subsequent slow reduction depending upon the clinical course and response to treatment, with maintenance therapy, usually on an alternate day basis, usually being required for months or years) is indicated. However, the addition of an immunosuppressive remedy such as azathioprine or cyclophosphamide may enhance the response and allow an earlier reduction in steroid dosage without loss of effect. In the event of acute relapse or severe disability, plasma exchange can sometimes be very beneficial while longer-term immunosuppression is taking effect. And in all cases of sensory neuropathy, appropriate steps must be taken to protect the extremities from physical injury and consequential trophic change, while if motor weakness is substantial, physiotherapy, occupational therapy and various appliances may be needed.

MYASTHENIA GRAVIS

The phenomenon of myasthenia consists of an abnormal degree of fatigability of skeletal muscle. If repeated contractions of an affected muscle are induced, either voluntarily or electrically, the power of these contractions becomes progressively less powerful. Hence patients with myasthenia usually find that they become weaker as the day wears on or after exceptional effort, and improve with rest. For some time it has been known in this disease that there is a defect of neuromuscular transmission which can be partially reversed by cholinesterase inhibitors such as edrophonium or neostigmine and its analogues. However, the discovery that the condition is autoimmune and that it is due to the presence of circulating antibodies against the acetylcholine receptor (AChR) of the muscle fibre, antibodies which coat the receptors and thus interfere with neuromuscular transmission, is much more recent. The exact part played by thymic lymphocytes (T cells) and by humoral factors in the elaboration of these antibodies and the nature of the primary process which stimulates their elaboration have yet to be fully explained. Methods for measuring circulating AChR antibodies are now generally available and are invaluable in diagnosis.

The myasthenic-myopathic (Lambert-Eaton) syndrome originally described in association with bronchogenic carcinoma differs from true myasthenia (see p. 300). Myasthenic fatigability is occasionally observed in polymyositis or muscular dystrophy, but it is much more common for myasthenia to occur alone without other evidence of disease in the skeletal muscles or elsewhere; this syndrome is referred to as myasthenia gravis, though the benign course of many cases belies the name. It occurs in association with thyrotoxicosis much more often than could be accounted for by chance and hence the exclusion of thyroid disease by means of thyroid function tests is an essential part of the investigation of myasthenic patients. It is seen in either sex but is much more common in females. In some patients the condition is associated with benign thymic hyperplasia, in a few with a thymoma (which may become malignant). Thymomas are commoner in patients with an older age of onset, and in cases with thymomas the sex incidence is equal. More than 90% of patients with thymomas have circulating antibodies against skeletal muscle. In females under the age of 40 there is an association with HLA A1, B8 and DRW3 in Caucasians (B12 in Japanese); in blacks and other non-Caucasians the association is with A1, B8 and DR5. In males over 40, A3, B7 and DRW2 (B10 in the Japanese) are the significant associations, while in older patients with thymomas there seems to be a weak association with A2 and A3. Only rarely does the disease affect more than one member of a family. It can begin at any age, in childhood, in adolescence, early adult life, or even in old age. An infant born of a myasthenic mother may suffer from neonatal myasthenia for the first few days of life, but then recovers; this results from AChR antibodies being conveyed across the placenta from mother to child.

This disease usually affects first the external ocular, pharyngeal or jaw muscles. In up to 10% of cases the condition remains limited to the extraocular muscles indefinitely and in such individuals the condition is benign. A common first symptom is ptosis, either unilateral or bilateral, and/or diplopia, which become worse towards the end of the day. Difficulty in swallowing or in chewing often follow, and sometimes the jaw becomes so fatigued after a meal that it hangs open. In other severe cases, there is similar fatigability of the neck, limb and trunk muscles, and respiratory paralysis is an important and sometimes fatal complication. After months or years permanent muscular weakness and wasting, uninfluenced by treatment, develop in some cases and the affected muscles show degenerative changes on histological examination. The triceps muscle is often selectively involved in this way. The tendon reflexes usually remain brisk in true myasthenia, while in the myasthenic syndrome they are usually lost; in the latter condition, too, the initial fatigability of an affected muscle during exercise is usually followed by a marked increase in strength.

A history of variable ptosis, diplopia, dysphagia, jaw or neck muscle weakness or weakness of the limbs should always raise the possibility of myasthenia and a diagnostic intravenous injection of 10 mg of edrophonium (Tensilon®), a drug with a rapid but transient effect, should be tried to see if the weakness is influenced thereby. It is wise to inject 2 mg initially and to await side-effects, before proceeding to give the entire 10 mg. Other diagnostic tests include measurement of the decrement observed in the amplitude of the evoked muscle action potential recorded in an appropriate muscle during repetitive stimulation of a peripheral nerve (usually the median or ulnar) during both slow and rapid rates of stimulation — but this test only gives diagnostic findings when the small hand muscles are affected by the disease, which is uncommon in the early stages (Fig. 18.7). Single fibre electromyography demonstrating increased 'jitter' and 'blocking' is more reliable. Ultimate confirmation of the diagnosis rests, in most cases, upon measurement of antibodies to the acetylcholine receptor in the circulating blood; however, it must be recognised that, for reasons which are still obscure, this assay gives negative results in 5–10% of patients subsequently shown to be suffering from the disease and the antibody titre cannot be precisely correlated with the clinical severity of the disease. In all cases it is essential to carry out posteroanterior and lateral chest X-rays to see whether there is any thymic enlargement, and if skeletal muscle antibodies are present in the serum a comprehensive CT scan of the anterior mediastinum is usually indicated because of the strong possibility of thymoma.

The prognosis is very variable; in the ocular cases the disease is benign, but acute generalised cases sometimes occur which, despite treatment, can be fatal within a few months. In cases of moderate severity, treatment may achieve adequate control of the muscular weakness and allow a reasonably active existence. Indeed, complete and permanent recovery can occur, especially after thymectomy (see below). Spontaneous remission, which can be heralded by reduced treatment requirements, is not uncommon and may last for months or years.

Treatment

Following the original clinical observation of Mary Walker that physosstigmine (eserine) temporarily reversed the manifestations of myasthenia, anticholinesterase drugs were for many years the mainstay of treatment. The remedy favoured in the earlier years was neostigmine but it was gradually supplanted by the longer-acting pyridostigmine bromide (Mestinon®), given in doses of 60 mg (in the adult) or 5–10 mg (in neonates), 10 mg in young children. This was given at first two, three or four times daily, and the dose was gradually increased until maximum benefit (relief of weakness) was obtained. Many patients needed two or three tablets every

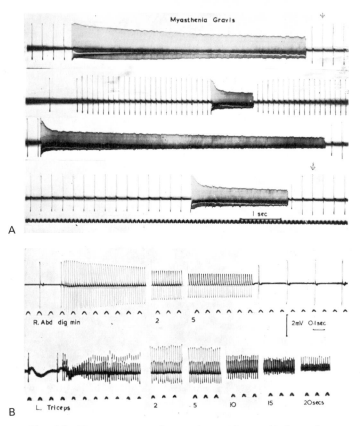

Fig. 18.7 Electromyograms from patients with myasthenia gravis. **A** Ulnar nerve at wrist stimulated with supramaximal shock, repeated 4, 8 and 50 times/s. Action potential recorded from abductor digiti minimi muscle by surface electrodes shows decrement ('fatigue') with fast tetanisation only. Note post-tetanic facilitation at arrows. **B** The classic response from abductor digiti minimi, but the triceps shows a temporary incremental response. (Reproduced with permission from Simpson 1988.)

four hours but individual requirements varied greatly. Often it was necessary to give atropine or propantheline hydrochloride twice daily to overcome the muscarinic side-effects. While patients with the disease generally became skilled in adjusting the level and timing of their medication to suit their individual needs, the principal hazard of this form of treatment was that of increasing cholinergic weakness (due to overdosage), often developing insidiously but sometimes terminating in crisis with diaphragmatic paralysis, respiratory insufficiency and a need for assisted ventilation. Theoretically it was always possible to distinguish myasthenic from cholinergic weakness by giving an injection of edrophonium which would improve persisting myasthenic and worsen cholinergic weakness, but practically the distinction was never so simple. Another problem was that of differential sensitivity of different muscles so that, for example, a

dose sufficient to produce maximum improvement in the external ocular muscles might cause cholinergic paralysis of the diaphragm.

With increasing experience it has become clear first that except perhaps in ocular cases or in elderly individuals in whom major surgery might be thought to be hazardous, thymectomy is the treatment of choice and is indeed obligatory in patients with thymoma (which can usually be demonstrated by CT scan of the anterior mediastinum; fewer than half are revealed by plain anteroposterior and lateral chest radiographs). In thymoma cases there is no evidence that preliminary radiotherapy is beneficial. A sternal splitting approach is preferred by most surgeons as by means of this approach visualisation of the anterior mediastinum with consequential removal of the entire gland and ectopic remnants is made easier. In severe and acute cases, plasma exchange prior to and after operation, thus 'washing out' circulating antibodies, appears to lessen pre-, peri- and post-operative risks but is not essential in all cases. It is in the pre-operative and post-operative periods that anti-cholinesterase drugs still find their most useful role in treatment. It must, however, be stressed that thymectomy should only be performed in units skilled and exper-ienced in the operative procedure and in pre- and post-operative care. With thymectomy, up to a third or more of all patients are cured and are eventually able to dis-continue all treatment, about 30–40% are much improved and require less drug treatment, while only about 20–30% are not improved; with increasing exper-ience the latter figure is decreasing steadily. While plasma exchange remains a most useful form of treat-ment in preparing seriously ill patients for operation and also in a myasthenic crisis (when assisted respiration in an intensive care unit may well be required) there is no convincing evidence that repeated exchanges are of any long-term benefit.

It is now clear that in ocular cases, in patients who are unfit for thymectomy and indeed in pre- and post-operative care of all patients with myasthenia gravis who require continuing treatment, steroid and/or immuno-suppressive drugs are now the treatment of choice save in those few cases in which trial and error shows no response to such treatment and a return to anticholinesterase medication must be adopted as a fall-back position. There also appear to be a few patients in whom pyridostigmine produces additional improvement once maximum bene-fit has been achieved with immunosuppression, but this number appears to be diminishing. Prednisone or pre-dnisolone remain the drugs of choice for initial treat-ment, given in standard dose, gradually reducing over weeks or months to a maintenance dose on alternate days which may have to be continued for months or years or even indefinitely. In mild and ocular cases alternate-day treatment may be appropriate from the outset. It is, however, important to be aware that some patients (as many as 80% in some series) who are given initially 50–100 mg daily of prednisone or prednisolone show a temporary sharp deterioration in symptoms and occasion-ally even respiratory failure, so that many authorities prefer to start with 2.5–5 mg daily and then to work up gradually to a full therapeutic dose. One must also be ready, if temporary deterioration occurs, to use plasma-pheresis or to add anticholinesterase drugs temporarily until improvement begins to result from the steroid treatment. Temporary deterioration appears to be due to a direct effect of the steroid on the ion channel of the acetylcholine receptor. Azathioprine is the preferred immunosuppressive agent and should probably be started at the same time as the steroids, first because it is slow to

act and secondly because as it begins to do so it may be possible to reduce the steroids more rapidly and to a lower maintenance level. Even among experts there is still much difference of opinion upon whether the steroids or the immunosuppressive agents should be reduced or eventually withdrawn and upon which, if either, should be continued in the long term. Thus treatment in this disease is still evolving.

CONGENITAL MYASTHENIA

Several rare forms of congenital myasthenia, sometimes sporadic, sometimes of presumed autosomal recessive inheritance, have been recognised in recent years. Ptosis, external ophthalmoplegia and variable weakness of facial and limb muscles, present from birth, are the predom-inant features and some improvement is usually pro-duced by anticholinesterase drugs. These conditions are not autoimmune and no circulating antibodies to the acetylcholine receptor are found; they are variously due to congenital defects of ACh synthesis or packaging, a deficiency of end-plate receptors for acetylcholine or of cholinesterase and a so-called 'slow channel' syndrome.

THE MYASTHENIC-MYOPATHIC (LAMBERT-EATON) SYNDROME

This disorder of neuromuscular transmission was first recognised in association with lung cancer. It is now known that the syndrome is autoimmune and that an IgG fraction in plasma reduces the number of voltage-gated calcium channels in the end-plate region, causing re-duced calcium entry during nerve terminal depolar-isation and a consequential reduction in transmitter release. In 50–60% of cases a small cell lung cancer is eventually found but in the remainder (who are usually, but not invariably, younger) no malignant disease is ever discovered. The predominant neurological manifest-ations are proximal lower limb weakness, depressed or absent tendon reflexes, an increase in muscle power induced by exercise with post-tetanic potentiation of evoked muscle action potentials, autonomic features (especially dryness of the mouth) and mild/moderate ptosis. Plasma exchange produces transient improvement but treatment with steroids and immunosuppressive remedies may be of longer-term benefit, especially in patients without cancer. Edrophonium and other anti-cholinesterase drugs produce only slight improvement but guanidine hydrochloride and 4-aminopyridine can increase strength; however, the latter remedies often produce unacceptable side-effects. Antiacetylcholine antibodies are not present in the blood.

MYOTONIA

The phenomenon of myotonia is one of apparent delay in relaxation of skeletal muscle, accompanied by a persistent electrical 'after-discharge', even when voluntary innervation of the muscle has ceased. The exact nature of the abnormality in such cases is still uncertain, although an abnormality of chloride conductance in the muscle fibre membrane has been demonstrated. A characteristic feature is that the patient, on taking a firm grasp of an object, is unable to let go, and typically a gradual uncurling of the clenched fingers, beginning in the index and middle fingers, is observed; the total period required for relaxation may be several seconds. The phenomenon can also be demonstrated by a firm tap upon the surface of a muscle, seen best in the tongue or thenar eminence, when a clear-cut 'dimple' or furrow appears and may persist for several seconds. The electromyogram (see p. 36) is diagnostic. Myotonia is accentuated by cold, and is usually reduced either by warmth or by repeated contraction of the affected muscles, which results in 'wearing-off' of the phenomenon. It can be partially or completely relieved by drugs such as quinine, procaine amide or phenytoin and by steroids.

There are two major clinical syndromes in which myotonia is observed. Both are usually inherited as autosomal dominant traits. However, one of these condi-tions, **myotonia congenita**, is transmitted in some families by an autosomal recessive mechanism. In the dominant form, Thomsen's disease, myotonia is generalised throughout the skeletal musculature, and is present from birth. Affected infants often have difficulty in feeding and a peculiarly 'strangled' cry. The principal symptom is stiffness of the muscles, with difficulty in beginning muscular activity and in relaxing afterwards; these features are accentuated by cold and can be 'worked-off' by exercise. Generalised hypertrophy of the skeletal muscles usually develops during adolescence, but weakness and atrophy of muscles is not usually observed, and most patients survive and remain active to a normal age. The milder, recessively-inherited form of myotonia congenita usually first produces symptoms in early childhood but is otherwise similar. In **dystrophia myotonica** (myotonia atrophica or Steinert's disease), by contrast, myotonia is usually apparent only in the hands and tongue, and may even be absent clinically, though it is almost invariably present electromyographically. The first symptoms usually develop in adolescence or adult life, although in occasional cases the condition causes hypotonia and developmental delay in infancy and is then only recognised as a rule when the fully-developed disease is identified in the affected parent who is almost invariably the mother. Facial weakness and an open mouth (Fig. 18.8) are typical. In the affected adult, in

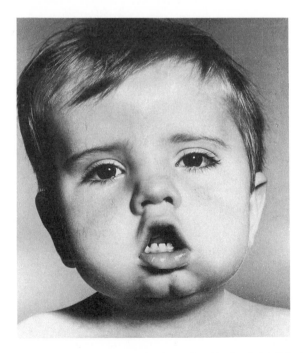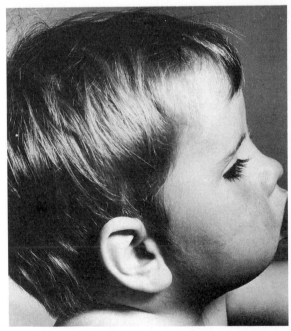

Fig. 18.8 Congenital muscular dystrophy, showing facial diplegia in a 2-year-old child. (Reproduced with permission from Harper 1988.)

addition to myotonia affecting the grip, there is progressive difficulty in walking. There are frontal baldness (in the male), impotence and testicular atrophy, cataracts, atrophy of the sternomastoids and of the facial and temporal muscles (Fig. 18.9), and weakness and wasting of the peripheral muscles of the limbs, involving especially long flexors and extensors but sparing, at least initially, the intrinsic muscles of the hands and feet; these changes are due to an associated muscular dystrophy which is an essential part of the disease process. Bilateral ptosis, and a typically long, lugubrious facies are usually seen. Many patients are of low intellect; the skull vault is thick, the sella small, the EEG may be abnormal, growth hormone output is diminished and there is excessive catabolism of immunoglobulin G. The condition is progressive and eventually results in severe disability leading to a wheel chair existence, with death from cardiac failure (due to myocardial degeneration) or from respiratory infection, in middle-life. Whereas the myotonia can be relieved by drugs, the dystrophic process

in the peripheral limb muscles, which is the principal cause of progressive disability, is uninfluenced by treatment.

Early diagnosis has depended in the past upon the detection of early posterior cortical cataracts by slit-lamp examination or upon the electromyographic detection of myotonic discharges before clinical myotonia is evident. However, the recent discovery of markers closely linked to the gene which lies on chromosome 19 has raised the possibility first of antenatal diagnosis with selective abortion of affected fetuses and secondly of discovering the missing gene product with the hope of subsequent gene replacement.

Paramyotonia is an uncommon disorder showing some affinities with myotonia congenita. In this condition the myotonia occurs only on exposure to cold and is then associated with attacks of generalised muscular weakness resembling closely those observed in cases of familial periodic paralysis but usually accompanied by a rise, rather than a fall, in the serum potassium (see below).

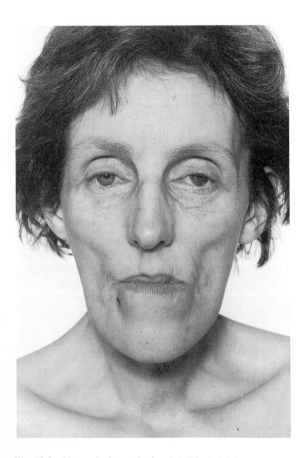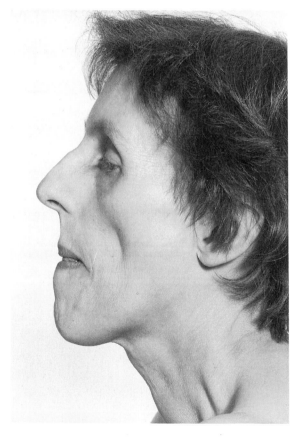

Fig. 18.9   Myotonic dystrophy in adult life: facial features, showing wasting of facial, jaw and sternomastoid muscles. (Reproduced with permission from Harper 1988.)

Myotonia paradoxa is a term given to cases in which the myotonia is accentuated and not improved by exertion. Some such cases constitute merely an unusual form of myotonia congenita, but many in which muscular pain and stiffness increase after exertion are suffering from one of the forms of myopathy which result from a defect in muscle glycogen breakdown such as McArdle's disease; some others are suffering from myxoedema, a disorder which can occasionally present with pain and stiffness on exertion with muscular hypertrophy (Hoffmann's syndrome) as well as slowness of both contraction and relaxation (pseudomyotonia).

PROGRESSIVE MUSCULAR DYSTROPHY

This condition, which causes progressive weakness and wasting of certain skeletal muscles, is the commonest form of genetically-determined primary degenerative myopathy. The pathological changes in the diseased muscles indicate a primary disorder of the muscle fibres and there is no conclusive evidence of disease in the central or peripheral nervous system. One rare variety of muscular dystrophy, **ocular myopathy**, gives progressive bilateral ptosis and eventually complete ophthalmoplegia and weakness of the orbicularis oculi; it is sometimes dominantly inherited, as is the rare oculopharyngeal variety which gives a similar clinical picture, but with dysphagia in addition. Many, but not all of the cases and families with the ocular and oculopharyngeal forms have been shown to have a mitochondrial myopathy rather than a true muscular dystrophy. Another dominantly inherited disease, **distal myopathy**, which is also very rare, except in Sweden, begins in the small muscles of the hands and feet and later spreads proximally in the limb muscles. Several rare varieties of **congenital dystrophy**, beginning at birth, have also been described, one of which, the Fukuyama type, associated with severe mental retardation, is especially prevalent in Japan.

The commonest forms of muscular dystrophy fall into several principal groups which are clinically and genetically distinct. All are progressive, and uninfluenced by any form of drug treatment. The first, the **Duchenne type,** exclusively affects young boys, being inherited via a sex-linked (X-linked) recessive mechanism; often several boys in a sibship develop the condition; occasional girls affected by a similar disorder have been described resulting from chromosomal translocations in which the X-chromosome has fractured, almost invariably at the Xp21 locus, and a portion of an autosome has become attached at the break point. This discovery ultimately led to localisation of the gene responsible for Duchenne dystrophy close to the Xp21 locus of the short arm of the X-chromosome, and to its characterisation and sequencing in 1987. Subsequently, a protein named dystrophin, bound to the sarcolemma of the muscle fibre in normal individuals, was found to be the missing gene product. The onset of Duchenne dystrophy is usually within the first three to five years of life; the child, who walked at the normal age, becomes clumsy in walking and running, has difficulty in climbing stairs, falls frequently and rises by 'climbing up his legs' (Fig. 18.10). He walks with his abdomen protruding (accentuated lumbar lordosis) and with a typical waddle. There is progressive weakness of the proximal upper and lower limb muscles; often firm rubbery enlargement (pseudo-hypertrophy, partly due to fatty infiltration and partly to actual increase in muscle bulk) of the calves, and sometimes of other muscles, is seen. The progress of the disease is inexorable. Often the child is unable to walk by the time he is eight to 12 years old and later progressive contractures of the weakened muscles develop with secondary skeletal deformity, to give a tragic terminal state, from which the child is carried off by respiratory infection or by cardiac failure due to associated cardiomyopathy, often before the age of 20. A less common variety, the **Becker type**, which resembles the Duchenne type clinically and which is also inherited as an X-linked trait, is seen in occasional families; its onset is later (at 5 to 15 years) and its course more benign so that many affected individuals survive into middle-life. This Becker variety is now known to be allelic with the Duchenne type but in such cases the deficiency of dystrophin is only partial. Another X-linked variety of dystrophy, the **Emery-Dreifuss type**, is a scapuloperoneal syndrome resembling scapuloperoneal muscular atrophy (p. 286) but giving in addition multiple contractures and cardiomyopathy; the gene responsible has been localised to the distal part of the long arm of the X-chromosome.

The **limb-girdle** variety (Erb-Leyden-Möbius) occurs equally in the two sexes and may begin at any age though it usually does so in adolescence or early adult life; it is usually inherited via an autosomal recessive gene. The disease may begin rarely in the pelvic girdle, giving difficulty in climbing stairs and a typical waddling gait, or more often in the shoulder girdle, resulting in inability to lift the arms above the shoulders. Sometimes the muscular involvement remains confined to the shoulders or pelvic girdle for many years, but later spreads to the other group. In the shoulder girdles the trapezii, serrati, pectorals, biceps and brachioradiales are commonly involved and the deltoids are spared, to give a characteristic clinical picture. Pseudohypertrophy of muscles is occasionally seen. The prognosis in these cases is much less grave than in the Duchenne variety, but nevertheless the disease is progressive, though sometimes intermittently

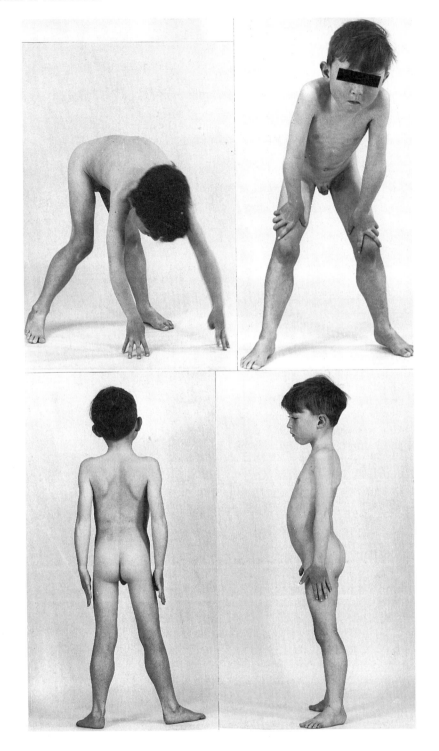

Fig. 18.10   The Duchenne type of muscular dystrophy: note the hypertrophy of the calves and the characteristic method of rising from the floor. (Reproduced with permission from Walton 1988.)

so; most patients are severely disabled, as a rule in middle-life, and few survive to a normal age. Up to half of all cases so diagnosed in the past are known to be suffering from benign spinal muscular atrophy (see p. 283) and some rare metabolic myopathies give a similar clinical picture so that diagnosis depends upon ancillary investigations. Indeed it has become more usual to speak of the limb-girdle syndrome, taking account of the fact that it is one of multiple aetiology. Nevertheless it is generally recognised that a true scapulohumeral form of muscular dystrophy and an uncommon pelvifemoral form (usually of late onset), both of autosomal recessive inheritance, can be identified. Also well characterised is an autosomal recessive form of **childhood muscular dystrophy**, resembling in many respects the Duchenne type but running a much more benign course. This condition, which is common in the Middle East, probably accounts, as does spinal muscular atrophy of the Kugelberg-Welander type, for many of the cases of so-called Duchenne dystrophy described in girls in previous years.

The **facioscapulohumeral form** (Landouzy-Dejerine) is often the most benign. It, too, may begin at any age (usually in adolescence or early adult life) and in either sex, but is generally inherited as an autosomal dominant trait. The facial muscles are first affected resulting in inability to close the eyes completely, a typical 'pout' of the lips and a 'transverse' smile. The shoulder girdle muscles are also involved, selectively as in some limb-girdle cases, and the disease may not spread to the pelvic girdle for many years, though the tibiales anterior are usually the first lower limb muscles to be involved. In some cases only a few muscles around the shoulders are involved and the disorder then arrests (abortive cases). Whereas the muscular weakness may progress unusually quickly causing a severe lumbar lordosis and progressive disablement in a few affected individuals, the advance of the disease is very slow in most, and some remain active, though with increasing disability, to a normal age. Recent evidence has shown that, as in the limb-girdle variety, this condition can be mimicked by spinal muscular atrophy. Scapuloperoneal muscular atrophy (see p. 286) also gives a similar clinical picture except that the facial muscles are not involved.

The diagnosis of muscular dystrophy, in an established case, is rarely difficult, but in the early stages, particularly in a young child, the history of clumsiness in walking or of inability to run as quickly as other children of comparable age is often attributed to flat feet or to laziness, unless this diagnosis is borne in mind. Estimation of the serum creatine kinase activity, which may be raised 300-fold in affected young boys, is especially useful in the diagnosis of the Duchenne type and less striking increases are seen in the other varieties. This test can be used to identify the disease in its preclinical stage in the young male sibs of affected boys and has also been useful in the diagnosis of the carrier state in their mothers and sisters. Carrier identification is particularly important for genetic counselling. About one-third of all new cases of Duchenne dystrophy arise as a result of genetic mutation but it has not been possible to be sure whether such a mutation first arose in the mother of the affected boy or in the maternal grandmother; if the former, then the mother would not be a carrier and the sisters of the dystrophic boy would probably not be either — but if the latter were the case, the mother would be a carrier and the patient's sisters would each have a 50:50 chance of being carriers. Each son of a female carrier has a 50:50 chance of being affected by the disease, each daughter a similar chance of being a carrier. If carriers are identified and do not have male children the number of dystrophic boys being born will diminish though some new cases will continue to result from genetic mutation. In known carriers who wish to have children, selective abortion of male fetuses (after identification of fetal sex by amniocentesis or chorionic villus biopsy) has been widely practised. Now that the Duchenne/Becker gene has been identified, carrier detection is becoming more precise with the aid of DNA recombinant techniques and so too is antenatal diagnosis, making possible abortion of only affected males. Carrier detection is impossible at present in relatives of limb-girdle and other autosomal recessive cases. In facioscapulohumeral dystrophy and other dominant conditions the condition is passed on only by affected individuals to half their children of either sex.

As so many other conditions may resemble muscular dystrophy, electromyography and muscle biopsy are also necessary for diagnosis. These procedures are of particular value in distinguishing muscular dystrophy from polymyositis (see below) and from spinal muscular atrophy and various metabolic myopathies with which the condition is most often confused. In the absence of any effective treatment, all that can be done is to keep the patients active with regular moderate exercise and avoidance of undue weight gain. Inactivity and bed rest are deleterious; every effort should be made to delay the development of contractures by passively stretching tendons which are shortening, but surgical lengthening of such tendons is not usually indicated unless the patient can be mobilised immediately afterwards. Attention should also be paid to the posture of the patients, particularly when confined to a wheelchair, and light spinal supports have often been used to prevent scoliosis. However, such supports are often poorly tolerated and ineffective and the Luque or other similar surgical procedures, if carried out at an appropriate stage, are much more satisfactory. With greatly improved management, both longevity and the quality of life for many patients have been greatly improved. The identification of the gene product, dystrophin, in Duchenne cases has raised the hope that some form of treatment circumventing its absence may be introduced pending gene replacement therapy.

POLYMYOSITIS AND DERMATOMYOSITIS

These names have been given to clinical syndromes produced by combined degenerative and inflammatory changes in skeletal muscle. They do not include suppurative and infective varieties of myositis which are comparatively rare, save for viral myositis (e.g. epidemic myalgia), which will be discussed below. In fact, suppurative myositis is not uncommon in some tropical countries (tropical myositis), and viruses other than Coxsackie B (which causes epidemic myalgia) sometimes give a self-limiting myositis; influenza is one example. The syndrome of polymyositis also excludes, conventionally, parasitic disorders such as trichinosis (due to eating pork contaminated with the *Trichinella spiralis*), toxoplasmosis and trypanosomiasis cruzi (South American Chagas' disease) and cysticercosis (causing muscular hypertrophy) which may also affect skeletal muscle. In some instances the skin and mucous membranes are also involved, in which case the condition is known as dermatomyositis, but often the main brunt of the disease process falls upon the skeletal muscles. Although the syndrome may embrace several diseases of varying aetiology, in most instances the pathological process is clearly one of so-called connective tissue disease. Until comparatively recently it has been customary to group together polymyositis and dermatomyositis but recent work has shown that in several respects the two conditions are different. Thus polymyositis is due to a lymphocyte-mediated autoimmune process in which sensitised T4 and T8 cells invade and destroy skeletal muscle; the typical histological picture is one of muscle fibre necrosis and regeneration with interstitial and perivascular infiltration with such cells, which can be identified in histological preparations with monoclonal antibodies. In dermatomyositis, the intramuscular blood vessels may be damaged by circulating immune complexes and the autoimmune process is humoral rather than cell-mediated. Histologically vasculitis is common and so too is perifascicular atrophy of muscle fibres.

The syndrome has been observed in patients of all ages and in both sexes. Acute polymyositis in adults is uncommon but dermatomyositis is much more so and sometimes occurs in childhood; it is characterised by generalised muscular pains and weakness of comparatively rapid progression, associated often with a widespread erythematous rash on the face, limbs and trunk. The proximal limb muscles are more severely affected than the distal. The affected muscles are tender and the patients are often ill and febrile; the respiratory muscles may be involved and the illness may end fatally within a few weeks or months. Subacute polymyositis is much more common. In such cases muscular pain and tenderness and symptoms of constitutional upset are often absent, and the presenting features are those of progressive weakness and moderate atrophy of the muscles of the shoulder and pelvic girdles. This clinical picture can resemble closely that of muscular dystrophy, save for the fact that in polymyositis all the proximal limb muscles are usually weakened, and the deltoid, for instance, is not spared; furthermore the neck muscles are often weak, dysphagia and a Raynaud phenomenon in the hands are common (though these two features occur more often in dermatomyositis), and the muscular weakness is often greater than the degree of atrophy would suggest. This form of subacute polymyositis is particularly common in middle- and late-life. When dermatomyositis occurs in childhood or adolescence there are often minor skin changes on the skin of the face and of the hands and fingers, resembling those of early systemic sclerosis or acrosclerosis. In some cases, the skin lesions resemble those of lupus erythematosus, while in others, there may be associated evidence of another 'collagen' disease such as rheumatoid arthritis. Subcutaneous and intramuscular calcification (calcinosis universalis) is not uncommon in childhood dermatomyositis. Another important point is that many cases of dermatomyositis in middle- and late-life develop in association with malignant disease in the lung or in some other organ. The relationship between adult polymyositis and malignant disease is much less striking and may not, indeed, be significant.

The prognosis of polymyositis and dermatomyositis is variable. Some of the acute cases are eventually fatal, despite modern methods of treatment. A few subacute cases in childhood have been known to remit spontaneously and even to recover incompletely; others enter a chronic stage with the development of fibrous contractures in the muscles and severe deformity (chronic myositis fibrosa). Most subacute cases occurring in adult life are progressive; very few if untreated arrest. Many cases remit completely or partially when treated with prednisone and immunosuppressive drugs (e.g. azathioprine, cyclophosphamide or methotrexate), but maintenance therapy may have to be continued for many years. Plasma exchange can be useful as a temporary measure in acute dermatomyositis, and in some intractable cases of polymyositis, whole body irradiation has been successful.

In diagnosis, a raised ESR may be helpful but this test

is normal in more than a third of all cases. The serum creatine kinase activity and immunoglobulins are also often raised, but in most cases final diagnosis depends upon a combination of the clinical findings on the one hand with the results of electromyography and muscle biopsy on the other.

Several rare forms of inflammatory myopathy resembling polymyositis have been identified. **Eosinophilic myositis** is clinically similar and is steroid-responsive, as are **granulomatous myositis** (resembling sarcoidosis of muscle) and **localised nodular myositis**, a focal form of polymyositis which causes painful swellings in one or more muscles. Somewhat different clinically is **inclusion body myositis**, possibly due to chronic mumps virus infection, which is commoner in the older age groups, often affects distal limb muscles predominantly and is insidiously progressive in most cases, usually being uninfluenced by steroids and immunosuppressive agents. Ringed vacuoles and intranuclear filamentous inclusions are characteristic of the latter condition histologically.

POLYMYALGIA RHEUMATICA

This is a disorder of middle-aged and elderly patients, of whom a few prove to be suffering from temporal or cranial arteritis. Typically it presents with diffuse muscle pain and aching which may restrict movement (getting out of the bath is often particularly difficult) but there is no muscular weakness or wasting. The ESR is invariably raised and the response to prednisone is dramatic. Maintenance treatment is often required for several months.

EPIDEMIC MYALGIA (BORNHOLM DISEASE)

This is a form of virus myositis, resulting from infection with Coxsackie B virus. It gives an acute febrile illness with severe pain in the upper abdomen and lower chest wall. Pain on breathing and coughing (pleurodynia) is a striking feature and the illness may simulate pleurisy or even an acute abdominal emergency. The condition is self-limiting, occurs in localised epidemics, and usually clears up without residual symptoms in three to five days.

PAROXYSMAL MYOGLOBINURIA

Myoglobin may appear in the urine in any condition which produces sudden destruction of muscle, and if the quantity released into the blood stream is large, death may result from renal failure due to blockage of renal tubules. Causes of myoglobinuria include massive crush injuries of muscle (crush syndrome), necrosis of the anterior tibial muscles in their tight fascial compartment after prolonged exertion (the anterior tibial syndrome), acute polymyositis, and paroxysmal myoglobinuria or rhabdomyolysis. In the latter, a condition of unknown aetiology, patients experience intermittent febrile episodes, each lasting a few days, during which they develop generalised muscular pain and weakness and pass dark brown urine containing myoglobin. The condition is uninfluenced by treatment, but even after repeated attacks, recovery is often complete, though death in an attack is a rare event. The disorder usually appears first in childhood and after repeated attacks some permanent muscular weakness and wasting may be found. Recently it has been shown that muscle pain and myoglobinuria developing after exercise can be due to an inherited deficiency of carnitine palmityl transferase.

FAMILIAL PERIODIC PARALYSIS

This uncommon condition of dominant inheritance affects patients of either sex, usually from birth. Sufferers experience attacks of generalised muscular weakness which vary in severity but may occasionally be so severe as to paralyse them almost completely. A common story is that the patient wakens from sleep to find that he is virtually unable to move. Although weakness of the skeletal musculature can be widespread and profound, swallowing is only occasionally disturbed, and respiratory muscle weakness is never sufficient to endanger life. The attacks vary in duration from one or two hours to as long as 48 hours. Commonly after a short period of total paralysis the patient is able to move but does so weakly and clumsily and may not be normal for several days. There are some cases in which the weakness is consistently localised to only a few muscle groups. The episodes are particularly likely to develop while the patient is resting after unusually heavy exertion, or after a heavy carbohydrate meal. Often they can be induced by the administration of insulin and glucose. Usually the serum potassium is low during the attacks and the weakness recovers slowly after the administration of 2–4 g of potassium chloride by mouth. Maintenance therapy with 4–5 g of potassium chloride daily and aldosterone antagonists have been used prophylactically but acetazolamide 250 mg three times daily has proved much more effective in most patients. Similar episodes can occur in patients whose serum potassium is lowered as a result of other causes, as in cases of potassium-losing nephritis, renal tubular acidosis, or aldosteronism.

In some cases and families, attacks which are characteristic of the syndrome described above occur in association with a high, and not a low, serum potassium. This syndrome has been called **adynamia episodica hereditaria** or **hyperkalaemic periodic paralysis**. The attacks are often less severe and of shorter duration than in the hypokalaemic type and may follow immediately after exertion, while some patients also have myotonia. Indeed it is still uncertain as to whether so-called myotonic periodic paralysis and paramyotonia congenita (p. 302) are different diseases or closely related variants. The paralysis in the hyperkalaemic cases is accentuated by potassium but can be terminated by the use of diuretics such as chlorothiazide or acetazolamide which promote potassium excretion; these drugs are often effective if given prophylactically, and paradoxically as indicated above, they may also prevent attacks of the hypokalaemic type. Yet a third variety of periodic paralysis, in which the serum potassium remains normal in the attacks and in which weakness is controlled by the administration of sodium and prevented by 9-α-fluorohydrocortisone 0.1 mg daily, has been described (**normokalaemic periodic paralysis**) but is probably a variant of the hyperkalaemic type. It has long been considered necessary in any individual experiencing attacks of this nature to estimate the serum potassium during an attack and to carry out other appropriate tests in order to identify the type of periodic paralysis from which he is suffering so that appropriate treatment may be given. However, the fact that acetazolamide is effective in prophylaxis of all varieties, and a number of inconsistencies in clinical pattern and biochemical findings even within families is now causing many authorities to question whether there is virtue in distinguishing the hypokalaemic from the hyperkalaemic cases. Muscle biopsies during attacks usually show large vacuoles within the muscle fibres. A form of periodic paralysis associated with thyrotoxicosis, which responds to treatment of the thyroid disease, is common in families of Chinese and Japanese descent.

ENDOCRINE MYOPATHIES

This group of disorders will be described in Chapter 19 (pp. 321–322).

OTHER METABOLIC MYOPATHIES

In the last 30 years the increasing use of new diagnostic techniques, such as biochemical, electrophysiological and histological methods (including histochemistry and electron microscopy) has led to the definition of many previously unrecognised disorders of muscle, most of which were previously thought to be forms of muscular dystrophy. Some of these are the specific varieties of congenital dystrophy giving rise to hypotonia and weakness in infancy and childhood, to be described below. Others have been shown to be due to genetically determined metabolic disorders. While all are rare, the commonest are disorders of glycogen storage, lipid storage diseases and conditions associated with abnormal mitochondria.

The commoner glycogen storage diseases are first **McArdle's disease** due to myophosphorylase deficiency and the clinically similar condition of phosphofructo-kinase deficiency (both autosomal recessive). These give muscle pain coming on after exertion, sometimes accompanied by myoglobinuria and physiological contracture and only slowly relieved by rest. No rise in blood lactate in the ante-cubital vein occurs after repeated contraction of forearm muscles with arterial occlusion by a tourniquet, and histochemical staining of a muscle biopsy is diagnostic. More recently, phosphoglycerate kinase deficiency (X-linked), phosphoglycerate mutase and lactate dehydrogenase deficiency (autosomal recessive) have also been identified. None of these can yet be influenced by any form of treatment but a form of myosin ATPase deficiency giving exercise-induced muscle pain responsive to verapamil has also been recognised. **Pompe's disease** due to acid maltase deficiency gives massive vacuolation of skeletal muscle sections due to glycogen deposition. It can give a severe diffuse cardiomyopathy which is rapidly fatal in infancy, or a subacute myopathy in adolescence or adult life. This condition is also due to an autosomal recessive gene.

Another vacuolar myopathy, usually presenting with a clinical picture of subacute muscular weakness like that of limb-girdle muscular dystrophy, but resulting from the deposition of neutral fat, especially in type I muscle fibres (as seen in frozen sections stained with Sudan Black), is due to autosomal recessive **carnitine deficiency;** clinical improvement in some cases follows the oral administration of carnitine. Cases in which the deficiency is confined to skeletal muscle tend to run a relatively benign course but systemic carnitine deficiency, which can also be secondary (as in Reye's syndrome, in some patients with an idiosyncratic response to sodium valproate therapy or in the renal Fanconi syndrome, to quote but a few examples) is much more severe and can cause severe vomiting with deepening stupor and coma which may end fatally.

Finally, a variety of disorders presenting either with hypermetabolism in the absence of hyperthyroidism, with ocular or oculopharyngeal muscular weakness or with a syndrome resembling limb-girdle or facioscapulo-humeral muscular dystrophy, has been shown to be associated with biochemical and morphological abnormalities of the muscle mitochondria (**mitochondrial myopathy**). Clusters of subsarcolemmal mitochondria may be identified in frozen sections of muscle stained histochemically with oxidative enzyme stains and are then predominant in type I (so-called 'ragged red') fibres.

But electron microscopy is needed to define the morphological changes in the mitochondria. In some families there is also retinal pigmentation and cerebellar ataxia with abnormal mitochondria in the cerebellum as well as in the muscles (the Kearns-Sayre syndrome). In others, many different specific enzyme defects of the cytochrome enzymes of the electron transport chain have been recognised and in some such cases lactic acidosis is a troublesome complication.

THE AMYOTONIA CONGENITA SYNDROME ('THE FLOPPY INFANT')

To determine the nature of the pathological changes responsible for widespread weakness and hypotonia of the skeletal muscles in infancy is often a difficult matter. In most cases which present with these manifestations in severe form the disease process is one of infantile progressive spinal atrophy type I (Werdnig-Hoffman disease), whether the illness begins at or before birth or during the first year of life. Infantile polyneuropathy can also cause widespread weakness and hypotonia but nerve conduction velocity is usually reduced in such cases and the CSF protein is raised. Dystrophia myotonica (see p. 301) and infantile myasthenia are other uncommon causes of hypotonia. In many cases, however, the child's hypotonia is a symptom of various infective, metabolic and neurological disorders which do not primarily affect the lower motor neurone or muscles. Thus weakness and hypotonia of some degree is common in infants recovering from acute infection, in cases of intestinal malabsorption, hypocalcaemia, mental handicap, and even initially in some of flaccid cerebral diplegia. Congenital heart disease may also be associated with generalised hypotonia, as may Pompe's disease (see above). There exists, however, a third group of cases in which the weakness and hypotonia are benign, though of unknown aetiology, and in which improvement and sometimes complete recovery may be expected. This syndrome was first described by Oppenheim under the title of myatonia congenita or amyotonia congenita, but this diagnosis was subsequently utilised to include all infants who showed severe generalised hypotonia soon after birth. As many of these proved to be suffering from progressive spinal atrophy, this title has been discarded, and the term **benign congenital or infantile hypotonia** is now preferred by many for cases which carry a relatively good prognosis. This condition is not a single disease entity but a syndrome of multiple aetiology, although many cases show no specific identifying features and the cause of the muscular weakness and hypotonia remains unknown. These children, though weak and 'limp' or 'floppy' from birth, are never as severely paralysed as those with Werdnig-Hoffman disease and show gradual improvement. They sit up late and often do not stand or walk until late in the second or in the third year of life. Some recover completely but others, who are more severely affected in early life, improve up to a point, but no further, and have small, weak muscles throughout life. The latter condition was once called 'congenital universal muscular hypoplasia' but **'benign congenital myopathy'** is now preferred. With the increasing use of electron microscopy to examine muscle biopsy sections, a specific morphological diagnosis is becoming possible in many more cases and relatively few now remain in this group, although there does appear to be a poorly defined non-progressive form of **congenital muscular dystrophy** which behaves in this way. In some cases of infantile hypotonia subsequently found to have generalised weakness and hypoplasia of muscles a curious defect of the centre of many muscle fibres can be demonstrated (**'central-core' disease**) while in yet others rod-shaped bodies derived from Z-bands are aggregated beneath the sarcolemma of many fibres (**'nemaline myopathy'**). A similar clinical picture occasionally results from mitochondrial myopathy (see above), or from congenital fibre type disproportion, in which there is a marked discrepancy in size between type I and type II fibres. Hypoplasia of the muscles is also seen in some individuals with long spidery fingers and a high arched palate (arachnodactyly). Another rare disorder identified in some weak and hypotonic infants by histology is **'myotubular or centronuclear myopathy'**, a condition in which external ocular as well as facial, limb and trunk muscles are involved and in which the muscle fibres show central chains of nuclei and superficially resemble fetal myotubes.

One final condition requires to be mentioned, namely **arthrogryposis multiplex congenita**. This is a condition of multiple contractures of skeletal muscle, combined with deformity of the limbs, which is present from birth. In some cases it appears to be due to a spinal muscular atrophy beginning in fetal life, in some to a severe myopathic process developing before birth (congenital muscular dystrophy), but in most, in which there is no evidence of disease in the motor nerves or muscles themselves, to excessive intra-uterine pressure, with abnormal posturing of the limbs.

REFERENCES

Albuquerque E X, Eldefrawi A T (eds) 1983 Myasthenia gravis. Chapman & Hall, New York
Bradley W G 1974 Disorders of peripheral nerves. Blackwell, Oxford
Brandt S 1950 Werdnig-Hoffmann's infantile progressive

muscular atrophy. Munksgaard, Copenhagen

Dubowitz V 1978 Muscle disorders in childhood. Major problems in clinical paediatrics, Vol XVI (Schaffer A J, Markowitz M, series eds). Saunders, London

Dubowitz V, Brooke M 1988 Muscle biopsy: a practical approach, 2nd edn. Saunders, London

Dyck P J, Thomas P K, Lambert E H 1984 Peripheral neuropathy, 2nd edn. Saunders, London

Engel A, Banker B Q 1986 Myology. McGraw-Hill, New York

Harper P S 1988 The myotonic disorders. In: Walton J N (ed) Disorders of voluntary muscle, 5th edn. Churchill Livingstone, Edinburgh

Harper P S 1989 Myotonic dystrophy, 2nd edn. Major problems in neurology, Vol 9 (Walton J N, series ed.). Saunders, London

Lisak R P, Barchi R L 1982 Myasthenia gravis. Major problems in neurology, Vol 11 (Walton J N, series ed.). Saunders, Philadelphia.

Mastaglia F L (ed) 1988 Inflammatory diseases of muscle. Blackwell, Oxford

Mastaglia F L, Walton J N (eds) 1983 Skeletal muscle pathology. Churchill Livingstone, Edinburgh

O'Neill J H, Murray N M F, Newsom-Davis J 1988 The Lambert-Eaton myasthenic syndrome. Brain 111: 577

Rose F C (ed) 1984 Research progress in motor neurone disease. Pitman, London

Simpson J A 1988 Myasthenia gravis and related syndromes. In: Walton J N (ed) Disorders of voluntary muscle, 5th edn. Churchill Livingstone, Edinburgh

Spillane J D, Spillane J A 1982 An atlas of clinical neurology, 3rd edn. Oxford University Press, Oxford

Walton J N 1985 Brain's Diseases of the nervous system, 9th edn. Oxford University Press, Oxford

Walton J N (ed) 1988 Disorders of voluntary muscle, 5th edn. Churchill Livingstone, Edinburgh

Walton J N, Adams R D 1958 Polymyositis. Livingstone, Edinburgh.

19. Metabolic disorders and the nervous system

Increasing interest has been taken of late in the group of diseases or symptom-complexes in which symptoms depend not so much upon recognisable structural changes occurring in the bodily tissues, but upon alterations in their chemical composition and metabolic activity. In many disorders physical changes eventually develop in the affected organs, but this is not always so, and the primary change is biochemical. Under this heading we may consider the so-called deficiency disorders which result either from an inadequate intake of certain foods, and particularly of vitamins, or from impaired absorption of them. Several of these disorders can disturb the functioning of the nervous system, as may abnormalities in the endocrine glands and some specific inborn errors of metabolism. The more common and important of these conditions will be described in this chapter. The effect of poisons upon the nervous system (neurotoxicology) and the influence of various forms of physical injury will also be considered, even though the latter is not strictly metabolic.

DEFICIENCY DISORDERS

Although many specific syndromes seen in man are ascribed to an insufficient dietary intake of certain vitamins, they are not solely dependent upon vitamin deficiency. Thus total starvation does not as a rule cause scurvy, pellagra or beri-beri, while manifestations of thiamine deficiency are greatly enhanced if the diet contains large amounts of carbohydrate. It thus appears that some food must be taken before typical clinical features of vitamin deficiency develop. Even so, the resultant clinical syndrome varies greatly in individual cases; it is not, for instance, clear why thiamine (vitamin B_1) deficiency produces Wernicke's encephalopathy in some cases, cardiac involvement with or without a peripheral neuropathy (wet beri-beri) or just a peripheral neuropathy (dry beri-beri) in others. A large carbohydrate intake associated with physical activity and a chronic degree of relative deficiency favour wet beri-beri, where-

as inactivity with a restricted carbohydrate intake seems to favour dry beri-beri. Conditions like pregnancy, or infective illness, which increase the body's demands for vitamins, may accentuate symptoms attributable to deficiency which were previously minimal. It is the vitamins of the B group, and particularly thiamine, nicotinic acid, pyridoxine and vitamin B_{12}, which are of greatest importance in relation to the nervous system. Clinical syndromes resulting from vitamin C deficiency (scurvy) and from lack of most of the fat-soluble vitamins (A, D and K) are not as a rule attended by symptoms of nervous disease but some recent evidence has emerged to implicate vitamin E deficiency in certain neurological syndromes.

Wernicke's encephalopathy

Wernicke's encephalopathy is characterised by mental disturbance, disorders of eye movement and ataxia, and results from thiamine deficiency. It occurs most often in chronic alcoholic patients in whom alcoholic beverages have gradually replaced other forms of food, and gastrointestinal irritation has contributed by producing anorexia. However, it can develop as a result of thiamine deficiency arising from any cause and has also been described as a consequence of repeated vomiting in pregnancy and as a sequel to gastrectomy. There is often an associated polyneuropathy. The principal pathological features are focal areas of haemorrhage and neuronal degeneration in the corpora mammillaria and upper midbrain. Although in severe cases consciousness may be impaired, the characteristic mental symptoms are first, transient delirium and hallucinations, occurring particularly in alcoholic patients and resulting from alcoholic withdrawal; secondly, apathy, listlessness and variable confusion; and thirdly, most typical of all, the Korsakoff syndrome (see p. 96). The principal abnormality in the latter is a memory defect giving inability to record new impressions, from which spring disorientation in time and place and confabulation (confabulatory amnesia); events from the patient's remote past are described elaborately, as if they had just happened. The principal neurological abnormalities accompanying these mental changes are coarse nystagmus, present in all directions of gaze, and ophthalmoplegia, which may consist merely of paralysis of both lateral recti or more often of disorders of conjugate ocular movement leading in some cases to total immobility of the eyes. A severe disequilibrium (truncal ataxia) is also present as a rule, even though signs of cerebellar inco-ordination in the limbs are often inconspicuous.

The diagnosis is made on these characteristic features and can be confirmed by measurement of the red cell transketolase activity. Once blood has been taken for confirmatory tests, the patient should be treated as soon as the diagnosis is suspected with intramuscular thiamine 50 mg a day for five days, followed by oral administration. Patients with Wernicke's encephalopathy are often deficient in other vitamins and the administration of thiamine should be combined with the other vitamins of the B group. A characteristic feature of Wernicke's disease is that the neurological abnormalities generally remit quickly with thiamine treatment, although the mental disturbances, and particularly those of the Korsakoff syndrome, may take weeks or months to resolve.

Subacute necrotising encephalomyelopathy (Leigh's disease)

This uncommon disorder, which is inherited as an autosomtal recessive trait, is an inborn error of metabolism mentioned here because the pathological changes in the affected infants resemble those of Wernicke's encephalopathy. The affected children show failure to thrive, hypotonia followed by spasticity and often convulsions, nystagmus, and optic atrophy. The condition usually begins in the first year of life; examination of the blood reveals an acidosis and a rise in the blood pyruvate due to a deficiency of pyruvate carboxylase which converts pyruvate to oxalacetate. The condition is usually fatal in six to 12 months but temporary improvement has followed the administration of lipoic acid or thiamine tetrafuryldisulphide. Rarely a more benign form of the disorder occurs in adults.

Beri-Beri

Although thiamine deficiency is clearly important in the aetiology of beri-beri, some additional factor is probably necessary in view of the rarity of the fully-developed syndrome in European or American chronic alcoholics and in view of the fact that it rarely occurs in its entirety except in populations fed upon milled rice. Polyneur-

opathy due to B-vitamin deficiency is, however, quite common in Western countries, not only in alcoholics, but in patients with prolonged anorexia due to mental disease and in elderly people living alone.

The principal clinical features of beri-beri are those of polyneuropathy (see p. 293). Apart from the distal muscular atrophy and sensory loss which are common to all varieties of peripheral neuropathy, a characteristic feature of this form is that the patients often complain of intense burning and tingling in the extremities and especially in the feet; touching the skin is often particularly unpleasant, so that walking becomes impossible, not as a result of muscular weakness, but because of sensory disturbance. In some individuals, these are the only manifestations ('dry' or 'neuritic' beri-beri) but generally there is also peripheral oedema, breathlessness, tachycardia and cardiac enlargement, indicating myocardial involvement. The administration of thiamine in large doses usually gives gradual improvement and eventual complete recovery.

The 'burning feet' syndrome

This syndrome commonly occurred in prisoner-of-war camps during the Second World War, particularly in the Far East, but has occurred at other times of similar deprivation. It seems clear that it is of nutritional origin and responds to large doses of vitamins and a proper diet, but the precise aetiology is unknown. The burning feet syndrome is characterised by predominantly sensory peripheral neuropathy, optic atrophy and oro-genital ulceration and in some patients a myelopathy.

Nutritional and toxic amblyopia

Optic atrophy is a rare complication of deficiency of the B group of vitamins but may be found in patients suffering from the more florid forms of deficiency, particularly as a complication of subacute combined degeneration of the cord due to vitamin B_{12} deficiency. It has also been described in vegans who refuse to eat any animal products. A more acute and often permanent blindness may occur as a result of methyl alcohol intoxication. However, the commonest cause is 'tobacco alcohol amblyopia'. The precise mechanism for this condition has not been determined, but it seems to be closely related to the high blood cyanide level that occurs in heavy smokers with impaired liver function due to alcohol. The diagnosis should be considered in patients at risk who complain of impaired visual acuity. Visual field charts show a centrocaecal scotoma. Prompt treatment with hydroxocobalamin and the avoidance of alcohol and tobacco usually result in significant improvement.

Tropical ataxic neuropathy

Optic atrophy due to cyanide toxicity also occurs in association with a predominantly sensory polyneuropathy due to the ingestion of cassava, the tuber of Manioc. This condition has been found in many parts of Africa, particularly in Nigeria (Nigerian neuropathy). The patients complain of painful tingling in the feet, followed by a progressive sensory ataxia due to impairment of vibration and joint position sense. Vision is impaired and optic atrophy eventually develops.

Tropical spastic paraplegia

A form of progressive spastic paraplegia now thought to be of infectious rather than nutritional origin has been observed both in the West Indies and in Southern India. Often there is associated evidence of posterior column dysfunction, and optic atrophy as well as nerve deafness are common. Inflammatory changes of granulomatous type have been found in the spinal cords of some patients in the West Indies but not in India and 80% of patients show evidence of infection with HTLV I. A similar clinical picture occurs in **lathyrism** due to the consumption of lathyrus peas.

Pyridoxine deficiency

Pyridoxine (vitamin B_6) deficiency may cause serious and intractable epilepsy in early infancy. Pyridoxine deficiency is an acquired disorder usually due to dietary insufficiency and there was one notable outbreak in the USA in infants fed on artificial milk which was deficient in this vitamin; it may also be drug-induced. Pyridoxine dependency is inherited as an autosomal recessive trait and these infants may have fits in utero and usually present with epilepsy shortly after birth. It is very important that this condition is recognised and treated at an early stage because without treatment cerebral damage results and infants may have repeated convulsions that eventually become unresponsive to pyridoxine. The diagnosis is made by an assay of the serum B_6 level, the finding of a low CSF GABA, but most conveniently with the EEG which is very abnormal in the untreated state and can be completely corrected within half a minute by an intravenous injection of pyridoxine. This response lasts 10 minutes or so before the EEG starts to become abnormal again. Pyridoxine deficiency may also cause a polyneuropathy, and the polyneuropathy which may complicate treatment with isoniazid is due to metabolic antagonism of pyridoxine.

Pellagra

Pellagra is generally attributed to dietary deficiency of nicotinic acid, but a secondary factor is often defective protein intake, as the amino acid tryptophan is a chemical precursor of nicotinic acid. Hence it occurs in individuals who are existing on a predominantly vegetable or cereal diet deficient in animal protein; it is not uncommon in vegans who refuse all foods derived from animal sources and also develops in some alcoholics. Commonly the skin lesions of pellagra, which consist initially of erythema on the face, hands and other exposed surfaces, and later give rise to vesiculation, pigmentation and thickening of the skin, are produced by exposure to sunlight. The symptoms of nervous dysfunction, which are almost invariable in such cases, are predominantly mental. Sometimes the clinical picture is that of a severe confusional state, while in other cases there is memory impairment, apathy, fatigue, depression and insomnia. Evidence of polyneuropathy is often found, but is probably due to an associated deficiency of other B-vitamins. In some cases of apparently uncomplicated pellagra there are manifestations of spinal cord involvement, with spastic paraparesis and with variable evidence of posterior column dysfunction.

Vitamin B_{12} deficiency

Vitamin B_{12} deficiency may be due to dietary deficiency or to a failure of absorption. Dietary deficiency is rare but may occur in strict vegans. Malabsorption may be due to lack of intrinsic factor in the gastric juice with which the vitamin normally combines. This can be due to a previous gastrectomy or to pernicious anaemia, in which case there is histamine-fast achlorhydria. The complex formed between vitamin B_{12} and intrinsic factor is absorbed from the distal ileum so that lesions in this part of the gut can affect absorption; these include Crohn's disease, small bowel resection and other malabsorption syndromes. B_{12} deficiency may also occur if it is taken up in the gut by bacteria as in the blind-loop syndrome or in patients infested with the fish tapeworm. Macrocytic anaemia is usually the first manifestation of B_{12} deficiency and may occur at blood levels below 300 ng/l, but neurological symptoms rarely occur until the level falls below 100 ng/l. Although the principal neurological symptoms and signs indicate disease of the spinal cord, there are occasional cases in which **cerebral symptoms** are predominant, at least initially. These symptoms include defects of intellect, of memory and of concentration, or episodes of confusion or paranoia; it may at times be difficult to distinguish these cerebral manifestations of vitamin B_{12} deficiency from the clinical features of early Alzheimer's disease or other forms of dementia or from those resulting from any organic confusional state. Occasionally, too, there is progressive bilateral visual loss with central scotomas and **optic atrophy** is found.

Subacute combined degeneration of the spinal cord

Symptoms and signs of involvement of the nervous system occur in about 80% of cases of pernicious anaemia. The principal sites of pathological change, in which initial loss of myelin with subsequent axonal degeneration occur, are the posterior columns and the pyramidal tracts. The disease process often also involves the posterior roots and peripheral nerves, giving clinical and pathological features of a predominantly sensory axonal polyneuropathy.

The clinical features of the illness depend upon which tracts of the spinal cord are principally affected. Since the lesions in the posterior columns usually predominate, the principal initial symptoms are generally paraesthesiae, tingling, numbness and pins and needles in the extremities. Commonly patients describe sensations as if a tight band of constriction were present around one toe, around a limb or about the waist, or say that the hands and feet feel swollen or as if encased in tight bandages; feelings suggesting that cold water is trickling down the legs may also occur. Physical signs may be slight but usually vibration sense is impaired early. The appreciation of position in the toes and fingers is defective and the threshold for two-point discrimination is raised. As evidence of posterior column involvement becomes more severe, so the patient develops sensory ataxia, so that locomotion or maintenance of the upright posture are particularly difficult in the dark or when the eyes are closed (Romberg's sign). Impairment of appreciation of light touch in the periphery of the limbs is sometimes seen, together with tenderness of the calves, and it is these features, along with depression or absence of tendon reflexes (usually the ankle jerks), as well as evidence of impaired sensory nerve conduction, which indicate involvement of peripheral nerves, the dorsal roots and the dorsal root entry zone. Rarely, pain and temperature sensation are impaired, due to changes in pain-conducting fibres of the peripheral nerves or in the spinothalamic tracts, and there may even be a sensory 'level' on the trunk but this is exceptional.

Disturbances of motor function result from damage to the pyramidal tracts. This gives the characteristic stiffness and slowness of the gait which develops in any case of spastic paraparesis, however caused. The abdominal reflexes are lost, and the lower limb reflexes may be exaggerated, with clonus, unless the lesions in the sensory pathways have interrupted the reflex arc; the plantar responses are usually extensor. The condition is, however, very variable in presentation. Usually sensory symptoms are predominant and the earliest signs may simply be those of a sensory neuropathy, but, on the other hand, there are some cases in which spasticity of the lower limbs is striking and signs of posterior column involvement, though present, are relatively slight. Hence this diagnosis should be seriously considered in any case of sensory neuropathy or spastic paraplegia which develops subacutely in adult life; even if examination of the blood and bone-marrow reveals no abnormality it is usually essential to estimate the level of vitamin B_{12} in the serum. A result of less than $100\mu\mu$g/ml of serum is virtually diagnostic of B_{12} deficiency. A Schilling test, examination of the gastric juice for histamine-fast achloryhydria, and estimation of gastric parietal-cell antibodies will then be necessary to confirm that B_{12} absorption is impaired and that the diagnosis is one of pernicious anaemia. When gastric acidity is normal and intestinal malabsorption or a small bowel 'blind-loop' syndrome is suspected, appropriate radiological and other studies will be needed. It is of the greatest importance to recognise B_{12} deficiency, as if the condition is treated early the neurological manifestations can resolve completely after giving parenteral vitamin B_{12}. Sensory symptoms and signs are usually the first to improve and may be relieved completely, but if there is a spastic paraplegia of moderate severity before treatment is begun, there is usually some persistent residual disability. Treatment should be started with intramuscular hydroxocobalamin 1000 μg daily for a few days and then 1000 μg should be given monthly for the rest of the patient's life.

Folate deficiency

A deficiency of folate caused by malabsorption or by the use of anticonvulsant drugs has long been known to cause megaloblastic anaemia. It has been noted that some patients with polyneuropathy and/or myelopathy, and even some with dementia, have serum folate levels of less than 2μg/ml. Treatment with folic acid (5 mg three times daily) has been recommended but the role of folate deficiency in the aetiology of these syndromes remains very uncertain.

Vitamin E deficiency

For many years no specific syndromes were attributed to vitamin E deficiency in man although a myopathy is well recognised to occur in many animal species deficient in this vitamin. However, a human form of spinocerebellar degeneration has now been shown to result from such a deficiency in patients with chronic fat malabsorption, and the administration of α-tocopherol has been shown to benefit many patients with the autosomal recessive disorder a β-lipoproteinaemia (p. 296). The low plasma concentration of vitamin E found in some patients with spinal muscular atrophy is of much more dubious significance.

Other neurological effects of malabsorption

While vitamin B_{12} deficiency may occur as a result of intestinal malabsorption, myopathy, peripheral neuropathy and, more rarely, myelopathy have all been described as uncommon complications of coeliac disease in childhood and of tropical and non-tropical sprue in adult life and are as yet largely unexplained.

NERVOUS DISORDERS DUE TO PHYSICAL AGENTS

There are a number of physical agents which, though influencing the metabolic behaviour of many of the tissues of the body, have a particular tendency to impair profoundly the functioning of the central and peripheral nervous system. Among the aetiological agents which are important in this connection are oxygen lack (anoxia, hypoxia), CO_2 intoxication, electricity, decompression sickness, and excessive heat or cold. Radiation injury, due either to excessive exposure to X-rays or to atomic explosions, has comparatively little effect upon the nervous system when compared with the severe damage which may be caused to the haematopoietic system. However, therapeutic irradiation of the neck or mediastinum is sometimes followed within six to 12 months by the development of a slowly progressive spastic paraparesis with sensory impairment in the lower limbs (**post-radiation myelopathy**). Similarly, the optic chiasm can be damaged by radiation for pituitary tumours and the brachial plexus following irradiation for carcinoma, either for lesions at the apex of the lung or for patients with carcinoma of the breast and spread to the supraclavicular nodes.

Anoxia

The commonest varieties of anoxia met with in clinical practice are those in which there is deficient oxygenation of the arterial blood due either to a failure of adequate quantities of oxygen to reach the lungs (high altitudes, drowning); or to diminished oxygenation resulting from pulmonary disease (emphysema); these cases are grouped together as **anoxic anoxia**. Mountain or high altitude sickness may be either acute or chronic. Acute mountain sickness occurs in subjects who ascend to altitudes of between eight and twelve thousand feet without proper acclimatisation, usually climbers, skiers and tourists who fly to high altitudes. There is a spectrum of symptoms ranging from headache, insomnia, lassitude and impaired concentration through to severe headache associated with drowsiness, features of raised intracranial pressure due to cerebral oedema with papilloedema and flame-shaped haemorrhages and epilepsy. This process may proceed to the death of the patient if oxygen is not provided promptly and the patient is not moved to lower altitudes. Chronic mountain sickness (Monge's disease) occurs in subjects accustomed to living at high altitude and results in fatigue, dyspnoea, finger clubbing, cyanosis and somnolence; these patients are usually found to have very high haematocrit levels. In **anaemic anoxia** there is a deficiency in circulating haemoglobin or a chemical alteration in the haemoglobin (as in carbon monoxide poisoning) which prevents it from carrying oxygen. Cardiac arrest occurring as a result of heart disease or during anaesthesia may also be followed by irreversible anoxic brain damage which is also sometimes seen as a complication of open-heart surgery. In the latter situation air or gas embolism is an additional hazard. Local anoxia of the tissues can of course be due to arterial disease producing **ischaemic anoxia**. Apart from local infarction of the brain, spinal cord or peripheral nerves, resulting from focal vascular occlusion due to atheroma, thrombosis or embolism, diffuse ischaemic anoxia can also be due to fat embolism (usually complicating multiple fractures of one or more long bones) or to widespread disease of small arteries and arterioles as in granulomatous arteritides and in thrombotic microangiopathy. Oxygen lack may have a profound effect upon the brain, but the spinal cord and peripheral nerves seem capable of resisting degrees of anoxia which produce irreversible cerebral damage. When the oxygen supply to the brain is moderately reduced over a long period, the most frequent symptoms are fatigue, drowsiness, apathy and failure of attention, followed later by impairment of judgement and of memory, ataxia and inco-ordination. Sudden profound anoxia produces almost instantaneous loss of the senses, and normally the brain cannot withstand more than a few minutes of total anoxia, after cardiac arrest. If the period of anoxia is much more prolonged, respiration ceases and death rapidly ensues. After a period of from five to 15 minutes of cardiac arrest, even if the circulation is re-established, the patient may survive for a time in a semicomatose decerebrate state but full intellectual function is never restored. After less prolonged periods of anoxia the patient may gain full control of his limbs, and consciousness is restored after several hours or days, but there is commonly some degree of permanent intellectual deficit; epileptic seizures of temporal-lobe type are a frequent sequel, resulting from the pathological changes which anoxia produces in Ammon's horn and in contiguous areas of the hippocampus. In some cases of carbon monoxide poisoning the patient is initially unconscious but then may regain his senses at least to some extent after 24 to 48 hours. A relatively lucid interval may then be followed by progressively deepening coma and death (**post-anoxic encephalopathy**). Many cases showing partial recovery from an anoxic insult, however caused, show not only permanent dementia and severe behaviour disorders but also cerebellar ataxia (due to Purkinje cell damage), variable extrapyramidal features superficially resembling those of parkinsonism, and spastic weakness of the limbs with extensor plantar responses. In occasional cases there may be a surprising degree of recovery even after prolonged unconsciousness so that the prognosis is difficult to predict in any single case.

Carbon dioxide intoxication

In some patients with chronic bronchitis and emphysema the respiratory centre appears to become increasingly insensitive to carbon dioxide, which is retained in the circulation as bicarbonate due to chronic alveolar hypoventilation. The syndrome can also result from chronic respiratory insufficiency in neuromuscular disorders such as motor neurone disease, poliomyelitis, polyneuropathy, muscular dystrophy or myasthenia, especially when the diaphragm is involved; morphine or other sedative drugs may have a similar effect. In some cases there are headache, drowsiness and confusion persisting over many months but sometimes an acute syndrome characterised by intense headache, vomiting, convulsions, and papilloedema develops and can be precipitated by the administration of oxygen. As in chronic CO_2 retention, the respiratory centre fails to react to the raised level of CO_2 and respiration is then maintained by the receptors which respond to oxygen lack. Administering oxygen then removes the stimulus to respiration, raises the blood CO_2 still further and hence causes coma. Steroid drugs and diuretics may reduce cerebral oedema in such cases but some patients require intermittent positive pressure respiration for a few weeks in order to blow off CO_2 and to restore the sensitivity of the respiratory centre.

Electrical injuries

Electrocution, occurring either as a result of accidental contact with an electrical supply or from being struck by lightning, can be immediately fatal due to cardiac arrest. In such cases there are extensive pathological changes in the brain, muscles and peripheral nerves, as well as in other tissues. Less severe and more localised injuries commonly produce extensive burning or electrical necrosis of the tissues. It is not uncommon in such cases for a temporary flaccid paralysis of the lower limbs to occur, with sensory loss; this usually passes off in 24 hours and is believed to be due to profound vasoconstriction in the arteries of the spinal cord. Other syndromes resulting from focal injury to the brain, spinal cord or peripheral nerves also occur in some cases.

Decompression sickness (caisson disease)

This condition, which is commonest in divers and in tunnel workers who work in an atmosphere of compressed air, is due to the release of bubbles of nitrogen into the blood stream during decompression. Many neurological symptoms, including hemiplegia, paraplegia, visual scotomas, vertigo and diplopia can occur in such cases, presumably as a result of gas embolism of the arteries of the brain or spinal cord. Symptoms of this type developing in a compressed-air worker demand immediate recompression in a hyperbaric chamber, a measure which almost invariably relieves the symptoms; subsequently decompression must be repeated much more slowly. Non-neurological symptoms include chest pain, dyspnoea, cough, aching in the limbs and infarction of bones, with subsequent arthropathy, particularly of the hip joints.

Heat stroke

In an individual exposed to a consistently high environmental temperature, the typical manifestations of heat stroke are a rapidly mounting temperature and a hot dry skin with total absence of sweating. The patient is at first apathetic, later stuporose or comatose, and convulsions are common. Circulatory collapse soon follows if rapid cooling is not instituted. Variable degrees of cerebral damage may persist even in those patients who recover; variable confusion, slurring dysarthria, and ataxia are common in the recovery phase. The Purkinje cells of the cerebellum are particularly sensitive to heat injury and a severe cerebellar ataxia may be a permanent sequel.

Malignant hyperpyrexia

This rare condition gives a rapid rise in body temperature during surgical anaesthesia and has often proved fatal. Although halothane and/or suxamethonium are the commonest precipitating agents, no anaesthetic has been shown to be absolutely safe. The susceptibility is often dominantly inherited and in many affected patients evidence of overt or subclinical myopathy is found. While the resting level of creatine kinase in the serum is often raised in susceptible individuals, muscle biopsy under local anaesthesia followed by in vitro study of the halothane-induced contracture may be needed to identify susceptible individuals. Dantrolene sodium, 1–2 mg/kg body weight given intravenously every 5–10 minutes up to 10 mg/kg, is a specific treatment and may also be of prophylactic value.

Hypothermia

Accidental hypothermia is usually due to prolonged exposure to cold or immersion in cold water. Hypothermic coma, is, however, an occasional complication of myxoedema and can occur in elderly people living in unheated rooms in cold weather. Diagnosis depends upon careful measurement of rectal temperature which may be less than 34^0C (90^0F). Hypothermia is commonly used as an adjunct to anaesthesia; this too may have important complications and sequelae. Unduly prolonged hypothermia can lead to convulsions, irreversible coma, cardiac arrest and death, while less severe and prolonged hypothermia can give sequelae similar to those of cerebral anoxia. Semicoma, confusion and alternating rigidity of the limbs with coarse myoclonic jerking are sometimes seen during recovery. Mild hypothermia can be treated with external warming; it may be dangerous to do this to patients with severe hypothermia where special precautions may be necessary to increase the core temperature at the same time as or before that of peripheral structures such as the limbs. Immersion foot is a syndrome of local hypothermia involving the lower limbs; it occurred in shipwreck survivors and in soldiers living in trenches whose feet were cold and wet for a prolonged period. This condition caused extensive pathological changes in peripheral nerves, muscles and blood vessels and the neurological symptoms and signs were those of a severe peripheral neuropathy sometimes associated with gangrene. In frost-bite, by contrast, the principal pathological changes are in the blood vessels, and symptoms and signs of peripheral nerve injury are unobtrusive.

DISORDERS DUE TO DRUGS AND OTHER CHEMICAL AGENTS

Whereas many drugs will, in excess, produce manifestations of disordered nervous activity, those most often encountered in clinical practice as a cause of poisoning or intoxication are alcohol, either ethyl or methyl, barbiturates, anticonvulsants, psychotropic drugs, opiates, amphetamine and its derivatives, and heavy metals. Intoxication may result from excessive and prolonged indulgence or may be acute, as in a suicidal attempt. In the case of heavy metals, it is usually due to accidental ingestion, often in the course of the patient's occupation but some such agents are still used occasionally in deliberate acts of poisoning whether for suicide or attempted murder. Not only are there important specific symptoms induced by some of these drugs, but a characteristic clinical syndrome may follow their sudden withdrawal.

Alcoholism

Chronic alcoholism due to excessive ethyl alcohol consumption is one form of drug addiction and as a rule has potent psychological causes. It can develop insidiously in an individual who is at first merely a social drinker. Gradually his or her intake of alcohol increases so that any excuse or opportunity, however trivial, is regarded as a reason for having a drink, or another drink. It is when the patient begins to drink alone, when alcoholic beverages replace his meals, and when he has a compulsive and irresistible urge to drink, no matter the time of day, that he becomes an alcoholic. The individual who indulges in occasional episodes of excessive drinking with intervals of abstinence is not strictly an alcoholic, though he may become so if the intervals between the episodes shorten progressively, or if his debauches last for days rather than hours (a 'lost weekend'). Only occasionally does alcoholism develop quickly due to acute emotional stress and this usually implies a basically insecure personality. Even small quantities of alcohol impair significantly the performance of skilled motor activity as well as mental functions. Although the individual who has taken one or two drinks may be elated, and may feel himself to be in a state of heightened perception, his reaction time is increased and his senses are dulled. Alcohol also increases renal water and electrolyte excretion and thus has a diuretic effect. Dehydration and gastrointestinal irritation are largely responsible for 'hangover' symptoms, including headache.

The symptoms of alcoholism are first gastrointestinal, and secondly nervous. The principal **gastrointestinal symptoms** are nausea, anorexia and diarrhoea, due to chronic gastritis and enteritis; these frequently contribute to malnutrition which in turn results in **polyneuropathy** and/or **Wernicke's encephalopathy** (see above). Alcoholic liver cirrhosis, generally a sequel of long-continued alcoholism, is probably a result of nutritional deficiency combined with the toxic effects of alcohol. The **nervous symptoms** can be divided into those of acute intoxication and those which follow alcohol withdrawal. The symptoms and signs of acute intoxication are well known. The speech is slurred, the gait unsteady and the patient is either jocular and inattentive, noisy and aggressive, or dulled, confused and retarded. More severe intoxication results in stupor or coma; the diagnosis must be made not only upon the flushed face and alcohol-laden breath, but upon the absence of signs of nervous disease; it must always be remembered that subarachnoid haemorrhage, for instance, or head injury, perhaps complicated by a subdural haematoma, can occur during an alcoholic debauch. Pure alcoholic coma, however, is rarely deep or prolonged, and there are no focal neurological signs. Although an estimation of blood-alcohol may indicate the amount of alcohol that the individual has consumed, this may not be closely related to the degree of clinical intoxication, as individual tolerance varies widely and depends to some extent upon habituation.

Many symptoms and physical signs may follow the **withdrawal of alcohol** after prolonged intoxication or after several days of heavy drinking. The commonest feature is a state of nervousness or **intense tremulousness** ('the shakes'), which is relieved by a further drink, but returns more severely when once again the patient abstains. He is alert, jumpy and easily startled, and has a marked tremor of the limbs. Sometimes these symptoms settle within a few days but occasionally there is a superadded **hallucinosis** in the form of visual experiences, or less commonly auditory hallucinations, such as voices, motor cars, radios and the like. Occasionally, too, a series of convulsions ('rum fits') occur either at the height of a drinking bout or on withdrawal. The most severe of all the syndromes of alcoholic withdrawal is **delirium tremens**. It commonly develops two to four days after the last drink, usually in individuals who have been excessive drinkers for several years. Often it is seen when the patient develops an intercurrent illness such as pneumonia or is admitted to hospital for an operation, or after an accident. He is typically restless, voluble and sleepless, living in a state of intense physical and mental activity both day and night. At the same time there are tremor of the limbs, intermittent muscular twitching, confusion and, as a rule, hallucinations. A fatal outcome, due to circulatory failure or even, in some cases, to exhaustion despite sedation, is not uncommon. Usually the illness lasts for three to four days, and the patient at last falls into a calm sleep and awakens lucid but amnestic, having no recollection of it.

Among the less common syndromes which result from alcoholism are **alcoholic cerebellar degeneration** (a progressive, symmetrical cerebellar ataxia of subacute type), and **degeneration of the corpus callosum** (Marchiafava-Bignami disease), a syndrome of progressive dementia with fits and eventual spastic paralysis, which develops almost exclusively in Italian wine-drinking males. Nonspecific **alcoholic dementia** is more common; a rare manifestation is **central pontine myelinolysis** (see p. 323) which gives pseudo-bulbar palsy and quadriparesis. Recently acute and chronic varieties of **alcoholic myopathy** have been described; the acute variety usually develops at the height of a debauch and may give myoglobinuria, while the subacute variety is more often progressive and resembles other metabolic varieties of muscle disease. Alcoholic polyneuropathy has already been considered (see p. 295).

The syndrome produced by the ingestion of **methyl alcohol**, which occurs in methylated-spirit drinkers and in others who consume home-made liquor containing wood alcohol, is characterised by an acute acidosis and by nausea, vomiting, visual loss, muscle pains and impairment of consciousness. If large quantities have been taken, death in coma is not infrequent. If recovery takes place, permanent visual loss due to optic nerve damage is common; some patients remain blind, while others show bilateral central scotomas.

Barbiturate intoxication

Barbiturates have largely been supplanted by other hypnotics, notably the benzodiazepines, both as tranquillisers and for night sedation and their prescription is now restricted within the United Kingdom so that accidental overdose with barbiturates or their use in suicide attempts is now relatively uncommon.

Symptoms of **acute barbiturate poisoning** depend upon the dose taken. Mild intoxication results from taking about two or three times the maximum recommended dose; the patient is drowsy, but easily awakened and often shows nystagmus, dysarthria and ataxia. When the dose is five to 10 times normal, the patient is semicomatose and can only be awakened by vigorous stimulation, when he may mutter a few words and will then lapse again into unconsciousness. The patient who has taken from 15 to 21 times the usual dose or more is comatose with shallow respiration, absent reflexes and extensor plantar responses; sometimes blisters develop on the feet and legs. When the patient is in this condition, which can be fatal, treatment is urgent (see p. 204).

The clinical features of **chronic barbiturate intoxication** and those of withdrawal are similar to those of alcoholism. Increasing tolerance can be considerable, so that the patient who is habituated can take many times the recommended dose with comparatively little effect.

Characteristically the addict is slow in his mental reactions, his perception is dulled and he is slovenly in dress and habits. The physical signs are nystagmus, dysarthria and cerebellar ataxia. Withdrawal of the drug is followed by a few hours of temporary improvement but later by tremulousness, nervousness, weakness and confusion. There may be a phase of delirium with hallucinations and delusions, and convulsions are very common after barbiturate withdrawal.

Other sedative and psychotropic drugs

Anticonvulsant drugs such as phenytoin produce slurred speech, nystagmus, blurred vision and ataxia in moderate overdosage, symptoms and signs comparable to those produced by the barbiturates in higher dosage. The **benzodiazepines** are much safer and seldom cause more than prolonged but reversible coma except in patients with emphysema, when overdosage may be fatal. Although very safe, the benzodiazepines are unfortunately associated with a high risk of dependency and this may develop after only a few weeks of regular medication. The withdrawal symptoms can be quite disabling and some patients have great difficulty in stopping these drugs. **Phenothiazines**, too, cause less respiratory depression and impairment of consciousness than other sedatives but may produce dystonic reactions in small doses, or hypotension, hypothermia, tachycardia, cardiac arrhythmia or fits when taken in larger quantities. The **tricyclic antidepressants** cause coma, a dry mouth, hypothermia, hyperreflexia, convulsions, pupillary dilatation, cardiac arrhythmia, respiratory failure and sometimes paralytic ileus or urinary retention.

Aspirin and other salicylates normally cause tinnitus, profuse perspiration and hyperventilation but rarely coma; the principal risk of **paracetamol** overdosage is liver damage and there are few if any neurological manifestations.

Amphetamine intoxication

Amphetamines and related compounds were increasingly used in the recent past not only for their stimulant and antidepressant effects, but also in order to reduce appetite in patients who were attempting to lose weight. Such individuals often increased the dose up to a point where symptoms of intoxication or chronic addiction appeared. Other related remedies, still extensively used as appetite suppressants, may carry very similar risks. The principal symptoms of overdosage are restlessness and overactivity, dryness of the mouth, tremor, palpitations and tachycardia, hallucinations, irritability and profound insomnia. Very heavy dosage can give fits, hypertension and

fatal ventricular arrhythmia. Withdrawal is followed by an acute delirious state with severe hallucinations and sometimes by a delusional psychosis which may last for days or weeks.

Marihuana (cannabis)

This drug, used for many centuries in the Orient, was introduced more recently into Western countries, often being smoked in cigarettes. It produces a temporary sense of well-being and is a drug of habituation rather than of addiction. Its use is illegal; its principal danger is that it may introduce the habituè to more harmful narcotic drugs and there is some evidence that long-continued use in high dosage may produce dementia and cerebral atrophy.

Hallucinogenic agents

The hallucinations induced by mescaline and lysergic acid (LSD) are often terrifying and rarely pleasurable; continued use may lead to irreversible psychosis. Addiction to these and related remedies is increasing.

Opiates

The drugs of the opiate group which occasionally cause symptoms of intoxication are opium itself and its tincture (laudanum), morphine, heroin (diacetylmorphine), dipipanone (Diconal®) and codeine (methylmorphinephine and their derivatives). Synthetic analgesics such as pethidine (demerol), methadone and dromoran are similar pharmacologically and can also be addictive; they can be considered together with the opiates.

Acute poisoning with these drugs is relatively uncommon except as a result of accidental ingestion, mistakes in dispensing or illicit use, as their issue is carefully controlled by law. The usual clinical features are stupor or coma, pin-point pupils, shallow respiration and bradycardia.

Chronic **opiate intoxication or addiction** is characterised by an initial phase of tolerance in which increasing doses of the drug are required to produce the desired effect, whether it be the pleasurable feeling of detachment which first encourages the eventual addict to use them, or the relief of symptoms for which they were initially prescribed. Prolonged therapeutic use of these drugs in illness is a potent cause of addiction, particularly in doctors and nurses. The phase of tolerance is followed by one of dependence, in which attempted withdrawal gives a series of characteristic symptoms. Some 12 hours or so after the last dose the patient begins to yawn repeatedly and there is lacrimation and running of the nose. This is followed by restlessness, insomnia, muscular twitching, generalised aching and shivering, and then by nausea, vomiting and diarrhoea. Commonly, these acute symptoms last for two or three days, but insomnia and weakness can persist for days or even weeks. Even when the stage of withdrawal and physical dependence has passed, emotional dependence or habituation remains and is an important cause of relapse. Physical, mental and moral dilapidation is invariable in the established addict, and most addicts will resort to any measure involving lying, feigning illness, stealing and many other subterfuges in order to obtain supplies.

Heavy metals

Whereas poisoning with many heavy metals is accompanied by symptoms of involvement of the nervous system, the most important in clinical practice are arsenic, lead, manganese, thallium and mercury.

Arsenical poisoning

The principal symptoms of acute arsenical poisoning are gastrointestinal, namely vomiting, diarrhoea and acute abdominal pain, though convulsions may occur. In chronic arsenical poisoning, however, whether resulting from criminal intent, from the excessive use of therapeutic arsenical preparations, or from contamination of food with arsenical insecticides, the main symptoms are neurological though hyperkeratosis, pigmentation and desquamation of the skin are also common. The nervous symptoms include headache, drowsiness, confusion and a symmetrical polyneuropathy which gives burning paraesthesiae in the extremities followed by muscular weakness and atrophy, distal sensory loss and absence of the tendon reflexes.

Lead poisoning

In children, the principal symptom of lead poisoning, which sometimes results from chewing painted objects covered with lead paint, is an encephalopathy giving somnolence, convulsions and coma. In adults, and particularly in painters using lead-containing paint, agonising colicky abdominal pain and anaemia are the commonest presenting symptoms. A peripheral neuropathy is also common, but is rarely symmetrical, and more often affects one limb. Thus a worker who is making batteries or accumulators may develop a unilateral wrist drop in the arm most often used, and the presence of a blue line on the gums and of punctate basophilia in the red blood cells will suggest that this is due to lead. Confirmation depends upon measurement of lead in the serum and in the urine. Sometimes lead in the bones gives a characteristic increased density in radiographs.

Manganese poisoning

This industrial disease, seen almost exclusively in manganese miners, results from inhalation of dust and is observed particularly in Chile. It gives a clinical syndrome very similar to that of parkinsonism but there is often associated lethargy and irritability. Marked improvement follows the use of levodopa (see p. 193).

Thallium poisoning

Thallium has been used in suicidal and homicidal attempts and causes severe mental confusion, sensorimotor polyneuropathy and depilation.

Mercury poisoning

Acute mercurial poisoning gives severe vomiting and diarrhoea followed by anuria and uraemia due to renal tubular necrosis. In infants, however, chronic mercurial poisoning due to excessive use of calomel teething powders probably caused most cases of pink disease (acrodynia). A syndrome of chronic mercurial poisoning in adults has been described, due either to the inhalation of mercury vapour in makers of thermometers, to the ingestion of fish which have fed on the effluent from a mercury factory (Minimata disease), or in police officers working with outdated mercurial finger-print powders. Sometimes this causes cerebellar ataxia, a syndrome characterised by excessive salivation, tremulousness, vertigo, irritability and depression or erethism (childish over-emotionalism) occurs. These are the manifestations of methyl mercury (organic mercury) poisoning; exposure to inorganic mercury vapour (as in chlor-alkali plant workers) can cause an axonal sensorimotor polyneuropathy.

An attempt has been made above to outline the symptoms of nervous dysfunction which can result from a variety of drugs and other poisons. There are many other poisons which give rise to neurological symptoms, but these are less often encountered in clinical practice. Thus atropine and related drugs in excess produce nervous excitation and confusion which may progress to mania; bromism, rarely observed nowadays, is characterised by drowsiness, lethargy, dysarthria and sometimes by psychosis. Chloral hydrate has an effect similar to alcohol, and antihistamine drugs too may produce lethargy or coma and sometimes convulsions in children. Long-continued use of phenothiazines may give drug-induced parkinsonism or irreversible facial and limb dyskinesias (see p. ■■■). For a full description of the effects of these and of the many other drugs which affect the nervous system if taken to excess, the reader is referred to textbooks of clinical pharmacology and toxicology.

NEUROLOGICAL COMPLICATIONS OF ENDOCRINE DISEASE

It has been increasingly recognised that neurological symptoms and signs may be produced by hormonal abnormalities resulting from disease of the ductless glands. Thus in **hypopituitarism**, leaving aside the local effects of the pituitary tumours (chromophobe adenomas) which sometimes produce this syndrome, widespread muscular weakness and atrophy may develop. These improve when the hypopituitarism is treated. In **Cushing's disease**, which is usually due to hyperadrenalism, and much less often to a basophil adenoma of the pituitary (a tumour which is rarely, if ever, large enough to produce local symptoms), mental symptoms, including depression, paranoid ideas and confusional episodes are not uncommon. A myopathy, often painful, and usually affecting thigh muscles predominantly to give weakness, atrophy and histological changes, has also been found in some patients with Cushing's disease, and resembles the steroid myopathy seen in some patients under treatment for long periods with steroid drugs (particularly triamcinolone). A subacute myopathy may also occur due to excess secretion of ACTH in patients who have undergone adrenalectomy for Cushing's disease, while a similar disorder accounts for muscular weakness in **acromegaly**.

The exact pathogenesis of **exophthalmic ophthalmoplegia, ophthalmic Graves' disease** or, as it is more often called, **inflammatory ophthalmopathy**, remains in some doubt. It was formerly thought to result from an excessive output of an exophthalmos-producing substance by the pituitary. However, more recent evidence favours an autoimmune pathogenesis as a circulating serum antibody against an ocular muscle soluble antigen can be found in most cases. Histologically there is striking oedema of the orbital muscles and connective tissue. The first symptom is usually pain in one eye followed by unilateral exophthalmos and diplopia, but patients may present with diplopia alone, often due to weakness of the superior rectus or superior oblique muscles and with no other features. A Hess chart may show involvement of other muscles. The intraocular pressure rises on attempted upward gaze and an orbital CT scan shows the markedly enlarged extraocular muscles. Although exophthalmos may be predominantly unilateral for some time, the other eye is eventually affected, and paresis of several extrinsic ocular muscles develops. Occasionally the exophthalmos is sufficiently severe for orbital decompression to be imperative but in less severe cases it can be reduced by steroids. The syndrome sometimes develops acutely after thyroidectomy. Often there are few if any symptoms of thyrotoxicosis and thyroid function tests (T3, T4 and TSH) are usually normal, though the TRI may be abnormal.

Thyrotoxicosis (primary Graves' disease) is occasionally sufficiently acute to produce a severe confusional state, but this is uncommon. It is sometimes associated with myasthenia gravis and a rare syndrome of thyrotoxic periodic paralysis, which resolves when the thyrotoxicosis is relieved, has been described, especially in Orientals. A more common complication is a myopathy of girdle and proximal limb muscles (thyrotoxic myopathy). This condition improves, and generally recovers completely, when the thyrotoxicosis is adequately treated. **Myxoedema** may be associated with a carpal tunnel syndrome and may rarely cause a cerebellar syndrome. When it is severe, hypothermic coma is an occasional complication due to lowering of the body temperature, while acute psychotic episodes (myxoedematous madness) and even a reversible syndrome of depression and mild dementia may occur. More often there is muscular pain and aching, accentuated by exertion, with slowness of muscular contraction and relaxation best seen as the calf muscles relax during and after eliciting an ankle reflex (pseudomyotonia). These symptoms respond to treatment with thyroxin.

In **diabetes mellitus**, polyneuropathy is a well-recognised complication (see p. 293). Isolated cranial nerve palsies of the third and sixth cranial nerves are also common, but usually clear up spontaneously within a few weeks or months. They appear to result from focal infarction of cranial nerve trunks. **Diabetic coma** is usually associated with ketoacidosis, a blood sugar higher than 15 mmol/l and massive ketonuria. Metabolic acidosis may also be due to lactic acid; the diagnosis depends on finding a low pH and sufficient lactate in the blood to account for it. This may occur either due to hypoxia or to a large number of other conditions, including intoxication with some drugs and specific enzyme defects. It can also occur in some diabetic subjects, especially during treatment with hypoglycaemic agents. The condition is associated with nausea, vomiting and rapid deep breathing and may progress to stupor or coma. Hyperosmolality due to hyperglycaemia (hyperglycaemic non-ketotic diabetic coma) has also been described, and a similar syndrome has been observed in non-diabetic subjects with severe burns. The patient is wasted, pale and dehydrated, the rate and amplitude of respiration are increased, ocular tension is low, the pulse rapid and feeble and there is also hypotension.

An important complication, not of diabetes itself, but of its treatment, is **hypoglycaemia**, resulting from excessive insulin administration. Excessively low blood-sugar readings are also seen in some cases of hypopituitarism, in patients with hyperinsulinism due to an adenoma of the islets of Langerhans, and sometimes in liver disease. The first symptom of hypoglycaemia is often profuse sweating and light-headedness followed by confusion and sometimes abnormal behaviour. Such episodes usually occur several hours after a meal and thus are most commonly experienced during the night or early in the morning. Vertigo, diplopia and many other nervous symptoms occasionally occur. Gradually the patient lapses into coma and is found, sweating profusely, with flaccid limbs and extensor plantar responses. If the coma is severe, generalised convulsions may develop. Diagnosis depends upon obtaining a blood sugar estimation during an attack. In suspected cases of organic hyperinsulinism a 48-hour fast may be needed to produce an episode, while insulin tolerance tests and/or plasma insulin assay may be helpful. A deep hypoglycaemic coma which lasts more than a few hours can produce permanent cerebral damage, with clinical after-effects and histopathological changes resembling those of anoxia. Even after several hours of unconsciousness, however, complete recovery is still possible, but often takes several days.

Lassitude and asthenia are salient clinical features of **Addison's disease**, resulting from hypoadrenalism, but in addition, muscular weakness and wasting (Addisonian myopathy) occur in some cases, while papilloedema due to cerebral oedema has also been described (see benign intracranial hypertension, p. 259). A myopathy, giving symptoms of generalised muscular weakness, is also an occasional feature of hypoparathyroidism, while paradoxically, muscular weakness, lassitude and polyuria can also be prominent in cases of **hyperparathyroidism** due to parathyroid adenoma. In both of these disorders of calcium metabolism, even when there is considerable evidence of proximal limb muscle weakness, the tendon reflexes usually remain brisk, a feature rarely seen in any other form of myopathy. In hypoparathyroidism following accidental operative removal of the parathyroid glands, or in **hypocalcaemia** due to any cause, there is excessive neuromuscular irritability, giving tetany and a positive Cvostek's sign. Idiopathic hypoparathyroidism is much less common, but in this condition, mental defect, recurrent major fits and calcification of the basal ganglia are constant features. The severity and frequency of the attacks of epilepsy are greatly reduced by treatment with calciferol or dihydrotachysterol.

DISORDERS OF THE HYPOTHALAMUS

Disorders of the hypothalamus can be divided into those concerned with the control of the anterior and posterior pituitary and other functions not mediated in this way. Control of the anterior pituitary from the hypothalamus is achieved by release of substances into the hypothalamic-pituitary portal system. These include thyrotrophin-releasing hormone (TRH) which stimulates the release of the thyroid-stimulating hormone which in turn controls the production of thyroxin from the thyroid gland. The gonadotrophin-releasing hormone (also known as the lutein-releasing hormone) controls the release of the follicular-stimulating hormone (FSH) and the luteinising hormone (LH). ACTH is secreted from the anterior pituitary and its control is very much more complicated and does not depend on the secretion of a single substance from the hypothalamus. Growth hormone (GH) is secreted from the pituitary in response to growth hormone-releasing factor produced from the hypothalamus and is inhibited by somatostatin. The production of prolactin from the pituitary is also controlled by releasing and inhibiting factors from the hypothalamus.

The hormones released from the posterior pituitary are synthesised in the hypothalamus and are transported via the tuber cinereum to the pituitary. The release of antidiuretic hormone (ADH) is determined by the osmolarity of the blood. Oxytocin appears to be concerned only with pregnancy and delivery.

Assessment of hypothalamic-pituitary function depends on measuring the production of these various hormones, or measuring their effects, and many protocols exist by means of which a comprehensive assessment of hypothalamic-pituitary function can be achieved. The clinical features associated with pituitary tumours have been considered elsewhere (see p. 256). The so-called 'empty sella syndrome' may be associated with normal pituitary function. These patients have a large sella and the pituitary, though of normal size, is surrounded by a large space filled with spinal fluid. Occasionally the optic chiasm may prolapse into this fluid-filled space and cause bitemporal hemianopia. The diagnosis is made by CT scanning which demonstrates that the major contents of the sella are of CSF density. The diagnosis can be confirmed with an iohexal cisternogram if necessary.

The release of ADH is regulated by osmoreceptors in the hypothalamus. Failure of this mechanism results in diabetes insipidus. These patients pass excessive volumes of urine (polyuria) which in turn leads to excessive thirst and, therefore, polydipsia. The diagnosis is confirmed by measurements of urinary and plasma osmolarities and their failure to respond to water deprivation. Conversely, inappropriate ADH secretion results in hyponatraemia from water retention. This syndrome may occur as a complication of some malignant diseases where ADH appears to be secreted by the tumour tissue; however, it may also occur in many non-malignant pulmonary conditions and in several disorders of the central nervous system including head injury, intracranial haemorrhage and infections, including bacterial and tuberculous meningitis. It can also occur as a result of treatment with a number of drugs including the tricyclic antidepressants and carbamazepine. The patient presents with lethargy and confusion which may lead to stupor and coma. The diagnosis can be confirmed by the low serum sodium concentration and low plasma osmolarity. Initial treatment is with fluid restriction.

The hypothalamus is concerned with a wide range of other functions not related to hormone production, but the most striking clinical feature of lesions in this region relates to the regulation of appetite. The hypothalamus may be damaged by a craniopharyngioma or other tumours growing in this region. Pinealomas (see p. 258) may also enroach upon the hypothalamus. Sarcoidosis usually affects the meninges, but the hypothalamus is the commonest site of intracerebral sarcoid granulomas. Hypothalamic involvement in any of these lesions is often associated with obesity. Some patients with genetically determined syndromes, including Frohlich's syndrome which is characterised by obesity and hypogonadism, may also have diabetes insipidus. Other rare syndromes affecting this area and associated with obesity include the Laurence-Moon-Biedl syndrome, which is characterised by hypogonadism, mental retardation, polydactyly and retinitis pigmentosa. The Prader-Willi syndrome, which is also characterised by obesity and hypogonadism, also includes mental retardation.

All these conditions are associated with some disturbance of appetite regulation which causes the obesity. The hypothalamus is also concerned with waking/sleeping cycles and patients with the Kleine-Levin syndrome show a combination of hypersomnolence with a voracious appetite and often aberrant sexual behaviour; these occur in recurrent bouts lasting from a few days to a few weeks with periods of normality between.

Central pontine myelinolysis

This condition is characterised clinically by rapidly evolving flaccid quadriplegia with facial and tongue weakness, dysphagia and anarthria, often leading to a fatal termination, though less severe cases occur. Pathologically there is massive demyelination in the central part of the brain stem. The condition was originally described in alcoholic and malnourished patients but subsequently has been reported in patients with Wernicke's encephalopathy, hepatic cirrhosis, Wilson's disease, leu-

kaemia and as a complication of uraemia and haemodialysis. Prolonged hyponatraemia sometimes resulting from iatrogenic over-hydration in the course of intravenous therapy is now known to be the principal cause and the condition can be recognised before death with CT or MRI scanning.

Porphyria

The term porphyria embraces a group of diseases which have in common the excessive urinary excretion of uroporphyrin and coproporphyrin and of porphyrin precursors (porphobilinogen).

Congenital porphyria is a rare inherited disorder in which there is excessive photosensitivity from birth. Any exposure to sunlight results in blistering of the skin, and porphyrins are laid down in the affected area to give pigmentation; eventually extensive scarring takes place. When a similar disorder develops in adult life it is known as **porphyria cutanea tarda**.

It is, however, in **acute intermittent porphyria** of the Swedish type, which is also the result of an inborn error of metabolism, that neurological manifestations occur. Attacks can be produced by the administration of drugs, particularly barbiturates and sulphonamides. They occur usually in early adult life and in either sex. The cardinal manifestations are attacks of abdominal pain which are often diagnosed initially as acute surgical emergencies, episodes of mental confusion, and a predominantly motor axonal polyneuropathy. Autonomic neuropathy accounts for the tachycardia and postural hypotension and for the sphincter disturbances which may develop in this condition. Bulbar paralysis occasionally occurs. During latent periods between attacks there is generally excessive porphobilinogen G and excess δ-amino-laevulinic acid in the urine, but in the acute episodes the urine is port-wine coloured and contains large quantities of porphyrins. Remissions invariably occur and can last weeks, months or years, but many patients are seriously disabled by the polyneuropathy, even though this, too, may remit. Intravenous haematin (4 mg/kg body weight) infused slowly over 30 minutes and repeated daily for several days may be very helpful in terminating acute attacks. The rare South African type is similar but the attacks are sometimes fatal and light sensitivity like that in the congenital type sometimes occurs.

SOME OTHER METABOLIC ENCEPHALOPATHIES

There are many **primary or endogenous metabolic encephalopathies,** most of which are inherited and which cause disorders of neuronal, glial or myelin structure whether due to storage of abnormal metabolites or abnormalities of development. Some of these are the leucodystrophies previously described, many others are associated with mental retardation and yet others give rise to the storage of abnormal lipids, proteins, amino acids, carbohydrates or mucopolysaccharides in the tissue of the nervous system. Some are due to identifiable single enzyme defects. To quote but one example not mentioned in this chapter or elsewhere, the X-linked **Lesch-Nyhan syndrome** of hyperuricaemia gives rise to severe mental retardation, self-mutilation, choreoathetosis and joint changes resembling those of gout. For details of the rare disorders not mentioned in this book the reader is referred to text-books of paediatric neurology. There remain to be considered, however, one of the more common of these disorders (hepatolenticular degeneration) and two types of **secondary or exogenous metabolic encephalopathy** in which an extracerebral disorder (such as uraemia or portal-systemic encephalopathy) affect the brain only secondarily.

Uraemic encephalopathy

The encephalopathy of chronic renal disease produces no specific neuropathological changes and is usually reversible by dialysis. Subacute delirium progressing to stupor or coma is usual and there is often multifocal myoclonus, while major convulsions are common. Acidosis and azotaemia are diagnostic but the picture may be complicated by concomitant hypertensive encephalopathy. **Dialysis encephalopathy**, often leading to dementia and often associated with bone disease, which was found to develop in some patients undergoing repeated dialysis in certain centres, was found to be due to a high concentration of aluminium as a trace element in the domestic water supply used for dialysis and has virtually disappeared since deionised water was used.

HEPATIC COMA (PORTAL-SYSTEMIC ENCEPHALOPATHY)

In patients with liver disease, whether acute hepatic necrosis, active chronic hepatitis, or chronic cirrhosis, certain characteristic neurological manifestations result from the fact that blood from the bowel, containing large amounts of nitrogenous substances, by-passes the liver through anastomoses between the portal and systemic arterial systems, and enters the systemic circulation. These nitrogenous substances, of which the level of blood ammonia is a useful index, can have a profound effect upon the brain. The early symptoms of 'hepatic coma' are confusion, apathy, difficulty in concentration and inappropriate behaviour. Gradually the patient may lapse

into coma. In some cases the patients enter a chronic phase characterised by episodic confusion and abnormal behaviour; this may last for weeks or months and may be wrongly attributed to cerebral atherosclerosis or to presenile dementia, if clinical evidence of liver disease is unobtrusive. Although exaggeration of tendon reflexes is common, the most important neurological sign, which is almost pathognomonic, is a flapping tremor of the outstretched hands (asterixis), a movement reminiscent of the flapping of a bird's wings. The EEG in such cases reveals diffuse slow activity, often with typical triphasic waves. Less often an acute choreiform syndrome is seen and in some patients, particularly following portacaval shunt operations, a progressive myelopathy (spastic paraparesis) develops. A mild demyelinating peripheral neuropathy has also been described.

Clearly the mechanism by which these conditions are produced is enhanced by surgical procedures which create artificial anastomoses between the portal and systemic circulations. Episodes of encephalopathy can follow a high-protein meal, or a gastrointestinal haemorrhage (due to absorption of blood products). Treatment consists of a low-protein diet and the regular administration of intestinal antibiotics (e.g. neomycin) which destroy bacterial flora and so reduce the absorption of protein derivatives.

HEPATOLENTICULAR DEGENERATION (WILSON'S DISEASE)

Hepatolenticular degeneration was first clearly defined by Kinnier Wilson in 1912, although similar cases were previously described by Westphal and Strumpell under the title pseudosclerosis. This condition, which affects either sex, is familial, being due to an autosomal recessive gene, so that it can affect several members of a sibship, but there is generally no history of the disease in previous generations. It usually begins in the first two decades and is characterised first by the appearance of symptoms indicating progressive degeneration of the basal ganglia, secondly by the development of liver cirrhosis, and thirdly by the presence of a ring of brown pigment around the margin of the cornea, the Kayser-Fleischer ring. The primary defect is one of copper metabolism and copper is deposited in the brain and liver as well as in the periphery of the cornea. Characteristic biochemical features include amino-aciduria, an excessive output of copper in the urine (normal upper limit $70\mu g/24$th), and a reduction of the serum copper level (normal range $75-100\mu g/100$ ml); the serum copper oxidase is also reduced. The primary defect appears to be a congenital deficiency of caeruloplasmin, the copper-binding fraction of the serum proteins; as there is too litle of this sub-stance available to absorb ingested copper, the latter is either deposited in the tissues or excreted in the urine.

The principal clinical manifestations are usually neurological although occasionally symptoms of liver disease (jaundice, ascites, splenomegaly) predominate. The neurological manifestations, which generally begin in adolescence, include facial grimacing, tremor, dys-arthria, ataxia and personality change. An alteration in the child's speech is often the first symptom. The tremor is usually of action type, but is sometimes present at rest, as in Parkinson's disease, or accentuated towards the end of movement, as in cerebellar ataxia. Sometimes there is a flapping or wing-beating movement of the outstretched hands, as in hepatic coma, and occasionally choreiform or athetoid posturing of the limbs, or plastic rigidity, are observed. Speech is invariably slurred, and facile euphoria or intellectual deterioration are frequent in the later stages. There are no changes in the reflexes or in sensation and the plantar responses are flexor. Often there is little clinical evidence of hepatic dysfunction, but spider naevi on the skin, 'liver palms', and splenomegaly are not infrequent, while gastrointestinal bleeding from oesophageal varices is an important complication, and liver function tests are usually grossly abnormal.

If untreated, the disease is usually fatal in five to 15 years from the onset; neurological disability is progressive, leading to immobility, emaciation and dementia, and death is usually due to intercurrent infection, gastrointestinal haemorrhage, or hepatic fail-ure. All traceable relatives of a patient with Wilson's disease should be screened for this condition by estim-ation of the serum caeruloplasmin, since early treatment may prevent overt manifestations of the disease. Treat-ment with chelating agents can modify the course of the disease, as these agents promote copper excretion. Dimercaprol and calcium EDTA, once used, have now been superseded by penicillamine (dimethylcysteine) which should be given continuously in a dose of 1–1.5 g daily. When toxic side-effects of penicillamine such as nephropathy and thrombocytopenia occur, triethyl tetra-mine 1–2 g daily is an effective alternative. If treated early enough the disease is completely controlled and affected individuals become virtually normal, both mentally and physically, and remain so.

REFERENCES

Adams R D, Victor M 1985 Principles of neurology, 3rd edn. McGraw-Hill, New York

Davies D M 1986 Textbook of adverse drug reactions, 3rd edn. Oxford University Press, Oxford

Harrison M J G (ed) 1984 Contemporary neurology. Butterworth, London

Pallis C, Lewis P D 1974 The neurology of gastrointestinal disease. Major problems in neurology, Vol 3 (Walton J N, series ed.). Saunders, London

Plum F (ed) 1974 Brain dysfunction in metabolic disorders. ARNMD, New York

Plum F, Posner J B 1980 The diagnosis of stupor and coma, 3rd edn. Blackwell, Oxford

Rosenberg R N 1986 Neurogenetics: principles and practice. Raven Press, New York

Spillane J D 1973 Tropical neurology. Oxford University Press, Oxford

Swash M, Kennard C (eds) 1985 Scientific basis of clinical neurology. Churchill Livingstone, Edinburgh

Walshe J M 1982 Treatment of Wilson's disease with trientine (triethylene tetramine) dihydrochloride. Lancet i: 643

Walton J N 1985 Brain's Diseases of the nervous system, 9th edn. Oxford University Press, Oxford

Walton J N 1987 Introduction to clinical neuroscience, 2nd edn. Baillière Tindall, London.

Index